ALSO BY ROBERT M. SAPOLSKY

A Primate's Memoir

The Trouble with Testosterone

Stress, the Aging Brain, and
the Mechanisms of Neuron Death

Why Zebras
Don't Get Ulcers

WHY ZEBRAS DON'T GET ULCERS

Third Edition

ROBERT M. SAPOLSKY

An Owl Book

HENRY HOLT AND COMPANY · NEW YORK

Owl Books
Henry Holt and Company, LLC
Publishers since 1866
175 Fifth Avenue
New York, New York 10010
www.henryholt.com

An Owl Book® and ® are registered trademarks of
Henry Holt and Company, LLC.

Library of Congress Cataloging-in-Publication Data
Sapolsky, Robert M.
    Why zebras don't get ulcers / Robert M. Sapolsky.—3rd ed.
        p.   cm.
    Includes index.
    ISBN-13: 978-0-8050-7369-0
    ISBN-10: 0-8050-7369-8
    1. Stress (Physiology)   2. Stress (Psychology)   3. Stress management.
I. Title.
    QP82.2.S8S266 2004
    616'.001'9—dc22   2004046044

Henry Holt books are available for special promotions and
premiums. For details contact: Director, Special Markets.

Originally published in 1994 by W. H. Freeman

First Owl Books Edition 2004

Designed by Victoria Tomaselli

Printed in the United States of America

5   7   9   10   8   6

For Lisa, my best friend,
who has made my life complete

CONTENTS

PREFACE

Perhaps you're reading this while browsing in a bookstore. If so, glance over at the guy down the aisle when he's not looking, the one pretending to be engrossed in the Stephen Hawking book. Take a good look at him. He's probably not missing fingers from leprosy, or covered with smallpox scars, or shivering with malaria. Instead, he probably appears perfectly healthy, which is to say he has the same diseases that most of us have—cholesterol levels that are high for an ape, hearing that has become far less acute than in a hunter-gatherer of his age, a tendency to dampen his tension with Valium. We in our Western society now tend to get different diseases than we used to. But what's more important, we tend to get different kinds of diseases now, with very different causes and consequences. A millennium ago, a young hunter-gatherer inadvertently would eat a reedbuck riddled with anthrax and the consequences are clear—she's dead a few days later. Now, a young lawyer unthinkingly decides that red meat, fried foods, and a couple of beers per dinner constitute a desirable diet, and the consequences are anything but clear—a half-century later, maybe he's crippled with cardiovascular disease, or maybe he's taking bike trips with his grandkids. Which outcome occurs depends on some obvious nuts-and-bolts factors, like what his liver does with cholesterol, what levels of certain enzymes are in his fat cells, whether he has any congenital weaknesses in the walls of his blood vessels. But the outcome will also depend heavily on such surprising factors as his personality, the amount of emotional stress he experiences over the years, whether he has someone's shoulder to cry on when those stressors occur.

There has been a revolution in medicine concerning how we think about the diseases that now afflict us. It involves recognizing the interactions between the body and the mind, the ways in which emotions and personality can have a tremendous impact on the functioning and health of virtually every cell in the body. It is about the role of stress in making some of us more vulnerable to disease, the ways in which some of us cope with stressors, and the critical notion that you cannot really understand a disease in vacuo, but rather only in the context of the person suffering from that disease.

This is the subject of my book. I begin by trying to clarify the meaning of the nebulous concept of stress and to teach, with a minimum of pain, how various hormones and parts of the brain are mobilized in response to stress. I then focus on the links between stress and increased risk for certain types of disease, going, chapter by chapter, through the effects of stress on the circulatory system, on energy storage, on growth, reproduction, the immune system, and so on. Next I describe how the aging process may be influenced by the amount of stress experienced over a lifetime. I then examine the link between stress and the most common and arguably most crippling of psychiatric disorders, major depression. As part of updating the material for this third edition, I have added two new chapters: one on the interactions between stress and sleep, and one on what stress has to do with addiction. In addition, of the chapters that appeared in the previous edition, I rewrote about a third to half of the material.

Some of the news in this book is grim—sustained or repeated stress can disrupt our bodies in seemingly endless ways. Yet most of us are not incapacitated by stress-related disease. Instead, we cope, both physiologically and psychologically, and some of us are spectacularly successful at it. For the reader who has held on until the end, the final chapter reviews what is known about stress management and how some of its principles can be applied to our everyday lives. There is much to be optimistic about.

I believe that everyone can benefit from some of these ideas and can be excited by the science on which they are based. Science provides us with some of the most elegant, stimulating puzzles that life has to offer. It throws some of the most provocative ideas into our arenas of moral debate. Occasionally, it improves our lives. I love science, and it pains me to think that so many are terrified of the subject or feel that choosing science means that you cannot also choose compassion, or the arts, or be awed by nature. Science is not meant to cure us of mystery, but to reinvent and reinvigorate it.

Thus I think that any science book for nonscientists should attempt to convey that excitement, to make the subject interesting and accessible even to those who would normally not be caught dead near the subject. That has been a particular goal of mine in this book. Often, it has meant simplifying complex ideas, and as a counterbalance to this, I include copious references at the end of the book, often with annotations concerning controversies and subtleties about material presented in the main text. These references are an excellent entrée for those readers who want something more detailed on the subject.

Many sections of this book contain material about which I am far from expert, and over the course of the writing, a large number of savants have been called for advice, clarification, and verification of facts. I thank them all for their generosity with their time and expertise: Nancy Adler, John Angier, Robert Axelrod, Alan Baldrich, Marcia Barinaga, Alan Basbaum, Andrew Baum, Justo Bautisto, Tom Belva, Anat Biegon, Vic Boff (whose brand of vitamins graces the cupboards of my parents' home), Carlos Camargo, Matt Cartmill, M. Linette Casey, Richard Chapman, Cynthia Clinkingbeard, Felix Conte, George Daniels, Regio DeSilva, Irven DeVore, Klaus Dinkel, James Doherty, John Dolph, Leroi DuBeck, Richard Estes, Michael Fanselow, David Feldman, Caleb Tuck Finch, Paul Fitzgerald, Gerry Friedland, Meyer Friedman, Rose Frisch, Roger Gosden, Bob Grossfield, Kenneth Hawley, Ray Hintz, Allan Hobson, Robert Kessler, Bruce Knauft, Mary Jeanne Kreek, Stephen Laberge, Emmit Lam, Jim Latcher, Richard Lazarus, Helen Leroy, Jon Levine, Seymour Levine, John Liebeskind, Ted Macolvena, Jodi Maxmin, Michael Miller, Peter Milner, Gary Moberg, Anne Moyer, Terry Muilenburg, Ronald Myers, Carol Otis, Daniel Pearl, Ciran Phibbs, Jenny Pierce, Ted Pincus, Virginia Price, Gerald Reaven, Sam Ridgeway, Carolyn Ristau, Jeffrey Ritterman, Paul Rosch, Ron Rosenfeld, Aryeh Routtenberg, Paul Saenger, Saul Schanburg, Kurt Schmidt-Nielson, Carol Shively, J. David Singer, Bart Sparagon, David Speigel, Ed Spielman, Dennis Styne, Steve Suomi, Jerry Tally, Carl Thoresen, Peter Tyak, David Wake, Michelle Warren, Jay Weiss, Owen Wolkowitz, Carol Worthman, and Richard Wurtman.

I am particularly grateful to the handful of people—friends, collaborators, colleagues, and ex-teachers—who took time out of their immensely busy schedules to read chapters. I shudder to think of the errors and distortions that would have remained had they not tactfully told me I didn't know what I was writing about. I thank them all sincerely: Robert Ader of the University of Rochester; Stephen Bezruchka of the University of Washington; Marvin Brown of the University of California, San Diego; Laurence Frank at the University of California, Berkeley; Craig Heller of Stanford University; Jay Kaplan of Bowman Gray Medical School; Ichiro Kawachi of Harvard University; George Koob of the Scripps Clinic; Charles Nemeroff of Emory University;

Seymour Reichlin of Tufts/New England Medical Center; Robert Rose of the MacArthur Foundation; Tim Meier of Stanford University; Wylie Vale of the Salk Institute; Jay Weiss of Emory University; and Redford Williams of Duke University.

A number of people were instrumental in getting this book off the ground and into its final shape. Much of the material in these pages was developed in continuing medical education lectures. These were presented under the auspices of the Institute for Cortext Research and Development, and its director, Will Gordon, who gave me much freedom and support in exploring this material. Bruce Goldman of the Portable Stanford series first planted the idea for this book in my head, and Kirk Jensen recruited me for W. H. Freeman and Company; both helped in the initial shaping of the book. Finally, my secretaries, Patsy Gardner and Lisa Pereira, have been of tremendous help in all the logistical aspects of pulling this book together. I thank you all, and look forward to working with you in the future.

I received tremendous help with organizing and editing the first edition of the book, and for that I thank Audrey Herbst, Tina Hastings, Amy Johnson, Meredyth Rawlins, and, above all, my editor, Jonathan Cobb, who was a wonderful teacher and friend in this process. Help in the second edition came from John Michel, Amy Trask, Georgia Lee Hadler, Victoria Tomaselli, Bill O'Neal, Kathy Bendo, Paul Rohloff, Jennifer MacMillan, and Sheridan Sellers. Liz Meryman, who selects the art for *Natural History* magazine, helping to merge the cultures of art and science in that beautiful publication, graciously consented to read the manuscript and gave splendid advice on appropriate artwork. In addition, I thank Alice Fernandes-Brown, who was responsible for making my idea for the cover such a pleasing reality. In this new edition help came from Rita Quintas, Denise Cronin, Janice O'Quinn, Jessica Firger, and Richard Rhorer at Henry Holt.

This book has been, for the most part, a pleasure to write and I think it reflects one of the things in my life for which I am most grateful—that I take so much joy in the science that is both my vocation and avocation. I thank the mentors who taught me to do science and, even more so, taught me to enjoy science: the late Howard Klar, Howard Eichenbaum, Mel Konner, Lewis Krey, Bruce McEwen, Paul Plotsky, and Wylie Vale.

A band of research assistants have been indispensable to the writing of this book. Steve Balt, Roger Chan, Mick Markham, Kelley Parker, Michelle Pearl, Serena Spudich, and Paul Stasi have wandered the basements of archival libraries, called strangers all over the world with questions, distilled arcane articles into coherency. In the line of duty, they have sought out drawings of opera castrati, the daily menu at Japanese-American internment camps, the causes of voodoo death, and the history of firing squads. All of their research was done with spectacular competence, speed, and humor. I am fairly certain this book could not have been completed without their help and am absolutely certain its writing would have been much less enjoyable. And finally, I thank my agent, Katinka Matson, and my editor, Robin Dennis, who have been just terrific to work with. I look forward to many more years of collaborations ahead.

Parts of the book describe work carried out in my own laboratory, and these studies have been made possible by funding from the National Institutes of Health, the National Institute of Mental Health, the National Science Foundation, the Sloan Foundation, the Klingenstein Fund, the Alzheimer's Association, and the Adler Foundation. The African fieldwork described herein has been made possible by the long-standing generosity of the Harry Frank Guggenheim Foundation. Finally, I heartily thank the MacArthur Foundation for supporting all aspects of my work.

Finally, as will be obvious, this book cites the work of a tremendous number of scientists. Contemporary lab science is typically carried out by large teams of people. Throughout the book, I refer to the work of "Jane Doe" or "John Smith" for the sake of brevity—it is almost always the case that such work was carried out by Doe or Smith along with a band of junior colleagues.

There is a tradition among stress physiologists who dedicate their books to their spouses or significant others, an unwritten rule that you are supposed to incorporate something cutesy about stress in the dedication. So, to Madge, who attenuates my stressors; for Arturo, the source of my eustress; for my wife who, over the course of the last umpteen years, has put up with my stress-induced hypertension, ulcerative colitis, loss of libido, and displaced aggression. I will forgo that style in the actual dedication of this book to my wife, as I have something simpler to say.

Why Zebras
Don't Get Ulcers

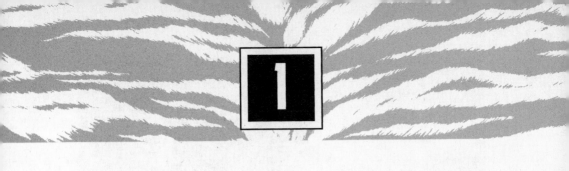

1

WHY DON'T ZEBRAS GET ULCERS?

It's two o'clock in the morning and you're lying in bed. You have something immensely important and challenging to do that next day—a critical meeting, a presentation, an exam. You have to get a decent night's rest, but you're still wide awake. You try different strategies for relaxing—take deep, slow breaths, try to imagine restful mountain scenery—but instead you keep thinking that unless you fall asleep in the next minute, your career is finished. Thus you lie there, more tense by the second.

If you do this on a regular basis, somewhere around two-thirty, when you're really getting clammy, an entirely new, disruptive chain of thought will no doubt intrude. Suddenly, amid all your other worries, you begin to contemplate that nonspecific pain you've been having in your side, that sense of exhaustion lately, that frequent headache. The realization hits you—I'm sick, fatally sick! Oh, why didn't I recognize the symptoms, why did I have to deny it, why didn't I go to the doctor?

When it's two-thirty on those mornings, I always have a brain tumor. These are very useful for that sort of terror, because you can attribute every conceivable nonspecific symptom to a brain tumor and justify your panic. Perhaps you do, too; or maybe you lie there thinking that you have cancer, or an ulcer, or that you've just had a stroke.

Even though I don't know you, I feel confident in predicting that you don't lie there thinking, "I just know it; I have leprosy." True? You are exceedingly unlikely to obsess about getting a serious case of dysentery if it starts pouring. And few of us lie there feeling convinced that our bodies are teeming with intestinal parasites or liver flukes.

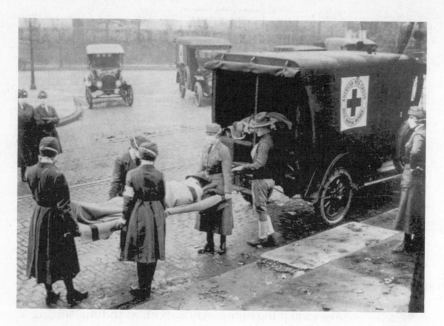

Influenza pandemic, 1918.

Of course not. Our nights are not filled with worries about scarlet fever, malaria, or bubonic plague. Cholera doesn't run rampant through our communities; river blindness, black water fever, and elephantiasis are third world exotica. Few female readers will die in childbirth, and even fewer of those reading this page are likely to be malnourished.

Thanks to revolutionary advances in medicine and public health, our patterns of disease have changed, and we are no longer kept awake at night worrying about infectious diseases (except, of course, AIDS or tuberculosis) or the diseases of poor nutrition or hygiene. As a measure of this, consider the leading causes of death in the United States in 1900: pneumonia, tuberculosis, and influenza (and, if you were young, female, and inclined toward risk taking, childbirth). When is the last time you heard of scads of people dying of the flu? Yet the flu, in 1918 alone, killed many times more people than throughout the course of that most barbaric of conflicts, World War I.

Our current patterns of disease would be unrecognizable to our great-grandparents or, for that matter, to most mammals. Put succinctly, we get different diseases and are likely to die in different ways from most of our ancestors (or from most humans currently living in the less privileged areas of this planet). Our nights are filled with worries about a different class of diseases; we are now living well enough and long enough to slowly fall apart.

The diseases that plague us now are ones of slow accumulation of damage—heart disease, cancer, cerebrovascular disorders. While none of these diseases is particularly pleasant, they certainly mark a big improvement over succumbing at age twenty after a week of sepsis or dengue fever. Along with this relatively recent shift in the patterns of disease have come changes in the way we perceive the disease process. We have come to recognize the vastly complex intertwining of our biology and our emotions, the endless ways in which our personalities, feelings, and thoughts both reflect and influence the events in our bodies. One of the most interesting manifestations of this recognition is understanding that extreme emotional disturbances can adversely affect us. Put in the parlance with which we have grown familiar, *stress can make us sick,* and a critical shift in medicine has been the recognition that many of the damaging diseases of slow accumulation can be either caused or made far worse by stress.

In some respects this is nothing new. Centuries ago, sensitive clinicians intuitively recognized the role of individual differences in vulnerability to disease. Two individuals could get the same disease, yet the courses of their illness could be quite different and in vague, subjective ways might reflect the personal characteristics of the individuals. Or a clinician might have sensed that certain types of people were more likely to contract certain types of disease. But since the twentieth century, the addition of rigorous science to these vague clinical perceptions has made stress physiology—the study of how the body responds to stressful events—a real discipline. As a result, there is now an extraordinary amount of physiological, biochemical, and molecular information available as to how all sorts of intangibles in our lives can affect very real bodily events. These intangibles can include emotional turmoil, psychological characteristics, our position in society, and how our society treats people of that position. And they can influence medical issues such as whether cholesterol gums up our blood vessels or is safely cleared from the circulation, whether our fat cells stop listening to insulin and plunge us into diabetes, whether neurons in our brain will survive five minutes without oxygen during a cardiac arrest.

This book is a primer about stress, stress-related disease, and the mechanisms of coping with stress. How is it that our bodies can adapt to some stressful emergencies, while other ones make us sick? Why are some of us especially vulnerable to stress-related diseases, and what does that have to do with our personalities? How can purely psychological turmoil make us sick? What might stress have to do with our vulnerability to depression, the speed at which we age, or how well our memories work? What do our patterns of stress-related diseases have to do with where we stand on the rungs of society's ladder? Finally, how can we increase the effectiveness with which we cope with the stressful world that surrounds us?

 ## SOME INITIAL CONCEPTS

Perhaps the best way to begin is by making a mental list of the sorts of things we find stressful. No doubt you would immediately come up with some obvious examples—traffic, deadlines, family relationships, money worries. But what if I said, "You're thinking like a speciocentric human. Think like a zebra for a second." Suddenly, new items might appear at the top of your list—serious physical injury, predators, starvation. The need for that prompting illustrates something critical— you and I are more likely to get an ulcer than a zebra is. For animals like zebras, the most upsetting things in life are *acute physical* crises. You are that zebra, a lion has just leapt out and ripped your stomach open, you've managed to get away, and now you have to spend the next hour evading the lion as it continues to stalk you. Or, perhaps just as stressfully, you are that lion, half-starved, and you had better be able to sprint across the savanna at top speed and grab something to eat or you won't survive. These are extremely stressful events, and they demand immediate physiological adaptations if you are going to live. Your body's responses are brilliantly adapted for handling this sort of emergency.

An organism can also be plagued by *chronic physical* challenges. The locusts have eaten your crops, and for the next six months, you have to wander a dozen miles a day to get enough food. Drought, famine, parasites, that sort of unpleasantness—not the sort of experience we have often, but central events in the lives of non-westernized humans and most other mammals. The body's stress-responses are reasonably good at handling these sustained disasters.

Critical to this book is a third category of ways to get upset—*psychological and social* disruptions. Regardless of how poorly we are getting along with a family member or how incensed we are about losing a parking spot, we rarely settle that sort of thing with a fistfight. Likewise, it is a rare event when we have to stalk and personally wrestle down our dinner. Essentially, we humans live well enough and long enough, and are smart enough, to generate all sorts of stressful events

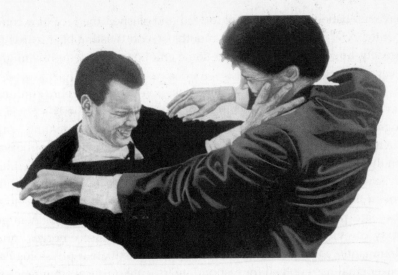

Robert Longo, Untitled Work on Paper, 1981. (Two yuppies contesting the last double latte at a restaurant?)

purely in our heads. How many hippos worry about whether Social Security is going to last as long as they will, or what they are going to say on a first date? Viewed from the perspective of the evolution of the animal kingdom, sustained psychological stress is a recent invention, mostly limited to humans and other social primates. We can experience wildly strong emotions (provoking our bodies into an accompanying uproar) linked to mere thoughts.* Two people can sit facing each other, doing nothing more physically strenuous than moving little pieces of wood now and then, yet this can be an emotionally taxing event: chess grand masters, during their tournaments, can place metabolic demands on their bodies that begin to approach those of athletes during the peak of a competitive event.† Or a person can do nothing more exciting than sign a piece of paper: if she has just signed the order to fire a hated rival after months of plotting and maneuvering, her physiological responses might be shockingly similar to those of a

---

* The neurologist Antonio Damasio recounts a wonderful study done on the conductor Herbert von Karajan, showing that the maestro's heart would race just as wildly when he was listening to a piece of music as when he was conducting it.

† Perhaps journalists are aware of this fact; consider this description of the Kasparov-Karpov chess tournament of 1990: "Kasparov kept pressing for a murderous attack. Toward the end, Karpov had to oppose threats of violence with more of the same and the game became a melee."

savanna baboon who has just lunged and slashed the face of a competitor. And if someone spends months on end twisting his innards in anxiety, anger, and tension over some emotional problem, this might very well lead to illness.

This is the critical point of this book: if you are that zebra running for your life, or that lion sprinting for your meal, your body's physiological response mechanisms are superbly adapted for dealing with such short-term physical emergencies. For the vast majority of beasts on this planet, stress is about a short-term crisis, after which it's either over with or you're over with. When we sit around and worry about stressful things, we turn on the same physiological responses—but they are potentially a disaster when provoked chronically. A large body of evidence suggests that stress-related disease emerges, predominantly, out of the fact that we so often activate a physiological system that has evolved for responding to acute physical emergencies, but we turn it on for months on end, worrying about mortgages, relationships, and promotions.

This difference between the ways that we get stressed and the ways a zebra does lets us begin to wrestle with some definitions. To start, I must call forth a concept that you were tortured with in ninth-grade biology and hopefully have not had to think about since—*homeostasis*. Ah, that dimly remembered concept, the idea that the body has an ideal level of oxygen that it needs, an ideal degree of acidity, an ideal temperature, and so on. All these different variables are maintained in homeostatic balance, the state in which all sorts of physiological measures are being kept at the optimal level. The brain, it has been noted, has evolved to seek homeostasis.

This allows us to generate some simple initial working definitions that would suffice for a zebra or a lion. A *stressor* is anything in the outside world that knocks you out of homeostatic balance, and the *stress-response* is what your body does to reestablish homeostasis.

But when we consider ourselves and our human propensity to worry ourselves sick, we have to expand on the notion of stressors merely being things that knock you out of homeostatic balance. A stressor can also be the *anticipation* of that happening. Sometimes we are smart enough to see things coming and, based only on anticipation, can turn on a stress-response as robust as if the event had actually occurred. Some aspects of anticipatory stress are not unique to humans—whether you are a human surrounded by a bunch of thugs in a deserted subway station or a zebra face to face with a lion, your heart is probably racing, even though nothing physically damaging has occurred (yet). But unlike less cognitively sophisticated species, we can turn on the stress-response by thinking about potential stressors that may throw us out of homeostatic balance far in the future. For example, think of the African farmer watching a swarm of locusts descend on his crops. He has eaten an adequate breakfast and is not suffering the homeostatic imbalance of starving, but that farmer will still be undergoing a stress-response. Zebras and lions may see trouble coming in the next minute and mobilize a stress-response in anticipation, but they can't get stressed about events far in the future.

And sometimes we humans can be stressed by things that simply make no sense to zebras or lions. It is not a general mammalian trait to become anxious about mortgages or the Internal Revenue Service, about public speaking or fears of what you will say in a job interview, about the inevitability of death. Our human experience is replete with psychological stressors, a far cry from the physical world of hunger, injury, blood loss, or temperature extremes. When we activate the stress-response out of fear of something that turns out to be real, we congratulate ourselves that this cognitive skill allows us to mobilize our defenses early. And these anticipatory defenses can be quite protective, in that a lot of what the stress-response is about is preparative. But when we get into a physiological uproar and activate the stress-response for no reason at all, or over something we cannot do anything about, we call it things like "anxiety," "neurosis," "paranoia," or "needless hostility."

Thus, the stress-response can be mobilized not only in response to physical or psychological insults, but also in expectation of them. It is this generality of the stress-response that is the most surprising—a physiological system activated not only by all sorts of physical disasters but by just thinking about them as well. This generality was first appreciated about sixty-five years ago by one of the godfathers of stress physiology, Hans Selye. To be only a bit facetious, stress physiology exists as a discipline because this man was both a very insightful scientist and lame at handling lab rats.

In the 1930s, Selye was just beginning his work in endocrinology, the study of hormonal communication in the body. Naturally, as a young, unheard-of assistant professor, he was fishing around for something with which to start his research career. A biochemist down the hall had just isolated some sort of extract from the ovary, and colleagues were wondering what this ovarian extract did to the body. So Selye obtained some of the stuff from the biochemist and set about studying its effects. He attempted to inject his rats daily, but apparently not with a great display of dexterity. Selye would try to inject the rats, miss them, drop them, spend half the morning chasing the rats around the room or vice versa, flailing with a broom to get them out from behind the sink, and so on. At the end of a number of months of this, Selye examined the rats and discovered something extraordinary: the rats had peptic ulcers, greatly enlarged adrenal glands (the source of two important stress hormones), and shrunken immune tissues. He was delighted; he had discovered the effects of the mysterious ovarian extract.

Being a good scientist, he ran a control group: rats injected daily with saline alone, instead of the ovarian extract. And, thus, every day they too were injected, dropped, chased, and chased back. At the end, lo and behold, the control rats had the same peptic ulcers, enlarged adrenal glands, and atrophy of tissues of the immune system.

Now, your average budding scientist at this point might throw up his or her hands and furtively apply to business school. But Selye, instead, reasoned through what he had observed. The physiological changes couldn't be due to the ovarian extract after all, since the same changes occurred in both the control and the experimental groups. What did the two groups of rats have in common? Selye reasoned that it was his less-than-trauma-free injections. Perhaps, he thought, these changes in the rats' bodies were some sort of nonspecific responses of the body to generic unpleasantness. To test this idea, he put some rats on the roof of the research building in the winter, others down in the boiler room. Still others were exposed to forced exercise, or to surgical procedures. In all cases, he found increased incidences of peptic ulcers, adrenal enlargement, and atrophy of immune tissues.

We know now exactly what Selye was observing. He had just discovered the tip of the iceberg of stress-related disease. Legend (mostly promulgated by Selye himself) has it that Selye was the person who, searching for a way to describe the nonspecificity of the unpleasantness to which the rats were responding, borrowed a term from physics and proclaimed that the rats were undergoing "stress." In fact, by the 1920s the term had already been introduced to medicine in roughly the sense that we understand it today by a physiologist named Walter Cannon. What Selye did was to formalize the concept with two ideas:

- The body has a surprisingly similar set of responses (which he called the general adaptation syndrome, but which we now call the stress-response) to a broad array of stressors.

- If stressors go on for too long, they can make you sick.

HOMEOSTASIS PLUS: THE MORE STRESS-APPROPRIATE CONCEPT OF ALLOSTASIS

The homeostasis concept has been modified in recent years in work originated by Peter Sterling and Joseph Eyer of the University of Pennsylvania and extended by Bruce McEwen of Rockefeller University.* They have produced a new framework that I steadfastly tried to ignore at first and have now succumbed to, because it brilliantly modernizes the homeostasis concept in a way that works even better in making sense of stress (although not all folks in my business have embraced it, using "old wine in a new bottle" imagery).

The original conception of homeostasis was grounded in two ideas. First, there is a single optimal level, number, amount for any given measure in the body. But that can't be true—after all, the ideal blood pressure when you're sleeping is likely to be different than when you're ski jumping. What's ideal under basal conditions is different than during stress, something central to allostatic thinking. (The field uses this Zen-ish sound bite about how allostasis is about "constancy through change." I'm not completely sure I understand what that means, but it always elicits meaningful and reinforcing nods when I toss it out in a lecture.)

The second idea in homeostasis is that you reach that ideal set point through some local regulatory mechanism, whereas allostasis recognizes that any given set point can be regulated in a zillion different ways, each with its own consequences. Thus, suppose there's a water shortage in California. Homeostatic solution: mandate smaller toilet tanks.† Allostatic solutions: smaller toilet tanks, convince people to conserve water, buy rice from Southeast Asia instead of doing water-intensive farming in a semi-arid state. Or suppose there's a water shortage in your body. Homeostatic solution: kidneys are the ones that figure this out, tighten things up there, produce less urine for water conservation. Allostatic solutions: brain figures this out, tells the kidneys to do their thing, sends signals to withdraw water from parts of your body where it easily evaporates (skin, mouth, nose), makes you feel thirsty. Homeostasis is about tinkering with this valve or that gizmo. Allostasis is about the brain coordinating body-wide changes, often including changes in behavior.

---

* McEwen and his work are going to pop up frequently in this book, as he is the giant of this field (as well as a wonderful man and, a long time ago, my thesis advisor).

† Physiologists actually spend a lot of time thinking about the inner workings of toilet bowls.

A final feature of allostatic thinking dovetails beautifully with thinking about stressed humans. The body doesn't pull off all this regulatory complexity only to correct some set point that has gone awry. It can also make allostatic changes in *anticipation* of a set point that is likely to go awry. And thus we hark back to the critical point of a few pages back—we don't get stressed being chased by predators. We activate the stress-response in anticipation of challenges, and typically those challenges are the purely psychological and social tumult that would make no sense to a zebra. We'll be returning repeatedly to what allostasis has to say about stress-related disease.

 ## WHAT YOUR BODY DOES TO ADAPT TO AN ACUTE STRESSOR

Within this expanded framework, a stressor can be defined as anything that throws your body out of allostatic balance and the stress-response is your body's attempt to restore allostasis. The secretion of certain hormones, the inhibition of others, the activation of particular parts of the nervous system, and so on. And regardless of the stressor—injured, starving, too hot, too cold, or psychologically stressed—you turn on the same stress-response.

It is this generality that is puzzling. If you are trained in physiology, it makes no sense at first glance. In physiology, one is typically taught that *specific* challenges to the body trigger *specific* responses and adaptations. Warming a body causes sweating and dilation of blood vessels in the skin. Chilling a body causes just the opposite—constriction of those vessels and shivering. Being too hot seems to be a very specific and different physiological challenge from being too cold, and it would seem logical that the body's responses to these two very different states should be extremely different. Instead, what kind of crazy bodily system is this that is turned on whether you are too hot or too cold, whether you are the zebra, the lion, or a terrified adolescent going to a high school dance? Why should your body have such a generalized and stereotypical stress-response, regardless of the predicament you find yourself in?

When you think about it, it actually makes sense, given the adaptations brought about by the stress-response. If you're some bacterium stressed by food shortage, you go into a suspended, dormant state. But if you're a starving lion, you're going to have to run after someone. If you're some plant stressed by someone intent on eating you, you stick poisonous chemicals in your leaves. But if you're a zebra being chased by that lion, you have to run for it. For us vertebrates, the core of the stress-response is built around the fact that your muscles are going to work like crazy. And thus the muscles need energy, right now, in the most readily utilizable form, rather than stored away somewhere in your fat cells for some building project next spring. One of the hallmarks of the stress-response is the rapid mobilization of energy from storage sites and the inhibition of further storage. Glucose and the simplest forms of proteins and fats come pouring out of your fat cells, liver, and muscles, all to stoke whichever muscles are struggling to save your neck.

If your body has mobilized all that glucose, it also needs to deliver it to the critical muscles as rapidly as possible. Heart rate, blood pressure, and breathing rate increase, all to transport nutrients and oxygen at greater rates.

Equally logical is another feature of the stress-response. During an emergency, it makes sense that your body halts long-term, expensive building projects. If there is a tornado bearing down on the house, this isn't the day to repaint the garage. Hold off on the long-term projects until you know there is a long term. Thus, during stress, digestion is inhibited—there isn't enough time to derive the energetic benefits of the slow process of digestion, so why waste energy on it? You have better things to do than digest breakfast when you are trying to avoid being someone's lunch. The same thing goes for growth and reproduction, both expensive, optimistic things to be doing with your body (especially if you are female). If the lion's on your tail, two steps behind you, worry about ovulating or growing antlers or making sperm some other time. During stress, growth and tissue repair is curtailed, sexual drive decreases in both sexes; females are less likely to ovulate or to carry pregnancies to term, while males begin to have trouble with erections and secrete less testosterone.

Along with these changes, immunity is also inhibited. The immune system, which defends against infections and illness, is ideal for spotting the tumor cell that will kill you in a year, or making enough antibodies to protect you in a few weeks, but is it really needed this instant? The logic here appears to be the same—look for tumors some other time; expend the energy more wisely now. (As we will see in chapter 8, there are some major problems with this idea that the immune system is suppressed during stress in order to save energy. But that idea will suffice for the moment.)

Another feature of the stress-response becomes apparent during times of extreme physical pain. With sufficiently sustained stress, our perception of pain can become blunted. It's the middle of a battle;

soldiers are storming a stronghold with wild abandon. A soldier is shot, grievously injured, and the man doesn't even notice it. He'll see blood on his clothes and worry that one of his buddies near him has been wounded, or he'll wonder why his innards feel numb. As the battle fades, someone will point with amazement at his injury—didn't it hurt like hell? It didn't. Such stress-induced analgesia is highly adaptive and well documented. If you are that zebra and your innards are dragging in the dust, you still have to escape. Now would not be a particularly clever time to go into shock from extreme pain.

Finally, during stress, shifts occur in cognitive and sensory skills. Suddenly certain aspects of memory improve, which is always helpful if you're trying to figure out how to get out of an emergency (Has this happened before? Is there a good hiding place?). Moreover, your senses become sharper. Think about watching a terrifying movie on television, on the edge of your seat at the tensest part. The slightest noise—a creaking door—and you nearly jump out of your skin. Better memory, sharper detection of sensations—all quite adaptive and helpful.

Collectively, the stress-response is ideally adapted for that zebra or lion. Energy is mobilized and delivered to the tissues that need them; long-term building and repair projects are deferred until the disaster has passed. Pain is blunted, cognition sharpened. Walter Cannon, the physiologist who, at the beginning of the century, paved the way for much of Selye's work and is generally considered the other godfather of the field, concentrated on the adaptive aspect of the stress-response in dealing with emergencies such as these. He formulated the well-known "fight-or-flight" syndrome to describe the stress-response, and he viewed it in a very positive light. His books, with titles such as *The Wisdom of the Body,* were suffused with a pleasing optimism about the ability of the body to weather all sorts of stressors.

Yet stressful events can sometimes make us sick. Why?

Selye, with his ulcerated rats, wrestled with this puzzle and came up with an answer that was sufficiently wrong that it is generally thought to have cost him a Nobel Prize for all his other work. He developed a three-part view of how the stress-response worked. In the initial (alarm) stage a stressor is noted; metaphorical alarms go off in your head, telling you that you are hemorrhaging, too cold, low on blood sugar, or whatever. The second stage (adaptation, or resistance) comes with the successful mobilization of the stress-response system and the reattainment of allostatic balance.

It is with prolonged stress that one enters the third stage, which Selye termed "exhaustion," where stress-related diseases emerge. Selye believed that one becomes sick at that point because stores of the hormones secreted during the stress-response are depleted. Like an army that runs out of ammunition, suddenly we have no defenses left against the threatening stressor.

It is very rare, however, as we will see, that any of the crucial hormones are actually depleted during even the most sustained of stressors. The army does not run out of bullets. Instead, the body spends so much on the defense budget that it neglects education and health care and social services (okay, so I may have a hidden agenda here). It is not so much that the stress-response runs out, but rather, with sufficient activation, that *the stress-response can become more damaging than the stressor itself*, especially when the stress is purely psychological. This is a critical concept, because it underlies the emergence of much stress-related disease.

That the stress-response itself can become harmful makes a certain sense when you examine the things that occur in reaction to stress. They are generally shortsighted, inefficient, and penny-wise and dollar-foolish, but they are the sorts of costly things your body has to do to respond effectively in an emergency. And if you experience every day as an emergency, you will pay the price.

If you constantly mobilize energy at the cost of energy storage, you will never store any surplus energy. You will fatigue more rapidly, and your risk of developing a form of diabetes will even increase. The consequences of chronically activating your cardiovascular system are similarly damaging: if your blood pressure rises to 180/100 when you are sprinting away from a lion, you are being adaptive, but if it is 180/100 every time you see the mess in your teenager's bedroom, you could be heading for a cardiovascular disaster. If you constantly turn off long-term building projects, nothing is ever repaired. For paradoxical reasons that will be explained in later chapters, you become more at risk for peptic ulcers. In kids, growth can be inhibited to the point of a rare but recognized pediatric endocrine disorder—stress dwarfism—and in adults, repair and remodeling of bone and other tissues can be disrupted. If you are constantly under stress, a variety of reproductive disorders may ensue. In females, menstrual cycles can become irregular or cease entirely; in males, sperm count and testosterone levels may decline. In both sexes, interest in sexual behavior decreases.

But that is only the start of your problems in response to chronic or repeated stressors. If you suppress immune function too long and too much, you are now more likely to fall victim to a number of infectious diseases, and be less capable of combating them once you have them.

Finally, the same systems of the brain that function more cleverly during stress can also be damaged by one class of hormones secreted during stress. As will be discussed, this may have something to do with how rapidly our brains lose cells during aging, and how much memory loss occurs with old age.

All of this is pretty grim. In the face of repeated stressors, we may be able to precariously reattain allostasis, but it doesn't come cheap, and the efforts to reestablish that balance will eventually wear us down. Here's a way to think about it: the "two elephants on a seesaw" model of stress-related disease. Put two little kids on a seesaw, and they can pretty readily balance themselves on it. This is allostatic balance when nothing stressful is going on, with the children representing the low levels of the various stress hormones that will be presented in coming chapters. In contrast, the torrents of those same stress hormones released by a stressor can be thought of as two massive elephants on the seesaw. With great effort, they can balance themselves as well. But if you constantly try to balance a seesaw with two elephants instead of two little kids, all sorts of problems will emerge:

- First, the enormous potential energies of the two elephants are consumed balancing the seesaw, instead of being able to do something more useful, like mowing the lawn or paying the bills. This is equivalent to diverting energy from various long-term building projects in order to solve short-term stressful emergencies.

- By using two elephants to do the job, damage will occur just because of how large, lumbering, and unsubtle elephants are. They squash the flowers in the process of entering the playground, they strew leftovers and garbage all over the place from the frequent snacks they must eat while balancing the seesaw, they wear out the seesaw faster, and so on. This is equivalent to a pattern of stress-related disease that will run through many of the subsequent chapters: it is hard to fix one major problem in the body without knocking something else out of balance (the very essence of allostasis spreading across systems throughout the body). Thus, you may be able to solve one bit of imbalance brought on during stress by using your elephants (your massive levels of various stress hormones), but such great quantities of those hormones can make a mess of something else in the process. And a long history of doing this produces wear and tear throughout the body, termed *allostatic load*.

- A final, subtle problem: when two elephants are balanced on a seesaw, it's tough for them to get off. Either one hops off and the other comes crashing to the ground, or there's the extremely delicate task of coordinating their delicate, lithe leaps at the same time. This is a metaphor for another theme that will run through subsequent chapters—sometimes stress-related disease can arise from turning off the stress-response too slowly, or turning off the different components of the stress-response at different speeds. When the secretion rate of one of the hormones of the stress-response returns to normal yet another of the hormones is still being secreted like mad, it can be the equivalent of one elephant suddenly being left alone on the seesaw, crashing to earth.*

The preceding pages should allow you to begin to appreciate the two punch lines of this book:

The first is that if you plan to get stressed like a normal mammal, dealing with an acute physical challenge, and you cannot appropriately *turn on* the stress-response, you're in big trouble. To see this, all you have to do is examine someone who cannot activate the stress-response. As will be explained in the coming chapters, two critical classes of hormones are secreted during stress. In one disorder, Addison's disease, you are unable to secrete one class of these hormones. In another, called Shy-Drager syndrome, it is the secretion of the second class of hormones that is impaired. People with Addison's disease or Shy-Drager syndrome are not more at risk for cancer or diabetes or any other such disorders of slow accumulation of damage. However, people with untreated Addison's disease, when faced with a major stressor such as a car accident or an infectious illness, fall into an "Addisonian" crisis, where their blood pressure drops, they cannot maintain circulation, they go into shock. In Shy-Drager syndrome, it is hard enough simply to stand up, let alone go sprinting after a zebra for dinner—mere standing causes a severe drop in blood pressure, involuntary twitching and rippling of muscles, dizziness, all sorts of unpleasantness. These two diseases teach something important, namely, that you need the stress-response during physical challenges. Addison's and Shy-Drager represent catastrophic failures of turning on the stress-response. In coming chapters, I will discuss some disorders that involve subtler undersecretion of stress hormones. These include chronic fatigue syndrome, fibromyalgia, rheumatoid arthritis, a subtype of depression, critically ill patients, and possibly individuals with post-traumatic stress disorder.

---

* If you find this analogy silly, imagine what it is like to have a bunch of scientists locked up together at a stress conference working with it. I was at a meeting where this analogy first emerged, and in no time there were factions pushing analogies about elephants on pogo sticks, elephants on monkey bars and merry-go-rounds, sumo wrestlers on seesaws, and so on.

That first punch line is obviously critical, especially for the zebra who occasionally has to run for its life. But the second punch line is far more relevant to us, sitting frustrated in traffic jams, worrying about expenses, mulling over tense interactions with colleagues. If you *repeatedly turn on* the stress-response, or if you *cannot turn off* the stress-response at the end of a stressful event, the stress-response can eventually become damaging. A large percentage of what we think of when we talk about stress-related diseases are disorders of excessive stress-responses.

A few important qualifications are necessary concerning that last statement, which is one of the central ideas of this book. On a superficial level, the message it imparts might seem to be that stressors make you sick or, as emphasized in the last few pages, that chronic or repeated stressors make you sick. It is actually more accurate to say that chronic or repeated stressors can *potentially* make you sick or can increase your *risk* of being sick. Stressors, even if massive, repetitive, or chronic in nature, do not automatically lead to illness. And the theme of the last section of this book is to make sense of why some people develop stress-related diseases more readily than others, despite the same stressor.

An additional point should be emphasized. To state that "chronic or repeated stressors can increase your risk of being sick" is actually incorrect, but in a subtle way that will initially seem like semantic nit-picking. It is never really the case that stress makes you sick, or even increases your risk of being sick. Stress increases your risk of getting *diseases* that make you sick, or if you have such a disease, stress increases the risk of your defenses being overwhelmed by the disease. This distinction is important in a few ways. First, by putting more steps between a stressor and getting sick, there are more explanations for individual differences—why only some people wind up actually getting sick. Moreover, by clarifying the progression between stressors and illness, it becomes easier to design ways to intervene in the process. Finally, it begins to explain why the stress concept often seems so suspect or slippery to many medical practitioners—clinical medicine is traditionally quite good at being able to make statements like "You feel sick because you have disease X," but is usually quite bad at being able to explain why you got disease X in the first place. Thus, medical practitioners often say, in effect, "You feel sick because you have disease X, not because of some nonsense having to do with stress; however, this ignores the stressors' role in bringing about or worsening the disease in the first place.

With this framework in mind, we can now begin the task of understanding the individual steps in this system. Chapter 2 introduces the hormones and brain systems involved in the stress-response: which ones are activated during stress, which ones are inhibited? This leads the way to chapters 3 through 10, which examine the individual systems of your body that are affected. How do those hormones enhance cardiovascular tone during stress, and how does chronic stress cause heart disease (chapter 3)? How do those hormones and neural systems mobilize energy during stress, and how does too much stress cause energetic diseases (chapter 4)? And so on. Chapter 11 examines the interactions between stress and sleep, focusing on the vicious circle of how stress can disrupt sleep and how sleep deprivation is a stressor. Chapter 12 examines the role of stress in the aging process and the disturbing recent findings that sustained exposure to certain of the hormones secreted during stress may actually accelerate the aging of the brain. As will be seen, these processes are often more complicated and subtle than they may seem from the simple picture presented in this chapter.

Chapter 13 ushers in a topic obviously of central importance to understanding our own propensity toward stress-related disease: why is psychological stress stressful? This serves as a prelude to the remaining chapters. Chapter 14 reviews major depression, a horrible psychiatric malady that afflicts vast numbers of us and is often closely related to psychological stress. Chapter 15 discusses what personality differences have to do with individual differences in patterns of stress-related disease. This is the world of anxiety disorders and Type A-ness, plus some surprises about unexpected links between personality and the stress-response. Chapter 16 considers a puzzling issue that lurks throughout reading this book—sometimes stress feels *good*, good enough that we'll pay good money to be stressed by a scary movie or roller-coaster ride. Thus, the chapter considers when stress is a good thing, and the interactions between the sense of pleasure that can be triggered by some stressors and the process of addiction.

Chapter 17 focuses above the level of the individual, looking at what your place in society, and the type of society in which you live, has to do with patterns of stress-related disease. If you plan to go no further, here's one of the punch lines of that chapter: if you want to increase your chances of avoiding stress-related diseases, make sure you don't inadvertently allow yourself to be born poor.

In many ways, the ground to be covered up to the final chapter is all bad news, as we are regaled with the evidence about new and unlikely parts of our bodies and minds that are made miserable by stress. The final chapter is meant to give some hope. Given the same external stressors, certain bodies and certain psyches deal with stress better than others. What are those folks doing right, and what can the rest of us learn from them? We'll look at the main principles of stress management and some surprising and exciting realms in which they have been applied with stunning success. While the intervening chapters document our numerous vulnerabilities to stress-related disease, the final chapter shows that we have an enormous potential to protect ourselves from many of them. Most certainly, all is not lost.

GLANDS, GOOSEFLESH, AND HORMONES

In order to begin the process of learning how stress can make us sick, there is something about the workings of the brain that we have to appreciate. It is perhaps best illustrated in the following rather technical paragraph from an early investigator in the field:

As she melted small and wonderful in his arms, she became infinitely desirable to him, all his blood-vessels seemed to scald with intense yet tender desire, for her, for her softness, for the penetrating beauty of her in his arms, passing into his blood. And softly, with that marvelous swoon-like caress of his hand in pure soft desire, softly he stroked the silky slope of her loins, down, down between her soft, warm buttocks, coming nearer and nearer to the very quick of her. And she felt him like a flame of desire, yet tender, and she felt herself melting in the flame. She let herself go. She felt his penis risen against her with silent amazing force and assertion, and she let herself go to him. She yielded with a quiver that was like death, she went all open to him.

Now think about this. If D. H. Lawrence is to your taste, there may be some interesting changes occurring in your body. You haven't just run up a flight of stairs, but maybe your heart is beating faster. The temperature has not changed in the room, but you may have just activated a sweat gland or two. And even though certain rather sensitive parts of your body are not being overtly stimulated by touch, you are suddenly very aware of them.

You sit in your chair not moving a muscle, and simply think a thought, a thought having to do with feeling angry or sad or euphoric or lustful, and suddenly your pancreas secretes some hormone. Your *pancreas*? How did you manage to do that with your pancreas? You don't even know where your pancreas is. Your liver is making an enzyme that wasn't there before, your spleen is text-messaging something to your thymus gland, blood flow in little capillaries in your ankles has just changed. All from thinking a thought.

We all understand intellectually that the brain can regulate functions throughout the rest of the body, but it is still surprising to be reminded of how far-reaching those effects can be. The purpose of this chapter is to learn a bit about the lines of communication between the brain and elsewhere, in order to see which sites are activated and which are quieted when you are sitting in your chair and feeling severely stressed. This is a prerequisite for seeing how the stress-response can save your neck during a sprint across the savanna, but make you sick during months of worry.

STRESS AND THE AUTONOMIC NERVOUS SYSTEM

The principal way in which your brain can tell the rest of the body what to do is to send messages through the nerves that branch from your brain down your spine and out to the periphery of your body. One dimension of this communication system is pretty straightforward and familiar. The voluntary nervous system is a conscious one. You decide to move a muscle and it happens. This part of the nervous system allows you to shake hands or fill out your tax forms or do a polka. It is another branch of the nervous system that projects to organs besides skeletal muscle, and this part controls the other interesting things your body does—blushing, getting gooseflesh, having an orgasm. In general, we have less control over what our brain says to our sweat glands, for example, than to our thigh muscles. (The workings of this automatic nervous system are not entirely out of our control, however; biofeedback, for example, consists of learning to alter this automatic function consciously. Potty training is another example of us gaining mastery. On a more mundane level, we are doing the same thing when we repress a loud burp during a wedding ceremony.) The set of nerve projections to places like sweat glands carry messages that are relatively involuntary and automatic. It is thus

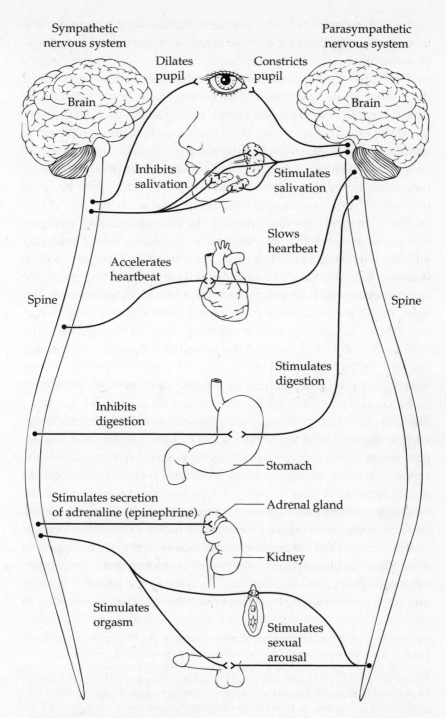

Sympathetic
nervous system

Parasympathetic
nervous system

Dilates
pupil

Constricts
pupil

Brain

Brain

Inhibits
salivation

Stimulates
salivation

Slows
heartbeat

Accelerates
heartbeat

Spine

Spine

Stimulates
digestion

Inhibits
digestion

Stomach

Stimulates secretion
of adrenaline (epinephrine)

Adrenal gland

Kidney

Stimulates
orgasm

Stimulates
sexual
arousal

Outline of some of the effects of the sympathetic and parasympathetic nervous systems on various organs and glands.

termed the *autonomic nervous system*, and it has everything to do with your response to stress. One half of this system is activated in response to stress, one half is suppressed.

The half of the autonomic nervous system that is turned on is called the *sympathetic nervous system*.* Originating in the brain, sympathetic projections exit your spine and branch out to nearly every organ, every blood vessel, and every sweat gland in your body. They even project to the scads of tiny little muscles attached to hairs on your body. If you are truly terrified by something and activate those projections, your hair stands on end; gooseflesh results when the parts of your body are activated where those muscles exist but lack hairs attached to them.

The sympathetic nervous system kicks into action during emergencies, or what you think are emergencies. It helps mediate vigilance, arousal, activation, mobilization. To generations of first-year medical students, it is described through the obligatory lame joke about the sympathetic nervous system mediating the four F's of behavior—flight, fight, fright, and sex. It is the archetypal system that is turned on at times when life gets exciting or alarming, such as during stress. The nerve endings of this system release adrenaline. When someone jumps out from behind a door and startles you, it's your sympathetic nervous system releasing adrenaline that causes your stomach to clutch. Sympathetic nerve endings also release the closely related substance noradrenaline. (*Adrenaline* and *noradrenaline* are actually British designations; the American terms, which will be used from now on, are *epinephrine* and *norepinephrine*.) Epinephrine is secreted as a result of the actions of the sympathetic nerve endings in your adrenal glands (located just above your kidneys); norepinephrine is secreted by all the other sympathetic nerve endings throughout the body. These are the chemical messengers that kick various organs into gear, within seconds.

The other half of the autonomic nervous system plays an opposing role. This parasympathetic component mediates calm, vegetative activities—everything but the four F's. If you are a growing kid and you have gone to sleep, your parasympathetic system is activated. It

---

* Where did this name come from? According to the eminent stress physiologist Seymour Levine, this goes back to Galen, who believed that the brain was responsible for rational thought and the peripheral viscera for emotions. Seeing this collection of neural pathways linking the two suggested that it allowed your brain to sympathize with your viscera. Or maybe for your viscera to sympathize with your brain. As we'll see shortly, the other half of the autonomic nervous system is called the parasympathetic nervous system. Para, meaning "alongside," refers to the not very exciting fact that the parasympathetic neural projections sit alongside those of the sympathetic.

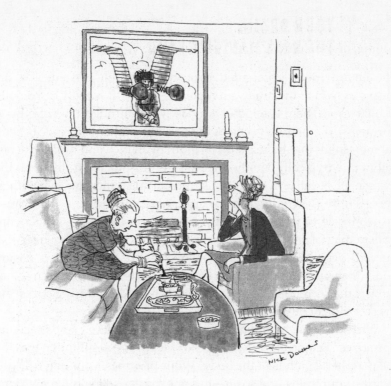

"Oh, that's Edward and his fight-or-flight mechanism."

promotes growth, energy storage, and other optimistic processes. Have a huge meal, sit there bloated and happily drowsy, and the parasympathetic is going like gangbusters. Sprint for your life across the savanna, gasping and trying to control the panic, and you've turned the parasympathetic component down. Thus, the autonomic system works in opposition: sympathetic and parasympathetic projections from the brain course their way out to a particular organ where, when activated, they bring about opposite results. The sympathetic system speeds up the heart; the parasympathetic system slows it down. The sympathetic system diverts blood flow to your muscles; the parasympathetic does the opposite. It's no surprise that it would be a disaster if both branches were very active at the same time, kind of like putting your foot on the gas and brake simultaneously. Lots of safety features exist to make sure that does not happen. For example, the parts of the brain that activate one of the two branches typically inhibit the other.

YOUR BRAIN:
THE REAL MASTER GLAND

The neural route represented by the sympathetic system is a first means by which the brain can mobilize waves of activity in response to a stressor. There is another way as well—through the secretion of hormones. If a neuron (a cell of the nervous system) secretes a chemical messenger that travels a thousandth of an inch and causes the next cell in line (typically, another neuron) to do something different, that messenger is called a neurotransmitter. Thus, when the sympathetic nerve endings in your heart secrete norepinephrine, which causes heart muscle to work differently, norepinephrine is playing a neurotransmitter role. If a neuron (or any cell) secretes a messenger that, instead, percolates into the bloodstream and affects events far and wide, that messenger is a hormone. All sorts of glands secrete hormones; the secretion of some of them is turned on during stress, and the secretion of others is turned off.

What does the brain have to do with all of these glands secreting hormones? People used to think, "Nothing." The assumption was that the peripheral glands of the body—your pancreas, your adrenal, your ovaries, your testes, and so on—in some mysterious way "knew" what they were doing, had "minds of their own." They would "decide" when to secrete their messengers, without directions from any other organ. This erroneous idea gave rise to a rather silly fad during the early part of the twentieth century. Scientists noted that men's sexual drive declined with age, and assumed that this occurs because the testicles of aging men secrete less male sex hormone, testosterone. (Actually, no one knew about the hormone testosterone at the time; they just referred to mysterious "male factors" in the testes. And in fact, testosterone levels do not plummet with age. Instead, the decline is moderate and highly variable from one male to the next, and even a decline in testosterone to perhaps 10 percent of normal levels does not have much of an effect on sexual behavior.) Making another leap, they then ascribed aging to diminishing sexual drive, to lower levels of male factors. (One may then wonder why females, without testes, manage to grow old, but the female half of the population didn't figure much in these ideas back then.) How, then, to reverse aging? Give the aging males some testicular extracts.

Soon, aged, monied gentlemen were checking into impeccable Swiss sanitariums and getting injected daily in their rears with testicular extracts from dogs, from roosters, from monkeys. You could even go out to the stockyards of the sanitarium and pick out the goat of

Advertisement, New York Therapeutic Review, *1893.*

your choice—just like picking lobsters in a restaurant (and more than one gentleman arrived for his appointment with his own prized animal in tow). This soon led to an offshoot of such "rejuvenation therapy," namely, "organotherapy"—the grafting of little bits of testes themselves. Thus was born the "monkey gland" craze, the term *gland* being used because journalists were forbidden to print the racy word *testes*. Captains of industry, heads of state, at least one pope—all signed up. And in the aftermath of the carnage of World War I, there was such a shortage of young men and such a surfeit of marriages of younger women to older men, that therapy of this sort seemed pretty important.

Naturally, the problem was that it didn't work. There wasn't any testosterone in the testicular extracts—patients would be injected with a water-based extract, and testosterone does not go into solution in water. And the smidgens of organs that were transplanted would die almost immediately, with the scar tissue being mistaken for a healthy graft. And even if they didn't die, they still wouldn't work—if aging testes are secreting less testosterone, it is not because the testes are failing, but because another organ (stay tuned) is no longer telling them to do so. Put in a brand-new set of testes and they should fail also, for lack of a stimulatory signal. But not a problem. Nearly everyone reported wondrous results anyway. If you're paying a fortune for painful daily injections of extracts of some beast's testicles, there's a certain incentive to decide you feel like a young bull. One big placebo effect.

With time, scientists figured out that the testes and other peripheral hormone-secreting glands were not autonomous, but were under the control of something else. Attention turned to the pituitary gland, sitting just underneath the brain. It was known that when the pituitary was damaged or diseased, hormone secretion throughout the body became disordered. In the early part of the century, careful experiments showed that a peripheral gland releases its hormone only if the pituitary first releases a hormone that kicks that gland into action. The pituitary contains a whole array of hormones that run the show throughout the rest of the body; it is the pituitary that actually knows the game plan and regulates what all the other glands do. This realization gave rise to the memorable cliché that the pituitary is the master gland of the body.

This understanding was disseminated far and wide, mostly in the *Reader's Digest*, which ran the "I Am Joe's" series of articles ("I Am Joe's Pancreas," "I Am Joe's Shinbone," "I Am Joe's Ovaries," and so on). By the third paragraph of "I Am Joe's Pituitary," out comes that master gland business. By the 1950s, however, scientists were already learning that the pituitary wasn't the master gland after all.

The simplest evidence was that if you removed the pituitary from a body and put it in a small bowl filled with pituitary nutrients, the gland would act abnormally. Various hormones that it would normally secrete were no longer secreted. Sure, you might say, remove any organ and throw it in some nutrient soup and it isn't going to be good for much of anything. But, interestingly, while this "explanted" pituitary stopped secreting certain hormones, it secreted others at immensely high rates. It wasn't just that the pituitary was traumatized and had shut down. It was acting erratically because, it turned out, the pituitary didn't really have the whole hormonal game plan. It would normally be following orders from the brain, and there was no brain on hand in that small bowl to give directions.

The evidence for this was relatively easy to obtain. Destroy the part of the brain right near the pituitary and the pituitary stops secreting some hormones and secretes too much of others. This tells you that the brain controls certain pituitary hormones by stimulating their release and controls others by inhibiting them. The problem was to figure out how the brain did this. By all logic, you would look for nerves to project from the brain to the pituitary (like the nerve projections to the heart and elsewhere), and for the brain to release neurotransmitters that called the shots. But no one could find these projections. In 1944, the physiologist Geoffrey Harris proposed that the brain was also a hormonal gland, that it released hormones that traveled to the pituitary and directed the pituitary's actions. In principle, this was not a crazy idea; a quarter-century before, one of the godfathers of the field, Ernst Scharrer, had shown that some other hormones, thought to originate from a peripheral gland, were actually made in the brain. Nevertheless, lots of scientists thought Harris's idea was bonkers. You can get hormones from peripheral glands like ovaries, testes, pancreas—but your *brain* oozing hormones? Preposterous! This seemed not only scientifically implausible but somehow also an unseemly and indecorous thing for your brain to be doing, as opposed to writing sonnets.

Two scientists, Roger Guillemin and Andrew Schally, began looking for these brain hormones. This was a stupendously difficult task. The brain communicates with the pituitary by a minuscule circulatory system, only slightly larger than the period at the end of this sentence. You couldn't search for these hypothetical brain "releasing hormones" and "inhibiting hormones" in the general circulation of blood; if the hormones existed, by the time they reached the voluminous general circulation, they would be diluted beyond detection. Instead, you would have to search in the tiny bits of tissue at the base of the brain containing those blood vessels going from the brain to the pituitary.

Not a trivial task, but these two scientists were up to it. They were highly motivated by the abstract intellectual puzzle of these hormones, by their potential clinical applications, by the acclaim waiting at the end of this scientific rainbow. Plus, the two of them loathed each other, which invigorated the quest. Initially, in the late 1950s, Guillemin and Schally collaborated in the search for these brain hormones. Perhaps one tired evening over the test tube rack, one of them dissed the other in some way—the actual events have sunk into historical obscurity; in any case a notorious animosity resulted, one enshrined in the annals of science at least on a par with the Greeks versus the Trojans, maybe even with Coke versus Pepsi. Guillemin and Schally went their separate ways, each intent on being the first to isolate the putative brain hormones.

How do you isolate a hormone that may not exist or that, even if it does, occurs in tiny amounts in a minuscule circulation system to which you can't gain access? Both Guillemin and Schally hit on the same strategy. They started collecting animal brains from slaughterhouses. Cut out the part at the base of the brain, near the pituitary. Throw a bunch of those in a blender, pour the resulting brain mash into a giant test tube filled with chemicals that purify the mash, collect the droplets that come out the other end. Then inject those droplets into a rat and see if the rat's pituitary changes its pattern of hormone release. If it does, maybe those brain droplets contain one of those imagined releasing or inhibiting hormones. Try to purify what's in the droplets, figure out its chemical structure, make an artificial version of it, and see if that regulates pituitary function. Pretty straightforward in theory. But it took them years.

One factor in this Augean task was the scale. There was at best a minuscule amount of these hormones in any one brain, so the scientists wound up dealing with thousands of brains at a time. The great slaughterhouse war was on. Truckloads of pig or sheep brains were collected; chemists poured cauldrons of brain into monumental chemical-separation columns, while others pondered the thimblefuls of liquid that dribbled out the bottom, purifying it further in the next column and the next. . . . But it wasn't just mindless assembly-line work. New types of chemistry had to be invented, completely novel ways of testing the effects in the living body of hormones that might or might not actually exist. An enormously difficult scientific problem, made worse by the fact that lots of influential people in the field believed these hormones were fictions and that these two guys were wasting a lot of time and money.

Guillemin and Schally pioneered a whole new corporate approach to doing science. One of our clichés is the lone scientist, sitting there at two in the morning, trying to figure out the meaning of a result. Here there were whole teams of chemists, biochemists, physiologists, and so on, coordinated into isolating these putative hormones. And it worked. A "mere" fourteen years into the venture, the chemical structure of the first releasing hormone was published.* Two years after

---

* "So," asks the breathless sports fan, "who won the race—Guillemin or Schally?" The answer depends on how you define "getting there first." The first hormone isolated was one that indirectly regulates the release of thyroid hormone (that is, it controls the way in which the pituitary regulates the thyroid). Schally and crew were the first to submit a paper for publication saying, in effect, "There really does exist a hormone in the brain that regulates thyroid hormone release, and its chemical structure is X." In a photo finish, Guillemin's team submitted a paper reaching the identical conclusion five weeks later. But as a complication, a number of months before, Guillemin and friends had been the first to publish a paper saying, in effect, "If you synthesize a chemical with structure X, it regulates thyroid hormone release and does so in a way similar to the way hypothalamic brain mash does; we don't know yet if whatever it is in the

that, in 1971, Schally got there with the sequence for the next hypothalamic hormone, and Guillemin published two months later. Guillemin took the next round in 1972, beating Schally to the next hormone by a solid three years. Everyone was delighted, the by-then-deceased Geoffrey Harris was proved correct, and Guillemin and Schally got the Nobel Prize in 1976. One of them, urbane and knowing what would sound right, proclaimed that he was motivated only by science and the impulse to help mankind; he noted how stimulating and productive his interactions with his co-winner had been. The other, less polished but more honest, said the competition was all that drove him for decades and described his relationship with his co-winner as "many years of vicious attacks and bitter retaliation."

So hooray for Guillemin and Schally; the brain turned out to be the master gland. It is now recognized that the base of the brain, the hypothalamus, contains a huge array of those releasing and inhibiting hormones, which instruct the pituitary, which in turn regulates the secretions of the peripheral glands. In some cases, the brain triggers the release of pituitary hormone X through the action of a single releasing hormone. Sometimes it halts the release of pituitary hormone Y by releasing a single inhibiting hormone. In some cases, a pituitary hormone is controlled by the coordination of both a releasing and an inhibiting hormone from the brain—dual control. To make matters worse, in some cases (for example, the miserably confusing system that I study) there is a whole array of hypothalamic hormones that collectively regulate the pituitary, some as releasers, others as inhibitors.

---

hypothalamus also has structure X, but we wouldn't be one bit surprised if it did." So Guillemin was the first to say, "This structure works like the real thing," and Schally was the first to say, "This structure is the real thing." As I have discovered firsthand many decades afterward, the battle-scarred veterans of the Guillemin-Schally prizefight years are still willing to get worked up as to which counts as the knockout.

One might wonder why something obvious wasn't done a few years into this insane competition, like the National Institutes of Health sitting the two down and saying, "Instead of us giving you all of this extra taxpayers' money to work separately, why don't you two work together?" Surprisingly, this wouldn't necessarily be all that great for scientific progress. The competition served an important purpose. Independent replication of results is essential in science. Years into a chase, a scientist triumphs and publishes the structure of a new hormone or brain chemical. Two weeks later the other guy comes forward. He has *every* incentive on earth to prove that the first guy was wrong. Instead, he is forced to say, "I hate that son of a bitch, but I have to admit he's right. We get the identical structure." That is how you know that your evidence is really solid, from independent confirmation by a hostile competitor. When everyone works together, things usually do go faster, but everyone winds up sharing the same assumptions, leaving them vulnerable to small, unexamined mistakes that can grow into big ones.

HORMONES OF THE STRESS-RESPONSE

As the master gland, the brain can experience or think of something stressful and activate components of the stress-response hormonally. Some of the hypothalamus-pituitary-peripheral gland links are activated during stress, some inhibited.

Two hormones vital to the stress-response, as already noted, are epinephrine and norepinephrine, released by the sympathetic nervous system. Another important class of hormones in the response to stress are called *glucocorticoids*. By the end of this book you will be astonishingly informed about glucocorticoid trivia, since I am in love with these hormones. Glucocorticoids are steroid hormones. (*Steroid* is used to describe the general chemical structure of five classes of hormones: androgens—the famed "anabolic" steroids like testosterone that get you thrown out of the Olympics—estrogens, progestins, mineralocorticoids, and glucocorticoids.) Secreted by the adrenal gland, they often act, as we will see, in ways similar to epinephrine. Epinephrine acts within seconds; glucocorticoids back this activity up over the course of minutes or hours.

Because the adrenal gland is basically witless, glucocorticoid release must ultimately be under the control of the hormones of the brain. When something stressful happens or you think a stressful thought, the hypothalamus secretes an array of releasing hormones into the hypothalamic-pituitary circulatory system that gets the ball rolling. The principal such releaser is called CRH (corticotropin releasing hormone), while a variety of more minor players synergize with CRH.* Within fifteen seconds or so, CRH triggers the pituitary to release the hormone ACTH (also known as *corticotropin*). After ACTH is released into the bloodstream, it reaches the adrenal gland and, within a few minutes, triggers glucocorticoid release. Together, glucocorticoids and the secretions of the sympathetic nervous system (epinephrine and norepinephrine) account for a large percentage of what

---

* For the three people on earth who are reading this book, read the prior edition, *and* remember anything from it, you may be wondering why the hormone previously known as CRF (corticotropin releasing factor) has been transformed into CRH. By the rules of endocrinology, a putative hormone is referred to as a "factor" until its chemical structure is confirmed, at which point it graduates into being a "hormone." CRF achieved that status in the mid-1980s, and my continued use of "CRF" as recently as the 1998 edition was merely a nostalgic and pathetic attempt on my part to hold on to those reckless days of my youth before CRF was tamed. After much painful psychological work, I have come to terms with this and will use "CRH" throughout.

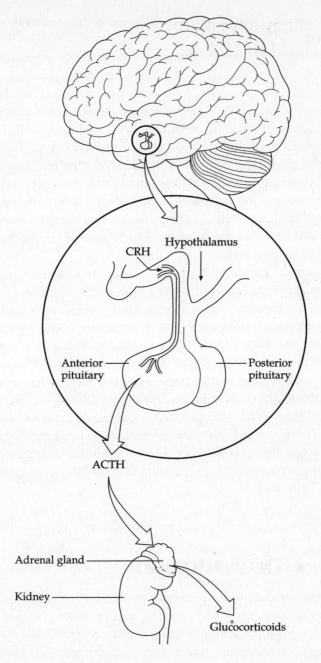

Outline of the control of glucocorticoid secretion. A stressor is sensed or antic-ipated in the brain, triggering the release of CRH (and related hormones) by the hypothalamus. These hormones enter the private circulatory system link-ing the hypothalamus and the anterior pituitary, causing the release of ACTH by the anterior pituitary. ACTH enters the general circulation and triggers the release of glucocorticoids by the adrenal gland.

happens in your body during stress. These are the workhorses of the stress-response.

In addition, in times of stress your pancreas is stimulated to release a hormone called *glucagon*. *Gluc*ocorticoids, *gluc*agon, and the sympathetic nervous system raise circulating levels of the sugar *gluc*ose. As we will see, these hormones are essential for mobilizing energy during stress. Other hormones are activated as well. The pituitary secretes prolactin, which, among other effects, plays a role in suppressing reproduction during stress. Both the pituitary and the brain also secrete a class of endogenous morphine-like substances called *endorphins* and *enkephalins,* which help blunt pain perception, among other things. Finally, the pituitary also secretes vasopressin, also known as *antidiuretic hormone,* which plays a role in the cardio-vascular stress-response.

Just as some glands are activated in response to stress, various hormonal systems are inhibited during stress. The secretion of various reproductive hormones such as estrogen, progesterone, and testosterone is inhibited. Hormones related to growth (such as growth hormone) are also inhibited, as is the secretion of insulin, a pancreatic hormone that normally tells your body to store energy for later use.

(Are you overwhelmed and intimidated by these terms, wondering if you should have bought some Deepak Chopra self-help book instead? Please, don't even dream of memorizing these names of hormones. The important ones are going to appear so regularly in the coming pages that you will soon be comfortably and accurately slipping them into everyday conversation and birthday cards to favorite cousins. Trust me.)

 A FEW COMPLICATIONS

This, then, is an outline of our current understanding of the neural and hormonal messengers that carry the brain's news that something awful is happening. Cannon was the first to recognize the role of epinephrine, norepinephrine, and the sympathetic nervous system. As noted in the previous chapter, he coined the phrase "fight-or-flight" response, which is a way of conceptualizing the stress-response as preparing the body for that sudden burst of energy demands. Selye pioneered the glucocorticoid component of the story. Since then the roles of the other hormones and neural systems have been recognized. In the dozen years since this book first came out, various new minor hormonal players have been added to the picture, and, undoubtedly, more are yet to be discovered. Collectively, these shifts in secretion and activation form the primary stress-response.

Naturally there are complications. As will be reiterated throughout the following chapters, the stress-response is about preparing the body for a major expenditure of energy—the canonical (or, perhaps, Cannonical) "fight-or-flight" response. Recent work by the psychologist Shelley Taylor of UCLA has forced people to rethink this. She suggests that the fight-or-flight response is what dealing with stress is about in males, and that it has been overemphasized as a phenomenon because of the long-standing bias among (mostly male) scientists to study males rather than females.

Taylor argues convincingly that the physiology of the stress-response can be quite different in females, built around the fact that in most species, females are typically less aggressive than males, and that having dependent young often precludes the option of flight. Showing that she can match the good old boys at coming up with a snappy sound bite, Taylor suggests that rather than the female stress-response being about fight-or-flight, it's about "tend and befriend"—taking care of her young and seeking social affiliation. As will be seen in the final chapter of the book, there are some striking gender differences in stress management styles that support Taylor's view, many of them built around the propensity toward social affiliation.

Taylor also emphasizes a hormonal mechanism that helps contribute to the "tend and befriend" stress-response. While the sympathetic nervous system, glucocorticoids, and the other hormones just reviewed are about preparing the body for major physical demands, the hormone *oxytocin* seems more related to the tend and befriend themes. The pituitary hormone plays a role in causing the female of various mammalian species to imprint on her child after birth, to stimulate milk production, and to stimulate maternal behavior. Moreover, oxytocin may be critical for a female to form a monogamous pair bond with a male (in the relatively few mammalian species that are monogamous).* And the fact that oxytocin is secreted during stress in females supports the idea that responding to stress may not just consist of preparing for a mad dash across the savanna, but may also involve feeling a pull toward sociality.

A few critics of Taylor's influential work have pointed out that sometimes the stress-response in females can be about fight-or-flight,

---

* A list of species that probably should not include humans, by a number of biological criteria. But that's another book.

rather than affiliation. For example, females are certainly capable of being wildly aggressive (often in the context of protecting their young), and often sprint for their lives or for a meal (among lions, for example, females do most of the hunting). Moreover, sometimes the stress-response in males can be about affiliation rather than fight-or-flight. This can take the form of creating affiliative coalitions with other males or, in those rare monogamous species (in which males typically do a fair amount of the child care), some of the same tending and befriending behaviors as seen among females. Nevertheless, amid these criticisms, there is a widespread acceptance of the idea that the body does not respond to stress merely by preparing for aggression or escape, and that there are important gender differences in the physiology and psychology of stress.

Some more complications arise. Even when considering the classic stress-response built around fight-or-flight, not all of its features work quite the same way in different species. For example, while stress causes a prompt decline in the secretion of growth hormone in rats, it causes a transient increase in growth hormone secretion in humans (this puzzle and its implication for humans are discussed in the chapter on growth).

Another complication concerns the time course in actions of epinephrine and glucocorticoids. A few paragraphs back, I noted that the former works within seconds, while the latter backs up epinephrine's activity over the course of minutes to hours. That's great—in the face of an invading army, sometimes the defensive response can take the form of handing out guns from an armory (epinephrine working in seconds), and a defense can also take the form of beginning construction of new tanks (glucocorticoids working over hours). But within the framework of lions chasing zebras, how many sprints across the grasslands actually go on for hours? What good are glucocorticoids if some of their actions occur long after your typical dawn-on-the-savanna stressor is over with? Some glucocorticoid actions do help mediate the stress-response. Others help mediate the *recovery* from the stress-response. As will be described in chapter 8, this probably has important implications for a number of autoimmune diseases. And some glucocorticoid actions *prepare* you for the next stressor. As will be discussed in chapter 13, this is critical for understanding the ease with which anticipatory psychological states can trigger glucocorticoid secretion.

Another complication concerns consistency of the stress-response when it is activated. Central to Selye's conceptualization was the belief that whether you are too hot or too cold, or are that zebra or that lion (or simply stressed by the repetitiveness of that phrase), you activate the same pattern of secretion of glucocorticoids, epinephrine, growth hormone, estrogen, and so forth for each of those stressors. This is mostly true, and this intertwining of the various branches of the stress-response into a package deal starts at the brain, where the same pathway can both stimulate CRH release from the hypothalamus and activate the sympathetic nervous system. Moreover, epinephrine and glucocorticoids, both secreted by the adrenal, can potentiate each other's release.

However, it turns out that not all stressors produce the exact same stress-response. The sympathetic nervous system and glucocorticoids play a role in the response to virtually all stressors. But the speed and magnitudes of the sympathetic and glucocorticoid branches can vary depending on the stressor, and not all of the other endocrine components of the stress-response are activated for all stressors. The orchestration and patterning of hormone release tend to vary at least somewhat from stressor to stressor, with there being a particular hormonal "signature" for a particular stressor.

One example concerns the relative magnitude of the glucocorticoid versus the sympathetic stress-responses. James Henry, who has done pioneering work on the ability of social stressors such as subordinance to cause heart disease in rodents, has found that the sympathetic nervous system is particularly activated in a socially subordinate rodent that is vigilant and trying to cope with a challenge. In contrast, it is the glucocorticoid system that is relatively more activated in a subordinate rodent that has given up on coping. Studies of humans have shown what may be a human analogue of that dichotomy. Sympathetic arousal is a relative marker of anxiety and vigilance, while heavy secretion of glucocorticoids is more a marker of depression. Furthermore, all stressors do not cause secretion of both epinephrine and norepinephrine, nor of norepinephrine from all branches of the sympathetic system.

In some cases, the stress signature sneaks in through the back door. Two stressors can produce identical profiles of stress hormone release into the bloodstream. So where's the signature that differentiates them? Tissues in various parts of the body may be altered in their *sensitivity* to a stress hormone in the case of one stressor, but not the other.

Finally, as will be the topic of chapter 13, two identical stressors can cause very different stress signatures, depending on the psychological context of the stressors. Thus, every stressor does not generate exactly the same stress-response. This is hardly surprising. Despite the dimensions common to various stressors, it is still a very different physiological challenge to be too hot or too cold, to be extremely anxious or deeply depressed. Despite this, the hormonal changes outlined in this chapter, which occur pretty reliably in the face of impressively different stressors, still constitute the superstructure of the neural and endocrine stress-response. We are now in a position to see how these responses collectively save our skins during acute emergencies but can make us sick in the long run.

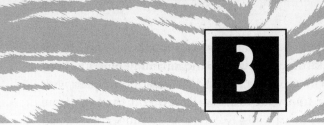

3

STROKE, HEART ATTACKS, AND VOODOO DEATH

It's one of those unexpected emergencies: you're walking down the street, on your way to meet a friend for dinner. You're already thinking about what you'd like to eat, savoring your hunger. Come around the corner and—oh no, a lion! As we now know, activities throughout your body shift immediately to meet the crisis: your digestive tract shuts down and your breathing rate skyrockets. Secretion of sex hormones is inhibited, while epinephrine, norepinephrine, and glucocorticoids pour into the bloodstream. And if your legs are going to save you, one of the most important additional things that better be going on is an increase in your cardiovascular output, in order to deliver oxygen and energy to those exercising muscles.

THE CARDIOVASCULAR STRESS-RESPONSE

Activating your cardiovascular system is relatively easy, so long as you have a sympathetic nervous system plus some glucocorticoids and don't bother with too many details. The first thing you do is shift your heart into higher gear, get it to beat faster. This is accomplished by turning down parasympathetic tone, and in turn activating the sympathetic nervous system. Glucocorticoids add to this as well, both by activating neurons in the brain stem that stimulate sympathetic arousal, and by enhancing the effects of epinephrine and norepineph-rine on heart muscle. You also want to increase the *force* with which your heart beats. This involves a trick with the veins that return blood to your heart. Your sympathetic nervous system causes them to constrict, to get more rigid. And that causes the returning blood to blast through those veins with more force. Blood returns to your heart with more force, slamming into your heart walls, distending them more than usual . . . and those heart walls, like a stretched rubber band, snap back with more force.

So your heart rate and blood pressure have gone up. The next task is to distribute the blood prudently throughout that sprinting body of yours. Arteries are relaxed—dilated—that lead to your muscles, increasing blood flow and energy delivery there. At the same time, there is a dramatic decrease in blood flow to nonessential parts of your body, like your digestive tract and skin (you also shift the pattern of blood flow to your brain, something that will be discussed in chapter 10). The decrease in blood flow to the gut was first noted in 1833, in an extended study of a Native American who had a tube placed in his abdomen after a gunshot wound there. When the man sat quietly, his gut tissues were bright pink, well supplied with blood. Whenever he became anxious or angry, the gut mucosa would blanch, because of decreased blood flow. (Pure speculation, perhaps, but one suspects that his transients of anxiety and anger might have been related to those white folks sitting around experimenting on him, instead of doing something useful, like sewing him up.)

There's one final cardiovascular trick in response to stress, involving the kidneys. As that zebra with its belly ripped open, you've lost a lot of blood. And you're going to need that blood to deliver energy to your exercising muscles. Your body needs to conserve water. If blood volume goes down because of dehydration or hemorrhage, it doesn't matter what your heart and veins are doing; your ability to deliver glucose and oxygen to your muscles will be impaired. What's the most likely place to be losing water? Urine formation, and the source of the water in urine is the bloodstream. Thus, you decrease blood flow to your kidneys and, in addition, your brain sends a message to the kidneys: stop the process, reabsorb the water into the circulatory system. This is accomplished by the hormone vasopressin (known as *antidiuretic hormone* for its ability to block diuresis, or urine formation), as well as a host of related hormones that regulate water balance.

A question no doubt at the forefront of every reader's mind at this point: if one of the features of the cardiovascular stress-response is to conserve water in the circulation, and this is accomplished by inhibition of urine formation in the kidneys, why is it that when we are *really* terrified, we wet our pants? I congratulate the reader for homing in on one of the remaining unanswered questions of modern science. In trying to answer it, we run into a larger one. Why do we have bladders? They are dandy if you are a hamster or a dog, because species like those fill their bladders up until they are just about to burst and then run around their territories, demarcating the boundaries—odoriferous little "keep out" signs to the neighbors.* A bladder is logical for scent-marking species, but I presume that you don't do that sort of thing.† For humans, it is a mystery, just a boring storage site. The kidneys, now those are something else. Kidneys are reabsorptive, bidirectional organs, which means you can spend your whole afternoon happily putting water in from the circulation and getting some back and regulating the whole thing with a collection of hormones. But once the urine leaves the kidneys and heads south to the bladder, you can kiss that stuff good-bye; the bladder is unidirectional. When it comes to a stressful emergency, a bladder means a lot of sloshy dead weight to carry in your sprint across the savanna. The answer is obvious: empty that bladder.‡

---

* One of my intrepid research assistants, Michelle Pearl, called up some of America's leading urologists to ask them why bladders evolved. One comparative urologist (as well as Jay Kaplan, whose research is discussed in this chapter) took the findings about territorial rodents having bladders to make scent trails and inverted the argument—maybe we have bladders so that we can avoid continual dribble of urine that would leave a scent trail so some predator could track us. The same urologist noted, however, that a weakness with his idea is that fish also have bladders, and they presumably don't have to worry about leaving scent trails. A number of urologists suggested that maybe the bladder acts as a buffer between the kidney and the outside world, to reduce the chance of kidney infections. However, it seems odd to develop an organ exclusively for the purpose of protecting another organ from infection. Pearl suggested that it may have evolved for male reproduction—the acidity of urine isn't very healthy for sperm (in ancient times, women would use half a lemon as a diaphragm), so perhaps it made sense to evolve a storage site for the urine. A remarkable percentage of the urologists questioned said something like, "Well, it would be an extreme social liability to not have a bladder," before realizing that they had just suggested that vertebrates evolved bladders tens of millions of years ago so that we humans wouldn't inadvertently pee on our party clothes. Mostly, however, the urologists said things like, "To be honest, I've never thought about this before," "I don't know and I talked to everyone here and they don't know anything either," and "Beats me."

The strangest thing about it all is that many animals may not actually take advantage of their bladder's storage capacity. In my vast experience watching baboons go about their urinary business, it is apparent that they very rarely hold it in when they have to go. Clearly, there's a lot of work to be done in this area.

† Well, maybe some humans do. When the Allies breached the Rhine River in Germany during World War II by putting up a pontoon bridge, General George Patton apparently walked across it, stopped in the middle, and, with cameras blazing, took a piss in the Rhine. "I've been waiting a long time for that," he said. Continuing this intersection of militarism, bodies of water, and scent-marking, during the Korean War, American troops would line up along the Yalu River, across from Chinese soldiers facing them, and urinate en masse into the river.

‡ It should be noted that in kids, while stress can increase the occurrence of enuresis (loss of control of the bladder), most kids who have nocturnal enuresis (bed-wetting)

THE FAR SIDE   By GARY LARSON

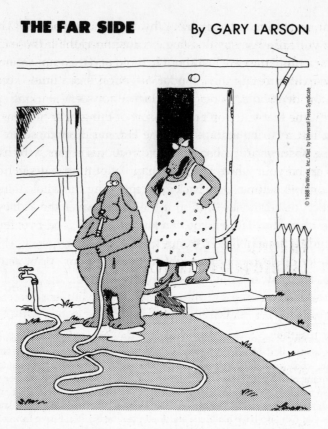

"So! Planning on roaming the neighborhood with some of your buddies today?"

Everything is great now—you have kept your blood volume up, it is roaring through the body with more force and speed, delivered where it is most needed. This is just what you want when running away from a lion. Interestingly, Marvin Brown of the University of California at San Diego and Laurel Fisher of the University of Arizona have shown that a different picture emerges when one is being vigilant—a gazelle crouching in the grass, absolutely quiet, as a lion passes nearby. The sight of a lion is obviously a stressor, but of a subtle sort; while having to remain as still as possible, you must also be prepared, physiologically, for a wild sprint across the grasslands with the briefest

---

are psychologically normal. This entire discussion raises that mysterious problem for guys as to why it is so difficult to urinate at a urinal when you are stressed by a crowd waiting in line behind you, all impatiently waiting to get back to their seats before the movie starts.

of warnings. During such vigilance, heart rate and blood flow tend to slow down, and vascular resistance throughout the body increases, including in the muscles. Another example of the complicating point brought up at the end of chapter 2 about stress signatures—you don't turn on the identical stress-response for every type of stressor.

Finally, the stressor is over, the lion pursues some other pedestrian, you can return to your dinner plans. The various hormones of the stress-response turn off, your parasympathetic nervous system begins to slow down your heart via something called the vagus nerve, and your body calms down.

 ## CHRONIC STRESS AND CARDIOVASCULAR DISEASE

So you've done all the right things during your lion encounter. But if you put your heart, blood vessels, and kidneys to work in this way every time someone irritates you, you increase your risk of heart disease. Never is the maladaptiveness of the stress-response during psychological stress clearer than in the case of the cardiovascular system. You sprint through the restaurant district terrified, and you alter cardiovascular functions to divert more blood flow to your thigh muscles. In such cases, there's a wonderful match between blood flow and metabolic demand. In contrast, if you sit and think about a major deadline looming next week, driving yourself into a hyperventilating panic, you still alter cardiovascular function to divert more blood flow to your limb muscles. Crazy. And, potentially, eventually damaging.

How does stress-induced elevation of blood pressure during chronic psychological stress wind up causing cardiovascular disease, the number one killer in the United States and the developed world? Basically, your heart is just a dumb, simple mechanical pump, and your blood vessels are nothing more exciting than hoses. The cardiovascular stress-response essentially consists of making them work harder for a while, and if you do that on a regular basis, they will wear out, just like any pump or hose you'd buy at Sears.

The first step in the road to stress-related disease is developing hypertension, chronically elevated blood pressure.* This one seems

---

* Resting blood pressure where systolic pressure—the upper number, reflecting the force with which blood is leaving your heart—is above 140, or when diastolic pressure—the lower number, reflecting the force with which blood returns to your heart—is above 90, is considered elevated.

obvious: if stress causes your blood pressure to go up, then chronic stress causes your blood pressure to go up chronically. Task accomplished, you've got hypertension.

It's a bit messier because a vicious cycle emerges at this point. The little blood vessels distributed throughout your body have the task of regulating blood flow to the local neighborhoods as a means of ensuring adequate local levels of oxygen and nutrients. If you chronically raise your blood pressure—chronically increase the force with which blood is coursing through those small vessels—those vessels have to work harder to regulate the blood flow. Think of the ease it takes to control a garden hose spritzing water versus a firehose with a hydrant's worth of force gushing through it. The latter takes more muscle. And that's precisely what happens at these small vessels. They build a thicker muscle layer around them, to better control the increased force of blood flow. But as a result of these thicker muscles, these vessels now have become more rigid, more resistant to the force of blood flow. Which tends to increase blood pressure. Which tends to further increase vascular resistance. Which tends . . .

So you've gotten yourself chronically high blood pressure. This isn't great for your heart. Blood is now returning to your heart with more force and, as mentioned, this makes for a greater impact upon the heart muscle wall that encounters that tsunami. Over time, that wall will thicken with more muscle. This is termed "left ventricular hypertrophy," which means increasing the mass of the left ventricle, the part of the heart in question. Your heart is now lopsided, in a sense, being overdeveloped in one quadrant. This increases the risk of developing an irregular heartbeat. And more bad news: in addition, this thickened wall of ventricular heart muscle may now require more blood than the coronary arteries can supply. It turns out that after controlling for age, having left ventricular hypertrophy is the single best predictor of cardiac risk.

The hypertension isn't good for your blood vessels, either. A general feature of the circulatory system is that, at various points, large blood vessels (your descending aorta, for example) branch into smaller vessels, then into even smaller ones, and so on, down to tiny beds of thousands of capillaries. This process of splitting into smaller and smaller units is called *bifurcation*. (As a measure of how extraordinarily efficient this repeated bifurcation is in the circulatory system, no cell in your body is more than five cells away from a blood vessel—yet the circulatory system takes up only 3 percent of body mass.) One feature of systems that branch in this way is that the points of bifurcation are particularly vulnerable to injury. The branch points in the vessel wall where bifurcation occurs bear the brunt of the fluid pressure slamming into them. Thus, a simple rule: when you increase the force with which the fluid is moving through the system, turbulence increases and those outposts of wall are more likely to get damaged.

With the chronic increase in blood pressure that accompanies repeated stress, damage begins to occur at branch points in arteries throughout the body. The smooth inner lining of the vessel begins to tear or form little craters of damage. Once this layer is damaged, you get an inflammatory response—cells of the immune system that mediate inflammation aggregate at the injured site. Moreover, cells full of fatty nutrients, called foam cells, begin to form there, too. In addition, during stress the sympathetic nervous system makes your blood more viscous. Specifically, epinephrine makes circulating platelets (a type of blood cell that promotes clotting) more likely to clump together, and these clumped platelets can get gummed up in these aggregates as well. As we'll see in the next chapter, during stress you're mobilizing energy into the bloodstream, including fat, glucose, and the "bad" type of cholesterol, and these can also add to the aggregate. All sorts of fibrous gunk builds up there, too. You've now made yourself an atherosclerotic plaque.

Therefore, stress can promote plaque formation by increasing the odds of blood vessels being damaged and inflamed, and by increasing the likelihood that circulating crud (platelets, fat, cholesterol, and so on) sticks to those inflamed injury sites. For years, clinicians have tried to get a sense of someone's risk of cardiovascular disease by measuring how much of one particular type of crud there is in the bloodstream. This is, of course, cholesterol, leading to such a skittishness about cholesterol that the egg industry has to urge us to give their cholesterol-filled products a break. High levels of cholesterol, particularly of "bad" cholesterol, certainly increase the risk for cardiovascular disease. But they're not a great predictor; a surprising number of folks can tolerate high levels of bad cholesterol without cardiovascular consequences, and only about half of heart attack victims have elevated cholesterol levels.

In the last few years, it is becoming clear that the amount of damaged, inflamed blood vessels is a better predictor of cardiovascular trouble than is the amount of circulating crud. This makes sense, in that you can eat eleventy eggs a day and have no worries in the atherosclerosis realm if there are no damaged vessels for crud to stick to; conversely, plaques can be forming even amid "healthy" levels of cholesterol, if there is enough vascular damage.

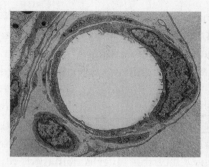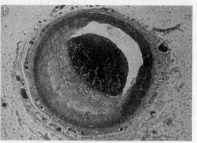

A healthy blood vessel (left), and one with an atherosclerotic plaque (right).

How can you measure the amount of inflammatory damage? A great marker is turning out to be something called C-reactive protein (CRP). It is made in the liver and is secreted in response to a signal indicating an injury. It migrates to the damaged vessel where it helps amplify the cascade of inflammation that is developing. Among other things, it helps trap bad cholesterol in the inflamed aggregate.

CRP is turning out to be a much better predictor of cardiovascular disease risk than cholesterol, even years in advance of disease onset. As a result, CRP has suddenly become quite trendy in medicine, and is fast becoming a standard endpoint to measure in general blood work on patients.

Thus, chronic stress can cause hypertension and atherosclerosis—the accumulation of these plaques. One of the clearest demonstrations of this, with great application to our own lives, is to be found in the work of the physiologist Jay Kaplan at Bowman Grey Medical School. Kaplan built on the landmark work of an earlier physiologist, James Henry (who was mentioned in the previous chapter), who showed that purely social stress caused both hypertension and atherosclerosis in mice. Kaplan and colleagues have shown a similar phenomenon in primates, bringing the story much closer home to us humans. Establish male monkeys in a social group, and over the course of days to months they'll figure out where they stand with respect to one another. Once a stable dominance hierarchy has emerged, the last place you want to be is on the bottom: not only are you subject to the most physical stressors but, as will be reviewed in chapter 13 on psychological stress, to the most psychological stressors as well. Such subordinate males show a lot of the physiological indices of chronically turning on their stress-responses. And often these animals wind up with atherosclerotic plaques—their arteries are all clogged up. As evidence that the atherosclerosis arises from the overactive sympathetic nervous system component of the stress-response, if Kaplan gave the monkeys at risk drugs that prevent sympathetic activity (beta-blockers), they didn't form plaques.

Kaplan showed that another group of animals is also at risk. Suppose you keep the dominance system *un*stable by shifting the monkeys into new groups every month, so that all the animals are perpetually in the tense, uncertain stage of figuring out where they stand with respect to everyone else. Under those circumstances, it is generally the animals precariously holding on to their places at the top of the shifting dominance hierarchy who do the most fighting and show the most behavioral and hormonal indices of stress. And, as it turns out, they have tons of atherosclerosis; some of the monkeys even have heart attacks (abrupt blockages of one or more of the coronary arteries).

In general, the monkeys under the most social stress were most at risk for plaque formation. Kaplan showed that this can even occur with a low-fat diet, which makes sense, since, as will be described in the next chapter, a lot of the fat that forms plaques is being mobilized from stores in the body, rather than coming from the cheeseburger the monkey ate just before the tense conference. But if you couple the social stress with a high-fat diet, the effects synergize, and plaque formation goes through the roof.

So stress can increase the risk of atherosclerosis. Form enough atherosclerotic plaques to seriously obstruct flow to the lower half of the body and you get *claudication,* which means that your legs and chest hurt like hell for lack of oxygen and glucose whenever you walk; you are then a candidate for bypass surgery. If the same thing happens to the arteries going to your heart, you can get coronary heart disease, myocardial ischemia, all sorts of horrible things.

But we're not done. Once you've formed those plaques, continued stress can get you in trouble another way. Again, increase stress and increase blood pressure, and, as the blood moves with enough force, increase the chances of tearing that plaque loose, rupturing it. So maybe you've had a plaque form in a huge aqueduct of a blood vessel, with the plaque being way too small to cause any trouble. But tear it loose now, form what is called a *thrombus,* and that mobile hairball can now lodge in a much smaller blood vessel, clogging it completely. Clog up a coronary artery and you've got a myocardial infarct, a heart attack (and this thrombus route accounts for the vast majority of heart attacks). Clog up a blood vessel in the brain and you have a brain infarct (a stroke).

But there's more bad news. If chronic stress has made a mess of your blood vessels, each individual new stressor is even more damaging, for

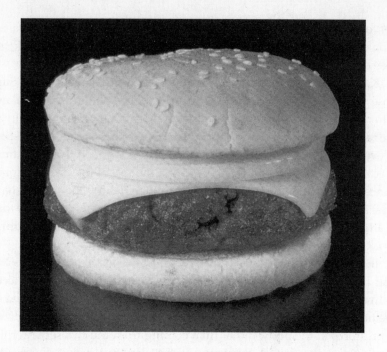

an additional insidious reason. This has to do with myocardial ischemia, a condition that arises when the arteries feeding your heart have become sufficiently clogged that your heart itself is partially deprived of blood flow and thus of oxygen and glucose.* Suppose something acutely stressful is happening, and your cardiovascular system is in great shape. You get excited, the sympathetic nervous system kicks into action. Your heart speeds up in a strong, coordinated fashion, and its contractive force increases. As a result of working harder, the heart muscle consumes more energy and oxygen and, conveniently, the arteries going to your heart dilate in order to deliver more nutrients and oxygen to the muscle. Everything is fine.

But if you encounter an acute stressor with a heart that has been suffering from chronic myocardial ischemia, you're in trouble. The

---

* It may initially seem illogical for the heart to need special arteries feeding it. When the walls of the heart—the heart muscle—require the energy and oxygen stores in the blood, you might imagine that these could simply be absorbed from the vast amounts of blood passing through the chambers of the heart. But instead it has evolved that heart muscle is fed by arteries coursing from the main aorta. As an analogy, consider people working at a city's water reservoir. Every time they get thirsty, they might go over to the edge of the reservoir with a bucket and pull up some water to drink. (Instead, the usual solution is to have a water fountain in the office, fed indirectly by that reservoir just outside.)

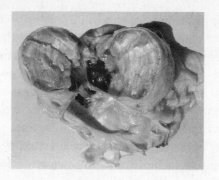

A necrotic heart.

coronary arteries, instead of vasodilating in response to the sympathetic nervous system, vaso*constrict.* This is very different from the scenario described at the beginning of the chapter, where you are constricting some big blood vessels that deliver blood to unessential parts of your body. Instead, these are the small vessels diverting blood right to your heart. Just when your heart needs more oxygen and glucose delivered through these already clogged vessels, acute stress shuts them down even more, producing a shortage of nutrients for the heart, *myocardial ischemia.* This is exactly the opposite of what you need. Your chest is going to hurt like crazy—angina pectoris. And it turns out that it takes only brief periods of hypertension to cause this vasoconstrictive problem. Therefore, chronic myocardial ischemia from atherosclerosis sets you up for, at the least, terrible chest pain whenever anything physically stressful occurs. This is the perfect demonstration of how stress is extremely effective at worsening a preexisting problem.

When cardiology techniques improved in the 1970s, cardiologists were surprised to discover that we are even more vulnerable to trouble in this realm than had been guessed. With the old techniques, you would take someone with myocardial ischemia and wire him (men are more prone to heart disease than women) up to some massive ECG machine (same as EKG), focus a huge X-ray camera on his chest, and then send him running on a treadmill until he was ready to collapse. Just as one would expect, blood flow to the heart would decrease and his chest would hurt.

Some engineers invented a miniature ECG machine that can be strapped on while you go about your daily business, and *ambulatory electrocardiography* was invented. Everyone got a rude surprise. There were little ischemic crises occurring all over the place in people at risk.

Most ischemic episodes turned out to be "silent"—they didn't give a warning signal of pain. Moreover, all sorts of psychological stressors could trigger them, like public speaking, pressured interviews, exams. According to the old dogma, if you had heart disease, you had better worry when you were undergoing physical stress and getting chest pains. Now it appears that, for someone at risk, trouble is occurring under all sorts of circumstances of psychological stress in everyday life, and you may not even know it. Once the cardiovascular system is damaged, it appears to be immensely sensitive to acute stressors, whether physical or psychological.

One last bit of bad news. We've been focusing on the stress-related consequences of activating the cardiovascular system too often. What about turning it off at the end of each psychological stressor? As noted earlier, your heart slows down as a result of activation of the vagus nerve by the parasympathetic nervous system. Back to the autonomic nervous system never letting you put your foot on the gas and brake at the same time—by definition, if you are turning on the sympathetic nervous system all the time, you're chronically shutting off the parasympathetic. And this makes it harder to slow things down, even during those rare moments when you're not feeling stressed about something.

How can you diagnose a vagus nerve that's not doing its part to calm down the cardiovascular system at the end of a stressor? A clinician could put someone through a stressor, say, run the person on a treadmill, and then monitor the speed of recovery afterward. It turns out that there is a subtler but easier way of detecting a problem. Whenever you inhale, you turn on the sympathetic nervous system slightly, minutely speeding up your heart. And when you exhale, the parasympathetic half turns on, activating your vagus nerve in order to slow things down (this is why many forms of meditation are built around extended exhalations). Therefore, the length of time between heartbeats tends to be shorter when you're inhaling than exhaling. But what if chronic stress has blunted the ability of your parasympathetic nervous system to kick the vagus nerve into action? When you exhale, your heart won't slow down, won't increase the time intervals between beats. Cardiologists use sensitive monitors to measure interbeat intervals. Large amounts of variability (that is to say, short interbeat intervals during inhalation, long during exhalation) mean you have strong parasympathetic tone counteracting your sympathetic tone, a good thing. Minimal variability means a parasympathetic component that has trouble putting its foot on the brake. This is the marker of someone who not only turns on the cardiovascular stress-response too often but, by now, has trouble turning it off.

 ## SUDDEN CARDIAC DEATH

The preceding sections demonstrate how chronic stress will gradually damage the cardiovascular system, with each succeeding stressor making the system even more vulnerable. But one of the most striking and best-known features of heart disease is how often that cardiac catastrophe hits during a stressor. A man gets shocking news: his wife has died; he's lost his job; a child long thought to be dead appears at the door; he wins the lottery. The man weeps, rants, exults, staggers about gasping and hyperventilating with the force of the news. Soon afterward, he suddenly grasps at his chest and falls over dead from sudden cardiac arrest. A strong, adverse emotion like anger doubles the risk of a heart attack during the subsequent two hours. For example, during the O. J. Simpson trial, Bill Hodgman, one of the prosecutors, got chest pains around the twentieth time he jumped up to object to something Johnnie Cochran was saying, and collapsed afterward (he survived). This sort of cardiac vulnerability to strong emotions has led Las Vegas casinos to keep defibrillators handy. It also is thought to have a lot to do with why exposure to New York City is a risk factor for a fatal heart attack.*

The phenomenon is quite well documented. In one study, a physician collected newspaper clippings on sudden cardiac death in 170 individuals. He identified a number of events that seemed to be associated with such deaths: the collapse, death, or threat of loss of someone

---

* This is for real, as was reported in a widely cited study published in 1999 by Nicholas Christenfeld and colleagues at the University of California at San Diego (what, you were expecting NYU?). The authors did a superb job of ruling out various confounding factors. They showed that this increased risk didn't occur in other urban areas in the country. It wasn't due to self-selection (i.e., who but stressed, heart disease–prone crazies choose to live in NYC?). It was not a function of socioeconomic status, race, ethnicity, or immigrant status. It was not due to people happening to be in NYC at the time of day when people get more heart attacks (i.e., commuters during work hours). It wasn't due to New York doctors having a tendency to mislabel other maladies as heart attacks. Instead, it was most plausibly a function of stress, excitement, fear, and more disruption of sleep/wake cycles than in most other places. And this was before 9/11. Naturally, like all the other native New Yorkers I know, I find this paper to be perversely pleasing and affirming.

close; acute grief; loss of status or self-esteem; mourning, on an anniversary; personal danger; threat of an injury, or recovery from such a threat; triumph or extreme joy. Other studies have shown the same. During the 1991 Persian Gulf war fewer deaths in Israel were due to SCUD missile damage than to sudden cardiac death among frightened elderly people. During the 1994 L. A. earthquake, there was similarly a big jump in heart attacks.*

The actual causes are obviously tough to study (since you can't predict what's going to happen, and you can't interview the people afterward to find out what they were feeling), but the general consensus among cardiologists is that sudden cardiac death is simply an extreme version of acute stress causing ventricular arrhythmia or, even worse, ventricular fibrillation plus ischemia in the heart.† As you would guess, it involves the sympathetic nervous system, and it is more likely to happen in damaged heart tissue than in healthy tissue. People *can* suffer sudden cardiac death without a history of heart disease and despite increased blood flow in the coronary vessels; autopsies have generally shown, however, that these people had a fair amount of atherosclerosis. Mysterious cases still occur, however, of seemingly healthy thirty-year-olds, victims of sudden cardiac death, who show little evidence of atherosclerosis on autopsy.

Fibrillation seems to be the critical event in sudden cardiac death, as judged by animal studies (in which, for example, ten hours of stress for a rat makes its heart more vulnerable to fibrillation for days afterward). As one cause, the muscle of a diseased heart becomes more electrically excitable, making it prone to fibrillation. In addition, activation of stimulatory inputs to the heart becomes disorganized during a massive stressor. The sympathetic nervous system sends two symmetrical nervous projections to the heart; it is theorized that during extreme emotional arousal, the two inputs are activated to such an extent that they become uncoordinated—major fibrillation, clutch your chest, keel over.

---

* I once received a letter from the chief medical examiner of Vermont describing his investigation of what he concluded to be a case of stress-induced cardiac arrest: an eighty-eight-year-old man with a history of heart disease, lying dead of a heart attack next to his beloved tractor, while just outside the house, at an angle where she could have seen him prone in the barn, was his eighty-seven-year-old wife, more recently dead of a heart attack (but with no history of heart disease and nothing obviously wrong found at autopsy). At her side was the bell she had used to summon him to lunch for who knows how many years.

† Don't panic at the jargon. In ventricular fibrillation the half of your heart called the *ventricles* begins to contract in a rapid, disorganized way that accomplishes nothing at all in terms of pumping blood.

FATAL PLEASURES

Embedded in the list of categories of precipitants of sudden cardiac death is a particularly interesting one: triumph or extreme joy. Consider the scenario of the man dying in the aftermath of the news of his winning the lottery, or the proverbial "at least he died happy" instance of someone dying during sex. (When these circumstances apparently claimed the life of an ex-vice president a few decades back, the medical minutiae of the incident received especially careful examination because he was not with his wife at the time.)

The possibility of being killed by pleasure seems crazy. Isn't stress-related disease supposed to arise from stress? How can joyful experiences kill you in the same way that sudden grief does? Clearly, because they share some similar traits. Extreme anger and extreme joy have different effects on reproductive physiology, on growth, most probably on the immune system as well; but with regard to the cardiovascular system, they have fairly similar effects. Once again, we deal with the central concept of stress physiology in explaining similar responses to being too hot or too cold, a prey or a predator: some parts of our body, including the heart, do not care in which direction we are knocked out of allostatic balance, but rather simply how much. Thus wailing and pounding the walls in grief or leaping about and shouting in ecstasy can place similarly large demands on a diseased heart. Put another way, your sympathetic nervous system probably has roughly the same effect on your coronary arteries whether you are in the middle of a murderous rage or a thrilling orgasm. Diametrically opposite emotions then can have surprisingly similar physiological underpinnings (reminding one of the oft-quoted statement by Elie Wiesel, the Nobel laureate writer and Holocaust survivor: "The opposite of love is not hate. The opposite of love is indifference."). When it comes to the cardiovascular system, rage and ecstasy, grief and triumph all represent challenges to allostatic equilibrium.

WOMEN AND HEART DISEASE

Despite the fact that men have heart attacks at a higher rate than women, heart disease is nonetheless the leading cause of death among women in the United States—500,000 a year (as compared to 40,000 deaths a year for breast cancer). And the rate is rising among women while cardiovascular death rates in men have been declining for decades. Moreover, for the same severity of heart attack, women are twice as likely as men to be left disabled.

What are these changes about? The increased rate of being disabled by a heart attack seems to be an epidemiological fluke. Women are still less subject to heart attacks than are men, with the onset of vulnerability delayed about a decade in women, relative to men. Therefore, if a man and woman both have heart attacks of the same severity, the woman is statistically likely to be ten years older than the man. And because of this, she is statistically less likely to bounce back afterward.

But what about the increasing incidence of heart disease in women? Various factors are likely to be contributing to it. Obesity is skyrocketing in this country, more so in women, and this increases the risk of heart disease (as discussed in the next chapter). Moreover, though smoking rates are declining in the country, they are declining more slowly among women than men.

Naturally, stress seems to have something to do with it as well. Kaplan and Carol Shively have studied female monkeys in dominance hierarchies and observe that animals chronically stuck in subordinate positions have twice the atherosclerosis as dominant females, even when on a low-fat diet. Findings with a similar theme of social subordination emerge among humans. This period of increasing rates of cardiovascular disease in women corresponds to a time when increasing percentages of women are working outside the home. Could the stressfulness of the latter have something to do with the former? Careful studies have shown that working outside the home does not increase the risk of cardiovascular disease for a woman. Unless she is doing clerical work. Or has an unsupportive boss. Go figure. And just to show what a myth it is that women working outside the home causes a shift toward men shouldering more of the burden of work at home, the other predictor of cardiovascular disease for women working outside the home is having kids back home.

So why does stress increase the risk of cardiovascular disease in female primates, human or otherwise? The answer is all the usual suspects—too much sympathetic nervous system arousal, too much secretion of glucocorticoids. But another factor is relevant, one that is wildly controversial, namely estrogen.

At the time of the previous edition of this book, estrogen was boring news. People had known for decades that estrogen protects against cardiovascular disease (as well as stroke, osteoporosis, and possibly Alzheimer's disease), mostly thanks to estrogen working as an antioxidant, getting rid of damaging oxygen radicals. This explained why women didn't start to get significant amounts of heart disease until after estrogen levels dropped with menopause. This was widely known and was one of the rationales for post-menopausal estrogen replacement therapy.

The importance of estrogen in protecting against cardiovascular disease came not just from statistics with human populations, but from careful experimental studies as well. As will be discussed in chapter 7, stress causes a decline in estrogen levels, and Kaplan's low-ranking female monkeys had estrogen levels as low as you would find in a monkey that had had her ovaries removed. In contrast, subject a female to years of subordinance but treat her with estrogen, raising her levels to those seen in dominant animals, and the atherosclerosis risk disappears. And remove the ovaries of a high-ranking female, and she was no longer protected from atherosclerosis. Studies like these seemed definitive.

Then in 2002 came a landmark paper, based on the Women's Health Initiative, a study of thousands of women. The goal had been to assess the effects of eight years of post-menopausal replacement therapy with estrogen plus progestin. The expectation was that this was going to be the gold-standard demonstration of the protective effects of such therapy against cardiovascular disease, stroke, and osteoporosis. And five years into it, the codes as to who was getting hormone and who placebo were cracked, and the ethics panel overseeing the mammoth project brought it to a halt. Because the benefits of estrogen plus progestin were so clear that it was unethical to give half the women placebo? No—because estrogen plus progestin was so clearly *increasing* the risk of heart disease and stroke (while still protecting against osteoporosis) that it was unethical to continue the study.

This was a bombshell. Front-page news everywhere. Similar trials were halted in Europe. Pharmaceutical stocks plummeted. And zillions of perimenopausal women wondered what they were supposed to do about estrogen replacement therapy.

Why such contradictory findings, with years of clinical statistics and careful laboratory studies on one side, and this huge and excellent study on the other? As one important factor, studies like those of Kaplan's involved estrogen, while this clinical trial was about estrogen *plus* progestin. This could well make a big difference. Then, as an example of the nit-picking that scientists love and which drives everyone else mad, the doses of hormones used probably made a difference, as did the type of estrogen (estradiol versus estriol versus estrone, and synthetic versus natural hormone). Finally, and this is an important point, the laboratory studies suggest that estrogen protects against the *formation* of atherosclerosis, rather than reverses atherosclerosis that is already there. This is quite relevant because, given our Western diets, people are probably just starting to form atherosclerotic plaques in their thirties, not in their post-menopausal fifties or sixties.

The jury is still out on this one. And though it may not turn out that post-menopausal estrogen protects against cardiovascular disease, it seems plausible that estrogen secreted by women themselves at much younger ages does. And stress, by suppressing such estrogen levels, could be contributing to cardiovascular disease through that route.

 ## VOODOO DEATH

The time has come to examine a subject far too rarely discussed in our public schools. Well-documented examples of voodoo death have emerged from all sorts of traditional non-westernized cultures. Someone eats a forbidden food, insults the chief, sleeps with someone he or she shouldn't have, does something unacceptably violent or blasphemous. The outraged village calls in a shaman who waves some ritualistic gewgaw at the transgressor, makes a voodoo doll, or in some other way puts a hex on the person. Convincingly soon, the hexed one drops dead.

The Harvard team of ethnobotanist Wade Davis and cardiologist Regis DeSilva reviewed the subject.* Davis and DeSilva object to the use of the term voodoo death, since it reeks of Western condescension toward non-Western societies—grass skirts, bones in the nose, and all that. Instead, they prefer the term *psychophysiological death,* noting that in many cases even that term is probably a misnomer. In some instances, the shaman may spot people who are already very sick and, by claiming to have hexed them, gain brownie points when the person kicks off. Or the shaman may simply poison them and gain kudos for his cursing powers. In the confound (that is, the source of confusion) that I found most amusing, the shaman visibly puts a curse on someone, and the community says, in effect, "Voodoo cursing works; this

---

* Wade Davis is the favorite ethnobotanist of horror movie fans far and wide. As detailed in the reference section, his prior research uncovered a possible pharmacological basis of how zombies (people in a deathlike trance with no will of their own) are made in Haiti. Davis's Harvard doctoral dissertation about zombification was first turned into a book, *The Serpent and the Rainbow,* and then a schlocky horror movie of the same name—a dream come true for every graduate student whose thesis is destined to be skimmed briefly by a distracted committee member or two.

person is a goner, so don't waste good food and water on him." The individual, denied food and water, starves to death; another voodoo curse come true, the shaman's fees go up.

Nevertheless, instances of psychophysiological death do occur, and they have been the focus of interest of some great physiologists in this century. In a great face-off, Walter Cannon (the man who came up with the fight-or-flight concept) and Curt Richter (a grand old man of psychosomatic medicine) differed in their postulated mechanisms of psychophysiological death. Cannon thought it was due to overactivity of the sympathetic nervous system; in that scheme, the person becomes so nervous at being cursed that the sympathetic system kicks into gear and vasoconstricts blood vessels to the point of rupturing them, causing a fatal drop in blood pressure. Richter thought death was due to too much *para*sympathetic activity. In this surprising formulation, the individual, realizing the gravity of the curse, gives up on some level. The vagus nerve becomes very active, slowing the heart down to the point of stopping—death due to what he termed a "vagal storm." Both Cannon and Richter kept their theories unsullied by never examining anyone who had died of psychophysiological death, voodoo or otherwise. It turns out that Cannon was probably right. Hearts almost never stop outright in a vagal storm. Instead, Davis and DeSilva suggest that these cases are simply dramatic versions of sudden cardiac death, with too much sympathetic tone driving the heart into ischemia and fibrillation.

All very interesting, in that it explains why psychophysiological death might occur in individuals who already have some degree of cardiac damage. But a puzzling feature about psychophysiological death in traditional societies is that it can also occur in young people who are extremely unlikely to have any latent cardiac disease. This mystery remains unexplained, perhaps implying more silent cardiac risk lurking within us than we ever would have guessed, perhaps testifying to the power of cultural belief. As Davis and DeSilva note, if faith can heal, faith can also kill.

PERSONALITY AND CARDIAC DISEASE: A BRIEF INTRODUCTION

Two people go through the same stressful social situation. Only one gets hypertensive. Two people go through a decade's worth of life's ups and downs. Only one gets cardiovascular disease.

These individual differences could be due to one person already having a damaged cardiovascular system—for example, decreased coronary blood flow. They could also be due to genetic factors that influence the mechanics of the system—the elasticity of blood vessels, the numbers of norepinephrine receptors, and so on. They could be the result of differences in how many risk factors each individual experiences—does the person smoke, eat a diet teeming with saturated fats? (Interestingly, individual differences in these risk factors explain less than half the variability in patterns of heart disease.)

Faced with similar stressors, whether large or small, two people may also differ in their risk for cardiovascular disease as a function of their personalities. In chapters 14 and 15 I will review some of these— how the risk of cardiovascular disease is increased by hostility, a Type-A personality, and by clinical depression. The bad news is that these personality risk factors are substantial in their impact. But the good news is that something can often be done about them.

This discussion has served as the first example of the style of analysis that will dominate the coming chapters. In the face of a short-term physical emergency, the cardiovascular stress-response is vital. In the face of chronic stress, those same changes are terrible news. These adverse effects are particularly deleterious when they interact with the adverse consequences of too much of a metabolic stress-response, the subject of the next chapter.

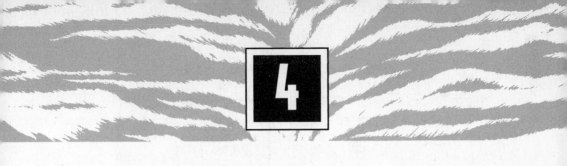

4

STRESS, METABOLISM, AND LIQUIDATING YOUR ASSETS

So you're sprinting down the street with the lion after you. Things looked grim for a moment there, but—your good luck—your cardiovascular system kicked into gear, and now it is delivering oxygen and energy to your exercising muscles. But what energy? There's not enough time to consume a candy bar and derive its benefits as you sprint along; there's not even enough time to digest food already in the gut. Your body must get energy from its places of storage, like fat or liver or non-exercising muscle. To understand how you mobilize energy in this circumstance, and how that mobilization can make you sick at times, we need to learn how the body stores energy in the first place.

PUTTING ENERGY IN THE BANK

The basic process of digestion consists of breaking down chunks of animals and vegetables so that they can then be transformed into chunks of human. We can't make use of the chunks exactly as they are; we can't, for example, make our leg muscles stronger by grafting on the piece of chicken muscle we ate. Instead, complex food matter is broken down into its simplest parts (molecules): amino acids (the building blocks of protein), simple sugars like glucose (the building blocks of more complex sugars and of starches [carbohydrates]), and free fatty acids and glycerol (the constituents of fat). This is

THE FOUR MAJOR FOOD GROUPS

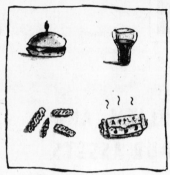

Regular:

Hamburger, cola, French fries, fruit pie.

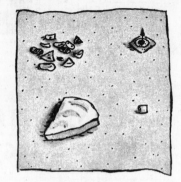

Company:

Cracker variety, canapé, "interesting" cheese, mint.

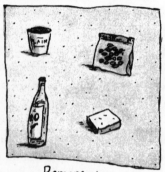

Remorse:

Plain yogurt, soybeans, mineral water, tofu.

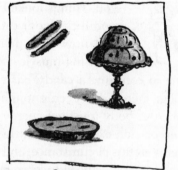

Silly:

Space-food sticks, gelatine mold with fruit salad in it, grasshopper pie.

R. Chast

accomplished in the gastrointestinal tract by enzymes, chemicals that can degrade more complex molecules. The simple building blocks thus produced are absorbed into the bloodstream for delivery to whichever cells in the body need them. Once you've done that, the cells have the ability to use those building blocks to construct the proteins, fats, and carbohydrates needed to stay in business. And just as important, those simple building blocks (especially the fatty acids and sugars) can also be burned by the body to provide the energy to do all that construction and to operate those new structures afterward.

It's Thanksgiving, and you've eaten with porcine abandon. Your bloodstream is teeming with amino acids, fatty acids, glucose. It's far more than you need to power you over to the couch in a postprandial daze. What does your body do with the excess? This is crucial to understand because, basically, the process gets reversed when you're later sprinting for your life.

To answer this question, it's time we talked finances, the works—savings accounts, change for a dollar, stocks and bonds, negative amortization of interest rates, shaking coins out of piggy banks—because the process of transporting energy through the body bears some striking similarities to the movement of money. It is rare today for the grotesquely wealthy to walk around with their fortunes in their pockets, or to hoard their wealth as cash stuffed inside mattresses. Instead, surplus wealth is stored elsewhere, in forms more complex than cash: mutual funds, tax-free government bonds, Swiss bank accounts. In the same way, surplus energy is not kept in the body's form of cash—circulating amino acids, glucose, and fatty acids—but stored in more complex forms. Enzymes in fat cells can combine fatty acids and glycerol to form triglycerides (see the table on page 60). Accumulate enough of these in the fat cells and you grow plump. Meanwhile, your cells can stick series of glucose molecules together. These long chains, sometimes thousands of glucose molecules long, are called *glycogen*. Most glycogen formation occurs in your muscles and liver. Similarly, enzymes in cells throughout the body can combine long strings of amino acids, forming them into proteins.

The hormone that stimulates the transport and storage of these building blocks into target cells is insulin. Insulin is this optimistic hormone that plans for your metabolic future. Eat a huge meal and insulin pours out of the pancreas into the bloodstream, stimulating the transport of fatty acids into fat cells, stimulating glycogen and protein synthesis. It's insulin that's filling out the deposit slips at your fat banks. We even secrete insulin when we are *about* to fill our bloodstream with all those nutritive building blocks: if you eat dinner each day at six o'clock, by five forty-five you're already secreting insulin in anticipation of the rising glucose levels in your bloodstream. Logically, it is the parasympathetic nervous system that stimulates the anticipatory secretion, and this ability to secrete insulin in preparation for the glucose levels that are about to rise is a great example of the anticipatory quality of allostatic balance.

What you stick in your mouth	How it winds up in your bloodstream	How it gets stored if you have a surplus	How it gets mobilized in stressful emergency
Proteins	→ Amino acids	→ Protein	→ Amino acids
Starch, sugars, carbohydrates	→ Glucose	→ Glycogen	→ Glucose
Fat	→ Fatty acids and glycerol	→ Triglycerides	→ Fatty acids, glycerol, ketone bodies

 ## EMPTYING THE BANK ACCOUNT: ENERGY MOBILIZATION DURING A STRESSOR

This grand strategy of breaking your food down into its simplest parts and reconverting it into complex storage forms is precisely what your body should do when you've eaten plenty. And it is precisely what your body should *not* do in the face of an immediate physical emergency. Then, you want to stop energy storage. Turn up the activity of the sympathetic nervous system, turn down the parasympathetic, and down goes insulin secretion: step one in meeting an emergency accomplished.

The body makes sure that energy storage is stopped in a second way as well. With the onset of the stressful emergency, you secrete glucocorticoids, which block the transport of nutrients into fat cells. This counteracts the effects of any insulin still floating around.

So you've made sure you don't do anything as irrational as store away new energy at this time. But in addition, you want your body to gain access to the energy *already* stored. You want to dip into your bank account, liquidate some of your assets, turn stored nutrients into your body's equivalent of cash to get you through this crisis. Your body reverses all of the storage steps through the release of the stress hormones glucocorticoids, glucagon, epinephrine, and norepinephrine. These cause triglycerides to be broken down in the fat cells and, as a result, free fatty acids and glycerol pour into the circulatory system. The same hormones trigger the degradation of glycogen to glucose in cells throughout the body, and the glucose is then flushed into the bloodstream. These hormones also cause protein in non-exercising muscle to be converted back to individual amino acids.

The stored nutrients have now been converted into simpler forms. Your body makes another simplifying move. Amino acids are not a very good source of energy, but glucose is. Your body shunts the circulating amino acids to the liver, where they are converted to glucose. The liver can also generate new glucose, a process called *gluconeogenesis*, and this glucose is now readily available for energy during the disaster.

As a result of these processes, lots of energy is available to your leg muscles. There's a burst of activity; you leave the lion in the dust and arrive at the restaurant only a smidgen late for your five forty-five anticipatory insulin secretion.

The scenario I've been outlining is basically a strategy to shunt energy from storage sites like fat to muscle during an emergency. But it doesn't make adaptive sense to automatically fuel, say, your arm muscles while you're running away from a predator if you happen to be an upright human. It turns out that the body has solved this problem. Glucocorticoids and the other hormones of the stress-response also act to block energy uptake into muscles and into fat tissue. Somehow the individual muscles that are exercising during the emergency have a means to override this blockade and to grab all the nutrients floating around in the circulation. The net result is that you shunt energy from fat and from *non*-exercising muscle to the exercising ones.

And what if you can't mobilize energy during a crisis? This is what occurs in Addison's disease, where people cannot secrete adequate amounts of glucocorticoids, or in Shy-Drager syndrome, where it is epinephrine and norepinephrine that are inadequate, having an inability to mobilize the body during energetic demands. Obviously, the lion is more likely to feast. And in a more subtle scenario, if you live in a westernized society and tend to have a somewhat underactive stress-response? Just as obviously, you'll have trouble mobilizing energy in response to the demands of daily life. And that is precisely what is seen in individuals with *chronic fatigue syndrome*, which is characterized by, among other things, too low levels of glucocorticoids in the bloodstream.

 ## SO WHY DO WE GET SICK?

You most definitely want to have a metabolic stress-response if you're evading a lion, and even if you are doing anything as taxing as walking up a flight of stairs (or even getting up in the morning, the time of day when our glucocorticoid levels normally peak). But what about the more typical scenario for us, one of turning on the stress-response too often, for months on end? We get into metabolic trouble for many of the same reasons that constantly running to the bank and drawing on your account is a foolish way to handle your finances.

On the most basic level, it's inefficient. Another financial metaphor helps. Suppose you have some extra money and decide to put it away for a while in a high-interest account. If you agree not to touch the money for a certain period (six months, two years, whatever), the bank agrees to give you a higher-than-normal rate of interest. And, typically, if you request the money earlier, you will pay a penalty for the early withdrawal. Suppose, then, that you happily deposit your money on these terms. The next day you develop the financial jitters, withdraw your money, and pay the penalty. The day after, you change your mind again, put the money back in, and sign a new agreement, only to change your mind again that afternoon, withdraw the money, and pay another penalty. Soon you've squandered half your money on penalties.

In the same way, every time you store energy away from the circulation and then return it, you lose a fair chunk of the potential energy. It takes energy to shuttle those nutrients in and out of the bloodstream, to power the enzymes that glue them together (into proteins, triglycerides, and glycogen) and the other enzymes that then break them apart, to fuel the liver during that gluconeogenesis trick. In effect, you are penalized if you activate the stress-response too often: you wind up expending so much energy that, as a first consequence, you tire more readily—just plain old everyday fatigue.

As a second consequence, your muscles can waste away, although this rarely happens to a significant degree. Muscle is chock-full of proteins. If you are stressed chronically, constantly triggering the breakdown of proteins, your muscles never get the chance to rebuild. While they atrophy ever so slightly each time your body activates this component of the stress-response, it requires a really extraordinary amount of stress for this to happen to a serious extent. As we will see in later chapters, sometimes clinicians give patients massive doses of synthetic glucocorticoids. In this scenario, significant amounts of *myopathy*—atrophy of muscle—can occur, of a type similar to that seen in people who are bedridden for long periods.

Finally, another problem with constantly mobilizing the metabolic stress-response was hinted at in the last chapter. You don't want to have tons of fat and glucose perpetually circulating in your bloodstream because, as we saw, that increases the chances of the stuff glomming on to some damaged blood vessel and worsening atherosclerosis. Cholesterol also plays into this. As is well understood, there is "bad" cholesterol, also known as low-density lipoprotein-associated cholesterol (LDL) and "good" cholesterol (high-density lipoprotein-associated cholesterol, HDL). LDL-cholesterol is the type that gets added to an atherosclerotic plaque, whereas HDL-cholesterol is cholesterol that has been removed from plaques and is on its way to be degraded in the liver. As a result of this distinction, your total level of cholesterol in the bloodstream is not actually a meaningful number. You want to know how much of each type you have, and lots of LDL and minimal HDL are independently bad news. We saw in the last chapter that the amount of vascular inflammation, as measured by CRP levels, is the best predictor out there of cardiovascular disease risk. Nonetheless, you don't want to have tons of LDL-cholesterol floating around and not enough HDL to counteract it. And during stress, you increase LDL-cholesterol levels and decrease HDL.*

Therefore, if you are stressed too often, the metabolic features of the stress-response can increase your risks of cardiovascular disease. This becomes particularly relevant with diabetes.

 ## JUVENILE DIABETES

There are multiple forms of diabetes, and two are relevant to this chapter. The first is known as juvenile diabetes (or type 1, insulin-dependent diabetes). For reasons that are just being sorted out, in some people the immune system decides that the cells in the pancreas that secrete insulin are, in fact, foreign invaders and attacks them (such "auto-immune" diseases will be discussed in chapter 8). This destroys those cells, leaving the person with little ability to secrete insulin. For equally mysterious reasons, this tends to hit people relatively early in life (hence the "juvenile" part of the name) although, to add to the mystery, in recent decades, the rate at which adults, even middle-aged adults, are getting diagnosed with juvenile diabetes is climbing.

Because the person can no longer secrete adequate amounts of insulin (if any), there is little ability to promote the uptake of glucose (and, indirectly, fatty acids) into target cells. Cells starve—big trouble,

---

* So it can be bad news to frequently boost LDL levels because of frequent stressors. But, independent from that, it is also not a good sign if, for any given stressor, you have a particularly *large* LDL increase. Studies have shown that the offspring of people with heart disease tend to have atypically large LDL responses to stress, suggesting a vulnerability factor that has been passed on to them.

not enough energy, organs don't function right. In addition, there's now all that glucose and fatty acid circulating in the bloodstream—oleaginous hoodlums with no place to go, and soon there's atherosclerotic trouble there as well. The circulating stuff gums up the blood vessels in the kidneys, causing them to fail. The same can occur in the eyes, causing blindness. Blood vessels elsewhere in the body are clogged, causing little strokes in those tissues and, often, chronic pain. With enough glucose in the circulation, it begins to stick to proteins, begins to Velcro proteins together that have no business being connected, knocking them out of business. None of this good.

And what is the best way to manage insulin-dependent diabetes? As we all know, by accommodating that dependency with insulin injections. If you're diabetic, you never want your insulin levels to get too low—cells are deprived of energy, circulating glucose levels get too high. But you don't want to take too much insulin. For complex reasons, this deprives the brain of energy, potentially putting you into shock or a coma and damaging neurons. The better the metabolic control in a diabetic, the fewer the complications and the longer the life expectancy. Thus, there's a major task for this type of diabetic to keep things just right, to keep food intake and insulin dosages balanced with respect to activity, fatigue, and so on. And this is an area where there has been extraordinary technological progress enabling diabetics to monitor blood glucose levels minute by minute and make minuscule changes in insulin dosages accordingly.

How does chronic stress affect this process? First, the hormones of the stress-response cause even more glucose and fatty acids to be mobilized into the bloodstream. For a juvenile diabetic, this increases the likelihood of the now-familiar pathologies of glucose and fatty acids gumming up in the wrong places.

Another, more subtle problem occurs with chronic stress as well. When something stressful happens, you don't just block insulin secretion. Basically, the brain doesn't quite trust the pancreas not to keep secreting a little insulin, so a second step occurs. As noted earlier, during stress, glucocorticoids act on fat cells throughout the body to make them less *sensitive* to insulin, just in case there's some still floating around. Fat cells then release some newly discovered hormones that get other tissues, like muscle and liver, to stop responding to insulin as well. Stress promotes insulin resistance. (And when people get into this diabetic state because they are taking large amounts of synthetic glucocorticoids [to control any of a variety of diseases that will be discussed later in the book] they have succumbed to "steroid diabetes.")

Why is this stress-induced insulin resistance bad for someone with juvenile diabetes? They have everything nice and balanced, with a healthy diet, a good sensitivity to their body's signals as to when a little insulin needs to be injected, and so on. But throw in some chronic stress, and suddenly insulin doesn't work quite as well, causing people to feel terrible until they figure out that they need to inject more of the stuff . . . which can make cells even more resistant to insulin, spiraling the insulin requirements upward . . . until the period of stress is over with, at which point it's not clear when to start getting the insulin dose down . . . because different parts of the body regain their insulin sensitivity at different rates. . . . The perfectly balanced system is completely upended.

Stress, including psychological stress, can wreak havoc with metabolic control in a juvenile diabetic. In one demonstration of this, diabetics were exposed to an experimental stressor (speaking in public) and their glucocorticoid secretion was monitored. Those who tended to have the largest stress-response under those circumstances were the ones least likely to have their diabetes well controlled. Moreover, in related studies, those who had the strongest emotional reactions to an experimental stressor tended to have the highest blood glucose levels.

Stress may sneak in another way. Some careful studies have shown higher rates of major stressors suffered by people during the three years before the onset of their juvenile diabetes than would be expected by chance. Does this mean that stress can make the immune system more likely to attack the pancreas? There is a little bit of evidence for this, which will be discussed in chapter 8 on immunity. A more likely explanation is built around the fact that once the immune system begins to attack the pancreas (that is, once the diabetes has started), it takes a while before the symptoms become apparent. By having all the adverse effects just talked about, stress can speed up the whole process, making the person notice sooner that he or she is just not feeling right.

Thus, frequent stress and/or big stress-responses might increase the odds of getting juvenile diabetes, accelerate the development of the diabetes, and, once it is established, cause major complications in this life-shortening disease.* Therefore, this is a population in which successful stress management is critical.

---

* A major challenge for diabetologists in their attempt to keep the disease under control in their patients is that juvenile diabetes is often occurring in juveniles who stress their system by behaving in ways that are, well, juvenile. Eating the wrong things, skipping meals, not getting enough sleep. A major management headache.

ADULT-ONSET DIABETES

In adult-onset diabetes (type 2, non-insulin-dependent diabetes), the trouble is not too little insulin, but the failure of the cells to *respond* to insulin. Another name for the disorder is thus insulin-*resistant* diabetes. The problem here arises with the tendency of many people to put on weight as they age. (However, if people do not put on weight as they age, they show no increased risk of this disease. This is the case among people in non-westernized populations. The disease is not, therefore, a normal feature of aging; instead, it is a disease of inactivity and fat surplus, conditions that just happen to be more common with age in some societies.) With enough fat stored away, the fat cells essentially get full; once you are an adolescent, the number of fat cells you have is fixed, so if you put on weight, the individual fat cells are distended. Yet another heavy meal, a burst of insulin trying to promote more fat storage by the fat cells, and the fat cells refuse—"Tough luck, I don't care if you are insulin; we're completely full." No room at the inn. The fat cells become less responsive to insulin trying to promote more fat storage, and less glucose is taken up by these cells.* The overstuffed fat cells even release hormones that trigger other fat cells and muscle into becoming insulin resistant.

Do the cells now starve? Of course not, the abundant amounts of fat stored in them was the source of the trouble in the first place. The body gets into trouble because of all that circulating glucose and fatty acids, damaging blood vessels. Same old problem. And if the adult-onset diabetes goes on for a while, an additional, miserable development can occur. Your body has become insulin-resistant. Your pancreas responds by secreting even more insulin than usual. You're still resistant. So the pancreas secretes even more. Back and forth, your pancreas pumping out ever higher levels of insulin, trying to be heard. Eventually, this burns out the insulin-secreting cells in the pancreas, actually destroying them. So you finally get your adult-onset diabetes under control, thanks to losing weight and exercising, and you discover you've now got juvenile diabetes, thanks to that damage to your pancreas.

---

* The careful reader may be confused at this point—if insulin regulates glucose uptake, why does it influence the amount of fat being stored in fat cells? For immensely complex reasons that I once understood for a few hours for a final exam, the storage of fat as triglycerides requires glucose uptake.

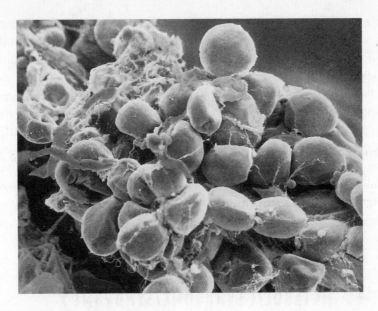

Photomicrograph of bloated fat cells.

How does chronic stress affect adult-onset diabetes? Once again, constantly mobilizing glucose and fatty acids into the bloodstream adds to the atherosclerotic glomming. And there's that problem of the stress-response involving your fat cells being instructed to become less responsive to insulin. Suppose that you're in your sixties, overweight, and just on the edge of insulin resistance. Along comes a period of chronic stress with those stress hormones repeatedly telling your cells what a great idea it is to be insulin-resistant. Enough of this and you pass the threshold for becoming overtly diabetic.

Why is any of this worth paying attention to? Because there is a worldwide epidemic of adult-onset diabetes going on, especially in our country. As of 1990, about 15 percent of Americans over age sixty-five had adult-onset diabetes. That was considered a health disaster then. As of a decade later, there's been a 33 percent increase above that, and among middle-aged adults as well. And this disease of aging is suddenly hitting far younger people as well—in the last decade, there's been a 70 percent increase in its incidence among thirty-year-olds. In addition, something like 20 million Americans are "pre-diabetic"—barreling toward a formal diagnosis. Adult-onset diabetes has even become more prevalent among kids than juvenile diabetes, which is pretty horrifying. Moreover, as people in the developing world are first being exposed to westernized diets, not only do they develop diabetes, they develop it at a faster rate than do westerners, for reasons that are probably both cultural and genetic. This once nonexistent disease afflicts an estimated 300 million people worldwide and killed 200,000 Americans last year.

What's this about? It's obvious. Despite the impression that everyone spends their days eating low-fat/carb/cholesterol/cardboard diets and power walking uphill while loudly reciting the writings of Atkins or Ornish, with each passing year, we are eating more food—more junk food—and exercising less. Twenty percent of Americans are now technically "obese" (versus 12 percent in 1990), and 54 percent are "overweight" (versus 44 percent then). To paraphrase the allostasis theorist Joseph Eyer, prosperity has become a cause of death.*

 ## METABOLIC SYNDROME/SYNDROME X

In the well-entrenched tradition of medical compartmentalizing, there's a whole set of things that can go wrong in you that would get you sent to a cardiologist, whereas a bunch of different problems would get you turfed to an internal medicine doc who specializes in diabetes. With any luck, they'd even confer with each other now and then. What should be obvious over the last two chapters is that your metabolic and cardiovascular systems are intimately interconnected. "Metabolic syndrome" (also known as Syndrome X) is a new term recognizing this interconnection. It's actually not so new, having been formalized in the late 1980s by Gerald Reaven of Stanford University. It's just become tremendously trendy in the past few years (so trendy that it's even been described in a population of wild baboons who forage through the desserts in a garbage dump at a tourist lodge in East Africa).

---

* If you learned your physiology sitting on the knee of Walter Cannon, none of this makes sense: "What's the deal with our bodies gaining all this weight, what happened to that 'Wisdom of the body' business?" you would ask. Peter Sterling points out that if the body worked by classical homeostatic principles of low-level, local feedback control, adult-onset diabetes shouldn't exist. It would be avoided with a simple regulatory issue—put on a certain amount of weight and fat cells tell appetite centers in the brain to stop being hungry. But it doesn't work that way—as we collectively keep putting on more weight, we collectively keep getting hungrier. Sterling points out the allostatic fact that there is a lot more to regulating appetite than simply how much fat you have stored, and that all sorts of higher level factors, including numerous societal ones, tend to override the efforts of fat cells to decrease appetite. This will be returned to in chapter 16.

Make a list of some of the things that can go wrong from the last two chapters: elevated insulin levels in the blood. Elevated glucose levels. Elevated systolic and diastolic blood pressure. Insulin resistance. Too much LDL-cholesterol. Too little HDL. Too much fat or cholesterol in the blood. Suffer from a subset of these, and you've got Metabolic syndrome (the formal diagnosis involves "one or more" from a list of some of these problems, and "two or more" from a list of the others).* The syndrome-ness is a way of stating that if you have a subset of those symptoms, you're probably heading toward the rest of them, since they're all one or two steps away from each other. Have elevated insulin levels, low HDL, and abdominal obesity and the chances are pretty good you're going to get insulin resistance. Elevated LDL-cholesterol, high blood pressure, and insulin resistance, and you're likely to be obese soon. Another bunch and they predict hypertension.

Subsets of these clusters of traits not only predict each other, they collectively predict major disease outcomes, like heart attacks or stroke, and mortality rates. This was shown with particular subtlety in an impressive study carried out by a team headed by Teresa Seeman of UCLA. Medicine normally works in diagnostic categories: have glucose levels above X, and it's official, you have hyperglycemia. Have blood pressure levels above Z, you're hypertensive. But how about if your glucose levels, blood pressure, HDL-cholesterol, and so on, are all in the normal range, but all of them are getting near the edge of where you have to start worrying? In other words, no measure is abnormal, but there's an abnormally large number of measures that are almost abnormal. Technically, nothing is wrong, amid it being obvious that things are not right. Take more than a thousand study subjects, all over age seventy, none of whom are certifiably sick—that is to say, where none of those measures are technically abnormal. Now, see how they're doing on all those Metabolic syndrome measures. Throw in some other measures as well—including resting levels of glucocorticoids, epinephrine, norepinephrine. Combine the insights into these measures mathematically and, collectively, this information was significantly predictive of who was going to have heart disease, a decline in cognitive or physical functioning, and mortality, far more predictive than subsets of those variables alone.

This is the essence of that "allostasis" concept, of keeping things in balance through interactions among different, far-flung systems in the

---

* I'm being a bit vague here because there doesn't seem to be a consensus, as far as I can tell, as to which are the exact set of symptoms to choose from to diagnose Metabolic syndrome.

body. This is also the essence of the wear-and-tear concept of allostatic "load," a formal demonstration that even if there's no single measure that's certifiably wrong, if there are enough things that are not quite right, you're in trouble. And, as the final, obvious point, this is also the essence of what stress does. No single disastrous effect, no lone gunman. Instead, kicking and poking and impeding, here and there, make this a bit worse, that a bit less effective. Thus making it more likely for the roof to cave in at some point.

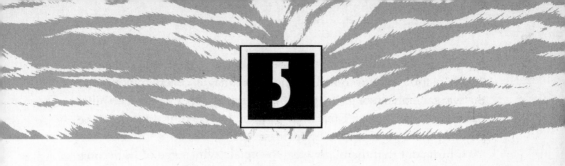

5

ULCERS, THE RUNS, AND
HOT FUDGE SUNDAES

 Not having enough food or water definitely counts as a stressor. If you're a human, having enough food and water for this meal, but not being sure where the next meal is coming from is a major stressor as well, one of the defining experiences of life outside the westernized world. And *choosing* not to eat to the point of starvation—anorexia—is a stressor as well (and one with an odd endocrine signature, harking back to chapter 2, in that glucocorticoids tend to be elevated while the sympathetic nervous system is unexpectedly inhibited). None of this is surprising. Nor is it surprising that stress changes eating patterns. This is well established. The question, of course, is in what way.

STRESS AND FOOD CONSUMPTION

From the previous chapter it's perfectly obvious where we're heading in terms of appetite. You're the zebra running for your life, don't think about lunch. That's the reason why we lose our appetites when we're stressed. Except for those of us who, when stressed, eat everything in sight, in a mindless mechanical way. And those who claim they're not hungry, are too stressed to eat a thing, and just happen to nibble 3,000 calories' worth of food a day. And those of us who really can't eat a thing. Except for chocolate-chocolate chip hot fudge sundaes. With whipped cream and nuts. The official numbers are that stress makes about two-thirds of people *hyper*phagic (eating more) and the rest *hypo*phagic.* Weirdly, when you stress lab rats, you get the same confusing picture, where some become hyperphagic, others hypophagic. So we can conclude with scientific certainty that stress can alter appetite. Which doesn't teach us a whole lot, since it doesn't tell us whether there's an increase or decrease.

It turns out that there are ways to explain why some of us become hyper- and others hypophagic during stress. To start, we extend the zebra scenario to the point of it surviving its encounter. During the stressor, appetite and energy storage were suppressed, and stored energy was mobilized. Thus, what's the logic during the post-stress period? Obvious—recover from that, reverse those processes. Block the energy mobilization, store the nutrients in your bloodstream, and get more of them. Appetite goes up.

This is accomplished through some endocrinology that is initially fairly confusing, but is actually really elegant. The confusing issue is that one of the critical hormones of the stress-response stimulates appetite, while another inhibits it. You might recall from earlier chapters that the hormone CRH is released by the hypothalamus and, by stimulating the pituitary to release ACTH, starts the cascade of events that culminates in adrenal release of glucocorticoids. Evolution has allowed the development of efficient use of the body's chemical messengers, and CRH is no exception. It is also used in parts of the brain to regulate other features of the stress-response. It helps to turn on the sympathetic nervous system, and it plays a role in increasing vigilance and arousal during stress. It also suppresses appetite. (Unsuccessful dieters should be warned against running to the neighborhood pharmacist for a bottle of CRH. It will probably help you lose weight, but you'll feel awful—as if you were always in the middle of an anxiety-provoking emergency: your heart racing; feeling jumpy, hyposexual, irritable. Probably better to just opt for a few more sit-ups.)

On the other side of the picture are glucocorticoids. In addition to the actions already outlined in response to stress, they appear to stimulate appetite. This is typically demonstrated in rats: glucocorticoids make these animals more willing to run mazes looking for food, more willing to press a lever for a food pellet, and so on. The hormone stimulates appetite in humans as well (although, to my knowledge, no one

---

* The jury remains out as to whether the folks who become hyperphagic after stress also develop a specific craving for carbohydrates. Clinical lore supports this picture, as do some laboratory studies. However, there's a problem here, which is that high-carb foods are typically easier to eat than low-carb foods, since the former tend to be snacks. So it's not clear if people really get a craving for carbohydrates, or if they get a craving for easy, mindless eating.

has stoked human volunteers on glucocorticoids and then quantified them scurrying up and down supermarket aisles). Scientists have a reasonably good idea where in the brain glucocorticoids stimulate appetite, which type of glucocorticoid receptors are involved, and so on.* What is really fascinating is that glucocorticoids don't just stimulate appetite—they stimulate it preferentially for foods that are starchy, sugary, or full of fat—and we reach for the Oreos and not the celery sticks.

Thus, we appear to have a problem here. CRH inhibits appetite, glucocorticoids do the opposite.† Yet they are both hormones secreted during stress. Timing turns out to be critical. When a stressful event occurs, there is a burst of CRH secretion within a few seconds. ACTH levels take about fifteen seconds to go up, while it takes many minutes for glucocorticoid levels to surge in the bloodstream (depending on the species). Thus, CRH is the fastest wave of the adrenal cascade, glucocorticoids the slowest. This difference in time course is also seen in the speed at which these hormones work on various parts of the body. CRH makes its effects felt within seconds, while glucocorticoids take minutes to hours to exert their actions. Finally, when the stressful event is over, it takes mere seconds for CRH to be cleared from the bloodstream, while it can take hours for glucocorticoids to be cleared.

Therefore, if there are large amounts of CRH in your bloodstream, yet almost no glucocorticoids, it is a safe bet that you are in the first few minutes of a stressful event. Good time to turn off appetite, and the combination of high CRH and low glucocorticoids accomplishes that.

Next, if there are large amounts of CRH *and* glucocorticoids in the bloodstream, you are probably in the middle of a sustained stressor. Also a good time to have appetite suppressed. You can pull this off only if the appetite-suppressing effects of CRH are stronger than the appetite-stimulating effects of glucocorticoids. And that's exactly how it works.

Finally, if there are substantial amounts of glucocorticoids in the circulation but little CRH, you have probably started the recovery period. That's exactly when digestion starts up again and your body

---

* The effect involves a recently discovered hormone called leptin. Very full fat cells secrete a lot of leptin, which works in the brain to decrease appetite. This fact caused entrepreneurial hysteria a while back, with all sorts of pharmaceutical companies thinking that giving people leptin was going to be the perfect diet drug. Hasn't worked, for some reason. In any case, glucocorticoids make the brain less sensitive to leptin, blunting its satiation signal. So you eat more.

† Beta-endorphins, released during stress, also increase appetite, but we're going to ignore that for the moment.

can begin to replenish those stores of energy consumed in that mad dash across the savanna. Appetite is stimulated. In chapter 4, we saw how glucocorticoids help to empty out the bank account of stored energy during a stressor. In this case, glucocorticoids would not so much serve as the mediator of the stress-response, but as the means of *recovering* from the stress-response.

Things now begin to make sense when you consider both the duration of a stressor and the recovery period combined. Suppose that something truly stressful occurs, and a maximal signal to secrete CRH, ACTH, and glucocorticoids is initiated. If the stressor ends after, say, ten minutes, there will cumulatively be perhaps a twelve-minute burst of CRH exposure (ten minutes during the stressor, plus the seconds it takes to clear the CRH afterward) and a two-hour burst of exposure to glucocorticoids (the roughly eight minutes of secretion during the stressor plus the much longer time to clear the glucocorticoids). So the period where glucocorticoid levels are high and those of CRH are low is much longer than the period of CRH levels being high. A situation that winds up stimulating appetite.

In contrast, suppose the stressor lasts for days, nonstop. In other words, days of elevated CRH and glucocorticoids, followed by a few hours of high glucocorticoids and low CRH, as the system recovers. The sort of setting where the most likely outcome is suppression of appetite.

The type of stressor is key to whether the net result is hyper- or hypophagia. Take some crazed, maze-running rat of a human. He sleeps through the alarm clock first thing in the morning, total panic. Calms down when it looks like the commute isn't so bad today, maybe he won't be late for work after all. Gets panicked all over again when the commute then turns awful. Calms down at work when it looks like the boss is away for the day and she didn't notice he was late. Panics all over again when it becomes clear the boss is there and did notice. So it goes throughout the day. And how would that person describe his life? "I am like, SO stressed, like totally, nonstop stressed, 24/7." But that's not really like totally nonstop stressed. Take a whole body burn. *That's* like totally nonstop stressed, 24/7. What this first person is actually experiencing is *frequent intermittent* stressors. And what's going on hormonally in that scenario? Frequent bursts of CRH release throughout the day. As a result of the slow speed at which glucocorticoids are cleared from the circulation, elevated glucocorticoid levels are close to nonstop. Guess who's going to be scarfing up Krispy Kremes all day at work?

So a big reason why most of us become hyperphagic during stress is our westernized human capacity to have intermittent psychological stressors throughout the day. The type of stressor is a big factor.

Another variable that helps predict hyperphagia or hypophagia during stress is how your body responds to a particular stressor. Put a bunch of subjects through the same experimental stressor (for example, a session on an exercise bicycle, a time-pressured set of math questions, or having to speak in public) and, not surprisingly, not everyone secretes the exact same amount of glucocorticoids. Furthermore, at the end of the stressor, everyone's glucocorticoid levels don't return to baseline at the same rate. The sources of these individual differences can be psychological—the experimental stressor may be an utter misery for one person and no big deal for another. Differences can also arise from physiology—one person's liver may be pokier at breaking down glucocorticoids than the next person's.

Elissa Epel of UCSF has shown that the glucocorticoid hypersecreters are the ones most likely to be hyperphagic after stress. Moreover, when given an array of foods to choose from during the post-stress period, they also atypically crave sweets. This is an effect that is specific to stress. The people who secrete excess glucocorticoids during stress don't eat any more than the other subjects in the absence of stress, and their resting, non-stressed levels of glucocorticoids aren't any higher than the others.

What else separates the stress hyperphagics from the stress hypophagics? Some of it has to do with your attitude toward eating. Lots of people eat not just out of nutritional need, but out of emotional need as well. These folks tend both to be overweight and to be stress-eaters. In addition, there's a fascinating literature concerning the majority of us, for whom eating is a regulated, disciplined task. At any given point, about two-thirds of us are "restrained" eaters. These are people who are actively trying to diet, who would agree with statements like, "In a typical meal, I'm conscious of trying to restrict the amount of food that I consume." Mind you, these are not people who are necessarily overweight. Plenty of heavy people are not dieting, plenty of everyone else is at any point. Restrained eaters are actively restricting their food intake. What the studies consistently show is that during stress, people who are normally restrained eaters are more likely than others to become hyperphagic.

This makes lots of sense. Things are a bit stressful—corporate thugs have looted your retirement savings, there's anthrax in the mail, and you've realized that you hate how your hair looks. That's exactly the

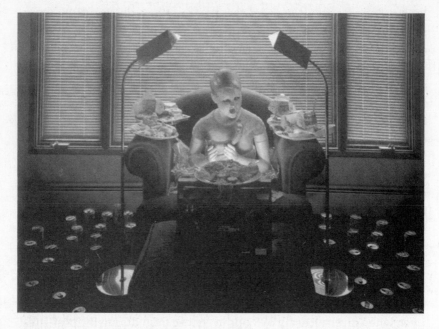

Mark Daughhetee, The Sin of Gluttony, *oil on silver print, 1985.*

time when most people decide that, as a coping device, as a means of being nice to themselves during a tough time, they need to ease up on something about which they're normally pretty regimented. So if you normally force yourself to watch *Masterpiece Theater* instead of reality TV as some sort of gesture of self-improvement, on goes *Survivor XII*. And if it's food intake that you're normally regimented about, out come the fudge brownies.

So we differ as to whether stress stimulates or inhibits our appetite, and this has something to do with the type and pattern of stressors, how reactive our glucocorticoid system is to stress, and whether eating is normally something that we keep a tight, superegoish lid on. It turns out that we also differ as to how readily we store food away after a stressor. And *where* in the body we store it.

 ## APPLES AND PEARS

Glucocorticoids not only increase appetite but, as an additional means to recover from the stress-response, also increase the storage of that ingested food. Mobilize all that energy during that mad dash across the savanna, and you're going to have to do a lot of energy storage during your recovery period. In order to have this effect, glucocorticoids trigger fat cells to make an enyzme that breaks down the circulating nutrients into their storage forms, ideal for storing them for next winter.

It's not just any fat cells that glucocorticoids stimulate. Time for one of the great dichotomies revered by fat cell aficionados: fat cells located in your abdominal area, around your belly, are known as "visceral" fat. Fill up those fat cells with fat, without depositing much fat elsewhere in your body, and you take on an "apple" shape.

In contrast, fat cells around your rear end form "gluteal" fat. Fill those up preferentially with fat and you take on a "pear" shape, being round-bottomed. The formal way to quantify these different types of fat deposition is to measure the circumference of your waist (which tells you about the amount of abdominal fat) and the circumference of your hips (a measure of gluteal fat). Apples have waists that are bigger than hips, producing a "waist-hip ratio" (WHR) that is bigger than 1.0, while pears have hips that are bigger than waists, producing a WHR that is less than 1.0.

It turns out that when glucocorticoids stimulate fat deposition, they do it preferentially in the abdomen, promoting apple-shaped obesity. This even occurs in monkeys. The pattern arises because abdominal fat cells are more sensitive to glucocorticoids than are gluteal fat cells; the former have more receptors that respond to glucocorticoids by activating those fat-storing enzymes. Furthermore, glucocorticoids only do this in the presence of high insulin levels. And once again, this makes sense. What does it mean if you have high glucocorticoid levels and low insulin levels in the bloodstream? As we know from chapter 4, you're in the middle of a stressor. High glucocorticoids and high insulin? This happens during the recovery phase. Pack away those calories to recover from the grassland sprint.

This stimulation of visceral fat deposition by glucocorticoids is not good news. This is because if you have to pack on some fat, you definitely want to become a pear, not an apple. As we saw in the chapter on metabolism, lots of fat is a predictor for Syndrome X. But it turns out that a large WHR is an even better predictor of trouble than being overweight is. Take some extremely applish people and some very peary ones. Match them for weight, and it's the apples who are at risk for metabolic and cardiovascular disease. Among other reasons, this is probably because fat released from abdominal fat cells more readily finds its way to the liver (in contrast to fat from gluteal fat stores, which gets dispersed more equally throughout the body), where it is converted into glucose, setting you up for elevated blood sugar and insulin resistance.

These findings lead to a simple prediction, namely that for the same stressor, if you tend to secrete more glucocorticoids than most, not only are you going to have a bigger appetite post-stressor, you're going to go apple, preferentially socking away more of those calories in your abdominal fat cells. And that's precisely what occurs. Epel has studied this in women and men across a range of ages, and she finds that a prolonged glucocorticoid response to novelty is a feature of applish people, not pears.

So with lots of stress, you get cravings for starchy comfort food and you pack it in the abdomen. One final distressing piece of information, based on some fascinating recent work by Mary Dallman from the University of California at San Francisco: consuming lots of those comfort foods and bulking up on abdominal fat are stress-reducers. They tend to decrease the size of the stress-response (both in terms of glucocorticoid secretion and sympathetic nervous system activity). Not only do the Oreos taste good, but by reducing the stress-response, they make you *feel* good as well.

There seems to be a huge number of routes by which obesity can occur—too much or too little of this or that hormone; too much or too little sensitivity to this or that hormone.* But another route appears to involve being the sort of person who secretes too many glucocorticoids, either because of too many stressors, too many perceived stressors, or trouble turning off the stress-response. And thanks to that weird new regulatory loop discovered by Dallman, it appears as if abdominal fat is one route for trying to tone down that overactive stress-response.

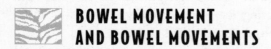

BOWEL MOVEMENT
AND BOWEL MOVEMENTS

Thanks to the preceding part of this chapter and to chapter 4, we've now sorted out how stress alters what you ingest, how it gets stored and mobilized. We have one last piece to fill in, which is getting food from your mouth to its digested form in your circulation. This is the

---

* The hormones involved obviously include the ones we've already heard of, like insulin, leptin, CRH, and glucocorticoids, plus other players like growth hormone, estrogen, and testosterone. But there's also an array of brand-new appetite-related hormones and neurotransmitters with names that are so hideous that I have no choice but to bury them in a footnote. Neuropeptide Y. Cholecystokinin. Melanocyte-stimulating hormone. Oleylethanolamide. Adiponectin. Hypocretin. Agouti-related protein. Ghrelin (yes, that's actually how you spell it; however, I have no idea how you pronounce it).

purview of the gastrointestinal (GI) tract—your esophagus, stomach, small intestines and large intestines (also known as the colon or the bowel).

When it comes to your GI tract, there's no such thing as a free lunch. You've just finished some feast, eaten like a hog—slabs of turkey, somebody's grandma's famous mashed potatoes and gravy, a bare minimum of vegetables to give a semblance of healthiness, and—oh, why not—another drumstick and some corn on the cob, a slice or two of pie for dessert, ad nauseam. You expect your gut to magically convert all that into a filtrate of nutrients in your bloodstream? It takes energy, huge amounts of it. Muscular work. Your stomach not only breaks down food chemically, it does so mechanically as well. It undergoes systolic contractions: the muscle walls contract violently on one side of your stomach, and hunks of food are flung against the far wall, breaking them down in a cauldron of acids and enzymes. Your small intestines do a snake dance of peristalsis (directional contraction), contracting the muscular walls at the top end in order to squeeze the food downstream in time for the next stretch of muscle to contract. After that, your bowels do the same, and you're destined for the bathroom soon. Circular muscles called *sphincters* located at the beginning and end of each organ open and close, serving as locks to make sure that things don't move to the next level in the system until the previous stage of digestion is complete, a process no less complicated than shuttling ships through the locks of the Panama Canal. At your mouth, stomach, and small intestines, water has to be poured into the system to keep everything in solution, to make sure that the sweet potato pie, or what's left of it, doesn't turn into a dry plug. By this time, the action has moved to your large intestines, which have to extract the water and return it to your bloodstream so that you don't inadvertently excrete all that fluid and desiccate like a prune. All this takes energy, and we haven't even considered jaw fatigue. All told, your run-of-the-mill mammals, including us, expend 10 to 20 percent of their energy on digestion.

So back to our by-now-familiar drama on the savanna: if you are that zebra being pursued by a lion, you can't waste energy on your stomach walls doing a rumba. There isn't time to get any nutritional benefits from digestion. And if you are that lion running after a meal, you haven't just staggered up from some all-you-can-eat buffet.

Digestion is quickly shut down during stress. We all know the first step in that process. If you get nervous, you stop secreting saliva and your mouth gets dry. Your stomach grinds to a halt, contractions stop, enzymes and digestive acids are no longer secreted, your small intestines stop peristalsis, nothing is absorbed. The rest of your body even knows that the digestive tract has been shut down—as we saw two chapters ago, blood flow to your stomach and gut is decreased so that the blood-borne oxygen and glucose can be delivered elsewhere, where they're needed. The parasympathetic nervous system, perfect for all that calm, vegetative physiology, normally mediates the actions of digestion. Along comes stress: turn off the parasympathetic, turn on the sympathetic, and forget about digestion.* End of stress; switch gears again, and the digestive process resumes.

As usual, this all makes wonderful sense for the zebra or the lion. And as usual, it is in the face of chronic stress that diseases emerge instead.

 BOWELS IN AN UPROAR

Regardless of how stressful that board meeting or examination is, we're not likely to soil our pants. Nevertheless, we are all aware of the tendency of immensely terrified people—for example, soldiers amid horrifying battle—to defecate spontaneously. (This reaction is consistent enough that in many states, prisoners are clothed in diapers before an execution.)

The logic as to why this occurs is similar to why we lose control of our bladders if we are very frightened, as described in chapter 3. Most of digestion is a strategy to get your mouth, stomach, bile ducts, and so forth to work together to break your food down into its constituent parts by the time it reaches the small intestines. The small intestines, in turn, are responsible for absorbing nutrients out of this mess and delivering them to the bloodstream. As is apparent to most of us, not much of what we eat is actually nutritious, and a large percentage of what we consume is left over after the small intestines pick through it. In the large intestines, the leftovers are converted to feces and eventually exit stage left.

Yet again, you sprint across the veld. All that stuff sitting in your large intestines, from which the nutritive potential has already been absorbed, is just dead weight. You have the choice of sprinting for

---

* Back to stress turning off salivation, an inhibition mediated by the sympathetic nervous system. What if you have to salivate for a living, if you are, say, an oboe player? Big audition comes along, good and nervous and—disaster—no spittle. Thus, many reed musicians wind up using drugs like beta-blockers that block the action of the sympathetic nervous system in order to slobber just in time for the big arpeggio.

your life with or without a couple of pounds of excess baggage in your bowels. Empty them.

The biology of this is quite well understood. The sympathetic nervous system is responsible. At the same time that it is sending a signal to your stomach to stop its contractions and to your small intestine to stop peristalsis, your sympathetic nervous system is actually stimulating muscular movement in your large intestine. Inject into a rat's brain the chemicals that turn on the sympathetic nervous system, and suddenly the small intestine stops contracting and the large intestine starts contracting like crazy.

But why, to add insult to injury, is it so frequently diarrhea when you are truly frightened? Relatively large amounts of water are needed for digestion, to keep your food in solution as you break it down so that it will be easy to absorb into the circulation when digestion is done. As noted, a job of the large intestine is to get that water back, and that's why your bowels have to be so long—the leftovers slowly inch their way through the large intestine, starting as a soupy gruel and ending up, ideally, as reasonably dry stool. Disaster strikes, run for your life, increase that large intestinal motility, and everything gets pushed through too fast for the water to be absorbed optimally. Diarrhea, simple as that.

 ## STRESS AND FUNCTIONAL GASTROINTESTINAL DISORDERS

Broadly, there are two types of gastrointestinal disorders. In the first, you feel terrible, something isn't working right, and the doctors find something wrong. These are "organic" GI disorders. A gaping hole in the wall of your stomach, in other words, a peptic ulcer, counts as there being something demonstrably wrong. We'll consider ulcers shortly. Out-of-control inflammation of tissue throughout your GI tract, which is what inflammatory bowel disease is, also counts as demonstrably wrong. This disorder will be briefly touched on in chapter 8.

But suppose you feel terrible, something isn't working right, and the docs can't find a thing wrong. Congratulations, you now have a "functional" GI disorder. These are immensely sensitive to stress. And this is not just the touchy-feely psychologists saying this. Papers about stress and functional GI disorders are even published in tough-guy meat-and-potato scientific journals with names like *Gut*.

The most common functional GI disorder, which will be considered here, is *irritable bowel syndrome* (IBS), which involves abdominal pain (particularly just after a meal) that is relieved by defecating and symptoms such as diarrhea or constipation, passage of mucus, bloating, and abdominal distention. Despite physicians checking you from every which end, they can't find anything wrong, which qualifies IBS as a functional disorder. IBS is among the most common of stress-sensitive disorders. Personally, all the major rites of passage in my life have been marked by pretty impressive cases of the runs a few days before—my bar mitzvah, going away to college, my doctoral defense, proposing marriage, my wedding. (Finally, here's that confessional tone obligatory to successful books these days. Now if I can only name some Hollywood starlet with whom I've taken diuretics, this may become a bestseller.)

Carefully conducted studies show that major chronic stressors increase the risk of the first symptoms of IBS appearing, and worsen preexisting cases. This makes sense. As we saw, what stress does is increase the contractions in the colon, getting rid of that dead weight. And IBS—also known as "spastic colon"—involves the colon being too contractile, an excellent way of producing diarrhea. (It is not clear why lots of stress-induced contractions of the colon can lead to constipation. As a possible explanation, the stress-induced contractions in the colon are directional, which is to say, they push the contents of the colon from the small intestinal end to the anus. And if they do that a lot, things get accelerated, resulting in diarrhea. However, in one plausible scenario, with long enough periods of stress, the contractions begin to get disorganized, lose their directionality, so that not much of anything moves toward the anus).

So people with IBS are disproportionately likely to be experiencing a lot of stressors. But in addition, IBS can be a disorder of too much gastrointestinal sensitivity to stress. This can be shown in experimental situations, where a person with IBS is subjected to a controlled stressor (keeping her hand in ice water for a while, trying to make sense of two recorded conversations at once, participating in a pressured interview). Contractions in the colon increase in response to these stressors more in IBS patients than in control subjects.

Another connection between stress and IBS concerns pain. As we'll see in chapter 9, stress can blunt the sort of pain you feel in your skin and skeletal muscles while increasing the sensitivity of internal organs like the intestines to pain (something called "visceral" pain). And that is the profile seen in IBS patients—less sensitivity to skin ("cutaneous") pain, and more visceral pain. Even more support for the stress/IBS link is that people with IBS don't typically have hypercontractility of their bowels when they are asleep. Gut spasticity is not something that's going on all the time—only when the person is awake, amid the opportunities to be stressed.

What's the physiology of this gut that is too contractile? As we saw earlier, the sympathetic nervous system is responsible for the increased large intestinal contractions during stress. And as would be expected, people with IBS have overactive sympathetic nervous systems (though it is less clear whether glucocorticoid levels are abnormal in IBS). And just to make the whole process worse, the pain of that gassy, distended, hypersensitive gut can stimulate sympathetic activation even further, making for a vicious circle.

So ongoing stress can be closely associated with IBS. Interestingly, traumatic stress early in life (abuse, for example) greatly increases the risk of IBS in adulthood. This implies that childhood trauma can leave an echo of vulnerability, a large intestine that is hyperreactive to stress, long afterward. Animal studies have shown that this occurs.

Despite these findings, there is a great deal of resistance to the link between stress and IBS (prompting some semi-irate letters to me from readers of earlier editions of this book). One reason for this is the linkage between IBS and certain personality types. In the cases of depression or anxiety, the connection is solid, but earlier linkages seem pretty suspect. These studies tended to focus on a lot of psychoanalytic gibberish (there, now I'll get myself into trouble with that crowd)—some hoo-ha about the person being stuck in the anal stage of development, a regression to the period of toilet training where going to the bathroom gained great acclaim and, suddenly, diarrhea was a symbolic reach for parental approval. Or the approval of the doctor as a parental surrogate. Or something or other. I'm not sure how they factored in constipation, but I'm sure they did.

Few gastroenterologists take these ideas seriously anymore. However, in less scientific circles, some still cling to these views. It is easy to see how someone suffering from IBS, who has just managed to clear up the perception that they're still having some potty-training issues, isn't enthused about getting fingered for not dealing well with stress.

Another reason why the stress/IBS connection is often viewed with suspicion is because there have been many studies that have failed to find a link. Why should this be?

First, both the severity of IBS symptoms and the intensity of stressors that someone is experiencing tend to wax and wane over time, and detecting a link between two such fluctuating patterns takes some very fancy statistics. (Typically, a technique called *time-series analysis*, a subject four classes more advanced than the statistics that most biomedical scientists have sort of learned. When my wife had to do a time-series analysis as part of her doctoral research, it made me nervous just to have a textbook on the subject in the house.) Such waxing and waning of stress and of symptoms is particularly difficult to track because most studies are *retrospective* (they look at people who already have IBS and ask them to identify stressors in their past) rather than *prospective* (in which people who do not have a disease are followed to see if stress predicts who is going to get it). The problem here is that people are terribly inaccurate at recalling information about stressors and symptoms that are more than a few months old, a point we're going to return to often in this book. Moreover, as was mentioned above, the sorts of stressors that can increase the risk of IBS can occur many years prior to the emergence of symptoms, making the link hard to detect even in prospective studies. Finally, "IBS" is probably a hodgepodge of diseases with multiple causes, and stress may be relevant to only some of them, and it takes some additional fancy statistics to detect those folks as a meaningful subset of the whole, instead of as just random noise in the data.

At later junctures in this book, we will see other supposed links between stress and some disease, and be in the same quandary—there definitely is a link in some patients, or clinical impressions strongly support a stress-disease link, yet hard-nosed studies fail to show the same thing. As we will see repeatedly, the trouble is that the supposedly hard-nosed studies are often asking a fairly unsophisticated, straightforward question: does stress cause the disease in the majority of sufferers? The far more sophisticated questions to ask are whether stress worsens preexisting disease, whether patterns of symptoms and of stressors fluctuate in parallel over time, and whether these links occur only in a subset of vulnerable individuals. When asked in those ways, the stress-disease link becomes far more solid.

 ## ULCERS

At last we arrive at the medical problem that started the stress concept on the road to fame and fortune. An ulcer is a hole in the wall of an organ, and ulcers originating in the stomach or in the organs immediately bordering it are termed *peptic ulcers*. The ones within the stomach are called *gastric ulcers*; those a bit higher up than the stomach are *esophageal,* and those at the border of the stomach and the intestine are *duodenal* (the most common of peptic ulcers).

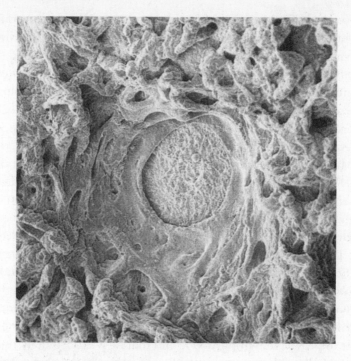

Photomicrograph of a stomach ulcer.

As will be recalled, peptic ulcers were among the trio of symptoms Selye noted more than sixty years ago when he exposed his rats to nonspecific unpleasantness. Since then, stomach ulcers have emerged as the disorder most recognized by the lay public as a stress-related disease: in this view, you have upsetting thoughts for a long period of time and holes appear in the walls of your stomach.

Most clinicians agree that there is a subtype of ulcers that forms relatively rapidly (sometimes over the course of days) in humans who are exposed to immensely stressful crises—hemorrhage, massive infection, trauma due to accident or surgery, burns over large parts of the body, and so on. Such "stress ulcers" can be life threatening in severe cases.

But where a lot of contention has appeared has been with the issue of gradually emerging ulcers. This used to be a realm where people, including physicians, would immediately think stress. But a revolution has dramatically changed thinking about ulcers.

That revolution came with the discovery in 1983 of a bacterium called *Helicobacter pylori*. This obscure microorganism was discovered by an obscure Australian pathologist named Robert Warren. He, in turn, interested an even more obscure younger colleague named Barry Marshall, who documented that this bacterium consistently turned up in biopsies of the stomachs of people with duodenal ulcers and stomach inflammation (gastritis). He theorized that it actually *caused* the inflammation and ulcers, announced this to the (gastroenterological) world at a conference, and was nearly laughed out of the room. Ulcers were caused by diet, genetics, stress—not bacteria. Everyone knew that. And besides, because the stomach is so incredibly acidic, owing to the hydrochloric acid in stomach juices, no bacteria could survive in there. People had known for years that the stomach was a sterile environment, and that any bacteria that might turn up were just due to contamination by some sloppy pathologist.

Marshall showed that the bacteria caused gastritis and ulcers in mice. That's great, but mice work differently than humans, everyone said. So, in a heroic, soon-to-be-a-movie gesture, he swallowed some *Helicobacter* bilge and caused gastritis in himself. Still, they ignored Marshall. Eventually, some folks in the field got tired of hearing him go on about the damn bacteria at meetings, decided to do some experiments to prove him wrong, and found that he was absolutely right.

Helicobacter pylori turns out to be able to live in the acidic stomach environment, protecting itself by having a structure that is particularly acid-resistant and by wrapping itself in a coat of protective bicarbonate. And this bacterium probably has a lot to do with 85 to 100 percent of ulcers in Western populations (as well as with stomach cancer). Nearly 100 percent of people in the developing world are infected with *Helicobacter*—it is probably the most common chronic bacterial infection in humans. The bacteria infect cells in the lining of the stomach, causing gastritis, which somehow compromises the ability of those cells lining the duodenum to defend themselves against stomach acids. Boom, under the right conditions, you've got a hole in that duodenal wall.

Many of the details remain to be sorted out, but the greatest triumph for Marshall and Warren has been the demonstration that antimicrobial drugs, such as antibiotics, turn out to be the greatest things since sliced bread for dealing with duodenal ulcers—they are as good at getting rid of the ulcers as are antacids or antihistamine drugs (the main prior treatments) and, best of all, unlike the aftermath of other treatments, ulcers now stay away (or at least until the next *Helicobacter* infection).

Once everybody in the field got used to the idea of Marshall and Warren being carried around on sedan chairs for their discovery, they embraced *Helicobacter* with a vengeance. It makes perfect sense, given the contemporary desire of medicine to move toward hard-nosed, reductive models of disease, rather than that wimpy psychosomatic stuff. The Center for Disease Control sent out educational pamphlets to every physician in America, advising them to try to disabuse their patients of the obsolete notion that stress has anything to do with peptic ulcers. Clinicians celebrated at never having again to sit down with their ulcer patients, make some serious eye contact, and ask them how their lives were going. In what one pair of investigators has termed the "Helicobacterization" of stress research on ulcers, the number of papers on stress as a component of the ulcer story has plummeted. Don't bother with this psychological stuff when we finally have gotten some real science here, complete with a bacterium that's got its own Latin name.

The trouble is that one bacterium can't be the whole story. For starters, up to 15 percent of duodenal ulcers form in people who aren't infected with *Helicobacter*, or with any other known bacterium related to it. More damning, only about 10 percent of the people infected with the bacteria get ulcers. It's got to be *Helicobacter pylori* plus something else. Sometimes, the something else is a lifestyle risk factor—alcohol, smoking, skipping breakfast habitually, taking a lot of nonsteroidal anti-inflammatory drugs like aspirin. Maybe the something else is a genetic tendency to secrete a lot of acid or to make only minimal amounts of mucus to protect stomach linings from the acid.

But one of the additional factors is stress. Study after study, even those carried out after the ascendancy of the bacteria, show that duodenal ulceration is more likely to occur in people who are anxious, depressed, or undergoing severe life stressors (imprisonment, war, natural disasters). An analysis of the entire literature shows that somewhere between 30 and 65 percent of peptic ulcers have psychosocial factors (i.e., stress) involved. The problem is that stress causes people to drink and smoke more. So maybe stress increases the risk of an ulcer merely by increasing the incidence of those lifestyle risk factors. But no—after you control for those variables, stress itself still causes a two- to threefold increase in the risk of an ulcer.

Helicobacter is relevant to ulcers, but it is only in the context of its interactions with these other factors, including stress. You can show this statistically if you study a zillion ulcer patients. Then, do a fancy mathematical analysis that takes into account bacterial load, lifestyle risk factors, and stress (something aptly called a *multivariate analysis*). You'll observe that ulcers can arise if you only have a little bit of one of the factors (bacterial load, stress, or lifestyle risks), so long as you have a lot of one or two of the others. As an example of that, if you expose lab rats to psychological stressors, they get ulcers—but not if they live in a germ-free environment that lacks *Helicobacter*.

So how does stress exacerbate the process of ulcer formation? Some sixty years after Selye first noticed his rats' ulcers, it is still not quite clear. There are some favorite scenarios, however.

Acid Rebound To understand this mechanism, we have to grapple with the grim reality of what bizarre things we are willing to eat and expect our stomachs to digest. The only way that the stomach is going to be able to handle some of this stuff is if it has powerful degradative weapons. The contractions certainly help, but the main weapon is the hydrochloric acid that pours into your stomach from the cells lining it. Hydrochloric acid is immensely acidic; all well and good, but it raises the obvious question of why your stomach is not itself digested by the digestive acids. Eat somebody else's stomach and your stomach disintegrates it. How do your own stomach walls remain unscathed? Basically, your stomach has to spend a fortune protecting itself. It builds many layers of stomach wall and coats them with thick, soothing mucus that buffers the acid. In addition, bicarbonate is secreted into the stomach to neutralize the acid. This is a wonderful solution, and you happily go about digestion.

Along comes a stressful period that lasts months. Your body cuts down on its acid secretion—there are now frequent times when digestion is being inhibited. During this period, your stomach essentially decides to save itself some energy by cutting corners. It cuts back a bit on the constant thickening of the stomach walls, undersecretes mucus and bicarbonate, and pockets the difference. Why not? There isn't much acid around during this stressful period anyway.

End of stressful period; you decide to celebrate by eating a large chocolate cake inscribed for the occasion, stimulate your parasympathetic nervous system, start secreting hydrochloric acid, and . . . your defenses are down. The walls have thinned, there isn't as thick a protective mucous layer as there used to be, the bicarbonate is overwhelmed. A couple of repeated cycles of stress and rebound with a bacterial infection that is already compromising the defenses and you've got an ulcer.

Suppose you are in the middle of a very stressful period, and you worry that you are at risk for an ulcer. What's the solution? You could make sure that you remain under stress every second for the rest of your life. You definitely will avoid ulcers caused by hydrochloric acid secretion, but of course you'll die for a zillion other reasons. The paradox is that, in this scenario, ulcers are not formed so much during the stressor as during the recovery. This idea predicts that several periods of transient stress should be more ulcerative than one long, continuous period, and animal experiments have generally shown this to be the case.

Decreased Blood Flow As we know, in an emergency, you want to deliver as much blood as possible to the muscles that are exercising. In response to stress, your sympathetic nervous system diverts blood from the gut to more important places—remember the man with a gunshot wound in the stomach, whose guts would blanch from decreased blood flow every time he became angry or anxious. If your stressor is one that involves a dramatic decrease in blood flow to the gut (for example, following a hemorrhage), it begins to cause little infarcts—small strokes—in your stomach walls, because of lack of oxygen. You develop small lesions of necrotic (dead) tissue, which are the building blocks of ulcers.

This condition probably arises for at least two reasons. First, with decreased blood flow, less of the acid that accumulates is being flushed away. The second reason involves another paradoxical piece of biology. We all obviously need oxygen and would turn an unsightly blue without it. However, running your cells on oxygen can sometimes produce an odd, dangerous class of compounds called *oxygen radicals.* Normally, another group of compounds (free radical quenchers, or scavengers) dispose of these villains. There is some evidence, however, that during periods of chronic stress, when blood flow (and thus oxygen delivery) to the gut decreases, your stomach stops making the scavengers that protect you from the oxygen radicals. Fine for the period of stress (since the oxygen radicals are also in shorter supply); it's a clever way to save energy during a crisis. At the end of stress, however, when blood flow chock-full of oxygen resumes and the normal amount of oxygen radicals is generated, the stomach has its oxidative pants down. Without sufficient scavengers, the oxygen radicals start killing cells in the stomach walls; couple that with cells already in trouble thanks to bacterial infection and you've got an ulcer. Note how similar this scenario is to the acid-rebound mechanism: in both cases, the damage occurs not during the period of stress but in its aftermath, and not so much because stress increases the size of an insult (for example, the amount of acid secreted or the amount of oxygen radicals produced), but because, during the stressful emergency, the gut scrimps on defenses against such insults.

Immune Suppression *Helicobacter* as a bacterium triggers your immune system into trying to defend against it.* As you will soon learn in sickening detail (chapter 8), chronic stress suppresses immunity, and in this scenario, lowered immune defenses equals more *Helicobacters* reproducing happily.

Insufficient Amounts of Prostaglandins In this scenario, micro-ulcers begin now and then in your gut, as part of the expected wear and tear on the system. Normally your body can repair the damage by secreting a class of chemicals called *prostaglandins,* thought to aid the healing process by increasing blood flow through the stomach walls. During stress, however, the synthesis of these prostaglandins is inhibited by the actions of glucocorticoids. In this scenario, stress does not so much cause ulcers to form as impair your body's ability to catch them early and repair them. It is not yet established how often this is the route for ulcer formation during stress. (Aspirin also inhibits prostaglandin synthesis, which is why aspirin can aggravate a bleeding ulcer.)

Stomach Contractions For unknown reasons, stress causes the stomach to initiate slow, rhythmic contractions (about one per minute); and for unknown reasons, these seem to add to ulcer risk. One idea is that during the contractions, blood flow to the stomach is disrupted, causing little bursts of ischemia; there's not much evidence for this, however. Another idea is that the contractions mechanically damage the stomach walls. The jury is still out on that mechanism.

Most of these mechanisms are pretty well documented routes by which ulcers can form; of those credible mechanisms, most can occur during at least certain types of stressors. More than one mechanism may occur simultaneously, and people seemingly differ as to how likely each mechanism is to occur in their gut during stress, and how likely it is to interact with bacterial infection. Additional mechanisms for stress's role in ulcer formation will no doubt be discovered, but for the moment these should be quite sufficient to make anyone sick.

Peptic ulcers are what the physician Susan Levenstein, the wittiest person on earth writing about gastroenterology, has termed "the very model of a modern etiology."† Stress doesn't cause peptic ulcers to

---

* And some scientists even think that *Helicobacter*, amid its disease-causing potential, is also beneficial insofar as it stimulates immunity.

† Admittedly, there's a small sample size of such writers. In one of my favorite essays of hers, she begins, "When I was in medical school, the reigning approach to the patient combined the paternal, the veterinary, and the priestly: interrogate, palpate, pontificate."

form. But it makes the biological villains that do cause ulcers to form more likely to occur, or more virulent, or impairs your ability to defend yourself against those villains. This is the classic interaction between the organic (bacteria, viruses, toxins, mutations) and the psychogenic components of disease.

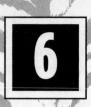

6

DWARFISM AND
THE IMPORTANCE OF MOTHERS

It still surprises me that organisms grow. Maybe I don't believe in biology as much as I claim. Eating and digesting a meal seems very real. You put a massive amount of something or other in your mouth, and, as a result, all sorts of tangible things happen—your jaw gets tired, your stomach distends, eventually something comes out the other end. Growth seems pretty tangible, too. Long bones get longer, kids weigh more when you heft them.

My difficulty is with the steps that connect digestion with growth. I know how it works; my university even allows me to teach impressionable students about it. But it just seems implausible. Someone ate a mountain of spaghetti, salad, garlic bread, and two slices of cake for dessert—and that has been transformed and is now partially inside this test tube of blood? And somehow it's going to be reconstructed into bone? Just think, your femur is made up of tiny pieces of your mother's chicken potpie that you ate throughout your youth. Ha! You see, you don't really believe in the process either. Maybe we're too primitive to comprehend the transmogrification of material.

HOW WE GROW

Nevertheless, growth does occur as a result of eating. And in a kid, it's not a trivial process. The brain gets bigger, the shape of the head changes. Cells divide, grow in size, and synthesize new proteins. Long bones lengthen as cartilaginous cells at the ends of bones migrate into the shaft and solidify into bone. Baby fat melts away and is replaced by muscle. The larynx thickens and the voice deepens, hair grows in all sorts of unlikely places on the body, breasts develop, testes enlarge.

From the standpoint of understanding the effects of stress on growth, the most important feature of the growth process is that, of course, growth doesn't come cheap. Calcium must be obtained to build bones, amino acids are needed for all that protein synthesis, fatty acids build cell walls—and it's glucose that pays for the building costs. Appetite soars, and nutrients pour in from the intestines. A large part of what various hormones do is to mobilize the energy and the material needed for all these civic expansion projects. Growth hormone dominates the process. Sometimes it works directly on cells in the body—for example, growth hormone helps to break down fat stores, flushing them into the circulation so they can be diverted to the growing cells. Alternatively, sometimes growth hormone must first trigger the release of another class of hormones called *somatomedins*, which actually do the job, such as promoting cell division. Thyroid hormone plays a role, promoting growth hormone release, making bones more responsive to somatomedins. Insulin does something similar as well. The reproductive hormones come into play around puberty. Estrogen promotes the growth of long bones, both by acting directly on bone and by increasing growth hormone secretion. Testosterone does similar things to long bones and, in addition, enhances muscle growth.

Adolescents stop growing when the ends of the long bones meet and begin to fuse, but for complex reasons, testosterone, by accelerating the growth of the ends of long bones, can actually speed the cessation of growth. Thus, pubescent boys given testosterone will, paradoxically, wind up having their adult stature blunted a bit. Conversely, boys castrated before puberty grow to be quite tall, with lanky bodies and particularly long limbs. Opera history buffs will recognize this morphology, as castrati were famed for this body shape.

 ## NEUROTIC PARENTS: BEWARE!

It is time to look at how stress disrupts normal development. As we'll see, this not only involves impairing skeletal growth (that is, how tall you grow to be), but also how stress early in life can alter your vulnerability to disease throughout your lifetime.

Now, before I launch into this, I have to issue a warning to anyone who is a parent, or who plans to be a parent, or who had parents.

There's nothing like parenthood to make you really neurotic, as you worry about the consequences of your every act, thought, or omission. I have young children, and here are some of the heinous things that my wife and I have done to irreparably harm them: there was the time we were desperate to placate them about something and allowed them to eat some sugar-bomb breakfast cereal we'd normally ban; then there was the loud concert we went to when our firstborn was a third-trimester fetus, causing him to kick throughout, no doubt in pained protest; and there was the time we messed up with our otherwise ceaseless vigilance and allowed ten seconds of a violent cartoon to show on the television while we fumbled with the Kumbaya-esque video we were attempting to insert. You only want perfection for the ones you love beyond words, so you get nutsy at times. This section will make you nutsier.

So keep this warning in mind, a point I will return to at the end.

 ## PRENATAL STRESS

What is childhood about? It is a time when you make assessments about the nature of the world. For example, "If you let go of something, it falls down, not up." Or, "If something is hidden underneath something else, it still exists." Or, ideally, "Even if Mommy disappears for a while, she will come back because Mommy always comes back."

Often, these assessments shape your view of the world forever. For example, as will be discussed in chapter 14, if you lose a parent to death while you are a child, your risk of major depression has increased for the rest of your life. I will suggest that this arises from having learned at a premature age a deep emotional lesson about the nature of life, namely, that this is a world in which awful things can happen over which you have no control.

It turns out that during development, beginning with fetal life, your body is also learning about the nature of the world and, metaphorically, making lifelong decisions about how to respond to the outside world. And if development involves certain types of stressors, some of these "decisions" cause a lifelong increase in the risk of certain diseases.

Consider a female who is pregnant during a famine. She's not getting enough calories, nor is her fetus. It turns out that during the latter part of pregnancy, a fetus is "learning" about how plentiful food is in that outside world, and a famine winds up "teaching" it that, jeez, there's not a whole lot of food out there, better store every smidgen of it. Something about the metabolism of that fetus shifts permanently, a feature called metabolic "imprinting" or "programming." Forever after, that fetus will be particularly good at storing the food it consumes, at retaining every grain of precious salt from the diet. Forever after, that fetus develops what has been termed a "thrifty" metabolism.

And what are the consequences of that? Suddenly we find ourselves back in the middle of chapters 3 and 4. Everything else being equal throughout life, even late in life, that organism is more at risk for hypertension, obesity, adult-onset diabetes, and cardiovascular disease.

Remarkably, things work precisely this way in rats, pigs, and sheep. And humans as well. The most dramatic and most cited example concerns the Dutch Hunger Winter at the end of World War II. The occupying Nazis were being pushed back on all fronts, the Dutch were trying to aid the Allies coming to liberate them, and, as punishment, the Nazis cut off all food transport. For a demarcated season, the Dutch starved. People consumed less than 1,000 calories a day, were reduced to eating tulip bulbs, and 16,000 people starved to death. Fetuses, going about their lifelong metabolic programming, learned some severe lessons about food availability during that winter of starvation. The result is a cohort of people with thrifty metabolisms and increased risks of Metabolic syndrome a half-century later. Seemingly, different aspects of metabolism and physiology get programmed at different points of fetal development. If you were a first-trimester fetus during the famine, that programs you for a greater risk of heart disease, obesity, and an unhealthy cholesterol profile, whereas if you were a second- or third-trimester fetus, that programs you for a greater diabetes risk.

The key to this phenomenon seems to be not only that you were undernourished as a fetus, but that after birth you had plenty of food and were able to recover from the deprivation quickly. Thus, from early in childhood, you not only were highly efficient at storing nutrients, but had access to plentiful nutrients.*

So avoid starving a fetus while you're pregnant. But this phenomenon also applies to less dramatic situations. Within the normal range of birth weights, the lower the weight of a baby (when adjusted for body length), the greater the risk of those Metabolic syndrome

---

* The Dutch example was ideal for this, in that once the country recovered from that winter, people had the benefit of plentiful food. In contrast, the same has not been seen among people who were fetuses during the Siege of Leningrad in World War II—food was not plentiful afterward.

problems in adulthood. Even after you control for adult body weight, low birth weight still predicts an increased risk of diabetes and hypertension.

These are big effects. When you compare those who were heaviest versus lightest at birth, you see an approximate eight-fold difference in the risk of pre-diabetes, and about an eighteen-fold difference in the risk of Metabolic syndrome. Among both men and women, compare those whose birth weights were in the lowest 25 percent versus those in the highest 25 percent, and the former have a 50 percent higher rate of death from heart disease.

This relationship between fetal nutritional events and lifelong risks of metabolic and cardiovascular disease was first described by the epidemiologist David Barker of Southampton Hospital in England, and now goes by the name Fetal Origins of Adult Disease (FOAD). And we're not done with this yet.

Starvation is clearly a stressor, raising the question of whether the metabolic programming occurs because of the nutritional consequences of the shortage of calories, and/or because of the stressfulness of the shortage of calories. Asked another way, do non-nutritional stressors during pregnancy also induce FOAD-like effects? The answer is, yes.

An extensive literature, stretching back decades, shows that stressing a female rat in any number of ways while she is pregnant will cause lifelong changes in the physiology of her offspring. Predictably, one set of changes involves glucocorticoid secretion. Once again, think of the fetal body "learning" about the outside world, this time along the lines of, "How stressful is it out there?" Fetuses can monitor signals of stress from the mother, insofar as glucocorticoids readily pass through to the fetal circulation, and lots of glucocorticoids "teach" the fetus that it is indeed a stressful world out there. The result? Be prepared for that stressful world: tend toward secreting excessive amounts of glucocorticoids. Prenatally stressed rats grow into adults with elevated glucocorticoid levels—depending on the study, elevated basal levels, a larger stress-response, and/or a sluggish recovery from the stress-response. The lifelong programming seems to be due to a permanent decrease in the number of receptors for glucocorticoids in one part of the brain. The brain region is involved in turning off this stress-response by inhibiting CRH release. Fewer glucocorticoid receptors there mean less sensitivity to the hormone's signal, which means less effective reining in of subsequent glucocorticoid secretion. The result is a lifelong tendency toward elevated levels.

Is it the glucocorticoid secretion by the stressed pregnant female that gives rise to these permanent changes in the offspring? Seemingly yes—the effect can be replicated in a number of species, including nonhuman primates, by injecting the pregnant female with high glucocorticoid levels, instead of stressing her.

A smaller but fairly solid literature shows that prenatal stress programs humans for higher glucocorticoid secretion in adulthood as well. In these studies, low birth weight (corrected for body length) is used as a surrogate marker for stressors during fetal life, and the lower the birth weight, the higher the basal glucocorticoid levels in adults ranging from age twenty to seventy; this relationship becomes even more pronounced when low birth weight is coupled with premature birth.*

The excessive glucocorticoid exposure of a stressful fetal life seems to contribute to the lifelong increase in the risk of Metabolic syndrome as well. As evidence, if you expose a fetal rat, sheep, or nonhuman primate to lots of synthetic glucocorticoids during late gestational life (by injecting the mother with them), that fetus will be more at risk for the symptoms of Metabolic syndrome as an adult. How does this arise? A plausible sequence is that the prenatal exposure to high glucocorticoid levels leads to the elevated glucocorticoid levels in adulthood, which increases the risk of Metabolic syndrome. Those readers who have memorized the book so far will have no trouble recalling exactly how an excess of glucocorticoids in adulthood can increase the odds of obesity, insulin-resistant diabetes, and hypertension. Despite those potential links, the elevated glucocorticoid levels in adulthood are probably only one of the routes linking prenatal stress with the adult Metabolic syndrome.

So now we have hypertension, diabetes, cardiovascular disease, obesity, and glucocorticoid excess in this picture. Let's make it worse. How about the reproductive system? An extensive literature shows that if you stress pregnant rats, you "demasculinize" the male fetuses. They are less sexually active as adults, and have less developed genitals. As we will see in the next chapter, stress decreases testosterone secretion, and it seems to do so in male fetuses as well. Furthermore, glucocorticoids and testosterone have similar chemical structures

---

* The seventy-year-olds were studied in Finland. As we will see at a couple of points in the book, studies like this one could only be carried out in Scandinavia, whose countries have a tradition of obsessively good record keeping about everything imaginable, including birth weights for large populations of people.

(they are both "steroid" hormones), and a lot of glucocorticoids in a fetus can begin to gum up and block receptors for testosterone, making it impossible for the testosterone to have its effects.

More FOADish problems. Seriously stress a pregnant rat and her offspring will grow up to be anxious. Now, how do you tell if a rat is anxious? You put it in a new (and thus, by definition, scary) environment; how long does it take for it to explore? Or take advantage of the fact that rats, being nocturnal, don't like bright lights. Take a hungry rat and put some food in the middle of a brightly lit cage; how long until the rat goes for the food? How readily can the rat learn in a novel setting, or socially interact with new rats? How much does the rat defecate in a novel setting?* Prenatally stressed rats, as adults, freeze up when around bright lights, can't learn in novel settings, defecate like crazy. Sad. As we will see in chapter 15, anxiety revolves around a part of the brain called the amygdala, and prenatal stress programs the amygdala into a lifelong profile that has anxiety written all over it. The amygdala winds up with more receptors for (that is, more sensitivity to) glucocorticoids, more of a neurotransmitter that mediates anxiety, and fewer receptors for a brain chemical that reduces anxiety.† Does prenatal stress in humans make for anxious adults? It's difficult to study this in humans, in that it is hard to find mothers who are anxious during pregnancy, or anxious while their child is growing up, but not both. So there's not a huge amount of evidence for this happening in humans.

Finally, chapter 10 will review how an excess of stress can have bad effects on the brain, particularly in the developing brain. Prenatally stressed rodents grow up to have fewer connections between the neurons in a key area of the brain involved in learning and memory, and have more impairments of memory in old age, while prenatally stressed nonhuman primates have memory problems and form fewer

---

* I kid you not, and this should make perfect sense after chapter 5. Anxious in a new environment? Increase large intestinal motility, defecate, and the grad student doing a thesis on rat anxiety counts the number of fecal pellets in the cage afterward for a remarkably informative measure of anxiety.

† Just to give away some of the information coming in chapter 15, the neurotransmitter that mediates anxiety via the amygdala is none other than CRH (recall from chapter 5 that CRH mediates other aspects of the stress-response than merely releasing ACTH). Meanwhile, the receptor for the brain chemical that inhibits anxiety is called a benzodiazepine receptor. What is a benzodiazepine? No one is exactly sure what the anxiety-reducing benzodiazepine is in the brain that normally binds to the receptor, but we all know about the synthetic benzodiazepines—these are Valium and Librium, the anxiety-reducing tranquilizers.

neurons as well. The human studies have been very hard to carry out for reasons similar to that of those examining whether prenatal stress increases the risk of anxiety. With that caveat, a number of studies have shown that such stress results in children born with a smaller head circumference (which certainly fits in with the picture of being underweight in general). However, it's not clear whether head circumference at birth predicts how many academic degrees the kid is going to have after her name thirty years later.

One final piece of the FOAD story is so intrinsically fascinating that it made me stop thinking like a worried parent for a few minutes and instead I just marveled at biology.

Suppose you have a fetus exposed to lots of stress, say, malnutrition, and who thus programs a thrifty metabolism. Later, as an adult, she gets pregnant. She consumes normal amounts of food. Because she has that thrifty metabolism, is so good at storing away nutrients in case that fetal famine ever comes back again, her body grabs a disproportionate share of the nutrients in her bloodstream for herself. In other words, amid consuming an average amount of food, her fetus gets a less than average share of it, producing mild malnutrition. And thus programs a milder version of a thrifty metabolism. And when that fetus eventually becomes pregnant. . . .

In other words, these FOADish tendencies can be transmitted across generations, without the benefit of genes. It's not due to shared genes, but to shared environment, namely, the intimately shared blood supply during gestation.

Amazing. This is precisely what is seen in the Dutch Hunger Winter population, in that their grandchildren are born with lower than expected birth weights. This is seen in other realms as well. Pick some rats at random and feed them on a diet that will make them become obese at the time of pregnancy. As a result, their offspring, despite being fed a normal diet, have an increased risk of obesity. As will their grandkids. Similarly, in humans, having insulin-resistant diabetes while pregnant increases the risk of the disorder in your offspring, after controlling for weight. Wait a second—going through a famine means less nutrients in the bloodstream, while having insulin-resistant diabetes means more. How can they produce the same thrifty metabolism in the fetus? Remember, you have elevated levels of glucose in the bloodstream in the case of diabetes because you can't store the stuff. Recall a one-sentence factoid from chapter 4—when overstuffed fat cells begin to become insulin-resistant, they release hormones that urge other fat cells and muscle to do the same. And those hormones get into the fetal circulation. So you have Mom, who is insulin-resistant because she has too much energy stored away, releasing hormones that make the normal-weight fetus bad at energy storage as well . . . and the fetus winds up underweight and with a thrifty metabolic view of the world.

So expose a fetus to lots of glucocorticoids and you are increasing its risk for obesity, hypertension, cardiovascular disease, insulin-resistant diabetes, maybe reproductive impairments, maybe anxiety, and impaired brain development. And maybe even setting up that fetus's eventual offspring for the same. Aren't you sorry now that the two of you had that argument over whether to videotape the delivery? Now on to the next realm of worries.

 POSTNATAL STRESS

The obvious question to begin this section is, does postnatal stress have lifelong adverse effects on development as well?

Of course it can. To begin, what's the most stressful thing that could happen to an infant rat? Being deprived of its mother (while still receiving adequate nutrition). Work done by Paul Plotsky at Emory University shows that maternal deprivation causes similar consequences in a rat as prenatal stress: increased levels of glucocorticoids during stress and an impaired recovery at the end of stress. More anxiety, and the same sorts of changes in the amygdala as were seen in prenatally stressed adults. And impaired development of a part of the brain relevant to learning and memory. Separate an infant rhesus monkey from its mother and it grows up to have elevated glucocorticoid levels as well.

How about something more subtle? What if your rat mom is around but is simply inattentive? Michael Meaney of McGill University has looked at the lifelong consequences for rats of having had a highly attentive or highly inattentive mother. What counts as attentiveness? Grooming and licking. Infants whose mothers groomed and licked the least produced kids who were milder versions of rats who were maternally deprived as infants, with elevated glucocorticoid levels.*

---

* While this clearly emphasizes the importance of being a well-groomed child if you are a rat, it's not quite obvious what the human equivalent would be.

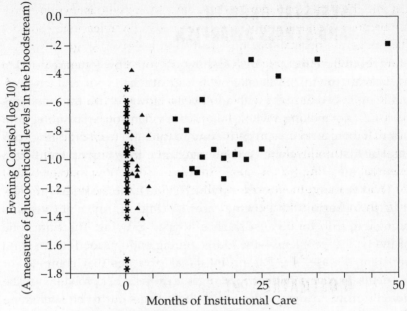

* Children reared with families of origin.
▲ Children adopted after less than four months of institutional care.
  Children adopted after more than eight months in orphanages in Romania.

What are the consequences of childhood stress for disease vulnerability during adulthood in humans? This has been studied only minimally, which is not surprising, given how difficult such studies are. A number of studies, mentioned earlier, show that loss of a parent to death during childhood increases the lifelong risk of depression. Another, discussed in chapter 5, shows that early trauma increases the risk of irritable bowel syndrome in adulthood, and similar animal studies show that early stress produces large intestines that contract to abnormal extents in response to stress.

Though the subject is still poorly studied, childhood stress may produce the building blocks for the sort of adult diseases we've been considering. For example, when you examine children who had been adopted more than a year before from Romanian orphanages, the longer the child spent in the orphanage, the higher the resting glucocorticoid levels.* Similarly, children who have been abused have elevated glucocorticoid levels, and decreased size and activity in the most highly evolved part of the brain, the frontal cortex.

---

* For those not familiar with these hellholes, Romanian orphanages have become the study subjects of choice for understanding the consequences of massive sensory, intellectual, and emotional deprivation in infants and children.

SKELETAL GROWTH
AND STRESS DWARFISM

How about the effects of stress on how tall you grow (often referred to as skeletal growth)? Skeletal growth is great when you are a ten-year-old lying in bed at night with a full belly. However, it's the usual scenario of it not making a whole lot of sense when you're sprinting from a lion. If there is no time to derive any advantages from digesting your meal at that point, there certainly isn't time to get any benefit from growth.

To understand the process by which stress inhibits skeletal growth, it helps to begin with extreme cases. A child of, say, eight years is brought to a doctor because she has stopped growing. There are none of the typical problems—the kid is getting enough food, there is no apparent disease, she has no intestinal parasites that compete for nutrients. No one can identify an organic cause of her problem; yet she doesn't grow. In many such cases, there turns out to be something dreadfully stressful in her life—emotional neglect or psychological abuse. In such circumstances, the syndrome is called stress dwarfism, or psychosocial or psychogenic dwarfism.*

A question now typically comes to mind among people who are below average height. If you are short, yet didn't have any obvious chronic diseases as a kid and can recall a dreadful period in your childhood, are you a victim of mild stress dwarfism? Suppose one of your parents had a job necessitating frequent moves, and every year or two throughout childhood you were uprooted, forced to leave your friends, moved off to a strange school. Is this the sort of situation associated with psychogenic dwarfism? Definitely not. How about something more severe? What about an acrimonious divorce? Stress dwarfism? Unlikely.

The syndrome is extremely rare. These are the kids who are incessantly harassed and psychologically terrorized by the crazy stepfather. These are the kids who, when the police and the social workers break down the door, are discovered to have been locked in a closet for

---

* Some clinical nomenclature: "maternal deprivation syndrome," "deprivation syndrome," and "nonorganic failure to thrive" usually refer to infants and invariably to the loss of the mother. "Stress dwarfism," "psychogenic dwarfism," and "psychosocial dwarfism" usually refer to children aged three years or older. However, some papers do not follow this age dichotomy; during the nineteenth century, infants dying of failure to thrive in orphanages were said to suffer from "marasmus," Greek for "wasting away."

extended periods, fed a tray of food slipped under the door. These are the products of vast, grotesque psychopathology. And they appear in every endocrinology textbook, standing nude in front of a growth chart. Stunted little kids, years behind their expected height, years behind in mental development, bruised, with distorted, flinching postures, haunted, slack facial expressions, eyes masked by the obligatory rectangles that accompany all naked people in medical texts. And all with stories to take your breath away and make you wonder at the potential sickness of the human mind.

Invariably, on the same page in the text is a surprising second photo—the same child a few years later, after having been placed in a different environment (or, as one pediatric endocrinologist termed it, having undergone a "parentectomy"). No bruises, maybe a tentative smile. And a lot taller. So long as the stressor is removed before the child is far into puberty (when the ends of the long bones fuse together and growth ceases), there is the potential for some degree of "catch-up" growth (although shortness of stature and some degree of stunting of personality and intellect usually persist into adulthood).

Despite the clinical rarity of stress dwarfism, instances pop up throughout history. One possible case arose during the thirteenth century as the result of an experiment by that noted endocrinologist, King Frederick II of Sicily. It seems that his court was engrossed in philosophic disputation over the natural language of humans. In an attempt to resolve the question, Frederick (who was apparently betting on Hebrew, Greek, or Latin) came up with a surprisingly sophisticated idea for an experiment. He commandeered a bunch of infants and had each one reared in a room of its own. Every day someone would bring the child food, fresh blankets, and clean clothes, all of the best quality. But they wouldn't stay and play with the infant, or hold it—too much of a chance that the person would speak in the child's presence. The infants would be reared without human language, and everyone would get to see what was actually the natural language of humans.

Of course, the kids did not spontaneously burst out of the door one day reciting poetry in Italian or singing opera. The kids didn't burst out of the door at all. None of them survived. The lesson is obvious to us now—optimal growth and development do not merely depend on being fed the right number of calories and being kept warm. Frederick "laboured in vain, for the children could not live without clappings of hands and gestures and gladness of countenance and blandishments," reported the contemporary historian Salimbene.

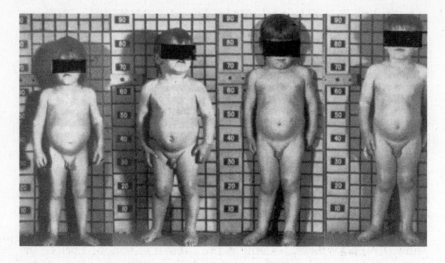

A child suffering from stress dwarfism: changes in appearance during hospitalization (left to right).

It seems quite plausible that these kids, all healthy and well fed, died of a nonorganic failure to thrive.*

Another study that winds up in half the textbooks makes the same point, if more subtly. The subjects of the "experiment" were children reared in two different orphanages in Germany after World War II. Both orphanages were run by the government; thus there were important controls in place—the kids in both had the same general diet, the same frequency of doctors' visits, and so on. The main identifiable difference in their care was the two women who ran the orphanages. The scientists even checked them, and their description sounds like a parable. In one orphanage was Fräulein Grun, the warm, nurturing mother figure who played with the children, comforted them, and spent all day singing and laughing. In the other was Fräulein Schwarz, a woman who was clearly in the wrong profession. She discharged her professional obligations, but minimized her contact with the children; she frequently criticized and berated them, typically among their assembled peers. The growth rates at the two orphanages

---

* Ol' King Fred was quite the budding scientist. Then there was the time he got interested in digestion. Frederick wondered whether digestion was faster when you rested after eating or if you exercised. He had two men brought from his prison, fed identical and sumptuous dinners, and sent one off to nap afterward, while the other went for a strenuous hunt. That phase of the experiment completed, he had both men returned to his court, disemboweled in front of him, and their innards examined. The sleeper had digested his food better.

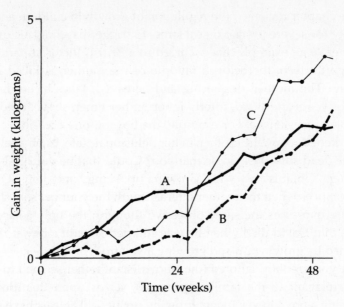

Growth rates in the two German orphanages. During the first 26 weeks of the study, growth rates in Orphanage A, under the administration of Fräulein Grun, were much greater than those in Orphanage B, with the stern Fräulein Schwarz. At 26 weeks (vertical line), Fräulein Grun left Orphanage A and was replaced by Fräulein Schwarz. The rate of growth in that orphanage promptly slowed; growth in Orphanage B, now minus the stern Fräulein Schwarz, accelerated and soon surpassed that of Orphanage A. A fascinating elaboration emerges from the fact that Schwarz was not completely heartless, but had a subset of children who were her favorites (Curve C), whom she had transferred with her.

were entirely different. Fräulein Schwarz's kids grew in height and weight at a slower pace than the kids in the other orphanage. Then, in an elaboration that couldn't have been more useful if it had been planned by a scientist, Fräulein Grun moved on to greener pastures and, for some bureaucratic reason, Fräulein Schwarz was transferred to the other orphanage. Growth rates in her former orphanage promptly increased; those in her new one decreased.

A final and truly disturbing example comes to mind. If you ever find yourself reading chapter after chapter about growth endocrinology (which I don't recommend), you will note an occasional odd reference to Peter Pan—perhaps a quotation from the play, or a snide comment about Tinker Bell. I'd long noted the phenomenon and finally, in a chapter in one textbook, I found the explanation for it.

The chapter reviewed the regulation of growth in children and the capacity for severe psychological stress to trigger psychogenic dwarfism. It gave an example that occurred in a British Victorian family. A son, age thirteen, the beloved favorite of the mother, is killed in an accident. The mother, despairing and bereaved, takes to her bed in grief for years afterward, utterly ignoring her other, six-year-old son. Horrible scenes ensue. For example, the boy, on one occasion, enters her darkened room; the mother, in her delusional state, briefly believes it is the dead son—"David, is that you? Could that be you?"—before realizing: "Oh, it is only you." Growing up, being "only you." On the rare instances when the mother interacts with the younger son, she repeatedly expresses the same obsessive thought: the only solace she feels is that David died when he was still perfect, still a boy, never to be ruined by growing up and growing away from his mother.

The younger boy, ignored (the stern, distant father seemed to have been irrelevant to the family dynamics), seizes upon this idea; by remaining a boy forever, by not growing up, he will at least have some chance of pleasing his mother, winning her love. Although there is no evidence of disease or malnutrition in his well-to-do family, he ceases growing. As an adult, he is just barely five feet in height, and his marriage is unconsummated.

And then the chapter informs us that the boy became the author of the much-beloved children's classic—*Peter Pan*. J. M. Barrie's writings are filled with children who didn't grow up, who were fortunate enough to die in childhood, who came back as ghosts to visit their mothers.

THE MECHANISMS UNDERLYING STRESS DWARFISM

Stress dwarfism involves extremely low growth hormone levels in the circulation. The sensitivity of growth hormone to psychological state has rarely been shown as clearly as in a paper that followed a single child with stress dwarfism. When brought to the hospital, he was assigned to a nurse who spent a great deal of time with him and to whom he became very attached. Row A in the table below shows his physiological profile upon entering the hospital: extremely low growth hormone levels and a low rate of growth. Row B shows his profile a few months later, while still in the hospital: growth hormone levels have more than doubled (without his having received any synthetic hormones), and the growth rate has more than tripled. The

A Demonstration of the Sensitivity of Growth to Emotional State

Condition	Growth hormone	Growth	Food intake
A. Entry into hospital	5.9	0.5	1663
B. 100 days later	13.0	1.7	1514
C. Favorite nurse on vacation	6.9	0.6	1504
D. Nurse returns	15.0	1.5	1521

Source: From Saenger and colleagues, 1977. Growth hormone is measured in nanograms of the hormone per milliliter of blood following insulin stimulation; growth is expressed as centimeters per 20 days. Food intake is expressed in calories consumed per day.

stress dwarfism is not a problem of insufficient food—the boy was eating more at the time he entered the hospital than a few months later, when his growth resumed.

Row C profiles the period when the nurse went on a three-week vacation. Despite the same food intake, growth hormone levels and growth plummeted. Finally, Row D shows the boy's profile after the nurse returned from vacation. This is extraordinary. To take a concrete, nuts and bolts feature of growth, the rate at which this child was depositing calcium in his long bones could be successfully predicted by his proximity to a loved one. You can't ask for a clearer demonstration that what is going on in our heads influences every cell in our bodies.

Why do growth hormone levels decline in these kids? Growth hormone is secreted by the pituitary gland, which in turn is regulated by the hypothalamus in the brain (see chapter 2). The hypothalamus controls the release of growth hormone through the secretion of a stimulatory hormone and an inhibitory one, and it looks as if stress dwarfism involves too much release of the inhibitory hormone. Stress-induced overactivity of the sympathetic nervous system may play some role in this. Furthermore, the body becomes less responsive to what little growth hormone is actually secreted. Therefore, even administering synthetic growth hormone doesn't necessarily solve the growth problem. Some stress dwarfism kids have elevated glucocorticoid levels, and the hormone blunts growth hormone release as well as responsiveness of the body to growth hormone.

Kids with stress dwarfism also have gastrointestinal problems, in that they're impaired at absorbing nutrients from their intestines.

This is probably because of the enhanced activity of their sympathetic nervous systems. As discussed in chapter 5, this will halt the release of various digestive enzymes, stop the muscular contractions of the stomach and intestinal walls, and block nutrient absorption.

This tells us something about which stress hormones shut down growth. But what is it about being reared under pathological conditions that causes a failure of skeletal growth? Cynthia Kuhn and Saul Schanberg of Duke University and, in separate studies, Myron Hofer of the New York State Psychiatric Institute, have examined that question in infant rats separated from their mothers. Is it the smell of Mom that would normally stimulate growth? Is it something in her milk? Do the rats get chilly without her? Is it the rat lullabies that she sings? You can imagine the various ways scientists test for these possibilities—playing recordings of Mom's vocalizations, pumping her odor into the cage, seeing what substitutes for the real thing.

It turns out to be touch, and it has to be active touching. Separate a baby rat from its mother and its growth hormone levels plummet. Allow it contact with its mother while she is anesthetized, and growth hormone is still low. Mimic active licking by the mother by stroking the rat pup in the proper pattern, and growth normalizes. In a similar set of findings, other investigators have observed that handling neonatal rats causes them to grow faster and larger.

The same seems to apply in humans, as demonstrated in a classic study. Tiffany Field of the University of Miami School of Medicine, along with Schanberg, Kuhn, and others, performed an incredibly simple experiment that was inspired both by the rat research and by the history of the dismal mortality rates in orphanages and pediatric wards, as discussed earlier. Studying premature infants in neonatology wards, they noted that the premature kids, while pampered and fretted over and maintained in near-sterile conditions, were hardly ever touched. So Field and crew went in and started touching them: fifteen-minute periods, three times a day, stroking their bodies, moving their limbs. It worked wonders. The kids grew nearly 50 percent faster, were more active and alert, matured faster behaviorally, and were released from the hospital nearly a week earlier than the premature infants who weren't touched. Months later, they were still doing better than infants who hadn't been touched. If this were done in every neonatology ward, this would not only make for a lot more healthy infants, but would save approximately a billion dollars annually. It's rare that the highest technology of medical instrumentation—MRI machines, artificial organs, pacemakers—has the potential for as much impact as this simple intervention.

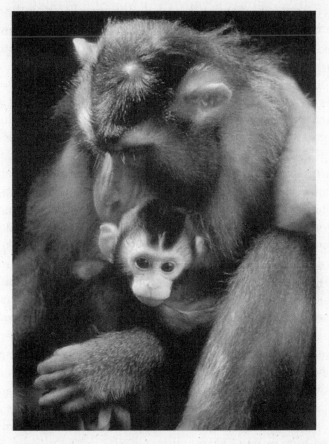

Pigtailed macaque mother and infant.

Touch is one of the central experiences of an infant. We readily think of stressors as consisting of various unpleasant things that can be done to an organism. Sometimes a stressor can be the failure to provide something essential, and the absence of touch is seemingly one of the most marked developmental stressors that we can suffer.

 ## STRESS AND GROWTH HORMONE SECRETION IN HUMANS

The pattern of growth hormone secretion during stress differs in humans from rodents, and the implications can be fascinating. But the subject is a tough one, not meant for the fainthearted. So feel free to go to the bathroom now and come back at the next commercial break.

When a rat is first stressed, growth hormone levels in the circulation decline almost immediately. If the stressor continues, growth hormone levels remain depressed. And as we have seen, in humans major and prolonged stressors cause a decrease in growth hormone levels as well. The weird thing is that during the period immediately following the onset of stress, growth hormone levels actually go up in humans and some other species. In these species, in other words, short-term stress actually stimulates growth hormone secretion for a time.

Why? As was mentioned, growth hormone has two classes of effects. In the first, it stimulates somatomedins to stimulate bone growth and cell division. This is the growing part of the story. But in addition, growth hormone works directly on fat cells, breaking down fat stores and flushing them into the circulation. This is the energy for the growth. In effect, growth hormone not only runs the construction site for the new building, but arranges financing for the work as well.

Now that business about breaking down stored energy and flushing it into the circulation should sound familiar—that's precisely what glucocorticoids, epinephrine, norepinephrine, and glucagon are doing during that sprint from the lion. So those direct growth hormone actions are similar to the energy mobilization that occurs during stress, while the somatomedin-mediated growth hormone actions are not what you want to be doing. During stress, therefore, it is adaptive to secrete growth hormone insofar as it helps to mobilize energy, but a bad move to secrete growth hormone insofar as it stimulates an expensive, long-term project like growth.

As noted, during stress, somatomedin secretion is inhibited, as is the sensitivity of the body to that hormone. This is perfect—you secrete growth hormone during stress and still get its energy-mobilizing effects, while blocking its more explicit growth-promoting effects. To extend the metaphor used earlier, growth hormone has just taken out cash from the bank, aiming to fund the next six months of construction; instead, the cash is used to solve the body's immediate emergency.

Given this clever solution—spare the growth hormone, block the somatomedins—why should growth hormone levels decline at all during stress (whether immediately, as in the rat, or after a while, as in humans)? It is probably because the system does not work perfectly—somatomedin action is not completely shut down during stress. Therefore, the energy-mobilizing effects of growth hormone might still be used for growth. Perhaps the timing of the decline of growth hormone levels in each species is a compromise between the trait triggered by the hormone that is good news during stress and the trait that is undesirable.

What impresses me is how careful and calculating the body has to be during stress in order to coordinate hormonal activities just right. It must perfectly balance the costs and benefits, knowing exactly when to stop secreting the hormone. If the body miscalculates in one direction and growth hormone secretion is blocked too early, there is relatively less mobilization of energy for dealing with the stressor. If it miscalculates in the other direction and growth hormone secretion goes on too long, stress may actually enhance growth. One oft-quoted study suggests that the second type of error occurs during some stressors.

In the early 1960s, Thomas Landauer of Dartmouth and John Whiting of Harvard methodically studied the rites of passages found in various non-Western societies around the world; they wanted to know whether the stressfulness of the ritual was related to how tall the kids wound up being as adults. Landauer and Whiting classified cultures according to whether and when they subjected their children to physically stressful development rites. Stressful rites included piercing the nose, lips, or ears; circumcision, inoculation, scarification, or cauterization; stretching or binding of limbs, or shaping the head; exposure to hot baths, fire, or intense sunlight; exposure to cold baths, snow, or cold air; emetics, irritants, and enemas; rubbing with sand, or scraping with a shell or other sharp object. (And you thought having to play the piano at age ten for your grandmother's friends was a stressful rite of passage.)

Reflecting the anthropological tunnel vision of the time, Landauer and Whiting only studied males. They examined eighty cultures around the world and carefully controlled for a potential problem with the data—they collected examples from cultures from the same gene pools, with and without those stressful rituals. For example, they compared the West African tribes of the Yoruba (stressful rituals) and Ashanti (nonstressful), and similarly matched Native American tribes. With this approach, they attempted to control for genetic contributions to stature (as well as nutrition, since related ethnic groups were likely to have similar diets) and to examine cultural differences instead.

Given the effects of stress on growth, it was not surprising that among cultures where kids of ages six to fifteen went through stressful maturational rituals, growth was inhibited (relative to cultures without such rituals, the difference was about 1.5 inches). Surprisingly, going through such rituals at ages two to six had no effect on growth. And most surprising, in cultures in which those rituals took place with kids under two years of age, growth was stimulated—adults were about 2.5 inches taller than in cultures without stressful rituals.

There are some possible confounds that could explain the results. One is fairly silly—maybe tall tribes like to put their young children through stressful rituals. One is more plausible—maybe putting very young children through these stressful rituals kills a certain percentage of them, and what doesn't kill you makes you stronger and taller. Landauer and Whiting noted that possibility and could not rule it out. In addition, even though they attempted to pair similar groups, there may have been differences other than just the stressfulness of the rites of passage—perhaps in diet or child-rearing practices. Not surprisingly, no one has ever measured levels of growth hormone or somatomedins, in, say, Shilluk or Hausa kids while they are undergoing some grueling ritual, so there is no direct endocrine evidence that such stressors actually stimulate growth hormone secretion in a way that increases growth. Despite these problems, these cross-cultural studies have been interpreted by many biological anthropologists as evidence that some types of stressors in humans can actually stimulate growth, amid the broader literature showing the growth-suppressing effects of stress.

 ENOUGH ALREADY

So there's a whole bunch of ways that prenatal or early childhood stress can have bad and long-term consequences. This can be anxiety provoking; it gets me into a storm of parental agitation just to write about this. Let's figure out what's worrisome and what's not.

First, can fetal or childhood exposure to synthetic glucocorticoids have lifelong, adverse effects? Glucocorticoids (such as hydrocortisone) are prescribed in vast amounts, because of their immunosuppressive or anti-inflammatory effects. During pregnancy, they are administered to women with certain endocrine disorders or who are at risk for delivering preterm. Heavy administration of them during pregnancy has been reported to result in children with smaller head circumferences, emotional and behavioral problems in childhood, and slowing of some developmental landmarks. Are these effects lifelong? No one knows. At this point, the experts have weighed in emphatically stating that a single round of glucocorticoids during either fetal or postnatal life has no adverse effects, though there is potential for problems with heavy use. But heavy doses of glucocorticoids are not administered unless there's a serious illness going on, so the most prudent advice is to minimize their use clinically but to recognize that the alternative, the disease that prompted the treatment in the first place, is most probably worse.

What about prenatal or postnatal stress? Does every little hiccup of stress leave an adverse scar forever after, unto multiple generations? Many times, some relationship in biology may apply to extreme situations—massive trauma, a whole winter's famine, and so on—but not to more everyday ones. Unfortunately, even the normal range of birth weights predicts adult glucocorticoid levels and the risk of Metabolic syndrome. So these appear not to be phenomena only of the extremes.

Next important question: How big are the effects? We've seen evidence that increasing amounts of fetal stress, over the normal range, predict increasing risk of Metabolic syndrome long afterward. That statement may be true and describes one of two very different scenarios. For example, it could be that the lowest levels of fetal stress result in a 1 percent risk of Metabolic syndrome, and each increase in stress exposure increases the risk until an exposure to a maximal fetal stress results in a 99 percent chance. Or the least fetal stress could result in a 1 percent risk, and each increase in stress exposure increases the risk until exposure to maximal fetal stress results in a 2 percent risk. In both cases, the endpoint is sensitive to small increments in the amount of stress, but the *power* of fetal stress to increase disease risk is vastly greater in the first scenario. As we will see in more detail in later chapters, early stress and trauma seem to have a tremendous power in increasing the risk of various psychiatric disorders many years later. Some critics of the FOAD literature seem to be of the opinion that it constitutes cool biology of the "Gee whiz, isn't nature amazing" variety, but is not a major source of worry. However, the risks of some of these adult diseases vary manyfold as a function of birth weight—so these strike me as big effects.

Next question: Regardless of how powerful these effects are, how *inevitable* are they? Lose it once in a crazed, sleepless moment at two in the morning and yell at your colicky infant and is that it, have you just guaranteed more clogging of her arteries in 2060? Not remotely. As discussed, stress dwarfism is reversible with a different environment. Studies have shown that the lifelong changes in glucocorticoid levels in prenatally stressed rats can be prevented with particular mothering styles postnatally. Much of preventative medicine is a demonstration that vast numbers of adverse health situations can be reversed—in fact, that is a premise of this book.

The Cornell anthropologist Merideth Small has written a wonderfully un-neurotic book, *Our Babies, Ourselves,* which looks at child-rearing practices across the planet. In a particular culture, how often is a child typically held by parents, by non-parents? Do babies sleep alone ever and, if so, starting at what age? What is the average length of time that a child cries in a particular culture before she is picked up and comforted?

In measure after measure, westernized societies and, in particular, the United States, come out at the extreme in these cross-cultural measures, with our emphasis on individuality, independence, and self-reliance. This is our world of both parents working outside the home, of single-parent households, of day care and latchkey kids. There is little evidence that any of these childhood experiences leave indelible biological scars, in contrast to the results of horrific childhood trauma. But whatever style of child-rearing is practiced, it will have its consequences. Small makes a profound point. You begin by reading her book assuming it is going to be an assortment box of prescriptions, that at the end, you'll emerge with a perfect combo for your kids, a mixture of the Kwakiutl Baby Diet, the Trobriand Sleeping Program, and the Ituri Pygmy Infant Aerobics Plan. But, Small emphasizes, there is no perfect, "natural" program. Societies raise their children so that they grow into adults who behave in a way valued by that society. As Harry Chapin sang in "Cat's in the Cradle," that ode to baby boomer remorse, "My boy was just like me."

 ## GROWTH AND GROWTH HORMONE IN ADULTS

Personally I don't grow much anymore, except wider. According to the textbooks, another half-dozen Groundhog Days or so and I'm going to start shrinking. Yet I, like other adults, still secrete growth hormone into my circulation (although much less frequently than when I was an adolescent). What good is it in an adult?

Like the Red Queen in *Alice in Wonderland,* the bodies of adults have to work harder and harder just to keep standing in the same place. Once the growth period of youth is finished and the edifice is complete, the hormones of growth mostly work at rebuilding and remodeling—shoring up the sagging foundation, plastering the cracks that appear here and there.

Much of this repair work takes place in bone. Most of us probably view our bones as pretty boring and phlegmatic—they just sit there, inert. In reality, they are dynamic outposts of activity. They are filled with blood vessels, with little fluid-filled canals, with all sorts of cell types that are actively growing and dividing. New bone is constantly being formed, in much the same way as in a teenager. Old bone is being broken down, disintegrated by ravenous enzymes (a process called resorption). New calcium is shuttled in from the bloodstream; old calcium is flushed away. Growth hormone, somatomedins, parathyroid hormone, and vitamin D stand around in hard hats, supervising the project.

Why all the tumult? Some of this bustle is because bones serve as the Federal Reserve for the body's calcium, constantly giving and collecting loans of calcium to and from other organs. And part is for the sake of bone itself, allowing it to gradually rebuild and change its shape in response to need. How else do cowboys' bow-legged legs get bowed from too much time on a horse? The process has to be kept well balanced. If the bones sequester too much of the body's calcium, much of the rest of the body shuts down; if the bones dump too much of their calcium into the bloodstream, they become fragile and prone to fracture, and that excess circulating calcium can start forming calcified kidney stones.

Predictably, the hormones of stress wreak havoc with the trafficking of calcium, biasing bone toward disintegration, rather than growth. The main culprits are glucocorticoids. They inhibit the growth of new bone by disrupting the division of the bone-precursor cells in the ends of bones. Furthermore, they reduce the calcium supply to bone. Glucocorticoids block the uptake of dietary calcium in the intestines (uptake normally stimulated by vitamin D), increase the excretion of calcium by the kidney, and accelerate the resorption of bone.

If you secrete excessive amounts of glucocorticoids, this increases the risk that your bones will eventually give you problems. This is seen in people with Cushing's syndrome (in which glucocorticoids are secreted at immensely high levels because of a tumor), and in people being treated with high doses of glucocorticoids to control some disease. In those cases, bone mass decreases markedly, and patients are at greater risk for osteoporosis (softening and weakening of bone).* Any situation that greatly elevates glucocorticoid concentrations in the bloodstream is a particular problem for older people, in whom bone

* JFK had a famously bad back, which his publicists always attributed to the injuries he sustained in the PT109 disaster in World War II. The recent opening of his sealed medical records indicate that it was probably due to severe osteoporosis, due to the massive levels of synthetic glucocorticoids he took for his Addison's disease and colitis.

resorption is already predominant (in contrast to adolescents, in whom bone growth predominates, or young adults, in which the two processes are balanced). This is especially a problem in older women. Tremendous attention is now being paid to the need for calcium supplements to prevent osteoporosis in postmenopausal women. Estrogen potently inhibits bone resorption, and as estrogen levels drop after menopause, the bones suddenly begin to degenerate.* A hefty regimen of glucocorticoids on top of that is the last thing you need.

These findings suggest that chronic stress can increase the risk of osteoporosis and cause skeletal atrophy. Most clinicians would probably say that the glucocorticoid effects on bone are "pharmacological" rather than "physiological." This means that normal (physiological) levels of glucocorticoids in the bloodstream, even those in response to normal stressful events, are not enough to damage bone. Instead, it takes pharmacological levels of the hormone (far higher than the body can normally generate), due to a tumor or to ingestion of prescription glucocorticoids, to cause these effects. However, work from Jay Kaplan's group has shown that chronic social stress leads to loss of bone mass in female monkeys.

 ## A FINAL WORD ABOUT THE L-WORD

In looking at research on how stress and understimulation can disrupt growth and increase the risks of all sorts of diseases, a theme pops up repeatedly: an infant human or animal can be well fed, maintained at an adequate temperature, peered at nervously, and ministered to by the best of neonatologists, yet still not thrive. Something is still missing. Perhaps we can even risk scientific credibility and detachment and mention the word *love* here, because that most ephemeral of phenomena lurks between the lines of this chapter. Something roughly akin to love is needed for proper biological development, and its absence is among the most aching, distorting stressors that we can suffer. Scientists and physicians and other caregivers have often been dim at recognizing its importance in the mundane biological processes by which organs and tissues grow and develop. For example, at the beginning of the twentieth century, the leading expert on child-rearing

---

* To reiterate a point from chapter 3, while right now it is wildly controversial whether estrogen protects from cardiovascular disease, it remains clear that it protects from osteoporosis.

was a Dr. Luther Holt of Columbia University, who warned parents of the adverse effects of the "vicious practice" of using a cradle, picking up the child when it cried, or handling it too often. All the experts believed that affection not only wasn't needed for development but was a squishy, messy thing that kept kids from becoming upright, independent citizens. Yet young organisms were able to teach about how these savants were wrong in a classic set of studies begun in the 1950s—studies that are, in my opinion, among the most haunting and troubling of all the pages of science.

The work was carried out by the psychologist Harry Harlow of the University of Wisconsin, a renowned and controversial scientist. Psychology at that time was dominated by either Freudians or a rather extreme school of thought called behaviorism, in which behavior (of an animal or a human) was thought to operate according to rather simple rules: an organism does something more frequently because it has been rewarded for it in the past; an organism does something less frequently because it has failed to be rewarded, or has even been punished for that behavior. In this view, just a few basic things like hunger, pain, or sex lie at the basis of reinforcement. Look at the behaviors, view organisms as machines responding to stimuli, and develop a predictive mathematics built around the idea of rewards and punishments.

Harlow helped to answer a seemingly obvious question in a non-obvious way. Why do infants become attached to their mothers? Because Mom supplies food. For behaviorists, this was obvious, as attachment was thought to arise solely from the positive reinforcement of food. For Freudians, it was also obvious—infants were thought to lack the "ego development" to form a relationship with any thing/one other than Mom's breast. For physicians influenced by the likes of Holt, it was obvious and convenient—no need for mothers to visit hospitalized infants—anyone with a bottle would supply attachment needs. No need to worry about preemies kept antiseptically isolated in incubators—regular feeding suffices for human contact. No need for children in orphanages to be touched, held, noted as individuals. What's love got to do with healthy development?

Harlow smelled a rat. He raised infant rhesus monkeys without mothers. Instead, he gave them a choice of two types of artificial "surrogate" mothers. One pseudo-mother had a monkey head constructed of wood and a wire-mesh tube resembling a torso. In the middle of the torso was a bottle of milk. This surrogate mother gave nutrition. The other surrogate mother had a similar head and wire-mesh torso. But instead of containing a milk bottle, this one's torso was wrapped in

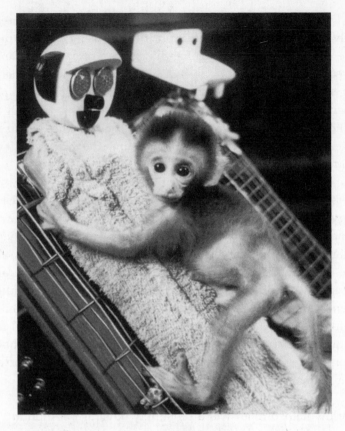

Infant monkey and cloth mother, in a Harlow study.

terry cloth. The behaviorists and the Freudians would be snuggling up to the milk-mom within seconds. But not the baby monkeys—they chose the terry-cloth mothers. Kids don't love their mothers because Mom balances their nutritive intake, these results suggested. They love them because, usually, Mom loves them back, or at least is someone soft to cling to. "Man cannot live by milk alone. Love is an emotion that does not need to be bottle- or spoon-fed," wrote Harlow.

Harlow and his work remain immensely controversial.* The controversy arises from the nature of his experiments and variations on them (for example, raising monkeys in complete social isolation, in which they never see another living animal). These were brutal studies, and they are often among the primary ones cited by those opposed to animal experimentation. Moreover, Harlow's scientific writing

---

* An excellent biography about Harlow, by the Pulitzer Prize–winning author Deborah Blum, is *Love at Goon Park: Harry Harlow and the Science of Affection* (Perseus 2002).

displayed an appalling callousness to the suffering of these animals—I remember as a student being moved to tears of rage by the savage indifference of his writing.

But at the same time, these studies have been extremely useful (although my feeling is that there should have been far fewer of them carried out). They have taught us the science of why we primates love individuals who treat us badly, why the mistreatment can at times increase the love. They have taught us about why being abused as a child increases the risk of your being an abusive adult. Other aspects of Harlow's work have taught us how repeated separations of infants from their mothers can predispose those individuals to depression when they are adults.

The irony is that it required Harlow's pioneering work to demonstrate the unethical nature of that work. But wasn't it obvious before? If you prick us, do we not bleed?; if you socially isolate us as infants, do we not suffer? Few in the know thought so. The main point of Harlow's work wasn't teaching what we might now wrongly assume to have been obvious then, namely that if you isolate an infant monkey, it is a massive stressor, and that she saddens and suffers for long after. It was to teach the utterly novel fact that if you do the same to a human infant, the same occurs.

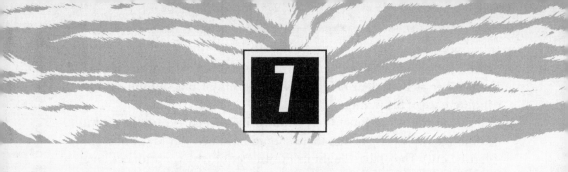

7

SEX AND REPRODUCTION

Kidneys and pancreas and heart are important, but what we really want to know is why, when we are being stressed, our menstrual cycles become irregular, erections are more difficult to achieve, and we lose our interest in sex. As it turns out, there are an astonishing number of ways in which reproductive mechanisms may go awry when we are upset.

MALES: TESTOSTERONE AND LOSS OF ERECTIONS

It makes sense to start simple, so let's initially consider the easier reproductive system, that of males. In the male, the brain releases the hormone LHRH (luteinizing hormone releasing hormone), which stimulates the pituitary to release LH (luteinizing hormone) and FSH (follicle-stimulating hormone).* LH, in turn, stimulates the testes to release testosterone. Since men don't have follicles to be stimulated by follicle-stimulating hormone, FSH instead stimulates sperm production. This is the reproductive system of your basic off-the-rack male.

With the onset of a stressor, the whole system is inhibited. LHRH concentrations decline, followed shortly thereafter by declines in LH and FSH, and then the testes close for lunch. The result is a decline in circulating testosterone levels. The most vivid demonstrations of this

---

* LHRH is also known as GnRH, or "gonadotropin releasing hormone."

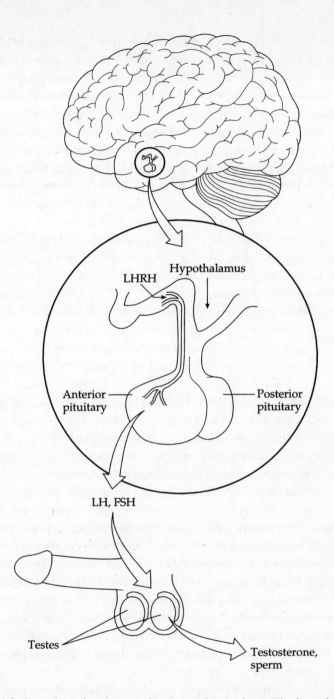

A simplified version of male reproductive endocrinology. The hypothalamus releases LHRH into the private circulatory system that it shares with the anterior pituitary. LHRH triggers the release by the pituitary of LH and FSH, which work at the testes to cause testosterone secretion and sperm production.

occur during physical stress. If a male goes through surgery, within seconds of the first slice of a scalpel through his skin, the reproductive axis begins to shut down. Injury, illness, starvation, surgery—all of these drive down testosterone levels. Anthropologists have even shown that in human societies in which there is constant energetic stress (for example, those of rural Nepalese villagers), there are significantly lower testosterone levels than among sedentary Bostonian controls.

But subtle psychological stressors are just as disruptive. Lower the dominance rank of a social primate and down go his testosterone levels. Put a person or a monkey through a stressful learning task and the same occurs. In a celebrated study several decades ago, U.S. Officer Candidate School trainees who underwent an enormous amount of physical and psychological stress were subjected to the further indignity of having to pee into Dixie cups so that military psychiatrists could measure their hormone levels. Lo and behold, testosterone levels were down; maybe not to the levels found in cherubic babies, but still it's worth keeping in mind the next time you see some leatherneck at a bar bragging about his circulating androgen concentrations.

Why do testosterone concentrations plunge with the onset of a stressor? For a variety of reasons. The first occurs at the brain. With the onset of stress, two important classes of hormones, the endorphins and enkephalins (mostly the former), act to block the release of LHRH from the hypothalamus. As will be discussed in chapter 9, endorphins play a role in blocking pain perception and are secreted in response to exercise (helping to account for the famed "runner's high" or "endorphin high" that hits many hardy joggers around the 30-minute mark). If males secrete endorphins when they are experiencing runner's high, and these compounds inhibit testosterone release, will exercise suppress male reproduction? Sometimes. Males who do extreme amounts of exercise, such as professional soccer players and runners who cover more than 40 or 50 miles a week, have less LHRH, LH, and testosterone in their circulation, smaller testes, less functional sperm. They also have higher levels of glucocorticoids in their bloodstreams, even in the absence of stress. (A similar decline in reproductive function is found in men who are addicted to opiate drugs.) To jump ahead to the female section, reproductive dysfunction is also seen in women athletes, and this is at least partially due to endorphin release as well. Up to half of competitive runners have menstrual irregularities, and highly athletic girls reach puberty later than usual. For example, in one study of fourteen-year-olds, approximately 95 percent of control subjects had started menstruating, whereas only 20 percent of gymnasts and 40 percent of runners had.

This brings up a broader issue important to our era of lookin' good. Obviously, if you don't exercise at all, it is not good for you. Exercise improves your health. And a lot of exercise improves your health a lot. But that doesn't mean that insanely large amounts of exercise are insanely good for your body. At some point, too much begins to damage various physiological systems. Everything in physiology follows the rule that too much can be as bad as too little. There are optimal points of allostatic balance. For example, while a moderate amount of exercise generally increases bone mass, thirty-year-old athletes who run 40 to 50 miles a week can wind up with decalcified bones, decreased bone mass, increased risk of stress fractures and scoliosis (sideways curvature of the spine)—their skeletons look like those of seventy-year-olds.

To put exercise in perspective, imagine this: sit with a group of hunter-gatherers from the African grasslands and explain to them that in our world we have so much food and so much free time that some of us run 26 miles in a day, simply for the sheer pleasure of it. They are likely to say, "Are you crazy? That's stressful." Throughout hominid history, if you're running 26 miles in a day, you're either very intent on eating someone or someone's very intent on eating you.

Thus, we have a first step. With the onset of stress, LHRH secretion declines. In addition, prolactin, another pituitary hormone that is released during major stressors, decreases the sensitivity of the pituitary to LHRH. A double whammy—less of the hormone dribbling out of the brain, and the pituitary no longer responding as effectively to it. Finally, glucocorticoids block the response of the testes to LH, just in case any of that hormone manages to reach them during the stressor (and serious athletes tend to have pretty dramatic elevations of glucocorticoids in their circulation, no doubt adding to the reproductive problems just discussed).

A decline in testosterone secretion is only half the story of what goes wrong with male reproduction during stress. The other half concerns the nervous system and erections. Getting an erection to work properly is so incredibly complicated physiologically that if men ever actually had to understand it, none of us would be here. Fortunately, it runs automatically. In order for a male primate to have an erection, he has to divert a considerable amount of blood flow to his penis, engorging it.*

---

* Weirdly, Da Vinci was the first to demonstrate (how!?) that erections arise from increased blood flow to the penis. He also wrote that, "The penis does not obey the order of its master. . . . [It] must be said to have a mind of its own." When combining his statement and scientific observation, it's only a few short steps to the famed wisecrack and near truism that a man can't have blood flow to his penis and brain simultaneously.

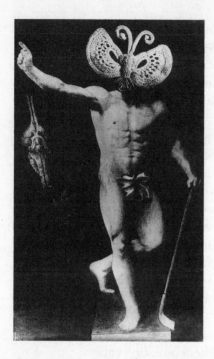 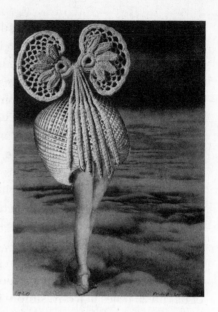

Overexercise can have a variety of deleterious effects. (Left) Max Ernst, Health Through Sport, *photographic enlargement of a photomontage mounted on wood, 1920; (right)* Above the Clouds Midnight Passes, *collage with fragments of photographs and pencil, 1920.*

This is accomplished by activating his parasympathetic nervous system. In other words, the guy has to be calm, vegetative, relaxed.

What happens next, if you are male? You are having a terrific time with someone. Maybe you are breathing faster, your heart rate has increased. Gradually, parts of your body are taking on a sympathetic tone—remember the four F's of sympathetic function introduced in chapter 2. After awhile, most of your body is screaming sympathetic while, heroically, you are trying to hold on to parasympathetic tone in that one lone outpost as long as possible. Finally, when you can't take it anymore, the parasympathetic shuts off at the penis, the sympathetic comes roaring on, and you ejaculate. (Incredibly complicated choreography between these two systems; don't try this unsupervised.) This new understanding generates tricks that sexual therapists advise—if you are close to ejaculating and don't want to yet, take a deep breath. Expanding the chest muscles briefly triggers a parasympathetic volley that defers the shift from parasympathetic to sympathetic.

What, then, changes during stress? One is that sufficient prior stress will damage and clog up your blood vessels—severe vascular disease can seriously impede blood flow. But what if you're stressed in that immediate situation? Well, obviously, if you're nervous or anxious, you're not calm or vegetative. First, it becomes difficult to establish parasympathetic activity if you are nervous or anxious. You have trouble having an erection. Impotency. And if you already have the erection, you get in trouble as well. You're rolling along, parasympathetic to your penis, having a wonderful time. Suddenly, you find yourself worrying about the strength of the dollar versus the euro and—shazaam—you switch from parasympathetic to sympathetic far faster than you wanted. Premature ejaculation.

It is extremely common for problems with impotency and premature ejaculation to arise during stressful times. Furthermore, this can be compounded by the fact that erectile dysfunction is a major stressor on its own, getting men into this vicious performance anxiety cycle of fearing fear itself. A number of studies have shown that more than half the visits to doctors by males complaining of reproductive dysfunction turn out to be due to "psychogenic" impotency rather than organic impotency (there's no disease there, just too much stress). How do you tell if it is organic or psychogenic impotency? This is actually diagnosed with surprising ease, because of a quirky thing about human males. As soon as they go to sleep and enter REM (rapid eye movement) dream sleep, they get erections. I've consulted with Earth's penis experts, and no one is sure why this should occur, but that's how it works.* So a man comes in complaining that he hasn't been able to have an erection in six months. Is he just under stress? Does he have some neurological disease? Take a handy little penile cuff with an electronic pressure transducer attached to it. Have him put it on just before he goes to sleep. By the next morning you may have your answer—if this guy gets an erection when he goes into REM sleep, his problem is likely to be psychogenic.†

---

* There's some great speculations, however: "To trigger sexual themes during dreams" (raising the question, of course, of what good is that). "So the body can practice at having erections, in preparation for the real thing." "Because."

† I've been told about an advance on this technology. Instead of having to use one of these fancy electronic cuffs that seems likely to electrocute you during the night, and thus constitutes a stressor on its own, here's what you do. Take a string of (I don't specify how many) postage stamps. Wrap it around the guy's penis, moisten the last one, tape it to the others, forming a postage stamp ring. The next morning, check: if the stamps have been pulled loose on one side or torn, the guy had a REM-stage erection during the night—fabulous, a lab result for a couple of bucks. The insurance people will hassle you about reimbursement for it, though.

Thus, stress will knock out erections quite readily. In general, the problems with erections are more disruptive than problems with testosterone secretion. Testosterone and sperm production have to shut down almost entirely to affect performance. A little testosterone and a couple of sperm wandering around and most males can muddle through. But no erection, and forget about it.*

The erectile component is exquisitely sensitive to stress in an incredible array of species. Nonetheless, there are some circumstances where stress does not suppress the reproductive system in a male. Suppose you're some big bull moose and it's mating season. You're spending all your time strutting your stuff and growing your antlers and snorting and having head-butting territorial disputes with the next guy and forgetting to eat right and not getting enough sleep and getting injured and worrying about the competition for some female moose's favors.† Stressful. Wouldn't it be pretty maladaptive if the male-male competitive behaviors needed to get the opportunity to mate were so stressful that when the opportunity came, you were sex-ually dysfunctional? Not a good Darwinian move.

Or suppose that in your species, sex is this wildly metabolically demanding activity, involving hours, even days of copulation at the cost of resting or feeding (lions fall in this category, for example). High energetic demands plus little eating or sleeping equals stress. It would be disadvantageous if the stress of mating caused erectile dysfunction.

It turns out that in a lot of species, stressors associated with mating season competition or with mating itself not only don't suppress the reproductive system, but can stimulate it a bit. In some species where this applies, the seeming stressor doesn't cause secretion of stress hor-mones; in other cases, the stress hormones are secreted but the repro-ductive system becomes insensitive to them.

And then there is one species which, regardless of whether it is mating season or not, breaks all the rules concerning the effects of stress on erectile function. It is time we had a little talk about hyenas.

---

* It is important to note that an inability to have an erection is not synonymous with an absence of desire. This is illustrated by a story I once read about Marx in his old age— Groucho in this case. A visitor to his home was admiring his various awards and com-memoratives of his career. Marx waved them away saying, I'd trade them all for one good erection. Stress can most certainly squelch desire, independent of disrupting erec-tions, through mechanisms that are poorly understood.

† Actually, I have no idea if moose grow antlers during mating season, or even if those things that Bullwinkle had on top of his head are technically *called* antlers or horns or what have you's, but you get the point—all this macho male display stuff.

OUR FRIEND, THE HYENA

The spotted hyena is a vastly unappreciated, misrepresented beast. I know this because over the years, in my work in East Africa, I have shared my campsite with the hyena biologist Laurence Frank of the University of California at Berkeley. For lack of distracting television, radio, or telephone, he has devoted his time with me to singing the hyena's praises. They are wondrous animals who have gotten a bad rap from the press.

We all know the scenario. It's dawn on the savanna. Marlin Perkins of Mutual of Omaha's *Wild Kingdom* is there filming lions eating something dead. We are delighted, craning to get a good view of the blood and guts. Suddenly, on the edge of our field of vision, we spot them—skulky, filthy, untrustworthy hyenas looking to dart in and steal some of the food. Scavengers! We are invited to heap our contempt on them (a surprising bias, given how few of the carnivorous among us ever wrestle down our meals with our canines). It wasn't until the Pentagon purchased a new line of infrared night-viewing scopes and decided to unload its old ones on various zoologists that, suddenly, researchers could watch hyenas at night (important, given that hyenas mostly sleep during the day). Turns out that they are fabulous hunters. And you know what happens? Lions, who are not particularly effective hunters, because they are big and slow and conspicuous, spend most of their time keying in on hyenas and ripping off their kills. No wonder when it's dawn on the savanna the hyenas on the periphery are looking cranky, with circles under their eyes. They stayed up all night hunting that thing, and who's having breakfast now?

Having established a thread of sympathy for these beasts, let me explain what is really strange about them. Among hyenas, females are socially dominant, which is fairly rare among mammals. They are more muscular and more aggressive, and have more of a male sex hormone (a close relative of testosterone called *androstenedione*) in their bloodstreams than males. It's also almost impossible to tell the sex of a hyena by looking at its external genitals.

More than two thousand years ago, Aristotle, for reasons obscure to even the most learned, dissected some dead hyenas, discussing them in his treatise *Historia Animalium*, VI, XXX. The conclusion among hyena savants at the time was that these animals were hermaphrodites—animals that possess all the machinery of both sexes. Hyenas are actually what gynecologists would call pseudohermaphrodites (they just look that way). The female has a fake scrotal sac made of

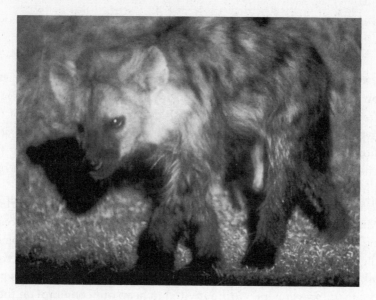

Behold, the female hyena.

compacted fat cells; she doesn't really have a penis but, instead, an enlarged clitoris that can become erect. The same clitoris, I might add, with which she has sex and through which she gives birth. It's pretty wild. Laurence Frank, who is one of Earth's experts on hyena genitals, will dart some animal and haul it, anesthetized, into camp. Excitement; we go to check it out, and maybe twenty minutes into examining it, he kind of thinks he knows what sex this particular one is. (Yes, the hyenas themselves know exactly who is which sex, most probably by smell.)

Perhaps the most interesting thing about hyenas is that there is a fairly plausible theory as to why they evolved this way, a theory complicated enough for me mercifully to relegate it to the endnotes. For our purposes here, what is important is that hyenas have evolved not only genitals that look unique, but also unique ways to use these organs for social communication. This is where stress comes into play.

Among many social mammals, males have erections during competitive situations as a sign of dominance. If you are having a dominance display with another male, you get an erection and wave it around in his face to show what a tough guy you are. Social primates do this all the time. However, among hyenas, an erection is a sign of social *subordinance*. When a male is menaced by a terrifying female, he gets an erection—"Look, I'm just some poor no-account male; don't hit me, I was just leaving." Low-ranking females do the same thing; if a low-ranking female is about to get trounced by a high-ranking one, she gets a conspicuous clitoral erection—"Look, I'm just like one of those males; don't attack me; you know you're dominant over me, why bother?" If you're a hyena, you get an erection *when you are stressed*. Among male hyenas, the autonomic wiring has got to be completely reversed in order to account for the fact that stress causes erections. This hasn't yet been demonstrated, but perhaps Berkeley scientists working on this, squandering tax dollars that could otherwise be going to Halliburton and Bechtel, will do it.

Thus the hyena stands as the exception to the rule about erectile functions being adversely affected by stress, a broader demonstration of the importance of looking at a zoological oddity as a means of better seeing the context of our own normative physiology, and a friendly word of warning before you date a hyena.

 ## FEMALES: LENGTHENED CYCLES AND AMENORRHEA

We now turn to female reproduction. Its basic outline is similar to that of the male. LHRH is released by the brain, which releases LH and FSH from the pituitary. The latter stimulates the ovaries to release eggs; the former stimulates ovaries to synthesize estrogen. During the first half of the menstrual cycle, the "follicular" stage, levels of LHRH, LH, FSH, and estrogen build up, heading toward the climax of ovulation. This ushers in the second half of the cycle, the "luteal" phase. Progesterone, made in the corpus luteum of the ovary, now becomes the dominant hormone on the scene, stimulating the uterine walls to mature so that an egg, if fertilized just after ovulation, can implant there and develop into an embryo. Because the release of hormones has the fancy quality of fluctuating rhythmically over the menstrual cycle, the part of the hypothalamus that regulates the release of these hormones is generally more structurally complicated in females than in males.

The first way in which stress disrupts female reproduction concerns a surprising facet of the system. There is a small amount of male sex hormone in the bloodstream of females, even non-hyena females. In human beings, this doesn't come from the ovaries (as in the hyenas), but from the adrenals. The amount of these "adrenal androgens" is only about 5 percent of that in males, but enough to cause trouble.* An

---

* Point of information: the adrenal androgens are usually not testosterone, but androstenedione.

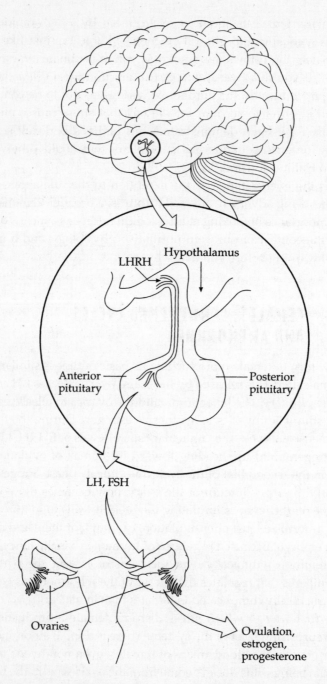

A simplified version of female reproductive endocrinology. The hypothalamus releases LHRH into the private circulatory system that it shares with the anterior pituitary. LHRH triggers the release by the pituitary of LH and FSH, which in turn bring about ovulation and hormone release from the ovaries.

enzyme in the fat cells of females usually eliminates these androgens by converting them to estrogens. Problem solved. But what if you are starving because the crops failed this year? Body weight drops, fat stores are depleted, and suddenly there isn't enough fat around to convert all the androgen to estrogen. Less estrogen, therefore, is produced. More important, androgen concentrations build up, which inhibits numerous steps in the reproductive system (it should be noted that this is but one of the mechanisms by which starvation inhibits reproduction).

Reproduction is similarly inhibited if you starve voluntarily. One of the hallmarks of anorexia nervosa is disruption of reproduction in the (typically) young women who are starving themselves. There's more to the reproduction cessation than just the weight loss, since cycling doesn't necessarily resume in women when they regain the weight unless the initial psychological stressors have been sorted out. But the weight loss still plays a critical, initiating role. And loss of body fat leading to androgen buildup is one of the mechanisms by which reproduction is impaired in females who are extremely active physically. As noted above, this has been best documented in young girls who are serious dancers or runners, in whom puberty can be delayed for years, and in women who exercise enormous amounts, in whom cycles can become irregular or cease entirely. Overall, this is a logical mechanism. In the human, an average pregnancy costs approximately 50,000 calories, and nursing costs about a thousand calories a day; neither is something that should be gone into without a reasonable amount of fat tucked away.

Stress also can inhibit reproduction in ways other than shrinkage of fat cells. Many of the same mechanisms apply as in the male. Endorphins and enkephalins will inhibit LHRH release (as discussed, this occurs in female athletes as readily as in males); prolactin and glucocorticoids will block pituitary sensitivity to LHRH; and glucocorticoids will also affect the ovaries, making them less responsive to LH. The net result is lowered secretion of LH, FSH, and estrogen, making the likelihood of ovulating decrease. As a result, the follicular stage is extended, making the entire cycle longer and less regular. At an extreme, the entire ovulatory machinery is not merely delayed, but shut down, a condition termed *anovulatory amenorrhea.*

Stress can also cause other reproductive problems. Progesterone levels are often inhibited, which disrupts maturation of the uterine walls. The release of prolactin during stress adds to this effect, interfering with the activity of progesterone. Thus, even if there is still enough hormonal action during the follicular period to cause ovulation, and the egg has become fertilized, it is now much less likely to implant normally.

The loss of estrogen with sustained stress has some consequences beyond the reproductive realm. For example, amid the controversies discussed in chapter 3 about whether estrogen protects against cardio-vascular disease, it is quite clear that it protects against osteoporosis, and stress-induced declines in estrogen levels have bad effects on bone strength.

Of all the hormones that inhibit the reproductive system during stress, prolactin is probably the most interesting. It is extremely power-ful and versatile; if you don't want to ovulate, this is the hormone to have lots of in your bloodstream. It not only plays a major role in the suppression of reproduction during stress and exercise, but it also is the main reason that breast feeding is such an effective form of contraception.

Oh, you are shaking your head smugly at the ignorance of this author with that Y chromosome; that's an old wives' tale; nursing isn't an effective contraceptive. On the contrary, nursing works fabulously. It probably prevents more pregnancies than any other type of contra-ception. All you have to do is do it right.

Breast feeding causes prolactin secretion. There is a reflex loop that goes straight from the nipples to the hypothalamus. If there is nipple stimulation for any reason (in males as well as females), the hypothala-mus signals the pituitary to secrete prolactin. And as we now know, prolactin in sufficient quantities causes reproduction to cease.

The problem with nursing as a contraceptive is how it is done in Western societies. During the six months or so that she breast-feeds, the average mother in the West allows perhaps half a dozen periods of nursing a day, each for 30 to 60 minutes. Each time she nurses, pro-lactin levels go up in the bloodstream within seconds, and at the end of the feeding, prolactin settles back to pre-nursing levels fairly quickly. This most likely produces a scalloping sort of pattern in prolactin release.

This is not how most women on earth nurse. A prime example emerged a few years ago in a study of hunter-gatherer Bushmen in the Kalahari Desert of southern Africa (the folks depicted in the movie *The Gods Must Be Crazy*). Bushman males and females have plenty of inter-course, and no one uses contraceptives, but the women have a child only about every four years. Initially, this seemed easy to explain. Western scientists looked at this pattern and said, "They're hunter-gatherers: life for them must be short, nasty, and brutish; they must all be starving." Malnutrition induces cessation of ovulation.

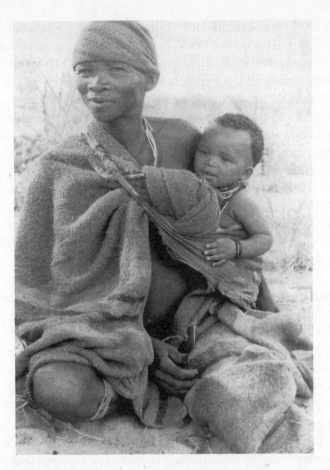

A Kalahari Bushman mother with her child in a hip sling.

However, when anthropologists looked more closely, they found that the Bushmen were anything but suffering. If you are going to be nonwesternized, choose to be a hunter-gatherer over being a nomadic pastoralist or an agriculturist. The Bushmen hunt and gather only a few hours a day, and spend much of the rest of their time sitting around chewing the fat. Scientists have called them the original affluent society. Out goes the idea that the four-year birth interval is due to malnutrition.

Instead, the lengthy interval is probably due to their nursing pattern. This was discovered by a pair of scientists, Melvin Konner and Carol Worthman.* When a hunter-gatherer woman gives birth, she

---

* The work and thinking of Konner, who was once my advisor at college, runs throughout this book, as he is the person who has had the greatest intellectual influence on my life.

begins to breast-feed her child for a minute or two approximately every fifteen minutes. Around the clock. For the next three years. (Suddenly this doesn't seem like such a hot idea after all, does it?) The young child is carried in a sling on the mother's hip so he can nurse easily and frequently. At night, he sleeps near his mother and will nurse every so often without even waking her (as Konner and Worthman, no doubt with their infrared night-viewing goggles and stopwatches, scribble away on their clipboards at two in the morning). Once the kid can walk, he'll come running in from play every hour or so to nurse for a minute.

When you breast-feed in this way, the endocrine story is very different. At the first nursing period, prolactin levels rise. And with the frequency and timing of the thousands of subsequent nursings, prolactin stays high for years. Estrogen and progesterone levels are suppressed, and you don't ovulate.

This pattern has a fascinating implication. Consider the life history of a hunter-gatherer woman. She reaches puberty at about age thirteen or fourteen (a bit later than in our society). Soon she is pregnant. She nurses for three years, weans her child, has a few menstrual cycles, becomes pregnant again, and repeats the pattern until she reaches menopause. Think about it: over the course of her life span, she has perhaps two dozen periods. Contrast that with modern Western women, who typically experience hundreds of periods over their lifetime. Huge difference. The hunter-gatherer pattern, the one that has occurred throughout most of human history, is what you see in nonhuman primates. Perhaps some of the gynecological diseases that plague modern westernized women have something to do with this activation of a major piece of physiological machinery hundreds of times when it may have evolved to be used only twenty times; an example of this is probably endometriosis (having uterine lining thickening and sloughing off in places in the pelvis and abdominal wall where it doesn't belong), which is more common among women with fewer pregnancies and who start at a later age.*

 ## FEMALES: DISRUPTION OF LIBIDO

The preceding section describes how stress disrupts the nuts and bolts of female reproduction—uterine walls, eggs, ovarian hormones, and so on. But what about its effects upon sexual behavior? Just

---

* Remarkably, the same is now being reported in zoo animals who, because of the circumstances of their captivity, reproduce far less often than those in the wild.

as stress does not do wonders for erections or for the desire of a male to do something with his erections, stress also disrupts female libido. This is a commonplace experience among women stressed by any number of circumstances, as well as among laboratory animals undergoing stress.

It is relatively easy to document a loss of sexual desire among women when they are stressed—just hand out a questionnaire on the subject and hope it is answered honestly. But how is sexual drive studied in a laboratory animal? How can one possibly infer a libidinous itch on the part of a female rat, for example, as she gazes into the next cage at the male with the limpid eyes and cute incisors? The answer is surprisingly simple—how often would she be willing to press a lever in order to gain access to that male? This is science's quantitative way of measuring rodent desire (or, to use the jargon of the trade, "proceptivity").* A similar experimental design can be used to measure proceptive behavior in primates. Proceptive and receptive behaviors fluctuate among female animals as a function of factors like the point in the reproductive cycle (both of these measures of sexual behavior generally peak around ovulation), the recency of sex, the time of year, or vagaries of the heart (who is the male in question). In general, stress suppresses both proceptive and receptive behaviors.

This effect of stress is probably rooted in its suppression of the secretion of various sex hormones. Among rodents, both proceptive and receptive behaviors disappear when a female's ovaries are removed, and the absence of estrogen after the ovariectomy is responsible; as evidence, injection of ovariectomized females with estrogen reinstates these sexual behaviors. Moreover, the peak in estrogen levels around ovulation explains why sexual behavior is almost entirely restricted to that period. A similar pattern holds in primates, but it is not as dramatic as in rodents. A decline in sexual behavior, although to a lesser extent, follows ovariectomy in a primate. For humans, estrogen plays a role in sexuality, but a still weaker one—social and interpersonal factors are far more important.

---

* Quick primer on how to describe animal sex the way professionals do: *attractivity* refers to how much the subject animal interests another animal. This can be operationally defined as how many times the other animal is willing to press a lever, for example, to gain access to the subject. *Receptivity* describes how readily the subject responds to the entreaties of the other animal. Among rats, this can be defined by the occurrence of the "lordosis" reflex, a receptive stance by the female in which she arches her back, making it easier for the male to mount. Female primates show a variety of receptive reflexes that facilitate male mounting, depending on the species. *Proceptivity* refers to how actively the subject pursues the other animal.

Estrogen exerts these effects both in the brain and peripheral tissue. Genitals and other parts of the body contain ample amounts of estrogen receptors and are made more sensitive to tactile stimulation by the hormone. Within the brain, estrogen receptors occur in areas that play a role in sexual behavior; through one of the more poorly understood mechanisms of neuroendocrinology, when estrogen floods those parts of the brain, salacious thoughts follow.

Surprisingly, adrenal androgens also play a role in proceptive and receptive behaviors; as evidence, sex drive goes down following removal of the adrenals and can be reinstated by administration of synthetic androgens. This appears to be more of a factor in primates and humans than in rodents. While the subject has not been studied in great detail, there are some reports that stress suppresses the levels of adrenal androgens in the bloodstream. And stress certainly suppresses estrogen secretion. As noted in chapter 3, Jay Kaplan has shown that the stressor of social subordinance in a monkey can suppress estrogen levels as effectively as removing her ovaries. Given these findings, it is relatively easy to see how stress disrupts sexual behavior in a female.

 ## STRESS AND THE SUCCESS OF HIGH-TECH FERTILIZATION

In terms of psychological distress, few medical maladies match infertility—the strain placed on a relationship with a significant other, the disruption of daily activities and ability to concentrate at work, the estrangement from friends and family, and the rates of depression.* Thus, circumventing infertility with recent high-tech advances has been a wonderful medical advance.

There is now a brave new world of assisted fertilization: *artificial insemination; in vitro fertilization* (IVF), in which sperm and egg meet in a petri dish, and fertilized eggs are then implanted in the woman; *preimplantation screening,* carried out when one of the couple has a serious genetic disorder; after eggs are fertilized, their DNA is analyzed, and only those eggs that do not carry the genetic disorder are

---

* Two of the most common subjects discussed in infertility support groups: (1) how to handle the damage done to friendships and family relations when you can no longer attend baby showers, can no longer join the family at holidays because of all those nieces and nephews just learning to walk, can no longer see the old friend who is pregnant; and (2) what happens to a relationship with one's significant other when sex has been turned into a medical procedure, especially an unsuccessful one.

implanted. Donor eggs, donor sperm. Injection of an individual sperm into an egg, when the problem is an inability of the sperm to penetrate the egg's membrane on its own.

Some forms of infertility are solved with some relatively simple procedures, but others involve extraordinary, innovative technology. There are two problems with that technology, however. The first is that it is an astonishingly stressful experience for the individuals who go through it. Furthermore, it's expensive as hell, and is often not paid for by insurance, especially when some of the fancier new experimental techniques are being tried. How many young couples can afford to spend ten to fifteen thousand dollars out of pocket each cycle they attempt to get pregnant? Next, most IVF clinics are located only near major medical centers, meaning that many participants have to spend weeks in a motel room in some strange city, far from friends and family. For some genetic screening techniques, only a handful of places in the world are available, thus adding a long waiting list to the other stress factors.

But those stress-induced factors pale compared with the stress generated by the actual process. Weeks of numerous, painful daily shots with synthetic hormones and hormone suppressors that can do some pretty dramatic things to mood and mental state. Daily blood draws, daily sonograms, the constant emotional roller-coaster of whether the day's news is good or bad: how many follicles, how big are they, what circulating hormone levels have been achieved? A surgical procedure and then the final wait to see whether you have to try the whole thing again.

The second problem is that it rarely works. It is very hard to figure out how often natural attempts at fertilization actually succeed in humans. And it is hard to find out what the success rates are for the high-tech procedures, as clinics often fudge the numbers in their brochures—"We don't like to publish our success rates, because we take on only the most difficult, challenging cases, and thus our numbers must superficially seem worse than those of other clinics that are wimps and take only the easy ones"—and thus, they say, it is hard to gauge just how bad the odds are for a couple with an infertility problem going this route. Nevertheless, going through one of those grueling IVF cycles has a pretty low chance of succeeding.

All that has preceded in this chapter would suggest that the first problem, the stressfulness of IVF procedures, contributes to the second problem, the low success rate. A number of researchers have specifically examined whether women who are more stressed during IVF cycles are the ones less likely to have successful outcomes. And the answer is a resounding maybe. The majority of studies do show that the more stressed women (as determined by glucocorticoid levels, cardiovascular reactivity to an experimental stressor, or self-report on a questionnaire) are indeed less likely to have successful IVFs. Why, then, the ambiguity? For one thing, some of the studies were carried out many days or weeks into the long process, where women have already gotten plenty of feedback as to whether things are going well; in those cases, an emerging unsuccessful outcome might cause the elevated stress-response, rather than the other way around. Even in studies in which stress measures are taken at the beginning of the process, the number of previous cycles must be controlled for. In other words, a stressed woman may indeed be less likely to have a successful outcome, but both traits may be due to the fact that she is an especially poor candidate who has already gone through eight unsuccessful prior attempts and is a wreck.

In other words, more research is needed. If the correlation does turn out to be for real, one hopes that the outcome of that will be something more constructive than clinicians saying, "And try not to be stressed, because studies have shown it cuts down the chances IVF will succeed." It would be kind of nice if progress in this area actually resulted in eliminating the stressor that initiated all these complexities in the first place, namely, the infertility.

 ## MISCARRIAGE, PSYCHOGENIC ABORTIONS, AND PRETERM LABOR

The link between stress and spontaneous abortion in humans prompted Hippocrates to caution pregnant women to avoid unnecessary emotional disturbances.* Since then, it is a thread that runs through some of our most florid and romantic interpretations of the biology of pregnancy. There's Anne Boleyn attributing her miscarriage to the shock of seeing Jane Seymour sitting on King Henry's lap, or Rosamond Vincy losing her baby when frightened by a horse in *Middlemarch*. In the 1990 movie *Pacific Heights* (which took the Reagan-Bush era to its logical extreme, encouraging us to root for the poor landlords being menaced by a predatory tenant), the homeowner,

---

* *Miscarriage* and *abortion* are used interchangeably in medical texts and will be so used throughout this section. In everyday clinical usage, however, spontaneous termination of a pregnancy when the fetus is close to being viable is more likely to be termed miscarriage than abortion.

played by Melanie Griffith, has a miscarriage in response to psychological harassment by the Machiavellian renter. And in the less literary and more mundane realm of everyday life, the stress of a high-demand/low-control job increases the risk of miscarriage among women.

Stress can cause miscarriages in other animals as well. This may occur, for example, when pregnant animals in the wild or in a corral have to be captured for some reason (a veterinary exam) or are stressed by being transported.

Studies of social hierarchies among animals in the wild have revealed one instance in which stress-induced miscarriages often occur. In many social species, not all males do equivalent amounts of reproducing. Sometimes the group contains only a single male (typically called a "harem male") who does all the mating; sometimes there are a number of males, but only one or a few dominant males reproduce.* Suppose the harem male is killed or driven out by an intruding male, or a new male migrates into the multi-male group and moves to the top of the dominance hierarchy. Typically, the now-dominant male goes about trying to increase his own reproductive success, at the expense of the prior male. What does the new guy do? In some species, males will systematically try to kill the infants in the group (a pattern called competitive infanticide and observed in a number of species, including lions and some monkeys), thus reducing the reproductive success of the preceding male. Following the killing, moreover, the female ceases to nurse and, as a result, is soon ovulating and ready for mating, to the convenient advantage of the newly resident male. Grim stuff, and a pretty strong demonstration of something well recognized by most evolutionists these days; contrary to what Marlin Perkins taught us, animals rarely behave "for the good of the species." Instead, they typically act for the good of their own genetic legacy and that of their close relatives. Among some species—wild horses and baboons, for example—the male will also systematically harass any pregnant females to the point of miscarriage, by the same logic.

This pattern is seen in a particularly subtle way among rodents. A group of females resides with a single harem male. If he is driven out by an intruder male who takes up residence, within days, females who have recently become pregnant fail to implant the fertilized egg. Remarkably, this termination of pregnancy does not require physical harassment on the part of the male. It is his new, strange odor that

---

* Although there is one august (female) primatologist who refers to single males, equally aptly, as "gigolo males."

causes the failed pregnancies by triggering a disruptive rise in pro-lactin levels. As proof of this, researchers can trigger this phenomenon (called the Bruce-Parkes effect) with merely the odor of a novel male. Why is it adaptive for females to terminate pregnancy just because a new male has arrived on the scene? If the female completes her pregnancy, the kids will promptly be killed by this new guy. So, mak-ing the best of a bad situation, evolution has sculpted this response to at least save the further calories that would be devoted to the futile pregnancy—terminate it and ovulate a few days later.*

Despite the drama of the Bruce-Parkes effect, stress-induced miscarriages are relatively rare among animals, particularly among humans. It is not uncommon to decide retrospectively that when something bad happens (such as a miscarriage), there was significant stress beforehand. To add to the confusion, there is a tendency to attribute miscarriages to stressful events occurring a day or so preced-ing them. In actuality, most miscarriages involve the expelling of a dead fetus, which has typically died quite a while before. If there was a stressful cause, it is likely to have come days or even weeks before the miscarriage, not immediately preceding it.

When a stress-induced miscarriage does occur, however, there is a fairly plausible explanation of how it happens. The delivery of blood to the fetus is exquisitely sensitive to blood flow in the mother, and anything that decreases uterine blood flow will be disruptive to the fetal blood supply. Moreover, fetal heart rate closely tracks that of the mother, and various psychological stimuli that stimulate or slow down the heart rate of the mother will cause a similar change a minute or so later in the fetus. This has been shown in a number of studies of both humans and primates.

Trouble seems to occur during stress as a result of repeated power-ful activation of the sympathetic nervous system, causing increased secretion of norepinephrine and epinephrine. Studies of a large num-ber of different species show that these two hormones will decrease blood flow through the uterus—dramatically, in some cases. Exposing animals to something psychologically stressful (for example, a loud noise in the case of pregnant sheep, or the entrance of a strange person into the room in which a pregnant rhesus monkey is housed) will

---

* Not to be outdone, females have evolved many strategies of their own to salvage reproductive success from these battling males. One is to go into a fake heat (in pri-mates, called pseudo-estrus) to sucker the new guy into thinking he's the father of the offspring she is already carrying. Given the appalling lack of knowledge about obstet-rics among most male rodents and primates, it usually works. Touché.

cause a similar reduction in blood flow, decreasing the delivery of oxygen (called *hypoxia*) to the fetus. This is certainly not a good thing, and this sort of prenatal stress returns us to all the issues of growth in chapter 6. The general assumption in the field is that it takes a number of these hypoxic episodes to cause asphyxiation.

Thus, severe stress can increase the likelihood of miscarriage. Furthermore, if one is at a late stage in pregnancy, stress can increase the risk of preterm birth, an effect that is probably due to elevated glucocorticoids. Certainly not a good thing, given what we saw in the last chapter about the metabolic imprinting consequences of low birth weight.

 ## HOW DETRIMENTAL TO FEMALE REPRODUCTION IS STRESS?

As we have seen, there is an extraordinary array of mechanisms by which reproduction can be disrupted in stressed females—fat depletion; secretion of endorphins, prolactin, and glucocorticoids acting on the brain, pituitary, and ovaries; lack of progesterone; excessive prolactin acting on the uterus. Moreover, possible blockage of implantation of the fertilized egg and changes in blood flow to the fetus generate numerous ways in which stress can make it less likely that a pregnancy will be carried to term. With all these different mechanisms implicated, it seems as if even the mildest of stressors would shut down the reproductive system completely. Surprisingly, however, this is not the case; collectively, these mechanisms are not all that effective.

One way of appreciating this is to examine the effects of chronic low-grade stress on reproduction. Consider traditional nonwesternized agriculturists with a fair amount of background disease (say seasonal malaria), a high incidence of parasites, and some seasonal malnutrition thrown in—farmers in Kenya, for example. Before family planning came into vogue, the average number of children born to a Kenyan woman was about eight. Compare this with the Hutterites, nonmechanized farmers who live a life similar to that of the Amish. Hutterites experience none of the chronic stressors of the Kenyan farmers, use no contraceptives, and have an almost identical reproductive rate—an average of nine children per woman. (It is difficult to make a close quantitative comparison of these two populations. The Hutterites, for example, delay marriage, decreasing their reproductive rate, whereas Kenyan agriculturists traditionally do not. Conversely, Kenyan agriculturists typically breast-feed for at least a year, decreasing their reproductive rate, in contrast to the Hutterites, who typically nurse far less. The main point, however, is that even with such different lifestyles, the two reproductive rates are nearly equal.)

How about reproduction during extreme stress? This has been studied in a literature that always poses problems for those discussing it: how to cite a scientific finding without crediting the monsters who did the research? These are the studies of women in the Third Reich's concentration camps, conducted by Nazi doctors. (The convention has evolved never to cite the names of the doctors, and always to note their criminality.) In a study of the women in the Theresienstadt concentration camp, 54 percent of the reproductive-age women were found to have stopped menstruating. This is hardly surprising; starvation, slave labor, and unspeakable psychological terror are going to disrupt reproduction. The point typically made is that, of the women who stopped menstruating, the majority stopped within their first month in the camps—before starvation and labor had pushed fat levels down to the decisive point. Many researchers cite this as a demonstration of how disruptive even psychological stress can be to reproduction.

To me, the surprising fact is just the opposite. Despite starvation, exhausting labor, and the daily terror that each day would be their last, only 54 percent of those women ceased menstruating. Reproductive mechanisms were still working in nearly half the women (although a certain number may have been having anovulatory cycles). And I would wager that despite the horrors of their situation, there were still many men who were reproductively intact. That reproductive physiology still operated in any individual to any extent, under those circumstances, strikes me as extraordinary.

Reproduction represents a vast hierarchy of behavioral and physiological events that differ considerably in subtlety. Some steps are basic and massive—the eruption of an egg, the diverting of rivers of blood to a penis. Others are as delicate as the line of a poem that awakens your heart or the whiff of a person's scent that awakens your loins. Not all the steps are equally sensitive to stress. The basic machinery of reproduction can be astoundingly resistant to stress in a subset of individuals, as evidence from the Holocaust shows. Reproduction is one of the strongest of biological reflexes—just ask a salmon leaping upstream to spawn, or males of various species risking life and limb for access to females, or any adolescent with that steroid-crazed look. But when it comes to the pirouettes and filigrees of sexuality, stress can wreak havoc with subtleties. That may not be of enormous consequence to a starving refugee or a wildebeest in the middle of a drought. But it matters to us, with our culture of multiple orgasms and minuscule refractory periods and oceans of libido. And while it is easy to make fun of those obsessions of ours, those nuances of sexuality, the *Cosmo*s and *GQ*s and other indices of our indulged lives, matter to us. They provide us with some of our greatest, if also our most fragile and evanescent, joys.

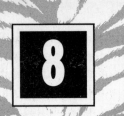

8

IMMUNITY, STRESS, AND DISEASE

The halls of academe are filling with a newly evolved species of scientist—the psychoneuroimmunologist—who makes a living studying the extraordinary fact that what goes on in your head can affect how well your immune system functions. Those two realms were once thought to be fairly separate—your immune system kills bacteria, makes antibodies, hunts for tumors; your brain makes you do the bunny hop, invents the wheel, has favorite TV shows. Yet the dogma of the separation of the immune and nervous systems has fallen by the wayside. The autonomic nervous system sends nerves into tissues that form or store the cells of the immune system and eventually enter the circulation. Furthermore, tissue of the immune system turns out to be sensitive to (that is, it has receptors for) all the interesting hormones released by the pituitary under the control of the brain. The result is that the brain has a vast potential for sticking its nose into the immune system's business.

The evidence for the brain's influence on the immune system goes back at least a century, dating to the first demonstration that if you waved an artificial rose in front of someone who is highly allergic to roses (and who didn't know it was a fake), they'd get an allergic response. Here's a charming and more recent demonstration of the brain influencing the immune system: take some professional actors and have them spend a day doing either a depressing negative scene, or an uplifting euphoric one. Those in the former state show decreased immune responsiveness, while those in the latter manifest an increase. (And where was such a study carried out? In Los Angeles, of course, at UCLA.) But the study that probably most solidified the link between the brain and the immune system used a paradigm called *conditioned immunosuppression.*

Give an animal a drug that suppresses the immune system. Along with it, provide, à la Pavlov's experiments, a "conditioned stimulus"— for example, an artificially flavored drink, something that the animal will associate with the suppressive drug. A few days later, present the conditioned stimulus by itself—and down goes immune function. In 1982 the report of an experiment using a variant of this paradigm, carried out by two pioneers in this field, Robert Ader and Nicholas Cohen of the University of Rochester, stunned scientists. The two researchers experimented with a strain of mice that spontaneously develop disease because of overactivity of their immune systems. Normally, the disease is controlled by treating the mice with an immunosuppressive drug. Ader and Cohen showed that by using their conditioning techniques, they could substitute the conditioned stimulus for the actual drug—and sufficiently alter immunity in these animals to extend their life spans.

Studies such as these convinced scientists that there is a strong link between the nervous system and the immune system. It should come as no surprise that if the sight of an artificial rose or the taste of an artificially flavored drink can alter immune function, then stress can, too. In the first half of this chapter, I discuss what stress does to immunity and how this might be useful during a stressful emergency. In the second half, I'll examine whether sustained stress, by way of chronic suppression of immunity, can impair the ability of a body to fight off infectious disease. This is a fascinating question, which can be answered only with a great deal of caution and many caveats. Although evidence is emerging that stress-induced immunosuppression can indeed increase the risk and severity of some diseases, the connection is probably relatively weak and its importance often exaggerated.

In order to evaluate the results of this confusing but important field, we need to start with a primer about how the immune system works.

 ## IMMUNE SYSTEM BASICS

The primary job of the immune system is to defend the body against infectious agents such as viruses, bacteria, fungi, and parasites. The process is dauntingly complex. For one thing, the immune system must tell the difference between cells that are normal parts of the body and cells that are invaders—in immunologic jargon, distinguishing between "self" and "non-self." Somehow, the immune system can remember what every cell in your body looks like, and any cells that lack your distinctive cellular signature (for example, bacteria) are attacked. Moreover, when your immune system does encounter a novel invader, it can even form an immunologic memory of what the infectious agent looks like, to better prepare for the next invasion—a process that is exploited when you are vaccinated with a mild version of an infectious agent in order to prime your immune system for a real attack.

Such immune defenses are brought about by a complex array of circulating cells called *lymphocytes* and *monocytes* (which are collectively known as *white blood cells; cyte* is a term for cells). There are two classes of lymphocytes: T cells and B cells. Both originate in the bone marrow, but T cells migrate to mature in the thymus (hence the *T*), while B cells mature in the bone marrow. B cells principally produce antibodies, but there are several kinds of T cells (T helper and T suppressor cells, cytotoxic killer cells, and so on).

The T and B cells attack infectious agents in very different ways. T cells bring about cell-mediated immunity (see the illustration on page 147). When an infectious agent invades the body, it is recognized by a type of monocyte called a macrophage, which presents the foreign particle to a T helper cell. A metaphorical alarm is now sounded, and T cells begin to proliferate in response to the invasion. This alarm system ultimately results in the activation and proliferation of cytotoxic killer cells, which, as their name implies, attack and destroy the infectious agent. It is this, the T-cell component of the immune system, that is knocked out by the AIDS virus.

By contrast, B cells cause antibody-mediated immunity (see the illustration on page 148). Once the macrophage–T helper cell collaboration has occurred, the T helper cells then stimulate B-cell proliferation. The main task of the B cells is to differentiate and generate antibodies, large proteins that will recognize and bind to some specific feature of the invading infectious agent (typically, a distinctive surface protein). This specificity is critical—the antibody formed has a fairly unique shape, which will conform perfectly to the shape of the distinctive feature of the invader, like the fit between a lock and key. In binding to the specific feature, antibodies immobilize the infectious agent and target it for destruction.

There is an additional twist to the immune system. If different parts of the liver, for example, need to coordinate some activity, they have

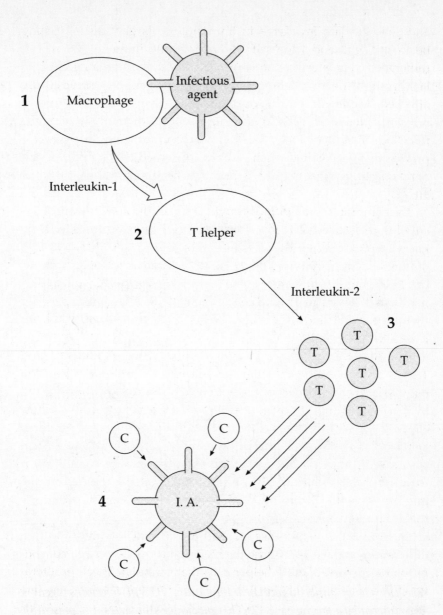

*The cascade of cell-mediated immunity. (1) An infectious agent is encoun-
tered by a type of monocyte called a macrophage. (2) This stimulates the
macrophage to present the infectious agent to a T helper cell (a type of white
blood cell) and to release interleukin-1 (IL-1), which stimulates T helper cell
activity. (3) The T helper cell, as a result, releases interleukin-2 (IL-2),
which triggers T-cell proliferation. (4) This eventually causes another type
of white blood cell, cytotoxic killer cells, to proliferate and destroy the
infectious agent.*

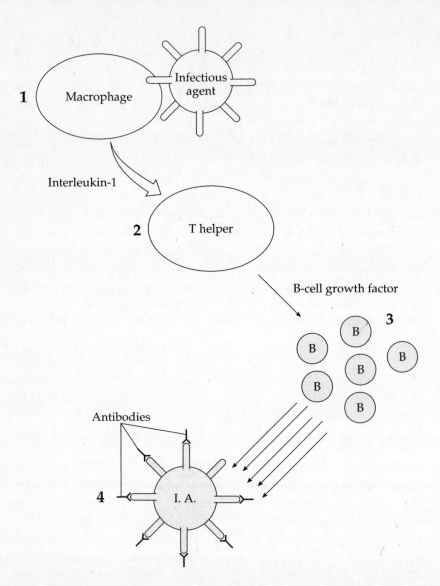

The cascade of antibody-mediated immunity. (1) An infectious agent is encountered by a macrophage. (2) This encounter stimulates it to present the infectious agent to a T helper cell and to release interleukin-1 (IL-1), which stimulates T helper cell activity. (3) The T helper cell then secretes B-cell growth factor, triggering differentiation and proliferation of another white blood cell, B cells. (4) The B cells make and release specific antibodies that bind to surface proteins on the infectious agent, targeting it for destruction by a large group of circulating proteins known as complement.

the advantage of sitting adjacent to each other. But the immune system is distributed throughout the circulation. In order to sound immune alarms throughout this far-flung system, blood-borne chemical messengers that communicate between different cell types, called *cytokines,* have evolved. For example, when macrophages first recognize an infectious agent, they release a messenger called *interleukin-1*. This triggers the T helper cell to release interleukin-2, which stimulates T-cell growth (to make life complicated, there are at least half a dozen additional interleukins with more specialized roles). On the antibody front, T cells also secrete B-cell growth factor. Other classes of messengers, such as interferons, activate broad classes of lymphocytes.

The process of the immune system sorting self and non-self usually works well (although truly insidious tropical parasites like those that cause schistosomiasis have evolved to evade your immune system by pirating the signature of your own cells). Your immune system happily spends its time sorting out self from non-self: red blood cells, part of us. Eyebrows, our side. Virus, no good, attack. Muscle cell, good guy. . . .

What if something goes wrong with the immune system's sorting? One obvious kind of error could be that the immune system misses an infectious invader; clearly, bad news. Equally bad is the sort of error in which the immune system decides something is a dangerous invader that really isn't. In one version of this, some perfectly innocuous compound in the world around you triggers an alarm reaction. Maybe it is something that you normally ingest, like peanuts or shellfish, or something airborne and innocuous, like pollen. But your immune system has mistakenly decided that this is not only foreign but dangerous, and kicks into gear. And this is an allergy.

In the second version of the immune system overreacting, a normal part of your own body is mistaken for an infectious agent and is attacked. When the immune system erroneously attacks a normal part of the body, a variety of horrendous "autoimmune" diseases may result. In multiple sclerosis, for example, part of your nervous system is attacked; in juvenile diabetes, it's the cells in the pancreas that normally secrete insulin. As we'll see shortly, stress has some rather confusing effects on autoimmune diseases.

So far in this overview of the immune system, we've been concentrating on something called *acquired immunity*. Suppose you're exposed to some novel, dangerous pathogen, pathogen X, for the first time. Acquired immunity has three features. First, you acquire the ability to target pathogen X specifically, with antibodies and cell-mediated immunity that specifically recognize that pathogen. This really works to your advantage—a bullet with pathogen X's name written on it. Second, it takes some time to build up that immunity when you are first exposed to pathogen X—this involves finding which antibody has the best fit and generating a zillion copies of it. Finally, while you will now be geared up to specifically go after pathogen X for a long time to come once that specific defense is on line, repeated exposure to pathogen X will boost those targeted defenses even more.

Such acquired immunity is a pretty fancy invention, and it is found only in vertebrates. But we also contain a simpler, more ancient branch of the immune system, one shared with species as distant as insects, called *innate* immunity. In this realm, you don't bother with acquiring the means to target pathogen X specifically with antibodies that will be different from those that would target, say, pathogen Y. Instead, the second any sort of pathogen hits your system, this nonspecific immune response swings into action.

This generalized immune response tends to occur at the beachhead where a pathogen gets its first foothold, like your skin, or moist *mucosal* tissue, like in your mouth or nose. As a first step, your saliva contains a class of antibodies that generically attack any sort of microbe that it encounters, instead of acquiring a means of targeting specific invaders. These antibodies are secreted and coat your mucosal surfaces like an antiseptic paint. In addition, at the site of infection, capillaries loosen up, allowing cells of the innate immune response to slip out of the circulation to infiltrate the immediate area of infection. These cells include *macrophages, neutrophils,* and *natural killer cells,* which then attack the microbe. The loosening of the capillaries also allows fluid containing proteins that can fight the invasive microbes to flow in from the circulation. And what happens as a result of that? The proteins fight the microbe, but the fluid also makes the area swell up, causing *edema*. This is your innate immune system leaping into action, causing inflammation.*

This gives us a broad overview of immune function. Time to see what stress does to immunity. Naturally, as it turns out, a lot more complicated things than used to be suspected.

---

* As just mentioned, the innate immune response involves proteins infiltrating into the area of injury. Among those proteins, fighting those microbes, is one we heard about in chapter 3 called "C-reactive protein." You will recall how gunk like cholesterol forms atherosclerotic plaques only at places where your blood vessels are injured. Thus, a measure of injury and inflammation at your blood vessels is a good predictor of atherosclerotic risk. C-reactive protein, as we learned, is the most reliable indicator of such inflammation.

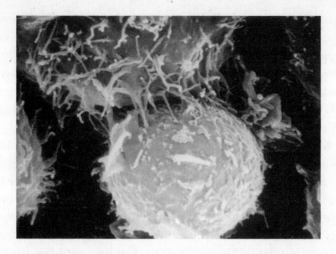

Photomicrograph of a natural killer T cell attacking a tumor cell.

 ## HOW DOES STRESS INHIBIT IMMUNE FUNCTION?

It's been almost sixty years since Selye discovered the first evidence of stress-induced immunosuppression, noting that immune tissues like the thymus gland atrophied among rats subjected to nonspecific unpleasantness. Scientists have learned more about the subtleties of the immune system since then, and it turns out that a period of stress will disrupt a wide variety of immune functions.

Stress will suppress the formation of new lymphocytes and their release into the circulation, and shorten the time preexisting lymphocytes stay in the circulation. It will inhibit the manufacturing of new antibodies in response to an infectious agent, and disrupt communication among lymphocytes through the release of relevant messengers. And it will inhibit the innate immune response, suppressing inflammation. All sorts of stressors do this—physical, psychological, in primates, rats, birds, even in fish. And, of course, in humans, too.

The best-documented way in which such immune suppression occurs is via glucocorticoids. Glucocorticoids, for example, can cause shrinking of the thymus gland; this is such a reliable effect that in olden days (circa 1960), before it was possible to measure directly the amount of glucocorticoids in the bloodstream, one indirect way of doing so was to see how much the thymus gland in an animal had shrunk. The smaller the thymus, the more glucocorticoids in the circulation. Glucocorticoids halt the formation of new lymphocytes in the thymus, and most of the thymic tissue is made up of these new cells, ready to be secreted into the bloodstream. Because glucocorticoids inhibit the release of messengers like interleukins and interferons, they also make circulating lymphocytes less responsive to an infectious alarm. Glucocorticoids, moreover, cause lymphocytes to be yanked out of the circulation and stuck back in storage in immune tissues. Most of these glucocorticoid effects are against T cells, rather than B cells, meaning that cell-mediated immunity is more disrupted than antibody-mediated immunity. And most impressively, glucocorticoids can actually kill lymphocytes. This taps into one of the hottest topics in medicine, which is the field of "programmed cell death."* Cells are programmed to commit suicide sometimes. For example, if a cell begins to become cancerous, there is a suicide pathway that gets activated to kill the cell before it starts dividing out of control; a few types of cancers involve the failure of the programmed cell death to occur. It turns out that glucocorticoids can trigger those suicide pathways into action in lymphocytes, through a variety of mechanisms.

Sympathetic nervous system hormones, beta-endorphin, and CRH within the brain also play a role in suppressing immunity during stress. The precise mechanisms by which this happens are nowhere near as well understood as with glucocorticoid-induced immune suppression, and these other hormones have traditionally been viewed as less important than the glucocorticoid part of the story. However, a number of experiments have shown that stressors can suppress immunity independently of glucocorticoid secretion, strongly implicating these other routes.

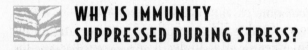

WHY IS IMMUNITY
SUPPRESSED DURING STRESS?

Figuring out exactly how glucocorticoids and the other stress hormones suppress immunity is a very hot topic these days in cell and molecular biology, especially the part about killing lymphocytes. But amid all this excitement about cutting-edge science, it would be

---

* Another trendy term in this field is *apoptosis,* which is derived from Latin for something like "falling off" (as in the falling off of leaves in the fall, an example of programmed death). There are great debates as to whether apoptosis equals programmed cell death or is just a subtype of it (I subscribe to the latter view), as well as, amazingly, whether you pronounce the second *p* in the word (I do, a pronunciation that is considered to have a rough-hewn man-in-the-street plebian air to it).

reasonable to begin to wonder *why* you should want your immune system suppressed during stress. In chapter 1, I offered an explanation for this; now that the process of stress-induced immunosuppression has been explained in a little more detail, it should be obvious that my early explanation makes no sense. I suggested that during stress it is logical for the body to shut down long-term building projects in order to divert energy for more immediate needs—this inhibition includes the immune system, which, while fabulous at spotting a tumor that will kill you in six months or making antibodies that will help you in a week, is not vital in the next few moments' emergency. That explanation would make sense only if stress froze the immune system right where it was—no more immune expenditures until the emergency is finished. However, that is not what happens. Instead, stress causes the active expenditure of energy in order to disassemble the preexisting immune system—tissues are shrunk, cells are destroyed. This cannot be explained by a mere halt to expenditures—you're *paying*, energetically, to take apart the immune system. So out goes this extension of the long-term versus short-term theory.

Why should evolution set us up to do something as apparently stupid as disassembling our immune system during stress? Maybe there isn't a good reason. This actually isn't as crazy of a response as you might think. Not everything in the body has to have an explanation in terms of evolutionary adaptiveness. Maybe stress-induced immunosuppression is simply a by-product of something else that is adaptive; it just came along for the ride.

This is probably not the case. During infections, the immune system releases the chemical messenger interleukin-1, which among other activities stimulates the hypothalamus to release CRH. As noted in chapter 2, CRH stimulates the pituitary to release ACTH, which then causes adrenal release of glucocorticoids. These in turn suppress the immune system. In other words, under some circumstances, the immune system will ask the body to secrete hormones that will ultimately suppress the immune system. For whatever reason the immunosuppression occurs, the immune system sometimes encourages it. It is probably not just an accident.*

---

* My tiny footnote in science: I was part of *the* group that discovered the fact that interleukin-1 stimulates CRH release. Or at least I thought I was. It was in the mid-1980s. The idea made some sense, and the lab I was in jumped on it under my prompting. We worked like maniacs, and at two o'clock one morning I had one of those moments of euphoria that scientists die for: looking at the printout from one of the machines and realizing, "Aha, I was right, it does work that way—interleukin-1 released CRH." We wrote up the findings, they were accepted by the prestigious journal *Science*, everyone

Various ideas have floated around over the years to explain why you actively disassemble immunity during stress with the willing cooperation of the immune system. Some seemed fairly plausible until people learned a bit more about immunity and could rule them out. Others were quite nutty, and I happily advocated a few of these in the first edition of this book. But in the last decade, an answer has emerged, and it really turns this field on its head.

 ## SURPRISE

It turns out that during the first few minutes (say, up to about thirty) after the onset of a stressor, you don't uniformly suppress immunity—you *enhance* many aspects of it (phase A on the accompanying graph). This is shown with all realms of immunity, but in particular for innate immunity. This makes sense—it may be helpful to activate parts of your immune system that are going to make some swell antibodies for you over the next few weeks, but it makes even more sense to immediately activate parts of the immune system that are going to help you out right now. More immune cells are rushed into the circulation and, in the injured nervous system, more inflammatory cells infiltrate the site of injury. Moreover, circulating lymphocytes are better at releasing and responding to those immune messengers. And more of those generic antibodies of the innate immune system are released into your saliva. This boosting of immunity doesn't occur only after some infectious challenge. Physical stressors, psychological stressors, all appear to cause an early stage of immune activation. Even more surprisingly, those immunosuppressive villains, glucocorticoids, appear to play a major role in this (along with the sympathetic nervous system).

So, with the onset of all sorts of stressors, your immune defenses are enhanced. And now we are ready for our usual other side of the two-edged sword, when the stress goes on longer. By the one-hour mark, more sustained glucocorticoid and sympathetic activation

---

was very excited, I called my parents, and so on. Paper gets published, and right next to it was an *identical* study from a group in Switzerland, sent in to the journal the same exact week. So I became *a* discoverer of this obscure fact. (To hark back to a theme of chapter 2, if you are a mature, confident individual—which unfortunately I am only rarely—you take pleasure in this sort of thing: two labs, working independently on opposite sides of the globe, come up with the same novel observation. It must be true. Science lurches forward an inch.)

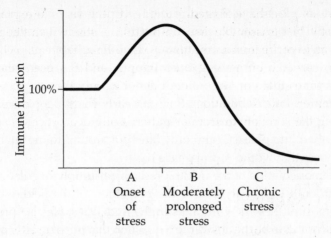

Stress turns out to transiently stimulate the immune system.

begins to have the opposite effect, namely, suppressing immunity. If the stressor ends around then, what have you accomplished with that immunosuppression? Bringing immune function back to where it started, back to baseline (phase B). It is only with major stressors of longer duration, or with really major exposure to glucocorticoids, that the immune system does not just return to baseline, but plummets into a range that really does qualify as immunosuppressing (phase C). For most things that you can measure in the immune system, sustained major stressors drive the numbers down to 40 to 70 percent below baseline.

The idea of temporarily perking up your immune system with the onset of a stressor makes a fair amount of sense (certainly at least as much as some of the convoluted theories as to why suppressing it makes sense). As does the notion that what goes up must come down. And as does the frequent theme of this book, namely, that if you have a stressor that goes on for too long, an adaptive decline back to baseline can overshoot and you get into trouble.

Why did it take people so long to figure this out? Probably for two reasons. First, because many of the techniques for measuring what's happening in the immune system have only recently become sensitive enough to pick up small, rapid differences, the thing needed to catch phase A, that fast immunostimulatory blip at the beginning of a stressor. Thus, for decades, people thought they were studying the immune response to stress, whereas they were actually studying the *recovery* of the immune response to stress. As a second reason, most scientists in this field study major, prolonged stressors, or administer major amounts of glucocorticoids for prolonged periods. This represents a reasonable bias in how experiments are done—start with a sledgehammer of an experimental manipulation. If nothing happens, pick a new field to study. If something does happen and it's been replicated enough times that you're confident about it, only then begin to think about more subtle elaborations. So in the early years, people were only studying the sorts of stressors or patterns of glucocorticoid exposure that pushed into phase C, and only later got around to the subtler circumstances that would reveal phase B.

This reorientation of the field represents a triumph for Allan Munck of Dartmouth University, one of the godfathers of the field, who predicted most of these new findings in the mid-1980s. He also predicted what turns out to be the answer to a question that pops up after a while. Why would you want to bring immune function back down to the pre-stress level (phase B in the diagram)? Why not just let it remain at the enhanced, improved level achieved in the first thirty minutes and get the benefits of an activated immune system all the time? Metaphorically, why not have your military that defends you always on maximal alert? For one thing, it costs too much. And, even more important, a system that's always on maximal, hair-trigger alert is more likely to get carried away at some point and shoot one of your own guys in a friendly fire accident. And that's what can happen with immune systems that are chronically activated—they begin to mistake part of you for being something invasive, and you've got yourself an autoimmune disease.

Such reasoning led Munck to predict that if you fail to have phase B, if you don't coast that activated immune system back down to baseline, you're more at risk for an autoimmune disease. This idea has been verified in at least three realms. First, artificially lock glucocorticoid levels in the low basal range in rats and then stress them. This produces animals that have phase A (mostly mediated by epinephrine), but there isn't the rise in glucocorticoids to fully pull off phase B. The rats are now more at risk for autoimmune disease. Second, doctors have to occasionally remove one of the two adrenal glands (the source of glucocorticoids) from a patient, typically because of a tumor. Immediately afterward, circulating glucocorticoid levels are halved for a period, until the remaining adrenal bulks up enough to take on the job of two. During that period of low glucocorticoid levels, people are more likely than normal to flare up with some autoimmune or inflammatory disease—there's not enough glucocorticoids around to pull off phase B when something stressful occurs. Finally, if you look at strains of rats or, weirdly, chickens, that spontaneously develop autoimmune diseases, they all turn out to have something wrong with

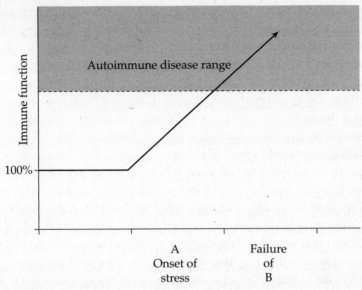

A schematic representation of how a failure to inhibit immune function during stress can bias you toward autoimmune disease.

the glucocorticoid system so that they have lower than normal levels of the hormone, or have immune and inflammatory cells that are less responsive than normal to glucocorticoids. Same for humans with autoimmune diseases like rheumatoid arthritis.

Thus, early on in the stress-response, the immune system is being activated, rather than inhibited, and a big thing that the stress-response does is make sure that immune activation doesn't spiral into autoimmunity.

So that has forced some revisionism in this field. But just to add to this, once stress has gone on long enough to begin to suppress immunity, some of what have classically been taken to be aspects of immune suppression are actually more subtle versions of immune enhancement.

This is seen in two ways. Give someone massive amounts of glucocorticoids, or a huge stressor that has gone on for many hours, and the hormones will be killing lymphocytes indiscriminately, just mowing them down. Have a subtle rise in glucocorticoid levels for a short time (like what is going on at the start of phase B), and the hormones kill only a particular subset of lymphocytes—older ones, ones that don't work as well. Glucocorticoids, at that stage, are helping to *sculpt* the immune response, getting rid of lymphocytes that aren't ideal for the immediate emergency. So that indirectly counts as a version of immune enhancement.

A second subtlety reflects reinterpretation of something people have known since the dawn of humans (or at least during Selye's prime). As noted, glucocorticoids not only kill lymphocytes, but also yank some remaining lymphocytes out of the circulation. Firdhaus Dhabhar of Ohio State University asked, Where do those immune cells go when they are pulled out of the circulation? The assumption in the field had always been that they all go into immune storage tissues (like the thymus gland)—they're taken out of action, so that they aren't much use to you. But Dhabhar's work shows that they don't all get mothballed. Instead, glucocorticoids and epinephrine are diverting many of those lymphocytes to the specific site of infection, such as the skin. The immune cells aren't being deactivated—they're being transferred to the front lines. And a consequence of this is that wounds heal faster.

Thus, early on during exposure to a stressor, glucocorticoids and other stress-responsive hormones transiently activate the immune system, enhancing immune defenses, sharpening them, redistributing immune cells to the scenes of infectious battle. Because of the dangers of the systems overshooting into autoimmunity, more prolonged glucocorticoid exposure begins to reverse these effects, bringing the system back to baseline. And during the pathological scenario of truly major, sustained stressors, immunity is suppressed below baseline.

These new findings help to explain one of the persistent paradoxes in this field. It concerns autoimmune diseases.

Two facts about autoimmunity:

1. Insofar as autoimmune diseases involve overactivation of the immune system (to the point of considering a healthy constituent of your body to actually be something invasive), the most time-honored treatment for such diseases is to put people "on steroids"—to give them massive amounts of glucocorticoids. The logic here is obvious: by dramatically suppressing the immune system it can no longer attack your pancreas or nervous system, or whatever is the inappropriate target of its misplaced zeal (and, as an obvious side effect to this approach, your immune system will also not be very effective at defending you against real pathogens). Thus, administration of large amounts of these stress hormones makes autoimmune diseases less damaging. Moreover, prolonged major stressors decrease the symptoms of autoimmune diseases in lab rats.

2. At the same time, it appears that stress can *worsen* autoimmune diseases. Stress is among the most reliable, if not the most reliable, factor to worsen such diseases. This has often been reported anecdotally by patients, and is typically roundly ignored by clinicians who know that stress hormones help reduce autoimmunity, not worsen

it. But some objective studies also support this view for autoimmune diseases such as multiple sclerosis, rheumatoid arthritis, Grave's disease, ulcerative colitis, inflammatory bowel disease, and asthma. There have been only a handful of such reports, and they suffer from the weakness of relying on patient-reported retrospective data, rather than on prospective data. Nevertheless, their findings are relatively consistent—there is a subset of patients whose initial onset of an autoimmune disease and, to an even greater extent, their intermittent flare-ups of bad symptoms are yoked to stress. Moreover, there is, by now, a pretty hefty literature showing that stress can worsen autoimmunity in animal models of these diseases.

So, do glucocorticoids and stress worsen or lessen the symptoms of autoimmunity? The graph below gives an answer that wasn't clear in earlier years. We've now seen two scenarios that increase the risk of autoimmune disease. First, it seems as if numerous transient stressors (that is, lots of phases A and B) increase the risk of autoimmunity—for some reason, repeated ups and downs ratchet the system upward, biasing it toward autoimmunity. Second, while it seems not to be great to have lots of instances of phase A followed by phase B, having phase A *not* followed by phase B increases the risk of autoimmunity as well. If you don't have an adequate phase B, that pushes the immune system spiral upward into autoimmunity (back to diagram on page 157).

As we would now expect, if you instead have massive prolonged stressors, or are administered big hefty doses of glucocorticoids, you put the system in phase C—dramatic immune suppression, which decreases the symptoms of autoimmunity. Supporting this summary

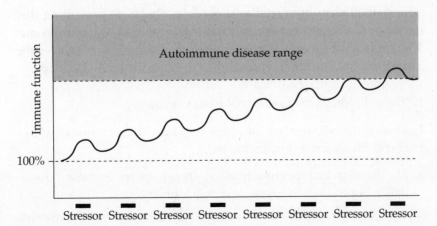

A schematic representation of how repeated stress increases the risk of autoimmune disease.

is the finding that while acute stress puts rats more at risk for a model of multiple sclerosis, chronic stress suppresses the symptoms of that autoimmune disease. The system apparently did not evolve for dealing with numerous repetitions of coordinating the various on-and-off switches, and ultimately something uncoordinated occurs, increasing the risk that the system becomes autoimmune.

 ## CHRONIC STRESS AND DISEASE RISK

A repeated theme in this book is how some physiological response to your average, run-of-the-mill mammalian stressor, if too long or too frequent, gets you into trouble. The ability of major stressors to suppress immunity below baseline certainly seems like a candidate for this category. How damaging is stress-induced immunosuppression when it actually occurs? As the AIDS virus has taught us, if you suppress the immune system sufficiently, a thirty-year-old will fester with cancers and pneumonias that doctors used to see once in an elderly patient during a fifty-year career. But can chronic stress suppress the immune system to the point of making you more susceptible to diseases you wouldn't otherwise get? Once you have a disease, are you now less capable of fighting it off?

Evidence pouring in from many quarters suggests that stress may indeed impair our immune systems and increase the risk of illness. But despite these striking findings, it remains far from clear just how much chronic stress makes you more vulnerable to diseases that would normally be fought off by the immune system. In order to appreciate the current disarray of the research, let us try to break down the findings into their component parts.

Essentially, all these studies show a link between something that increases or decreases stress and some disease or mortality outcome. The approach of many psychoneuroimmunologists is based on the assumption that this link is established through the following steps:

1. The individuals in question have been stressed,

2. causing them to turn on the stress-response (the secretion of glucocorticoids, epinephrine, and so on).

3. The duration and magnitude of the stress-response in these individuals is big enough to suppress immune function,

4. which increases the odds of these individuals getting some infectious disease, and impairs their ability to defend themselves against that disease once they have it.

Thus, suppose you see that a certain immune-related disease is more common in circumstances of stress. You now have to ask two critical questions. First, can you show that steps 1 to 4 occurred in those stressed individuals with that disease? Second, is there some alternative route that explains starting with stress and getting to the disease?

Let's begin by analyzing those four separate steps, in order to see how tough it is to demonstrate that all four have occurred.

Step 1, "The individuals in question have been stressed." In studies of nonhuman animals, the general consensus is that with enough stress, you are going to get to steps 2 through 4. But a problem in extrapolating to humans is that the experimental stressors used in animal studies are usually more awful than what we typically experience. Not only that, but we differ tremendously among ourselves as to what we experience as truly stressful—the whole realm of individual differences that will be the focus of the last chapter of this book. Therefore, if you try to study the effects of stressors on people's immune systems, you must wrestle with the problem of whether these things actually seem stressful to a given individual or not. What that winds up meaning is that step 1 is probably satisfied in stress/immune-related disease studies that involve events that most everyone would consider pretty awful—the death of a loved one, divorce, financially threatening unemployment. But if the external reality is one that a lot of people would not consider to be stressful, you can't automatically accept that you're at step 1.

There is another problem with step 1: it's often not clear whether humans are really exposed to the stressors to which they claim they're exposed. We tend to be notoriously bad reporters of what goes on in our lives. An imaginary experiment: take one hundred lucky people and slip them a drug that will give them bad stomachaches for a few days. Then send them to a doctor secretly participating in this experiment, who tells them that they have developed stomach ulcers. The doctor asks innocently, "Have things been particularly stressful for you recently?" Perhaps ninety of those subjects will come up with something or other putatively stressful to which they will now attribute the ulcer. In retrospective studies, people confronted with an illness are very likely to decide there were stressful events going on.

When you rely heavily on retrospective studies with humans, you are likely to get a falsely strong link between stress and disease; and the trouble is, most studies in this field are retrospective (a problem that popped up in the chapter on digestive disorders as well). The expensive and lengthy prospective studies are only recently becoming more common—pick a bunch of healthy people and follow them for decades to come, recording as an objective outsider when they are being exposed to stressors and whether they become sick.

We move to the next step: from the stressor to the stress-response (step 1 to step 2). Again, if you give an organism a massive stressor, it will reliably have a strong stress-response. With more subtle stressors, we have more subtle stress-responses.

The same thing holds for the move from step 2 to step 3. In experimental animal studies, large amounts of glucocorticoids will cause the immune system to hit the floor. The same occurs if a human has a tumor that causes massive amounts of glucocorticoids to be secreted (Cushing's syndrome), or if a person is taking huge doses of synthetic glucocorticoids to control some other disease. But as we now know, the moderate rises in glucocorticoid levels seen in response to many more typical stressors stimulate the immune system, rather than suppress it. Moreover, in a few types of cancers elevated levels of glucocorticoids should be protective. As we saw in the last chapter, very high levels of glucocorticoids will suppress levels of estrogens in females and testosterone in males, and certain types of cancers are stimulated by these hormones (most notably "estrogen-sensitive" forms of breast cancer and "androgen-sensitive" prostate cancers). In these cases, lots of stress equals lots of glucocorticoids equals less estrogen or testosterone equals slower tumor growth.

Moving from step 3 to step 4, how much does a change in immune profile alter patterns of disease? The odd thing is that immunologists are not sure about this. If your immune system is massively suppressed, you are more likely to get sick, no doubt about that. People taking high doses of glucocorticoids as medication, who are thus highly immunocompromised, are vulnerable to all sorts of infectious diseases, as are people with Cushing's syndrome. Or AIDS.

The more subtle fluctuations in immunity are less clear in their implications, however. Few immunologists would be likely to assert that "for every tiny decrease in some measure of immune function, there is a tiny increase in disease risk." Their hesitancy is because the relationship between immune competence and disease may be nonlinear. In other words, once you pass a certain threshold of immunosuppression, you are up the creek without a paddle; but before that, immune fluctuations may not really matter much. The immune system is so complex that being able to measure a change in one little piece of it in response to stress may mean nothing about the system as a whole. Thus, the link between relatively minor immune fluctuation and patterns of disease in humans winds up being relatively weak.

There is another reason why it may be difficult to generalize from findings in the laboratory to the real world. In the laboratory, you might be studying the effects of steps 1, 2, and 3 on disease outcome 4. It is inconvenient for most scientists to manipulate a rat's levels of stress, glucocorticoids, or immunity and then wait for the rest of the rat's lifetime to see if it is more likely to become ill than is a control rat. That's slow and expensive. Typically, instead, scientists study induced diseases. Manipulate step 1, 2, or 3 in a rat that has been exposed to a certain virus; then see what happens. When you do that, you get information about steps 1 through 3 that have to do with step 4 when dealing with severe, artificially induced disease challenges. But it should be obvious that an approach like this misses the point that we don't get sick because some scientist deliberately exposes us to disease. Instead, we spend our lives passing through a world filled with scattered

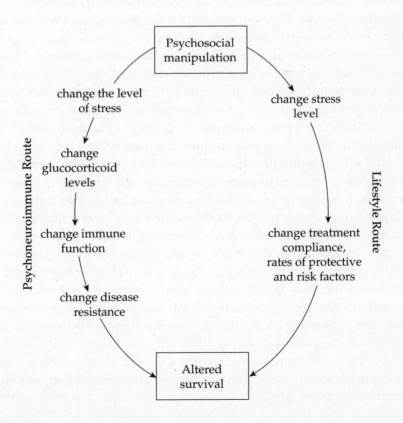

carcinogenic substances, occasional epidemics, someone sneezing from across the room. Relatively few experimental animal studies have looked at spontaneous diseases, rather than induced ones.

These are a lot of caveats. Let's consider some areas where there are links between stress and diseases associated with immune dysfunction. This will let us evaluate to what extent these links are a function of progressing from steps 1 through 4, what we will call the "Psychoneuroimmune Route," which links stress and disease. In each case, we'll consider if there is an alternative sequence, what we'll loosely call the "Lifestyle Route," which can link stress and immune-related disease while bypassing the sequence of steps 1 to 4.

 ## TESTING THE STRESS-DISEASE LINK

Social Support and Social Isolation

What the data show: the fewer social relationships a person has, the shorter his or her life expectancy, and the worse the impact of various infectious diseases. Relationships that are medically protective can take the form of marriage, contact with friends and extended family, church membership, or other group affiliations. This is a fairly consistent pattern that cuts across a lot of different settings. Moreover, these general findings are based on some careful prospective studies and are seen in both sexes and in different races, in American and European populations living in both urban and rural areas. Most important, this effect is big. The impact of social relationships on life expectancy appears to be at least as large as that of variables such as cigarette smoking, hypertension, obesity, and level of physical activity. For the same illness, people with the fewest social connections have approximately two-and-a-half times as much chance of dying as those with the most connections, after controlling for such variables as age, gender, and health status.

Very exciting. And what might explain this relationship? Maybe it's through the Psychoneuroimmune Route of steps 1 to 4, which would run something like: socially isolated people are more stressed for lack of social outlets and support (step 1); this leads to chronic activation of stress-responses (step 2); leading to immune suppression (step 3); and more infectious diseases (step 4).

Let's see what support there is for each of these steps. First, just because someone is socially isolated doesn't mean they are stressed by it—there are lots of hermits who would be happy to pass on yet another crowded Twister party. Social isolation as a stressor is a subjective assessment. In many of these studies, however, the subjects who fit the bill as socially isolated rate themselves as lonely, certainly a negative emotion. So we can check off step 1. On to step 2—do these people have chronically overactive stress-responses? We have little evidence for or against that.

How about step 3—is social isolation associated with damping down some aspect of immune function? There's a lot of evidence for that: lonelier, more socially isolated individuals having less of an antibody response to a vaccine in one study; in another study of people with AIDS, having a faster decline in a key category of lymphocytes; in another, of women with breast cancer, having less natural killer cell activity.

Then on to step 4—can you actually show that that degree of immune suppression played a role in the disease occurring? The facts are relatively weak. Some studies show social isolation and step 3; others show isolation and step 4, but few show both and also explicitly show that the magnitude of step 3 has something to do with the transition to step 4.

Still, there is relatively good evidence for this pathway being relevant. What about the Lifestyle Route? What if the problem is that socially isolated people lack that special someone to remind them to take their daily medication? It is known that isolated people are less likely to comply with a medical regime. What if they're more likely to subsist on reheated fast food instead of something nutritious? Or more likely to indulge in some foolish risk-taking behavior, like smoking, because there's no one to try to convince them to stop? Many lifestyle patterns could link social isolation with more infectious disease, bypassing this sequence of steps. Or what if the causality is reversed— what if the linkage occurs because sickly people are less likely to be able to maintain stable social relationships?

Numerous studies have controlled for these lifestyle risk factors like smoking, diet, or medication compliance and have shown that the isolation/poor health outcome relationship is still there. Moreover, critically, you can show the same in nonhuman primates, who don't confound their health with Big Macs, alcohol, and smoking. Infect monkeys with SIV (the simian equivalent of HIV) and more socially isolated animals had higher glucocorticoid levels, fewer antibodies against the virus, more virus in their system, and a greater mortality rate—in other words, steps 1 to 4.

Overall, I'd say a pretty good case can be made that social isolation can impact health through the effects of stress on immunity. But the case isn't airtight.

Bereavement

Bereavement, an extreme version of social isolation, is, of course, the loss of a loved one. An extensive literature shows that while bereavement often coincides with depression, it is distinct from it. A common belief is that the one left behind—the grieving spouse, the bereft parent, even the masterless pet—now pines away to an early death. A number of studies suggest that bereavement does indeed increase the risk of dying, although the effect is not all that strong. This is probably because the risk occurs only in a subset of grievers, amid those people who have an additional physiological or psychological risk factor coupled with the bereavement. In one careful prospective study, the parents of all the Israeli soldiers who died in the Lebanese war were followed for ten years afterward. Loss of a child did not affect mortality rates in the population of grieving parents in general. However, significantly higher mortality rates occurred among parents who were already widowed or divorced. In other words, this stressor is associated with increased mortality in the subset of parents with the added risk factor of minimal social support.

Thus, we are turfed back to the subject of social isolation. Again, the evidence for the Psychoneuroimmune Route occurring is decent but, again, there are many potential Lifestyle Routes—grieving people are unlikely to be eating, sleeping, exercising in a healthy manner. Sometimes the confound is more subtle. People tend to marry people who are ethnically and genetically quite similar to themselves. Intrinsic in this trend toward "homogamy" is a tendency of married couples to have higher-than-random chances of sharing environmental risk factors (as well as to disproportionately share disease-related genes, making this component of the Lifestyle Route not really related to lifestyle). This makes it more likely that they will get sick around the same time. Nonetheless, amid those confounds, the Psychoneuroimmune Route's steps 1 to 4 are probably relevant to the increased mortality rates among bereaved individuals lacking social support.

The Common Cold

Everybody knows that being stressed increases your chances of getting a cold. Just think back to being run down, frazzled, and sleep-deprived during final exams, and, sure enough, there's that cough and runny nose. Examine the records at university health services and you'll see the same thing—students succumbing to colds left and right around exam period. Many of us continue to see the same pattern decades later—burn the candle at both ends for a few days and, suddenly, there's that scratchy throat.

Psychoneuroimmune Route steps 1 to 4 seem quite plausible. Some of the studies involve some pretty hefty external events that most people would consider stressful, like financially disastrous unemployment (step 1). But few have looked at the magnitude of the stress-response (step 2). Changes in relevant immune measures have been documented, however—for example, in studies in which stress increases the risk of a cold, those same individuals are shown to have less of the cold-fighting class of antibodies that are secreted in your saliva and nasal passageways (steps 3 and 4).

But we have to consider some possible Lifestyle Route confounds. Maybe the disruptive effects of stress on memory (stay tuned for chapter 10) cause us to forget to button up our overcoats. Or maybe when we are under stress due to social isolation, we are more willing to consort with people who sneeze recklessly without covering their faces.

Okay, maybe those aren't confounds you have to worry about too much. But stress changes lifestyle and different lifestyles mean differing degrees of exposure to the viruses that cause colds.

That possibility has been controlled for in a celebrated series of studies. In one version, some cheerfully compliant volunteers were housed under conditions where some major lifestyle confounds were controlled for. They then filled out questionnaires regarding how stressed they were. Subjects were then spritzed up their noses with equal amounts of rhinovirus, the bug that causes the common cold. Note that everyone was exposed to the same amount of pathogen. And the results? (Fanfare.) More stress equaled about three times the likelihood of succumbing to a cold after being exposed to the virus. Prolonged stressors more than a month long that were social in nature provided the greatest risk.* Moreover, the same thing works in

---

* These studies came out of the famed Common Cold Unit of the Medical Research Council in Salisbury, England, which recruited volunteers for their frequent two-week experiments about various aspects of coming down with and recovering from the common cold. Apparently quite an experience: all expenses covered plus a small salary, many recreational activities in the peaceful Salisbury countryside, daily blowing of noses into collection tubs for the staff, questionnaires to fill out, and being spritzed up the nose with either placebo or a cold-causing virus. One in three chance, on average, of getting a cold while there. People would compete for slots as volunteers; couples have

laboratory mice and nonhuman primates—spritz them with rhino-virus, and it is the stressed, socially subordinate animals who get their species' equivalent of the sniffles.

Collectively, it seems pretty convincing that stress makes the common cold more common at least partially along the Psychoneuro-immune Route.

 ## AIDS

Given that AIDS is a disease of profound immunosuppression, and that major stressors suppress the immune system, can stress increase the likelihood that someone who is HIV positive develops AIDS? And once AIDS is established, can stress worsen its course?

These questions have been aired since the AIDS epidemic began. Since the last edition of this book, the triple combination antiretroviral therapy has turned AIDS from a fatal disease to an often manageable chronic one, making these questions even more relevant.*

There is some good indirect evidence to think that stress can alter the course of AIDS. Suppose you grow human lymphocytes in a petri dish and expose them to HIV. If you expose the cells to glucocorticoids as well, they become more likely to be infected with the virus. Moreover, norepinephrine can also make it easier for the virus to invade a lymphocyte and, once inside, enhances replication of the virus. Support also comes from a study with nonhuman primates, discussed earlier, which suggests that steps 1 to 4 might apply to HIV. To reiterate, the monkeys were infected with SIV, the simian version of HIV. The authors then showed that the monkeys who were more socially isolated (step 1) had higher glucocorticoid levels (step 2), fewer antibodies against the virus (step 3), and a higher mortality rate (step 4). How about humans?

---

met there, married, returned for honeymoons; folks with connections would maneuver for return visits, making it an annual paid vacation. (All was not idyllic sniffling heaven at the Cold Unit, however. An occasional group would be involved in studies showing that, for example, being chilled and damp does not cause colds, and would have to stand around for hours in wet socks.) Unfortunately, because of budget limitations, the unit has been closed. This paradise lost has been chronicled in at least one scholarly book, plus articles with titles like, "How I Blew My Summer Vacation."

* Assuming you are one of the lucky few with AIDS who has enough money, or whose country has enough money, to afford the medications.

To begin, starting with the same amount of HIV in your system, a faster decline and a higher mortality rate occur, on average, among people who have any of the following: (a) a coping style built around denial; (b) minimal social support; (c) a socially inhibited temperament; (d) more stressors, particularly loss of loved ones. These are not huge effects but, nevertheless, there seems a fair consistency in the findings on this. So that seems to qualify for step 1.

Do these individuals also have overactive stress-responses (step 2)? Glucocorticoid levels are not particularly predictive of the course of HIV. However, the more at-risk people with the socially inhibited temperaments have elevated activity of their sympathetic nervous system, and the extent of that overactivity is an even better predictor of decline than is the personality itself. So that seems to get us to step 2.

Does lots of stress, an inhibited temperament, denial, or lack of social support not only predict higher mortality rates (step 4) but a faster decline of immune function (step 3)? That seems to be the case as well.

So AIDS seems to follow the Psychoneuroimmune Route. How about the Lifestyle Route? The medication regimes for dealing with HIV can be enormously complex, and it is quite plausible that people who are more stressed are less likely to take their antiviral medication, or to take it correctly. My sense is that lifestyle risk factors have not been all that well controlled for in these studies. How about if the connection runs in the opposite direction—what if having a faster decline with the disease makes you more socially inhibited, makes for fewer social connections? That seems quite plausible but, as an important control, the personality style has been shown to predict immune profiles many months later.

In summary, psychoneuroimmune aspects could well contribute to a link between stress and worsening of aspects of AIDS. But more research needs to be done to examine how much stress influences whether people comply with their treatment regimes, versus how well their treatment regimes work.

Latent Viruses

After rhinoviruses and the AIDS virus, there is one last category of viruses—those that, after initially infecting you, can go latent. "Latency" means that the virus, once burrowing into some cells of yours, goes into hibernation for a while, just lurking near your own cellular DNA, but not yet replicating itself. At some later point, something triggers the dormant virus out of latency and it reactivates. After going through a couple of rounds of replication the by now larger number of viral particles burrow in and go latent again. The classic example are herpes viruses which, after infecting some of your neurons, can go latent for years, even decades, before flaring up out of latency.

This is a clever tactic that viruses have evolved. Infect some cells, replicate, burst the cells open in the process, make the sort of mess of things that sets off all sorts of alarms in the immune system and, just as those activated immune cells are about to pounce, burrow into another round of cells. While the immune cells are cleaning up, the virus goes latent again.

The next clever thing that viruses have done? They don't reactivate at any old time. They wait until the immune system of the host organism is lousy, and then gun for some quick rounds of replication. And when are immune systems often at their lousiest? You got it. It's been endlessly documented that latent viruses like herpes flare up during times of physical or psychological stress in all sorts of species. It's the same thing with some other viruses that go latent, like Epstein-Barr virus and varicella-zoster (which causes chicken pox and shingles).

So hats off to these highly evolved viruses. Now a key question. How does a latent herpes virus that, after all, is just some unschooled little stretch of DNA sitting mothballed inside a bunch of your neurons, know that you are immunosuppressed? One possibility is that herpes is always attempting to come out of latency and, if your immune system is working fine, it snuffs out the attempt. A second possibility is that herpes can somehow measure how the immune system is doing.

Amazingly, the answer has emerged in the last few years. Herpes doesn't measure how your immune system is doing. It measures something else that, for its purposes, gives it the information it needs—it measures your glucocorticoid levels. Herpes DNA contains a stretch that is sensitive to elevated glucocorticoid signals, and when levels are up, that DNA sensor activates the genes involved in coming out of latency. Epstein-Barr and varicella-zoster contain this glucocorticoid-sensitive stretch as well.

And now for something even more fiendishly clever. You know what else herpes can do once it infects your nervous system? It causes your hypothalamus to release CRH which releases ACTH which raises glucocorticoid levels. Unbelievable, huh? So you don't even need a stressor. Herpes infects you, artificially pushes you to step 2 with your elevated glucocorticoid levels, which gets you to step 3, and allows the virus to come out of latency. Moreover, elevated glucocorticoid levels impair your immune defenses against activated herpes. This leads to step 4—a cold sore flare-up. And we think we're so clever with our big brains and opposable thumbs.

We've now looked at several favorite topics in psychoneuroimmunology, and can see that stress can increase the likelihood, the severity, or both of some immune-related diseases. All of this is a prelude for considering the most contentious subject in this whole field. The punch line is one of the most important in this book, and runs counter to what is distressingly common folk wisdom.

 ## STRESS AND THE BIG C

What does stress have to do with getting cancer?

The first piece of evidence suggesting stress may increase the risk of a cancer diagnosis comes from animal studies. There is, by now, a reasonably convincing animal-experimentation literature showing that stress affects the course of some types of cancer. For example, the rate at which some tumors grow in mice can be affected merely by what sort of cages the animals are housed in—the more noisy and stressful, the faster the tumors grow. Other studies show that if you expose rats to electric shocks from which they can eventually escape, they reject transplanted tumors at a normal rate. Take away the capacity to escape, yet give the same total number of shocks, and the rats lose their capacity to reject tumors. Stress mice by putting their cages on a rotating platform (basically, a record player), and there is a tight relationship between the number of rotations and the rate of tumor growth. Substitute glucocorticoids for the rotation stressor, and tumor growth is accelerated as well. These are the results of very careful studies performed by some of the best scientists in the field.

Does stress work through the Psychoneuroimmune Route in these animals? Seemingly at least partially. These stressors raise glucocorticoid levels in these studies. And these glucocorticoids directly influence tumor biology through both immune and non-immune realms. As a first mechanism, the immune system contains a specialized class of cells (most notably, natural killer cells) that prevent the spread of tumors. Stress suppresses the numbers of circulating natural killer cells in these studies. A second route is probably non-immunologic. Once a tumor starts growing, it needs enormous amounts of energy, and one of the first things that tumors do is send a signal to the nearest blood vessel to grow a bush of capillaries into the tumor. Such *angio-genesis* allows for the delivery of blood and nutrients to the hungry tumor. Glucocorticoids, at the concentration generated during stress, aid angiogenesis. A final route may involve glucose delivery. Tumor cells are very good at absorbing glucose from the bloodstream. Recall the zebra sprinting away from the lion: energy storage has stopped in order to increase concentrations of circulating glucose to be used by the muscles. But, as my own lab reported some years back, when cir-culating glucose concentrations are elevated in rats during stress, at least one kind of experimental tumor can grab the glucose before the muscle does. Your storehouses of energy, intended for your muscles, are being emptied and inadvertently transferred to the ravenous tumor instead.

So we have some stress-cancer links in animals, and some psy-choneuroimmune mechanisms to explain those effects. Does this apply to humans? Two big features of these animal studies dramati-cally limit their relevance to us. First, these were studies of *induced* tumor, where tumorous cells are injected or transplanted into the ani-mal. So we're not looking at stress *causing* cancer in these animals, we're looking at stress altering the course of cancers introduced by artificial routes. No animal studies to my knowledge have shown that stress increases the incidence of spontaneous tumors. Furthermore, most of these studies have relied on tumors that are caused by viruses. In such cases, viruses take over the replication machinery of a cell and cause it to start dividing and growing out of control. In humans most cancers arise from genetic factors or exposure to environmental car-cinogens, rather than from viruses, and those have not been the subject of study with laboratory animals. So a cautionary note from the animal studies: stress can accelerate the growth of a number of tumors, but these are types of cancers of limited relevance to humans, and intro-duced through completely artificial means.

Thus, we turn our attention to humans. Our first, simplest ques-tion: Is a history of major stressors associated with an increased risk of having cancer somewhere down the line?

A number of studies seemed to show this, but they all suffered from the same problem, namely, that they were retrospective. Again, someone with a cancer diagnosis is more likely to remember stress-ful events than someone with a bunion. How about if you do a retro-spective study where you rely upon a history of verifiable stressors, like the death of a family member, loss of a job, or a divorce? A couple of studies have reported a link between such major stressors and the onset of colon cancer five to ten years later. A number of studies, especially of breast cancer patients, have had a "quasi-prospective" design, assessing stress histories of women at the time that they are having a biopsy for a breast lump, comparing those who get a cancer diagnosis with those who don't. Some of these studies have shown a stress-cancer link, and this should be solid—after all, there can't be a retrospective bias, if the women don't know yet if they have cancer. What's the problem here? Apparently, people can guess whether it will turn out to be cancer at a better than chance rate, possibly reflecting knowledge of a family history of the disease, or personal exposure to risk factors. Thus, such quasi-prospective studies are already quasi-retrospective, and of the least reliable kind.

When you rely on the rare prospective studies, there turns out not to be good evidence for a stress-cancer link. For example, as we will see in chapter 14 on depression, having a major depression is closely linked to both stress and excessive glucocorticoid secretion, and one famous study of two thousand men at a Western Electric plant showed that depression was associated with doubling the risk of cancer, even up to decades later. But a careful reexamination of those data showed that the depression-cancer link was attributable to a subset of men who were depressed as hell because they were stuck working with some major carcinogens.

Subsequent prospective studies of other populations have shown either no depression/cancer link, or a tiny one that is biologically meaningless. Moreover, these studies have not ruled out the alternative Lifestyle Route, in that depressed people smoke and drink more, two routes to increase the risk of cancer. Similar findings emerge from the careful prospective studies of bereavement as a stressor—no link with subsequent cancer.

Thus, we shift to a different literature. We'll be seeing in chapter 11 how sleep deprivation and altered sleep patterns (such as with night shifts) are major stressors. In searching for a link between stress and increased risk of cancer, it may not be surprising to find that women who have spent long periods (decades in these studies) working night shifts have an increased risk of breast cancer. However, the most plausible explanation here has nothing to do with stress. Instead, a shifted day/night schedule dramatically decreases the level of a light-responsive hormone called melatonin, and depletion of this hormone greatly increases the risk of a number of types of cancer, including breast cancer.

More suggestive links go by the wayside as well. As discussed earlier, individuals who get organ transplants are at risk for rejecting them, and one of the prevention strategies is to give them glucocorticoids in order to suppress the immune system past the point of being able to reject the organ. In a small subset of such individuals, there is an increased incidence of a few types of skin cancer (of the less serious, non-melanoma kind). Moreover, as noted, if someone's immune system is massively suppressed because of AIDS, there is an increased incidence of a handful of types of cancers. So do these findings tighten the links between cancer and stress? No. This is because: (a) stress never suppresses the immune system to that extent; (b) even when the immune system is suppressed that much, only a small subset of organ transplant or AIDS patients get cancer; and (c) it is only a tiny subset of cancers that now become more common.

So besides those two reports about colon cancer, there is no particular support for the idea that stress increases the risk of cancer (and, it should be noted, this conclusion includes numerous studies of breast cancer, the type of cancer most frequently assumed by people to be stress related). But is there a subset of individuals who have a particular (and poor) style of coping with stress that puts them more at risk for cancer? We already saw, in chapter 5, the notion of there being personality types that are more prone toward functional gastrointestinal disorders. Is there a cancer-prone personality, and can it be interpreted in the context of coping poorly with stress?

Some scientists think so. Much of the work in this area has been done with breast cancer, in part because of the prevalence and seriousness of the disease. However, the same pattern has been reported for other cancers as well. The cancer-prone personality, we're told, is one of repression—emotions held inside, particularly those of anger. This is a picture of an introverted, respectful individual with a strong desire to please—conforming and compliant. Hold those emotions inside and it increases the likelihood that out will come cancer, according to this view.

Most of these studies have been retrospective or quasi-prospective, and we have seen the problems endemic to such studies. Nonetheless, the prospective studies have shown there to be some link, though a small one.

Are we in the realm of Psychoneuroimmune Route steps 1 through 4? No one has shown that yet, in my opinion. As we will see in chapter 15, a repressed personality is associated with elevated glucocorticoid levels, so we're in the range of step 2. But, to my knowledge, no one has shown evidence for step 3—some sort of immune suppression—occurring, let alone it being of a magnitude relevant to cancer. In addition, none of the good prospective studies have ruled out the Lifestyle Route (such as smoking, drinking, or, in the case of breast cancer, more fat consumption). So the jury remains out on this one.

So collectively, we have, with the exception of two studies concerning one type of cancer, no overall suggestion that stress increases the risk of cancer in humans.

Stress and Cancer Relapse

What if your cancer has been cured? Does stress increase the risk of it coming back? The handful of studies on this subject don't suggest that there's a connection—a few say yes, an equal number, no.

Stress and the Course of Cancer

Now on to the most complex and controversial issue of all. Sure, stress may not have anything to do with whether you come down with cancer, but once you have cancer, will stress make a tumor grow faster, increasing your risks of dying from the disease? And can stress reduction slow down tumor growth, extending survival times?

As we saw above, stress will accelerate tumor growth in animals, but those types of instigated tumors and their biology are of limited relevance to the way humans get cancer. So we have to look at studies of humans. And here the subject is a mess.

We begin by looking at whether different coping styles predict different cancer outcomes. When you compare patients who respond to their cancer with a "fighting spirit" (that is, they are optimistic and assertive) with those who collapse into depression, denial, and repression, the former live longer, after controlling for cancer severity.

Findings like these prompted studies in which clinicians attempted to intervene, to reduce stress and inculcate more of that fighting spirit in people, in order to influence the patient's cancer outcome. The landmark study of this type was carried out in the late 1970s by the psychiatrist David Spiegel of Stanford University. Women who had just gotten a metastatic breast cancer diagnosis were randomly assigned to either a group that received standard medical care or a group that, in addition, had intensive supportive group psychotherapy with other breast cancer patients. As Spiegel has emphasized in his accounts of this famous study, he went into it anticipating that the group therapy intervention might decrease psychological distress in patients, but he certainly didn't expect that it would affect the biology of the cancer. Amid his skepticism, what he found was that the group therapy intervention extended life span an average of eighteen months, a whopping great effect.

This made front-page news. But there's been a big problem since then—it's just not clear if a psychosocial intervention actually works. Since the Spiegel study, there have been roughly a dozen others, and they are evenly split as to whether there is any protective effect from group therapy. In what was probably the most thorough attempt at a replication of Spiegel's findings, a study published in 2001 in the prestigious *New England Journal of Medicine*, there was no effect on survival time.

Why has this finding been so difficult to replicate? Spiegel and others give a plausible explanation, having much to do with the massive changes that have occurred over the years in the "culture of cancer." Not that many decades ago, getting cancer had a weirdly shameful quality to it—doctors wouldn't want to tell their patients about the embarrassing and hopeless diagnosis; patients would hide having the disease. As one example, in a 1961 survey, a boggling 90 percent of American physicians said they did not typically reveal a cancer diagnosis to their patients; within two decades, the number was down to 3 percent. Moreover, over the years, doctors have come to consider the psychological well-being of their patients as essential to fighting the cancer, and see the course of medical treatment as a collaboration between themselves and the patient. As Spiegel says, when he began his work in the 1970s, the biggest challenge was to get patients in the "experimental" group to be willing to waste their time with something as irrelevant as group therapy. In contrast, by the 1990s versions of these studies, the biggest challenge was to convince the "control" subjects to forgo group therapy. In this view, it has become difficult to show that introducing a stress-reducing psychosocial intervention extends cancer survival over control subjects because everyone, including control subjects, now recognizes the need to reduce stress during cancer treatment, and seeks psychosocial support all over the place, even if it doesn't come with an official stamp of "twice weekly group psychotherapy."

Let's assume this explanation is correct, and I do find it to be convincing. Thus we accept the premise that psychosocial interventions that reduce stress do extend cancer survival. Let's grind through the steps of the Psychoneuroimmune Route to see if we can understand why the group therapy has such an effect. Are the psychosocial interventions perceived as being stress reducing by the patients (step 1)? There are striking individual exceptions, but the studies, overall, show this resoundingly to be the case.

Are those psychosocial interventions associated with a damping of the stress-response (step 2)? A few studies have shown that psychosocial interventions can lower glucocorticoid levels. Flip the question the other way—does having an overactive stress-response predict shorter cancer survival? No. In the most detailed study of this, following a subsequent population of Spiegel's metastatic breast cancer patients, having high glucocorticoid levels around the time of diagnosis didn't predict a shorter survival time.*

So while psychosocial interventions can reduce glucocorticoid levels, there's little evidence that elevated glucocorticoid levels predict shorter cancer survival. But do cancer patients with more psychosocial support have better immune function (step 3)? Seemingly. Breast cancer patients who reported more stress had lower activities of those natural killer cells, while there's higher NK cell activity in women who report more social support or who received some sort of group therapy intervention. Were those immune changes relevant to the change in survival time (step 4)? Probably not, since someone's levels of NK cell activity didn't predict survival times in these studies.

So there's not much evidence for a Psychoneuroimmune Route. How about the Lifestyle Route? There are lots of reasons to think lifestyle plays a key role in the link between stress and the course of cancer, but it's very hard to show, for a subtle reason. One of the great confounds in cancer therapy is that about a quarter of cancer patients don't take their medications as often as prescribed, or miss chemotherapy appointments. Go figure, when these treatments make you feel so so awful. And what happens in a group therapy setting, when you're surrounded by people going through the same hell as you? "You can go the extra round of chemo, I know you can—yeah, I felt awful the whole time during mine, but you can do it, too," or "Have you eaten today? I know, I have no appetite either, but we're going to get something to eat right after this," or "Have you taken your meds today?" Compliance goes up. Any sort of intervention that increases compliance will increase the success rates of treatments. And because a cancer patient, reasonably, would often be very uncomfortable about admitting that she's not completely complying with a treatment regime, it's hard to detect accurately whether any of the protective effects of psychosocial therapy are kicking in through this route.[†]

---

* Instead, independent of the absolute levels of glucocorticoids, patients whose glucocorticoid levels lacked a 24-hour rhythm at the time had a shorter survival time. Given how much this section is, perhaps, reading like a critical dissection of this field, I think it is worth noting that I was a coauthor on this study. We're still utterly puzzled as to why the loss of the daily rhythmic fluctuation in glucocorticoid levels predicted a bad outcome. A possibility is that the loss of the glucocorticoid rhythm is irrelevant, a red herring, and the key thing is that the daily rhythm of some other hormone, like melatonin, has been lost. This is something that is now being investigated.

† The whole issue of compliance is something Spiegel raises in his writings. His renowned study is endlessly misinterpreted as explicitly supporting a Psychoneuroimmune Route of protection, and I respect him enormously for resisting that bandwagon on which he'd be given a front-row seat.

What we have here are some extremely interesting but murky waters. There appears to be virtually no link between a history of a lot of stress and a greater incidence of cancer, or a greater risk of relapse out of remission. There seems to be a link between a certain personality type and a somewhat greater cancer risk, but no studies have shown where stress physiology fits into that story, nor have lifestyle confounds been ruled out. Next, the findings are about evenly divided as to whether psychosocial interventions that reduce stress improve cancer outcomes. Finally, when considering the cases where psychosocial intervention is effective, there's little support for a Psychoneuroimmune Route to explain the efficacy, and good reasons to think that an alternative route involving issues of lifestyle and compliance is important.

What does one do with these findings? Right on cue—more research, of course. Lots more. However, it is time to discuss what one should *not* do with these findings in the meantime.

 ## CANCER AND MIRACLES

This leads to a tirade. Once we recognize that psychological factors, stress-reducing interventions, and so on can influence something like cancer, it is often a hopeful, desperate leap to the conclusion that such factors can control cancer. When that proves to be false, there is a corrosive, poisonous flip side: if you falsely believe you had the power to prevent or cure cancer through positive thinking, you may then come to believe that it is your own fault if you are dying of the disease.

The advocates of a rather damaging overstatement of these psychology-health relationships are not always addled voices from the lunatic fringe. They include influential health practitioners whose medical degrees appear to lend credence to their extravagant claims. I will focus my attention here on the claims of Bernie S. Siegel, a Yale University surgeon who has been wildly effective at disseminating his ideas to the public as the author of a bestseller.

The premise of Siegel's still-popular magnum opus, *Love, Medicine and Miracles* (New York: Harper & Row, 1986), is that the most effective way of stimulating the immune system is through love, and that miraculous healing happens to patients who are brave enough to love. Siegel purports to demonstrate this.

As the book unfolds, you note that it is a strange world that Siegel inhabits. When operating on anesthetized patients, "I also do not hesitate to ask the [anesthetized] patient not to bleed if circumstances call for it," he asserts (p. 49). In his world, deceased patients come back as birds (p. 222), there are unnamed countries in which individuals consistently live for a century (p. 140), and best of all, people who have the right spirituality not only successfully fight cancer but can drive cars that consistently break down for other people (p. 137).

This is relatively benign gibberish, and history buffs may even feel comforted by those among us who live the belief system of medieval peasants. Where the problems become appallingly serious is when Siegel concentrates on the main point of his book. No matter how often he puts in disclaimers saying that he's not trying to make people feel guilty, the book's premise is that (a) cancer can be caused by psychosocial factors in the person; (b) cancer (or any other disease, as far as I can tell) is curable if the patient has sufficient courage, love, and spirit; (c) if the patient is not cured, it is because of insufficient amounts of those admirable traits. As we have just seen, this is not how cancer works, and a physician simply should not go about telling seriously ill people otherwise.

His book is full of descriptions of people who get cancer because of their uptightness and lack of spirituality. He speaks of one woman who was repressed in her feelings about her breasts: "*Naturally* [my emphasis], Jan got breast cancer" (p. 85)—this seems an indication that Siegel is aware of the literature on cancer-prone personality, but this constitutes a caricature of those mostly careful studies. Of another patient: "She held all her feelings inside and developed leukemia" (p. 164). Or, in an extraordinary statement: "Cancer generally seems to appear in response to loss . . . I believe that, if a person avoids emotional growth at this time, the impulse behind it becomes misdirected into malignant physical growth" (p. 123).

Naturally, those who do have enough courage, love, and spirit can defeat cancer. Sometimes it takes a little prodding from Siegel. He advises on page 108 that people with serious diseases consider the ways in which they may have wanted their illness because we are trained to associate sickness with reward; Siegel cites our receiving cards and flowers on page 110. Sometimes Siegel has to be a bit more forceful with a recalcitrant cancer patient. One woman was apparently inhibited about drawing something Siegel requested her to, being embarrassed about her poor drawing skills. "I asked [her] how she expected to get over cancer if she didn't even have the courage to do a picture" (p. 81). You know whose fault it was if she eventually died.

But once the good patients overcome their attitude problems and get with the program, miracles just start popping up everywhere you look. One patient with the proper visualizing techniques cured his cancer, his arthritis, and, as long as he was at it, his twenty-year problem with impotency as well (p. 153). Of another, Siegel writes: "She chose the path of life, and as she grew, her cancer shrank" (p. 113). Consider the following exchange (p. 175):

I came in, and he said, "Her cancer's gone."

"Phyllis," I said, "Tell them what happened."

She said, "Oh, you know what happened."

"I know that I know," I said, "But I'd like the others to know."

Phyllis replied, "I decided to live to be a hundred and leave my troubles to God."

I really could end the book here, because this peace of mind can heal anything.

Thus, presumably, people who die from cancer never got around to deciding to live to be a hundred. According to Siegel, cancer is curable with the right combination of attributes, and those people without them may get cancer and die of it. An incurable disease is the fault of the victim. He tries to soften his message now and then: "Cancer's complex causes aren't all in the mind," he says (p. 103), and on page 75 he tells us he's interested in a person gaining understanding of his or her role in a disease rather than in creating guilt. But when he gets past his anecdotes about individual patients and states his premise in its broadest terms, its toxicity is unmistakable: "The fundamental problem most patients face is an inability to love themselves" (p. 4); "I feel that all disease is ultimately related to a lack of love" (p. 180).

Siegel has a special place in his book for children with cancer and for the parents of those children trying to understand why it has occurred. After noting that developmental psychologists have learned that infants have considerably greater perceptual capacities than previously believed, Siegel says he "wouldn't be surprised if cancer in early childhood was linked to messages of parental conflict or disapproval perceived even in the womb" (p. 75). In other words, if your child gets cancer, consider the possibility that you caused it.*

And perhaps most directly: "There are no incurable diseases, only incurable people" (p. 99). (Compare the statement by the late stress researcher Herbert Weiner: "Diseases are mere abstractions; they can-

---

* This was something that inflamed me when first reading this book fifteen years ago as a puerile single guy; it does so to an indescribable extent now that I am a father of young children, and have peers suffering the hell of a seriously ill child.

not be understood without appreciating the person who is ill." Superficially, Siegel's and Weiner's notions bear some resemblance to each other. The latter, however, is a scientifically sound statement of the interactions between diseases and individual makeups of sick people; the former seems to me an unscientific distortion of those interactions.)

Since at least the Middle Ages, there has been a philosophical view of disease that is "lapsarian" in nature, characterizing illness as the punishment meted out by God for sin (all deriving from humankind's lapse in the Garden of Eden). Its adherents obviously predated any knowledge about germs, infection, or the workings of the body. This view has mostly passed (although see the endnote for this page for an extraordinary example of this thinking that festered in the Reagan administration), but as you read through Siegel's book, you unconsciously wait for its reemergence, knowing that disease has to be more than just not having enough groovy New Age spirituality, that God is going to be yanked into Siegel's world of blame as well. Finally, it bubbles to the surface on page 179: "I suggest that patients think of illness not as God's will but as our deviation from God's will. To me it is the absence of spirituality that leads to difficulties." Cancer, thus, is what you get when you deviate from God's will.

Oh, and one other thing about Siegel's views. He founded a cancer program called Exceptional Cancer Patients, which incorporates his many ideas about the nature of life, spirit, and disease. To my knowledge there have been only two published studies of his program and its effects on survival time. Both reported that the program has no significant effect on survival. And one last word from the good doctor (p. 185), washing his hands of the first study (the second had not yet been published when he wrote his book): "I prefer to deal with individuals and effective techniques, and let others take care of the statistics."

Why is it worth going on at length about this subject, to pay so much attention to a more-than-fifteen-year-old book? Because of how influential Siegel's style of thinking has been. Here is but one chilling example: in one study, breast cancer patients were asked what they thought had caused their cancer. Among the hundreds of participants, answers came back such as genetics, environment, hormones, diet, and breast trauma. And what was the most common attribution, by a wide margin? Stress. This, in a paper published in 2001, at the dawn of our new millennium.

This topic is one that I will return to in the final chapter of the book when I discuss stress management theories. Obviously, a theme of this book is just how many things can go wrong in the body because of stress and how important it is for everyone to recognize this. However, it would be utterly negligent to exaggerate the implications of this idea. Every child cannot grow up to be president; it turned out that merely by holding hands and singing folk songs we couldn't end all war, and hunger does not disappear just by visualizing a world without it. Everything bad in human health now is not caused by stress, nor is it in our power to cure ourselves of all our worst medical nightmares merely by reducing stress and thinking healthy thoughts full of courage and spirit and love. Would that it were so. And shame on those who would profit from selling this view.

 ## POSTSCRIPT: A GROTESQUE PIECE OF MEDICAL HISTORY

The notion that the mind can influence the immune system, that emotional distress can change resistance to certain diseases, is fascinating; psychoneuroimmunology exerts a powerful pull. Nevertheless, it sometimes amazes me just how many psychoneuroimmunologists are popping up. They are even beginning to speciate into subspecialties. Some study the issue only in humans, others in animals; some analyze epidemiological patterns in large populations, others study single cells. During breaks at scientific conferences, you can even get teams of psychoneuroimmunological pediatricians playing volleyball against the psychoneuroimmunological gerontologists. I am old enough, I confess frankly, to remember a time when there was no such thing as a psychoneuroimmunologist. Now, like an aging Cretaceous dinosaur, I watch these new mammals proliferating. There was even a time when it was not common knowledge that stress caused immune tissues to shrink—and as a result, medical researchers carried out some influential studies and misinterpreted their findings, which indirectly led to the deaths of thousands of people.

By the nineteenth century, scientists and doctors were becoming concerned with a new pediatric disorder. On certain occasions parents would place their apparently perfectly healthy infant in bed, tuck the blankets in securely, leave for a peaceful night's sleep—and return in the morning to find the child dead. "Crib death," or sudden infant death syndrome (SIDS), came to be recognized during that time. When it happened, one initially had to explore the unsettling possibility that there was foul play or parental abuse, but that was usually eliminated, and one was left with the mystery of healthy infants dying in their sleep for no discernible reason.

Today, scientists have made some progress in understanding SIDS. It seems to arise in infants who, during the third trimester of fetal life, have some sort of crisis where their brains do not get enough oxygen, causing certain neurons in the brain stem that control respiration to become especially vulnerable. But in the nineteenth century, no one had a clue as to what was going on.

Some pathologists began a logical course of research in the 1800s. They would carefully autopsy SIDS infants and compare them with the normal infant autopsy material. Here is where the subtle, fatal mistake occurred: "normal infant autopsy material." Who gets autopsied? Who gets practiced on by interns in teaching hospitals? Whose bodies wind up being dissected in gross anatomy by first-year medical students? Usually, it has been poor people.

The nineteenth century was the time when men with strong backs and a nocturnal bent could opt for a career as "resurrectionists"— grave robbers, body snatchers, who would sell corpses to anatomists at the medical schools for use in study and teaching. Overwhelmingly, the bodies of the poor, buried without coffins in shallow mass graves in potter's fields, were taken; the wealthy, by contrast, would be buried in triple coffins. As body-snatching anxiety spread, adaptations evolved for the wealthy. The "patent coffin" of 1818 was explicitly and expensively marketed to be resurrectionist-proof, and cemeteries of the gentry would offer a turn in the dead-house, where the well-guarded body could genteelly putrefy past the point of interest to the dissectors, at which time it could be safely buried. This period, moreover, gave rise to the verb *burking,* named after one William Burke, the aging resurrectionist who pioneered the practice of luring beggars in for a charitable meal and then strangling them for a quick sale to the anatomists. (Ironic-ending department: Burke and his sidekick, after their execution, were handed over to the anatomists. Their dissection included particular attention to their skulls, with an attempt to find phrenological causes of their heinous crimes.)

All very helpful for the biomedical community, but with some drawbacks. The poor tended to express a riotous displeasure with the medico–body snatcher complex (to coin a phrase). Frenzied crowds lynched resurrectionists who were caught, attacked the homes of anatomists, burned hospitals. Concerned about the mayhem caused by unregulated preying on the bodies of the poor, governments moved decisively to supervise the preying. In the early nineteenth century, various European governments acted to supply adequate bodies to the anatomists, put the burkers and resurrectionists out of business, and keep the poor in line—all with one handy little law: anyone who died destitute in a poorhouse or a pauper's hospital would now be turned over to the dissectors.

Doctors were thus trained in what the normal human body looked like by studying the bodies and tissues of the poor. Yet the bodies of poor people are changed by the stressful circumstances of their poverty. In the "normal" autopsy population of six-month-olds, the infants had typically died of chronic diarrheal disorders, malnutrition, tuberculosis. Prolonged, stressful diseases. Their thymus glands had shrunk.

We now return to our pathologists, comparing the bodies of SIDS infants with those of "normal" dead infants. By definition, if children had been labeled as having died of SIDS, there was nothing else wrong with them. No prior stressors. No shrinking of the thymus gland. The researchers begin their studies and discover something striking: SIDS kids had thymuses much larger than those of "normal "dead infants. This is where they got things backward. Not knowing that stress shrinks the thymus gland, they assumed that the thymuses in the "normal" autopsy population were normal. They concluded that some children have an *abnormally* large thymus gland, and that SIDS is caused by that large thymus pressing down on the trachea and one night suffocating the child. Soon this imaginary disorder had a fancy name, "status thymicolymphaticus."

This supposed biological explanation for SIDS provided a humane substitute for the usual explanation at the time, which was to assume that the parents were either criminal or incompetent, and some of the most progressive physicians of the time endorsed the "big thymus" story (including Rudolph Virchow, a hero of chapter 17). The trouble was, the physicians decided to make some recommendations for how to *prevent* SIDS, based on this nonsense. It seemed perfectly logical at the time. Get rid of that big thymus. Maybe do it surgically, which turned out to be a bit tricky. Soon, the treatment of choice emerged: shrink the thymus through irradiation. Estimates are that in the ensuing decades it caused tens of thousands of cases of cancers in the thyroid gland, which sits near the thymus. When I lecture on this subject, I regularly encounter people whose parents, as late as the 1950s, had their throats irradiated for this reason.

What recommendations does one offer from the history of status thymicolymphaticus? I could try for some big ones. That so long as all people are not born equal and certainly don't get to live equally, we should at least be dissected equally. How about something even more grandiose, such as that something should be done about infants getting small thymuses from economic inequality.

Okay, I'll aim for something on a more manageable scientific scale. For example, while we expend a great deal of effort doing extraordinary things in medical research—say, sequencing the human genome—we still need smart people to study some of the moronically simple problems, like "how big is a normal thymus?" Because they are often not so simple. Maybe another lesson is that confounds can come from unexpected quarters—bands of very smart public health researchers wrestle with that idea for a living. Perhaps the best moral is that when doing science (or perhaps when doing anything at all in a society as judgmental as our own), be very careful and very certain before pronouncing something to be the norm—because at that instant, you have made it supremely difficult to ever again look objectively at an exception to that supposed norm.

STRESS AND PAIN

 In Joseph Heller's classic novel about World War II, *Catch-22*, the antihero, Yossarian, has an unlikely argument with someone about the nature of God. Unlikely because they are both atheists, which would presumably lead to agreement about the subject. However, it turns out that while Yossarian merely does not believe in the existence of a God and is rather angry about the whole concept, the God that she does not believe in is one who is good and warm and loving, and thus she is offended by the vehemence of his attacks.

"How much reverence can you have for a Supreme Being who finds it necessary to include such phenomena as phlegm and tooth decay in His divine system of creation? What in the world was running through that warped, evil, scatological mind of His when He robbed old people of the power to control their bowel movements? Why in the world did He ever create pain?"

"Pain?" Lieutenant Scheisskopf's wife pounced upon the word victoriously. "Pain is a useful symptom. Pain is a warning to us of bodily dangers."

"And who created the dangers?" Yossarian demanded. He laughed caustically. "Oh, He was really being charitable to us when He gave us pain! Why couldn't He have used a doorbell instead to notify us, or one of his celestial choirs? Or a system of blue-and-red neon tubes right in the middle of each person's forehead. Any jukebox manufacturer worth his salt could have done that. Why couldn't He?"

"People would certainly look silly walking around with red neon tubes in the middle of their foreheads."

"They certainly look beautiful now writhing in agony or stupefied with morphine, don't they?"

Unfortunately, we lack neon lights in the middle of our foreheads, and in the absence of such innocuous signs, we probably do need pain perception. Pain can hurt like hell, but it can inform us that we are sitting too close to the fire, or that we should never again eat the novel item that just gave us food poisoning. It effectively discourages us from trying to walk on an injured limb that is better left immobilized until it heals. And in our westernized lives, it is often a good signal that we had better see a doctor before it is too late. People who congenitally lack the ability to feel pain (a condition known as *pain asymbolia*) are a mess; because they can't feel pain when they step down with too much force, their feet may ulcerate, their knee joints may disintegrate, and their long bones may crack; they burn themselves unawares; in some cases, they even lose a toe without knowing it.

Pain is useful to the extent that it motivates us to modify our behaviors in order to reduce whatever insult is causing the pain, because invariably that insult is damaging our tissues. Pain is useless and debilitating, however, when it is telling us that there is something dreadfully wrong that we can do nothing about. We must praise the fact that we have evolved a physiological system that lets us know when our stomachs are empty. Yet at the same time we must deeply rue our evolving physiological system that can wrack a terminal cancer patient with unrelenting pain.

Pain, until we get the lights on our foreheads, will remain a necessary but highly problematic part of our natural physiology. What is surprising is how malleable pain signals are—how readily the intensity of a pain signal is changed by the sensations, feelings, and thoughts that coincide with the pain. One example of this modulation, the blunting of pain perception during some circumstances of stress, is the subject of this chapter.

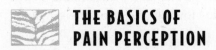 ## THE BASICS OF PAIN PERCEPTION

The sensation of pain originates in receptors located throughout our body. Some are deep within the body, telling us about muscle aches, fluid-filled, swollen joints, or damage to organs. Or even something as

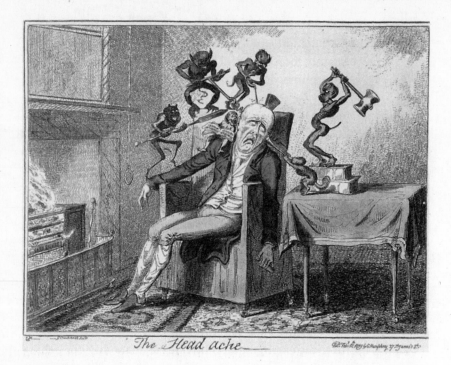

George Cruikshank, The Headache, *hand-colored etching, 1819.*

mundane as a distended bladder. Others, in our skin, can tell us that we have been cut, burned, abraded, poked, or compressed.* Often, these skin receptors respond to the signal of local tissue damage. Cut yourself with a paring knife, and you will slice open various cells of microscopic size that then spill out their proverbial guts; and, typically, within this cellular soup now flooding out of the area of injury is a variety of chemical messengers that trigger pain receptors into action. The tissue injury also triggers an influx of cells of the immune system, which are there to scarf up and dispose of those sliced-up cells. The swelling around the injury site because of this infiltration is what we call inflammation, and those inflammatory cells release chemicals that make pain receptors more sensitive.

Some pain receptors carry information only about pain (for example, the ones responding to cuts); others carry information about both pain and everyday sensations. How are the two differentiated?

---

* Great factoids: the pain receptors that respond to heat contain receptors for something called capsaicin. What is capsaicin? A compound found in red chilies. That's why spicy food tastes hot. And what other type of receptor is found in those same neurons? One that responds to the key component of horseradish, wasabi, and mustard.

By intensity. For example, by way of various tactile receptors on my back, I am greatly pleased to have my back scratched and rubbed by my wife. However, as evidence that there are limits to all good things, I would not at all enjoy it if she vigorously scratched my back with coarse sandpaper. Similarly, we may be pleased to have our thermal receptors stimulated by warm sunlight but not by boiling water. Sometimes pain consists of everyday sensations writ large.

Regardless of the particular type of pain and the particular receptor activated, all these receptors send nerve projections to the spinal cord. This can activate a *spinal reflex*, where spinal neurons rapidly send commands to your muscles (and thus, for example, you jerk your finger away from the flame). Information about the painful stimulus is also sent up to the brain (a lot more on this later).

SENSORY MODULATION OF PAIN PERCEPTION

A striking aspect of the pain system is how readily it can be modulated by other factors. The strength of a pain signal, for example, can depend on what other sensory information is funneled to the spine at the same time. This, it turns out, is why it feels great to have a massage when you have sore muscles. Chronic, throbbing pain can be inhibited by certain types of sharp, brief sensory stimulation.

The physiology behind this is one of the most elegant bits of wiring I know of in the nervous system, a circuit sorted out some decades ago by the physiologists Patrick Wall and Ronald Melzack. It turns out that the nervous projections—the fibers carrying pain information from your periphery to the spinal cord—are not all of one kind. Instead, they come in different classes. Probably the most relevant dichotomy is between fibers that carry information about acute, sharp, sudden pain and those that carry information about slow, diffuse, constant, throbbing pain. Both project to spinal cord neurons and activate them, but in different ways (see part A of the figure on page 190).

Two types of neurons found in the spinal cord are being affected by painful information (see part B of the illustration). The first (X) is the same neuron diagrammed before, which relays pain information to the brain. The second neuron (Y) is a local one called an *interneuron*. When Y is stimulated, it inhibits the activity of X.

As things are wired up, when a sharp, painful stimulus is felt, the information is sent on the fast fiber. This stimulates both neurons X and Y. As a result, X sends a painful signal up the spinal cord, and an

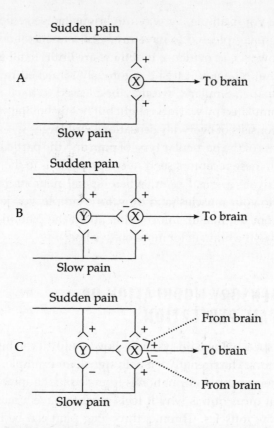

The Wall-Melzack model of how pain information is passed to the brain, and how it can be modulated by the brain. (A) A neuron (X) in the spinal cord sends a signal to the brain that something painful has happened, once it is stimulated by a pain fiber. Such pain fibers can carry information about sudden pain or slow, diffuse pain. (B) A more realistic version of how the system actually works, showing why sudden and slow pain information is differentiated. In the case of sudden pain, the sudden pain fiber stimulates neuron X, causing a pain signal to be relayed to the brain. The sudden pain fiber also stimulates an interneuron (Y) that inhibits neuron X, after a brief delay. Thus, neuron X sends a pain signal to the brain for only a short time. In contrast, the slow pain fiber stimulates neuron X and inhibits interneuron Y. Thus, Y does not inhibit X, and X continues to send a pain signal to the brain, producing a slow, diffuse pain. (C) Both stimulatory and inhibitory fibers come from the brain and send information to neuron X, modulating its sensitivity to incoming pain information. Thus, the brain can sensitize neuron X to a painful signal, or blunt its sensitivity.

instant later, Y kicks in and shuts X off. Thus the brain senses a brief, sharp burst of pain, such as after stepping on a tack.

By contrast, when a dull, throbbing pain is felt, the information is sent on the slow fiber. It communicates with both neurons X and Y, but differently from the way it does on the fast fiber. Once again the X neuron is stimulated and lets the brain know that something painful has occurred. This time, however, the slow fiber *inhibits* the Y neuron from firing. Y remains silent, X keeps firing, and your brain senses a prolonged, throbbing pain, the type you'd feel for hours or days after you've burned yourself. The pain physiologist David Yeomans has framed the functions of the fast and slow fibers in a way that fits perfectly with this book: what the fast fibers are about is getting you to move as quickly as possible (from the source of the piercing pain). What the slow fibers are about is getting you to hunker down, immobile, so you can heal.

The two classes of fibers can interact, and we often intentionally force them to. Suppose that you have some sort of continuous, throbbing pain—sore muscles, an insect bite, a painful blister. How can you stop the throbbing? Briefly stimulate the fast fiber. This adds to the pain for an instant, but by stimulating the Y interneuron, you shut the system down for a while. And that is precisely what we often do in all of those circumstances. Experiencing a good vigorous mauling massage inhibits the dull throbbing pain of sore muscles for a while. An insect bite throbs and itches unbearably, and we often scratch hard right around it to dull the pain. Or we'll pinch ourselves. In all these cases, the slow chronic pain pathway is shut down for up to a few minutes.

This model has had important clinical implications. For one thing, it has allowed scientists to design treatments for people with severe chronic pain syndromes (for example, a patient who has had a nerve root crushed in his back). By implanting a little electrode into the fast pain pathway and attaching it to a stimulator on the person's hip, they enable the patient to buzz that pathway now and then to turn off the chronic pain; works wonders in many cases.

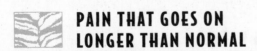

PAIN THAT GOES ON LONGER THAN NORMAL

If someone pokes you over and over, you will continue to feel pain each time. Similarly, if you get an injury that causes days of inflammation, there are likely to be days of pain as well. But sometimes, something goes wrong with pain pathways somewhere between those pain receptors and your spine, and you feel pain long after the noxious stimulus has stopped or the injury has healed, or you feel pain in response to stimuli that shouldn't be painful at all. Now you've got problems—*allodynia*, which is feeling pain in response to a normal stimulus.

Some versions of allodynia can arise down at the level of the pain receptors themselves. Recall how when there is tissue injury, inflammatory cells infiltrate into the area and release chemicals that make those local pain receptors more excitable, more easily stimulated. Now those inflammatory cells are pretty indiscriminate as to where they dump these chemicals, and some of them can leach over in the direction of receptors outside the area of injury, thereby making them more excitable. And suddenly the perfectly healthy tissue surrounding the injured area starts to hurt as well.

Allodynia can also occur when neurons in the pain pathway are injured. If nerve endings are severed near the pain receptors, those inflammatory cells release growth promoting factors that prompt the nerves to regenerate. Sometimes the regeneration is bollixed up so that the nerve endings rewire into a tangle called a neuroma, which tends to be hyperexcitable, sending pain signals from perfectly healthy tissue. And if the nerve projections carrying pain information are severed near the spine, this can lead to a cascade of inflammatory events that results in a hyperexcitable spinal cord. A mere touch now feels excruciating.

The Wall-Melzack pathway model on page 190 explains another instance of allodynia, as seen in severe cases of both types of diabetes. As we saw in chapter 4, elevated levels of glucose in the bloodstream can increase the risk of atherosclerotic plaques, clogging up blood vessels. As a result, insufficient energy gets through those vessels, potentially damaging nerves that depend on that energy. In general it is the fast fibers, which take more energy to operate than the lower-maintenance slow fibers, that are damaged. Thus, the person loses the ability to shut down the Y interneuron in that pathway, and what would be a transient pain for anyone else becomes a constant throbbing one for a diabetic.

 NO BRAIN, NO PAIN

We started with pain receptors scattered all over the body, and have gotten as far as the spinal cord receiving projections from them. From there, a lot of those spinal neurons that are activated by pain send projections up into the brain. This is where things become really interesting.

Consider three scenarios involving pain. First, a soldier is in the middle of some appalling battle, people being slaughtered all around. He is injured—not life-threatening, but serious enough to warrant evacuation. Second, consider someone with advanced liver cancer, administered an experimental drug. Within a few days, her gut hurts like hell, a sign of the drug killing the tumor cells. Or third, someone is abrading their rear end raw while enthusiastically having sex on a rough carpet. What do they all have in common? Their pain's not going to seem all that painful—the war's over for me; the drug's working; what carpet? The brain's interpretation of pain can be extremely subjective.

A study conducted in the 1980s provides a striking example of this subjectivity. A scientist examined a decade's worth of records at a suburban hospital, noting how many painkillers were requested by patients who had just had gallbladder surgery. It turned out that patients who had views of trees from their windows requested significantly less pain medication than those who looked out on blank walls. Other studies of chronic pain patients show that manipulating psychological variables such as the sense of control over events also dramatically changes the quantity of painkillers that they request (this important finding will be elaborated upon in the final chapter of the book).

This is because the brain is not a mindless pain-ometer, simply measuring units of ouchness. Certainly some parts of the brain allow you to make some objective assessments ("Whoa, this water is WAY too hot for the baby's bath"). And there are factors that can modulate how much those pain-ometer areas register pain—for example, oxytocin, the hormone released in connection with birth and maternal behavior in mammals, will blunt pain responsiveness in these pathways. But most of what the brain's responses to pain are about is generating emotional responses and giving contextual interpretations about the pain. This is how being shot in the thigh, gasping in pain, can also leave you gasping in euphoric triumph—I've survived this war, I'm going home.

Three important things about the emotional ways the brain interprets and responds to pain:

First, the emotional/interpretative level can be dissociated from the objective amount of pain signal that is coursing up to the brain from the spine. In other words, how much pain you feel, and how unpleasant that pain feels, can be two separate things. That's implicit in the war, cancer, and tush-abrading scenarios. An elegant study shows it more explicitly. In it, volunteers dipped their hands into hot water before and after being given a hypnotic suggestion that they feel no pain. During both hand dips, brain imaging was carried out to show which parts of the brain were becoming active. The sensation-processing part of the cortex (kind of a pain-ometer in this case) was activated to identical extents in both cases, reflecting the similar number of heat-sensitive pain receptors being triggered to roughly the equivalent extent in both cases. But the more emotional parts of the brain activated only in the pre-hypnosis case. The pain was the same in both cases; the response to it was not.

As a second point, those more emotive parts of the brain not only can alter how you respond to pain information coming up the spinal cord; those areas of the brain can alter how the spinal cord *responds* to pain information.

And the third point: this is where stress comes in big time.

 ## STRESS-INDUCED ANALGESIA

Chapter 1 recounted anecdotal cases of people who, highly aroused during battle, did not notice a severe injury. This is certainly a useful thing for a soldier, or a zebra, who still needs to function despite those circumstances. One of the first to document this phenomenon of stress-induced analgesia was an anesthesiologist, Henry Beecher, who examined injured soldiers as a battlefront medic in World War II and compared them with civilian populations. He found that for injuries of similar severity, approximately 80 percent of civilians requested morphine, while only a third of the soldiers did.

Few of us experience stress-induced analgesia in the midst of battle. For us, it is more likely to happen during some sporting event where, if we are sufficiently excited and involved in what we are doing, we can easily ignore an injury. On a more everyday level, stress-induced analgesia is experienced by the droves who exercise. Invariably the first stretch is agony, as you search for every possible excuse to stop before you suffer the coronary that you now fear. Then suddenly, about half an hour into this self-flagellation, the pain melts away. You even start feeling oddly euphoric. The whole venture seems like the most pleasant self-improvement conceivable, and you plan to work out like this daily until your hundredth birthday (with all vows, of course, forgotten the next day when you start the painful process all over again).*

Traditionally many hard-nosed laboratory scientists, when encountering something like stress-induced analgesia, would relegate it to the "psychosomatic" realm, dismissing it as some fuzzy aspect of "mind over matter." The analgesia, however, is a real biological phenomenon.

One bit of evidence for that assertion is that stress-induced analgesia occurs in other animals as well, not just in humans emotionally invested in the success of their nation's army or their office's softball team. This can be shown in animals with the "hot-plate test." Put a rat on a hot plate; then turn it on. Carefully time how long it takes for the rat to feel the first smidgen of discomfort, when it picks up its foot for the first time (at which point the rat is removed from the hot plate). Now do the same thing to a rat that has been stressed—forced to swim in a tank of water, exposed to the smell of a cat, whatever. It will take longer for this rat to notice the heat of the plate: stress-induced analgesia.

The best evidence that such analgesia is a real phenomenon is the neurochemistry that has been discovered to underlie it. The tale begins in the 1970s, with the subject that interested every ambitious, cutting-edge neurochemist of the time. It concerned the various opiate drugs that were being used recreationally in vast numbers: heroin, morphine, opium, all of which have similar chemical structures. In the early 1970s, three groups of neurochemists almost simultaneously demonstrated that these opiate drugs bound to specific opiate receptors in the brain. And these receptors tended to be located in the parts of the brain that process pain perception. This turned out to solve the problem of how opiate drugs block pain—they activate those descending pathways that blunt the sensitivity of the X neuron shown in the illustration on page 190.

Terrific—but two beats later, something puzzling hits you. Why should the brain make receptors for a class of compounds synthesized in poppy plants? The realization rushes in; there must be some chemical—a neurotransmitter? a hormone?—made in the body that is

---

* A recent study that I find fascinating: Take a bunch of jocks, of both genders, let them compete at their sport, and you'll find that they've developed stress-induced analgesia as a result (as measured by, say, their ability to keep their hand in a bucket of ice water for a longer period after the athletics than before). For the women, the key variable is the exercise, in that the analgesia will also be produced by time on an exercise bike. In contrast, for the men, the key variable is the competition, in that the analgesia is also induced by a competitive video game.

structurally similar to opiates. Some kind of endogenous morphine must occur naturally in the brain.

Neurochemists went wild at this point looking for endogenous morphine. Soon they found exactly what they were looking for: endogenous compounds with chemical structures reminiscent of the opiate drugs. They turned out to come in three different classes— enkephalins, dynorphins, and the most famous of them all, *endorphins* (a contraction for "endogenous morphines"). The opiate receptors were discovered to bind these endogenous opioid compounds, just as predicted. Furthermore, the opioids were synthesized and released in parts of the brain that regulated pain perception, and they would make some of the neurons that relay pain signals in the spine less excitable. (*Opiate* refers to analgesics not normally made by the body, such as heroin or morphine. *Opioid* refers to those made by the body itself. Because the field began with the study of the opiates—since no one had discovered the opioids as yet—the receptors found then were called *opiate receptors*. But clearly, their real job is to bind the opioids.)

Chapter 7 introduced the finding that the endorphins and enkephalins also regulate sex hormone release. An additional intriguing finding concerning opioid action emerged: release of these compounds explained how acupuncture worked. Until the 1970s, many Western scientists had heard about the phenomenon, but most had written it off, dumping it into a bucket of anthropological oddities—inscrutable Chinese herbalists sticking needles into people, Haitian shamans killing with voodoo curses, Jewish mothers curing any and all diseases with their secret-recipe chicken soup. Then, right around the time of the explosion in opiate research, Nixon ventured to China, and documentation started coming out from there about the reality of acupuncture. Furthermore, scientists noted that Chinese veterinarians used acupuncture to do surgery on animals, thereby refuting the argument that the painkilling characteristic of acupuncture was one big placebo effect ascribable to cultural conditioning (no cow on earth will go along with unanesthetized surgery just because it has a heavy investment in the cultural mores of the society in which it dwells). Then, as the corker, a prominent Western journalist (James Reston of the *New York Times*) got appendicitis in China, underwent surgery, and was administered acupuncture for pain relief. He survived just fine. Hey, this stuff must be legit—it even works on white guys.

Acupuncture stimulates the release of large quantities of endogenous opioids, for reasons no one really understands. The best demonstration of this is what is called a subtraction experiment: block the activity of endogenous opioids by using a drug that blocks the opiate receptor (most commonly a drug called naloxone). When such a receptor is blocked, acupuncture no longer effectively dulls the perception of pain.

Endogenous opioids turn out to be relevant to explaining placebos as well. A placebo effect occurs when a person's health improves, or the person's assessment of their health improves, merely because they believe that a medical procedure has been carried out on them, regardless of whether it actually has. This is where patients in a study either get the new medicine being tested or, without knowing it, merely a sugar pill, and sugar pill folks get somewhat better. Placebo effects remain controversial. A highly publicized paper in the *New England Journal of Medicine* a few years back surveyed the efficacy of placebo treatments across the board in all realms of medicine. The authors examined the results of 114 different studies, and concluded that, overall, receiving a placebo treatment had no significant effects. The study irritated me no end, because the authors included all sorts of realms where it seemed crazy to expect a placebo effect to occur. For example, the study informed us that believing you've received an effective medical treatment when you actually have not has no beneficial effects for epilepsy, elevated cholesterol levels, infertility, a bacterial infection, Alzheimer's disease, anemia, or schizophrenia.

Thus, the placebo effect got trashed and, amid the triumphant chest-thumping by all sorts of dead-white-male elements of the medical establishment, what was lost in that paper was a clear indication that placebo effects are highly effective against pain.

This makes a great deal of sense, given what we have now seen about pain processing in the brain. As an example of such a placebo effect, IV infusion of painkillers is more effective if the patient sees the infusion occurring than if it is done on the sly—knowing that a pain-reducing procedure is being carried out adds to its effectiveness. I saw a great example of this a few years back when my then two-year-old daughter came down with an ear infection. She was miserable beyond consolation, clearly in tons of pain. Off to the pediatrician and, amid much wailing and protestations of pain, she had her ears examined. Yup, she's got a huge infection, both ears, said the doc, disappearing to get an injection of antibiotics. We turn to find our daughter looking serene. "My ears feel much better now that the doctor fixed them," she announced. Placeboed by having some instrument stuck in her ears.

Not surprisingly, it turns out that they work by releasing endogenous opioids. As but one example of the evidence for that, block opiate receptors with naloxone, and placebos no longer work.

All of this is a prelude to the discovery that stress releases opioids as well. This finding was first reported in 1977 by Roger Guillemin. Fresh from winning the Nobel Prize for the discoveries described in chapter 2, he demonstrated that stress triggers the release of one type of endorphin, beta-endorphin, from the pituitary gland.

The rest is history. We all know about the famed runner's high that kicks in after about half an hour and creates that glowing, irrational euphoria, just because the pain has gone away. During exercise, beta-endorphin pours out of the pituitary gland, finally building up to levels in the bloodstream around the 30-minute mark that will cause analgesia. The other opiates, especially the enkephalins, are mobilized as well, mostly within the brain and spine. They activate the descending pathway originating in the brain to shut off the X neurons in the spinal cord, and they work directly at the spinal cord to accomplish the same thing. Moreover, they also work at the pain receptors in the skin and organs, blunting their sensitivity. All sorts of other stressors produce similar effects. Surgery, low blood sugar, exposure to cold, examinations, spinal taps, childbirth—all do it.* Certain stressors also cause analgesia through "nonopioid-mediated" pathways. No one is quite sure how those work, nor whether there is a systematic pattern as to which stressors are opioid-mediated.

So stress blocks pain perception, enabling you to sprint away from the lion despite your mauling, or at least to put up with the muscle ache of smiling obsequiously non-stop during the stressful meeting with the boss. This explains everything. Unless it happens to be the sort of stressful situation that makes pain *worse* instead of better.

 ## WHY IS MUZAK IN THE DENTIST'S OFFICE PAINFUL?

All that stress-induced analgesia stuff may be swell for that disemboweled zebra, but what if you're the sort of person where just seeing the nurse taking the cap off the hypodermic needle for the blood draw makes your arm throb? What we've got now is stress-induced *hyper*algesia.

The phenomenon is well documented, if studied less than stress-induced analgesia. What is known about it makes perfect sense, in that

---

* It should be obvious to anyone who has gone through childbirth or at least observed it at close quarters—as I have twice since the previous edition's version of this chapter was written—that those opiates do squat once those contractions really get going.

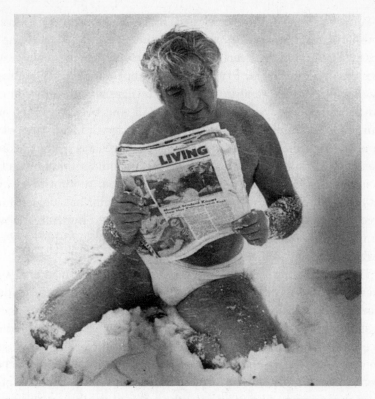

Vic Boff, New York Polar Bear Club member known as "Mr. Iceberg," sitting in the snow after a swim during the blizzard of 1978.

stress-induced hyperalgesia does not actually involve more pain perception, and has nothing to do with pain receptors or the spinal cord. Instead, it involves more emotional reactivity to pain, interpreting the same sensation as more unpleasant. So stress-induced hyperalgesia is just in your head. On the other hand, so is stress-induced analgesia, just a different part of your head. The pain-ometer parts of your brain respond to pain normally in people with stress-induced hyperalgesia. It's the more emotional parts of the brain that are hyperreactive, the parts of the brain that are the core of our anxieties and fears.

This can be shown with brain-imaging studies, showing what parts of pain circuitry in the brain become overly active during such hyperalgesia. Moreover, anti-anxiety drugs like Valium and Librium block stress-induced hyperalgesia. People who score high on tests for neuroticism and anxiety are most prone toward hyperalgesia during stress. Amazingly, so are rat strains that have been bred for high anxiety.

So we're at one of those crossroads that makes science look kind of lame. Just like, "Stress can increase appetite. And it can decrease it, too," we've got, "Stress can blunt pain perception. But sometimes it does the opposite." How to combine these opposing effects of stress? My sense from the literature is that the analgesia arises more in circumstances of massive, physical injury. Half your body is burned and your ankle's sprained, and you're trying to carry a loved one out of some inferno—that's when stress-induced analgesia is going to dominate. Discover some weirdo growth on your shoulder that hurts a bit, decide in a panic that you've got fatal melanoma, be informed by an unsympathetic answering machine that your doctor has just left for a three-day weekend. That's when the stress-induced hyperalgesia will dominate, as you lie awake for three nights, thanks to how painful you've now decided the spot feels.

This brings up a subject that needs to be treaded on carefully. So carefully in fact that in the last edition of the book, I bravely made a point of not mentioning a word about it. Fibromyalgia. This is the mysterious syndrome of people having markedly reduced pain tolerance and multiple tender spots throughout the body, often paralyzing extents of pain, and no one can find anything wrong—no pinched nerve, no arthritis, no inflammation. Mainstream medicine has spent decades consigning fibromyalgia to the realm of psychosomatic medicine (that is, "Get out of my office and go see a shrink"). It doesn't help that fibromyalgia is more likely to strike people with anxious or neurotic personalities. There's nothing wrong, is the typical medical conclusion. But this may not quite be the case. For starters, sufferers have abnormally high levels of activity in parts of the brain that mediate the emotional/contextual assessments of pain, the same areas activated in stress-induced hyperalgesia. Moreover, their cerebral spinal fluid contains elevated levels of a neurotransmitter that mediates pain (called Substance P). And, as noted in chapter 2, unexpectedly, glucocorticoid levels are below normal in people with fibromyalgia. Maybe these are highly stressed people with some sort of defect in glucocorticoid secretion, and because of that deficiency, instead of getting stress-induced analgesia, they get hyperalgesia.* I don't know. No one knows, as far as I can tell. But there is increasing evidence that there is something biologically real going on in these cases. There, I've broken the ice on this subject; stay tuned for the next edition.

---

* However, just to complicate that speculation, glucocorticoids are not particularly involved in stress-induced analgesia.

PAIN AND CHRONIC STRESS

Time now for our usual question. What happens with pain perception when there is chronic stress? With stress-induced hyperalgesia, the answer seems to be, the pain just keeps going, maybe even worsens. But what about stress-induced analgesia? In the acute, lion-mauling scenario, it is adaptive. To follow the structure laid out in previous chapters, this represents the good news. So what's the bad news? How does an excess of opioid release make us sick in the face of the chronic psychological stressors that we specialize in? Does chronic stress make you an endogenous opioid addict? Does it cause so much of the stuff to be released that you can't detect useful pain anymore? What's the downside in the face of chronic stress?

Here the answer is puzzling because it differs from all the other physiological systems examined in this book. When Hans Selye first began to note that chronic stress causes illness, he thought that illness occurs because an organism runs out of the stress-response, that the various hormones and neurotransmitters are depleted, and the organism is left undefended to the pummelings of the stressor. As we've seen in previous chapters, the modern answer is that the stress-response doesn't become depleted; instead, one gets sick because the stress-response itself eventually becomes damaging.

Opioids turn out to be the exception to the rule. Stress-induced analgesia does not go on forever, and the best evidence ascribes this to depletion of opioids. You are not permanently out of business, but it takes a while for supply to catch up with demand.

Thus, to my knowledge, there is no stress-related disease that results from too much opioid release during sustained stressors. From the standpoint of this book and our propensity toward chronic psychological stressors, that is good news—one less stress-related disease to worry about. From the standpoint of pain perception and the world of real physical stressors, the eventual depletion of the opioids means that the soothing effects of stress-induced analgesia are just a short-term fix. And for the elderly woman agonizing through terminal cancer, the soldier badly injured in combat, the zebra ripped to shreds but still alive, the consequence is obvious. The pain will soon return.

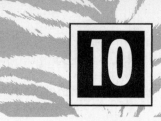

10

STRESS AND MEMORY

I'm old now, very old. I've seen a lot of things in my time and by now, I've forgotten a lot of them but, I tell you, that was one day that I'll remember forever like it was yesterday. I was twenty-four, maybe twenty-five. It was a cold spring morning. Raw, gray. Gray sky, gray slush, gray people. I was looking for a job again and not having much luck, my stomach complaining about the bad rooming house coffee that was last night's dinner and today's breakfast. I was feeling pretty hungry, and I suspect I was starting to look pretty hungry too, like some half-starved animal that picks through a garbage can, and that couldn't make much of an impression in an interview. And neither could the shabby jacket I was wearing, that last one I hadn't hocked.

I was plodding along, lost in my thoughts, when some guy comes sprinting around the corner, yelling with excitement, hands up in the air. Before I could even get a good look at him, he was shouting in my face. He was babbling, yelling about something being "classic," something called "classic." I couldn't understand what he was talking about, and then he sprinted off. What the hell, crazy guy, I thought.

But round the next corner, I see more people running around, yelling. Two of them, a man and woman, come running up to me and, by now, I tell you, I knew that something was up. They grabbed me by the arms, shouting "We won! We won!! We're getting it back!" They were pretty excited but at least making more sense than the first guy, and I finally figured out what they were saying. I couldn't believe it. I tried to speak, but I got all choked up, so I hugged them as if they were my brother and sister. The three of us ran into the street, where a big crowd was forming—people coming out of the office buildings, people stopping their cars, jumping out. Everyone screaming and crying and laughing, people shouting, "We won! We won!" Somebody told me a pregnant woman had gone right into labor, another that some old man had fainted right away. I saw a bunch of Navy guys, and one of them stepped right up and kissed this woman, a total stranger, leaning her way back—someone snapped a picture of them kissing, and I heard it became famous afterward.

The weird thing is how long ago this was—the couple who first told me are probably long gone, but I can still see their faces, remember how they were dressed, the smell of the guy's aftershave, the feel of the breeze that was blowing the confetti that people were tossing out the windows above. Still vivid. The mind's a funny thing. Well anyway, as I was saying, that's a day I'll always remember—the day they brought back the original Coke.

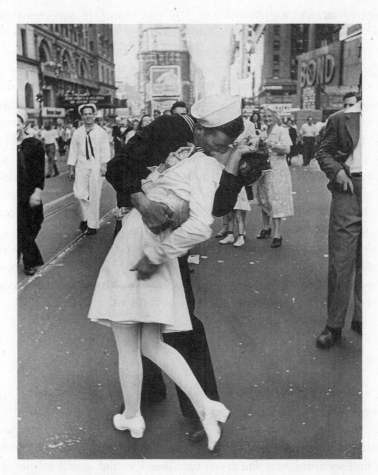

A day to remember!

We've all had similar experiences. Your first kiss. Your wedding ceremony. The moment when the war ended. And the same for the bad moments as well. The fifteen seconds when those two guys mugged you. The time the car spun out of control and just missed the oncoming truck. Where you were when the earthquake hit, when Kennedy was shot, on 9/11. All etched forever in your mind, when it's inconceivable that you can recall the slightest thing about incidents in the twenty-four hours before that life-changing event. Arousing, exciting, momentous occasions, including stressful ones, get filed away readily. Stress can enhance memory.

At the same time, we've all had the opposite experience. You're in the middle of the final exam, nervous and frazzled, and you simply can't remember a fact that would come effortlessly at any other time. You're in some intimidating social circumstance, and, of course, at the critical moment, you can't remember the name of the person you have to introduce. The first time I was "brought home" to meet my future wife's family, I was nervous as hell; during a frantically competitive word game after dinner, I managed to blow the lead of the team consisting of my future mother-in-law and me by my utter inability at one critical juncture to remember the word *casserole*. And some of these instances of failed memory revolve around infinitely greater traumas—the combat vet who went through some unspeakable battle catastrophe, the survivor of childhood sexual abuse—for whom the details are lost in an amnesiac fog. Stress can disrupt memory.

By now, this dichotomy should seem quite familiar. If stress enhances some function under one circumstance and disrupts it under another, think time course, think 30-second sprints across the savanna versus decades of grinding worry. Short-term stressors of mild to moderate severity enhance cognition, while major or prolonged stressors are disruptive. In order to appreciate how stress affects memory, we need to know something about how memories are formed (consolidated), how they are retrieved, how they can fail.

 ## A PRIMER ON HOW MEMORY WORKS

To begin, memory is not monolithic, but instead comes in different flavors. One particularly important dichotomy distinguishes short-term versus long-term memories. With the former, you look up a phone number, sprint across the room convinced you're about to forget it, punch in the number. And then it's gone forever. Short-term memory is your brain's equivalent of juggling some balls in the air for 30 seconds. In contrast, long-term memory refers to remembering what you had for dinner last night, the name of the U.S. president, how many grandchildren you have, where you went to college. Neuropsychologists are coming to recognize that there is a specialized subset of long-term memory. Remote memories are ones stretching back to your childhood—the name of your village, your native language, the smell of your grandmother's baking. They appear to be stored in some sort of archival way in your brain separate from more recent long-term memories. Often, in patients with a dementia that devastates most long-term memory, the more remote facets can remain intact.

Another important distinction in memory is that between *explicit* (also known as *declarative*) memory and *implicit* (which includes an important subtype called *procedural* memory) memory. Explicit memory concerns facts and events, along with your conscious awareness of knowing them: I am a mammal, today is Monday, my dentist has thick eyebrows. Things like that. In contrast, implicit procedural memories are about skills and habits, about knowing how to *do* things, even without having to think consciously about them: shifting the gears on a car, riding a bicycle, doing the fox-trot. Memories can be transferred between explicit and implicit forms of storage. For example, you are learning a new, difficult passage from a piece of piano music. Each time that stretch approaches, you must consciously, explicitly remember what to do—tuck your elbow in, bring your thumb way underneath after that trill. And one day, while playing, you realize you just barreled through that section flawlessly, without having to think about it: you did it with implicit, rather than explicit, memory. For the first time, it's as if your hands remember better than your brain does.

Memory can be dramatically disrupted if you force something that's implicit into explicit channels. Here's an example that will finally make reading this book worth your while—how to make neurobiology work to your competitive advantage at sports. You're playing tennis against someone who is beating the pants off of you. Wait until your adversary has pulled off some amazing backhand, then offer a warm smile and say, "You are a fabulous tennis player. I mean it; you're terrific. Look at that shot you just made. *How* did you do that? When you do a backhand like that, do you hold your thumb this way or that, and what about your other fingers? And how about your butt, do you scrunch up the left side of it and put your weight on your right toes, or the other way around?" Do it right, and the next time that shot is called for, your opponent/victim will make the mistake of thinking about it explicitly, and the stroke won't be any-where near as effective. As Yogi Berra once said, "You can't think and hit at the same time." Imagine descending a flight of stairs in an explicit manner, something you haven't done since you were two years old—okay, bend my left knee and roll the weight of my toes for-ward while shifting my right hip up slightly—and down you go down the stairs.

Just as there are different types of memory, there are different areas of the brain involved in memory storage and retrieval. One critical site is the cortex, the vast and convoluted surface of the brain. Another is a region tucked just underneath part of the cortex, called the *hippocam-pus*. (That's Latin for "sea horse," which the hippocampus vaguely resembles if you've been stuck inside studying neuroanatomy for too long instead of going to the seashore. It actually looks more like a jelly roll, but who knows the Latin term for that?) Both of these are regions vital to memory—for example, it is the hippocampus and cortex that are preferentially damaged in Alzheimer's disease. If you want a totally simplistic computer metaphor, think of the cortex as your hard drive, where memories are stored, and your hippocampus as the keyboard, the means by which you place and access memories in the cortex.

There are additional brain regions relevant to a different kind of memory. These are structures that regulate body movements. What do these sites, such as the cerebellum, have to do with memory? They appear to be relevant to implicit procedural memory, the type you need to perform reflexive, motor actions without even consciously thinking about them, where, so to speak, your body remembers how to do something before you do.

The distinction between explicit and implicit memory, and the neuroanatomical bases of that distinction, was first really appreciated because of one of the truly fascinating, tragic figures in neurology, perhaps the most famous neurological patient of all time. This man, known in the literature only by his initials, is missing most of his hippocampus. As an adolescent in the 1950s, "H.M." had a severe form of epilepsy that was centered in his hippo-campus and was resistant to drug treatments available at that time. In a desperate move, a famous neurosurgeon removed a large part of H.M.'s hippocampus, along with much of the sur-rounding tissue. The seizures mostly abated, and in the after-math, H.M. was left with a virtually complete inability to turn new short-term memories into long-term ones—mentally utterly frozen in time.* Zillions of studies of H.M. have been carried out since, and it has slowly become apparent that despite this profound amnesia, H.M. can still learn how to do some things. Give him some mechanical puzzle to master day after day, and he learns to put it together at the same speed as anyone else, while steadfastly denying each time that he has ever seen it before. Hippocampus and explicit memory are shot; the rest of the brain is intact, as is his ability to acquire a procedural memory.

This shifts us to the next magnification of examining how the brain handles memories and how stress influences the process—what's going on at the level of clusters of neurons within the cortex and hippocampus? A long-standing belief among many who studied the cortex was that each individual cortical neuron would, in effect, turn out to have a single task, a single fact that it knew. This was prompted by some staggeringly important work done in the 1960s by David Hubel and Torstein Wiesel of Harvard on what was, in retrospect, one of the simpler outposts of the cortex, an area that processed visual information. They found a first part of the visual cortex in which each neuron responded to one thing and one thing only, namely a single dot of light on the retina. Neurons that responded to a sequence of adjacent dots of light would funnel their projections to one neuron in the next layer. And thus, what was this neuron responding to? A straight line. A series of these neurons would project to the next level in a way that each neuron in that cortical level would respond to a particular moving line of light. This led people to believe that there would be a fourth level, where each neuron responded to a particular collection of lines, and a fifth and sixth layer, all the way up until, at the umpteenth layer, there would be a neuron that responded to one thing and one thing only, namely your grandmother's face at a particular angle (and next to it would be a neuron that recognized her face at a slightly different angle, and then the next one . . .). People went looking for what were actually called "grandmother" neurons—neurons way up in the layers of the cortex that "knew" one thing and one thing only, namely a complexly integrated bit of sensory stimulation. With time, it became apparent that there could be very few such neurons in the cortex, because you simply don't have enough neurons to go around to allow each one to be so narrow-minded and overspecialized.

---

* Brush with fame department: I met H.M. once—he won't remember me of course (ba-dum dum), and it was astonishing. You could stand there all day with him repeatedly introducing himself.

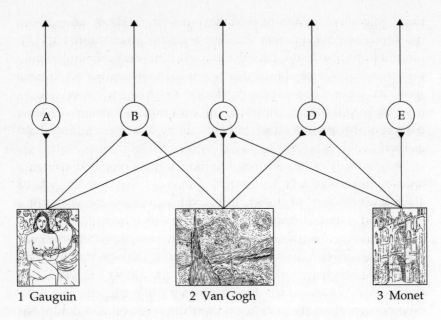

1 Gauguin   2 Van Gogh   3 Monet

A highly hypothetical neural network involving a neuron that "knows" about Impressionist paintings.

Rather than memory and information being stored in single neurons, they are stored in the patterns of excitation of vast arrays of neurons—in trendy jargon, in neuronal "networks." How does one of these work? Consider the wildly simplified neural network shown in the diagram above.

The first layer of neurons (neurons 1, 2, and 3) are classical Hubel and Wiesel type neurons, which is to say that each one "knows" one fact for a living. Neuron 1 knows how to recognize Gauguin paintings, 2 recognizes van Gogh, and 3 knows Monet. (Thus, these hypothetical neurons are more "grandmotherly"—specializing in one task—than any real neurons in the brain, but help illustrate well what neural networks are about.) Those three neurons project—send information to— the second layer in this network, comprising neurons A to E. Note the projection pattern: 1 talks to A, B, and C; 2 talks to B, C, and D; 3 talks to C, D, and E.

What "knowledge" does neuron A have? It gets information only from neuron 1 about Gauguin paintings. Another grandmotherly neuron. Similarly, E gets information only from neuron 3 and knows only about Monet. But what about neuron C; what does it know about? It knows about *Impressionism,* the features that these three painters had in common. It's the neuron that, metaphorically, says, "I can't tell you the painter, certainly not the painting, but it's one of those Impressionists." It has knowledge that does not come from any single informational input, but emerges from the convergence of information feeding into it. Neurons B and D are also Impressionism neurons, but they're just not as good at it as neuron C, because they have fewer examples to work with. Most neurons in your cortex process memory like neurons B through D, not like A or E.

We take advantage of such convergent networks whenever we are trying to pull out a memory that is almost, almost there. Continuing our art history theme, suppose you're trying to remember the name of a painter, that guy, what's his name. He was that short guy with a beard (activating your "short guy" neural network, and your "bearded guy" network). He painted all those Parisian dancers; it wasn't Degas (two more networks pulled in). My high school art appreciation teacher loved that guy; if I can remember her name, I bet I can remember his . . . wow, remember that time I was at the museum and there was that really cute person I tried to talk to in front of one of his paintings . . . oh, what was the stupid pun about that guy's name, about the train tracks being too loose. With enough of those nets being activated, you finally stumble into the one fact that is at the intersection of all of them: Toulouse-Lautrec, the equivalent of a neuron C.

That's a rough approximation of how a neural network operates, and neuroscientists have come to think of both learning and storing of memories as involving the "strengthening" of some branches rather than others of a network. How does such strengthening occur? For that, we switch to a final level of magnification, to consider the tiny gaps between the thready branches of two neurons, gaps called *synapses*. When a neuron has heard some fabulous gossip and wants to pass it on, when a wave of electrical excitation sweeps over it, this triggers the release of chemical messengers—neurotransmitters—that float across the synapse and excite the next neuron. There are dozens, probably hundreds, of different kinds of neurotransmitters, and synapses in the hippocampus and cortex disproportionately make use of what is probably the most excitatory neurotransmitter there is, something called *glutamate*.

Besides being superexcitatory, "glutamatergic" synapses have two properties that are critical to memory. The first is that these synapses are nonlinear in their function. What does this mean? In a run-of-the-mill synapse, a little bit of neurotransmitter comes out of the first neuron and causes the second neuron to get a little excited; if a smidgen more neurotransmitter is released, there is a smidgen more excitation, and so on. In glutamatergic synapses, some glutamate is released and nothing happens. A larger amount is released, nothing happens. It isn't until a certain threshold of glutamate concentration is passed that, suddenly, all hell breaks loose in the second neuron and there is a massive wave of excitation. This is what learning something is about. A professor drones on incomprehensibly in a lecture, a fact goes in one ear and out the other. It is repeated again—and, again, it fails to sink in. Finally, the hundredth time it is repeated, a lightbulb goes on, "Aha!" and you get it. On a simplistic level, when you finally get it, that nonlinear threshold of glutamate excitation has just been reached.

The second feature is even more important. Under the right conditions, when a synapse has just had a sufficient number of superexcitatory glutamate-driven "aha's," something happens. The synapse becomes persistently more excitable, so that next time it takes less of an excitatory signal to get the aha. That synapse just learned something; it was "potentiated," or strengthened. The most amazing thing is that this strengthening of the synapse can persist for a long time. A huge number of neuroscientists flail away at figuring out how this process of "long-term potentiation" works.

There's increasing evidence that the formation of new memories might also sometimes arise from the formation of new connections between neurons (in addition to the potentiating of pre-existing ones) or, even more radically, the formation of new neurons themselves. This latter, controversial idea is discussed below. For the moment, this is all you need to know about how your brain remembers anniversaries and sports statistics and the color of someone's eyes and how to waltz. We can now see what stress does to the process.

 ## IMPROVING YOUR MEMORY DURING STRESS

The first point, of course, is that mild to moderate short-term stressors enhance memory. This makes sense, in that this is the sort of optimal stress that we would call "stimulation"—alert and focused. This effect has been shown in laboratory animals and in humans. One particularly elegant study in this realm was carried out by Larry Cahill and James McGaugh at the University of California at Irvine. Read a fairly unexciting story to a group of control subjects: a boy and his mother walk through their town, pass this store and that one, cross the street and enter the hospital where the boy's father works, are shown the

X-ray room . . . and so on. Meanwhile, the experimental subjects are read a story that differs in that the central core of it contains some emotionally laden material: a boy and his mother walk through their town, pass this store and that one, cross the street where . . . the boy is hit by a car! He's rushed to the hospital and taken to the X-ray room. . . . Tested weeks later, the experimental subjects remember their story better than do the controls, but only the middle, exciting part. This fits with the picture of "flashbulb memory," in which people vividly remember some highly aroused scene, such as a crime they witnessed. Memory for the emotional components is enhanced (although the accuracy isn't necessarily all that good), whereas memory for the neutral details is not.

This study also indicated how this effect on memory works. Hear the stressful story and a stress-response is initiated. As we by now well know, this includes the sympathetic nervous system kicking into gear, pouring epinephrine and norepinephrine into the bloodstream. Sympathetic stimulation appears to be critical, because when Cahill and McGaugh gave subjects a drug to block that sympathetic activation (the beta-blocker propranolol, the same drug used to lower blood pressure), the experimental group did not remember the middle portion of their story any better than the controls remembered theirs. Importantly, it's not simply the case that propranolol disrupts memory formation. Instead, it disrupts stress-enhanced memory formation (in other words, the experimental subjects did as well as the controls on the boring parts of the story, but simply didn't have the boost in memory for the emotional middle section).

The sympathetic nervous system pulls this off by indirectly arousing the hippocampus into a more alert, activated state, facilitating memory consolidation. This involves an area of the brain that is going to become central to understanding anxiety when we get to chapter 15, namely the *amygdala*. The sympathetic nervous system has a second route for enhancing cognition. Tons of energy are needed for all that explosive, nonlinear, long-term potentiating, that turning on of lightbulbs in your hippocampus with glutamate. The sympathetic nervous system helps those energy needs to be met by mobilizing glucose into the bloodstream and increasing the force with which blood is being pumped up into the brain.

These changes are quite adaptive. When a stressor is occuring it is a good time to be at your best in memory retrieval ("How did I get out of this mess last time?") and memory formation ("If I survive this, I'd better remember just what I did wrong so I don't get into a mess like

THE FAR SIDE   By GARY LARSON

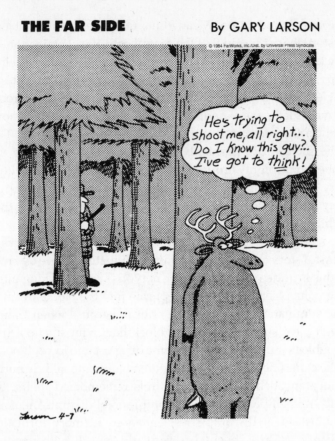

this again."). So stress acutely causes increased delivery of glucose to the brain, making more energy available to neurons, and therefore better memory formation and retrieval.

Thus, the sympathetic arousal during stress indirectly fuels the expensive process of remembering the faces of the crowd chanting ecstatically about Classic Coke. In addition, a mild elevation in glucocorticoid levels (the type you would see during a moderate, short-term stressor) helps memory as well. This occurs in the hippocampus, where those moderately elevated glucocorticoid levels facilitate long-term potentiation. Finally, there are some obscure mechanisms by which moderate, short-term stress makes your sensory receptors more sensitive. Your taste buds, your olfactory receptors, the cochlear cells in your ears all require less stimulation to get excited under moderate stress and pass on the information to your brain. In that special circumstance, you can pick up the sound of a can of soda being opened hundreds of yards away.

ANXIETY: SOME FORESHADOWING

What we've just seen is how moderate and transient stress can enhance the sort of explicit memories that are the purview of the hippocampus. It turns out that stress can enhance another type of memory. This is one relevant to emotional memories, a world apart from the hippocampus and its dull concern with factoids. This alternative type of memory, and its facilitation by stress, revolves around that brain area mentioned before, the amygdala. The response of the amygdala during stress is going to be critical to understanding anxiety and post-traumatic stress disorder in chapter 15.

 ## AND WHEN STRESS GOES ON FOR TOO LONG

With our "sprinting across the savanna" versus "worrying about a mortgage" dichotomy loaded and ready, we can now look at how the formation and retrieval of memories goes awry when stressors become too big or too prolonged. People in the learning and memory business refer to this as an "inverse-U" relationship. As you go from no stress to a moderate, transient amount of stress—the realm of stimulation— memory improves. As you then transition into severe stress, memory declines.

The decline has been shown in numerous studies with lab rats, and with an array of stressors—restraint, shock, exposure to the odor of a cat. The same has been shown when high levels of glucocorticoids are administered to rats instead. But this may not tell us anything interesting. Lots of stress or of glucocorticoids may just be making for a generically messed-up brain. Maybe the rats would now be lousy at tests of muscle coordination, or responsiveness to sensory information, or what have you. But careful control studies have shown that other aspects of brain function, such as implicit memory, are fine. Maybe it's not so much that learning and memory are impaired, as much as the rat being so busy paying attention to that cat smell, or so agitated by it, that it doesn't make much headway solving whatever puzzle is in front of it. And within that realm of explicit memory problems, the retrieval of prior memories seems more vulnerable to stress than the formation of new ones. Similar findings have been reported with nonhuman primates.

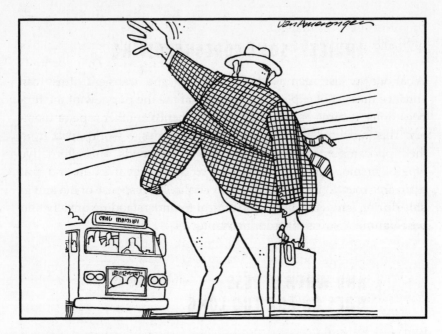

Hard-charging businessman Billy Sloan is about to learn that continued stress does inhibit one's memory.

What about humans? Much the same. In a disorder called Cushing's syndrome, people develop one of a number of types of tumors that result in secretion of tons of glucocorticoids. Understand what goes wrong next in a "Cushingoid" patient and you understand half of this book—high blood pressure, diabetes, immune suppression, reproductive problems, the works. And it's been known for decades that they get memory problems, specifically explicit memory problems, known as *Cushingoid dementia*. As we saw in chapter 8, synthetic glucocorticoids are often administered to people to control autoimmune or inflammatory disorders. With prolonged treatment, you see explicit memory problems as well. But maybe this is due to the disease, rather than to the glucocorticoids that were given for the disease. Pamela Keenan of Wayne State University has studied individuals with these inflammatory diseases, comparing those treated with steroidal anti-inflammatory compounds (that is, glucocorticoids) and those getting nonsteroidals; memory problems were a function of getting the glucocorticoids, not of the disease.

As the clearest evidence, just a few days of high doses of synthetic glucocorticoids impairs explicit memory in healthy volunteers. As one problem in interpreting these studies, these synthetic hormones work a bit differently from the real stuff, and the levels administered produce higher circulating glucocorticoid levels than the body normally produces, even during stress. Importantly, stress itself, or infusion of stress levels of the type of glucocorticoid that naturally occurs in humans, disrupts memory as well. As with the nonhuman studies, implicit memory is fine, and it's the recall, the retrieval of prior information, that is more vulnerable than the consolidation of new memories.

There are also findings (although fewer in number) showing that stress disrupts something called "executive function." This is a little different from memory. Rather than this being the cognitive realm of storing and retrieving facts, this concerns what you do with the facts— whether you organize them strategically, how they guide your judgments and decision making. This is the province of a part of the brain called the prefrontal cortex. We'll be returning to this in considerable detail in chapter 16 when we consider what stress may have to do with decision making and impulse control.

 ## THE DAMAGING EFFECTS OF STRESS IN THE HIPPOCAMPUS

How does prolonged stress disrupt hippocampal-dependent memory? A hierarchy of effects have been shown in laboratory animals:

First, hippocampal neurons no longer work as well. Stress can disrupt long-term potentiation in the hippocampus even in the absence of glucocorticoids (as in a rat whose adrenal glands have been removed), and extreme arousal of the sympathetic nervous system seems responsible for this. Nonetheless, most of the research in this area has focused on the glucocorticoids. Once glucocorticoid levels go from the range seen for mild or moderate stressors to the range typical of big-time stress, the hormone no longer enhances long-term potentiation, that process by which the connection between two neurons "remembers" by becoming more excitable. Instead, glucocorticoids now disrupt the process. Furthermore, similarly high glucocorticoid levels enhance something called *long-term depression,* which might be a mechanism underlying the process of forgetting, the flip side of hippocampal aha-ing.

How can it be that increasing glucocorticoid levels a little bit (during moderate stressors) does one thing (enhances the potentiation of communication between neurons), while increasing glucocorticoid levels a lot does the opposite? In the mid-1980s, Ron de Kloet of the University of Utrecht in the Netherlands discovered the very elegant answer. It turns out that the hippocampus has large amounts of two different types of receptors for glucocorticoids. Critically, the hormone is about ten times better at binding to one of the receptors (thus termed a "high-affinity" receptor) than the other. What that means is that if glucocorticoid levels only rise a little bit, most of the hormone effect in the hippocampus will be mediated by that high-affinity receptor. In contrast, it is not until you are dealing with a major stressor that the hormone activates a lot of the "low-affinity" receptor. And, logically, it turns out that activation of the high-affinity receptor enhances long-term potentiation, while activation of the low-affinity one does the opposite. This is the basis of the "inverse-U" property mentioned above.

In the previous section, I noted that the brain region called the amygdala plays a central role in the types of emotional memories involved in anxiety. But the amygdala is relevant here as well. The amygdala gets highly activated during major stressors and sends a large, influential neuronal projection to the hippocampus. Activation of this pathway seems to be a prerequisite for stress to disrupt hippocampal function. Destroy a rat's amygdala, or sever its connection to the hippocampus, and stress no longer impairs the kind of memory that the hippocampus mediates, even amid the usual high glucocorticoid levels. This explains a finding that harks back to the subject of stress "signatures," and also demonstrates that some activities can represent a challenge to physical allostasis without being psychologically

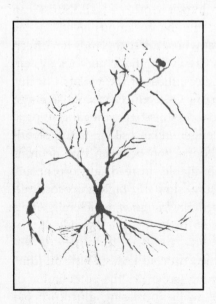 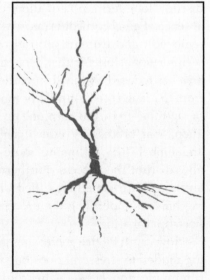

Neurons of the hippocampus of a rat. On the left, healthy neurons; on the right, neurons with their projections atrophied by sustained stress.

aversive. For example, sex raises glucocorticoid levels in a male rat—without activating the amygdala and without disrupting hippocampal function.

Second, neural networks get disconnected. If you look back at the diagram on the "Impressionism neuron" (see page 208), you'll see that there are symbols indicating how one neuron talks to another, "projects" to it. As mentioned a few paragraphs after that, those projections are quite literal—long multibranched cables coming out of neurons that form synapses with the multibranched cables of other neurons. These cables (known as *axons* and *dendrites*) are obviously at the heart of neuronal communication and neuronal networks. Bruce McEwen has shown that, in a rat, after as little as a few weeks of stress or of exposure to excessive glucocorticoids, those cables begin to shrivel, to atrophy and retract a bit. Moreover, the same can occur in the primate brain. When that happens, synaptic connections get pulled apart and the complexity of your neural networks declines. Fortunately, it appears that at the end of the stressful period, the neurons can dust themselves off and regrow those connections.

This transient atrophy of neuronal processes probably explains a characteristic feature of memory problems during chronic stress. Destroy vast acres of neurons in the hippocampus after a massive stroke or late terminal stage Alzheimer's disease, and memory is profoundly impaired. Memories can be completely lost, and never again will these people remember, for example, something as vital as the names of their spouses. "Weaken" a neural network during a period of chronic stress by retracting some of the complex branches in those neuronal trees, and the memories of Toulouse-Lautrec's name are still there. You simply have to tap into more and more associative cues to pull it out, because any given network is less effective at doing its job. Memories are not lost, just harder to access.

Third, the birth of new neurons is inhibited. If you learned your introductory neurobiology any time in the last thousand years, one fact that would be hammered in repeatedly is that the adult brain doesn't make new neurons. In the last decade, it has become clear that this is utterly wrong.* As a result, the study of "adult neurogenesis" is now, arguably, the hottest topic in neuroscience.

Two features about such neurogenesis are highly relevant to this chapter. First, the hippocampus is one of only two sites in the brain

---

* Actually, the evidence for new neurons in the adult brain was first reported in the 1960s by a handful of heretics who were generally ignored or hounded out of science. The field has finally caught up with them.

where these new neurons originate.* Second, the rate of neurogenesis can be regulated. Learning, an enriched environment, exercise, or exposure to estrogen all increase the rate of neurogenesis, while the strongest inhibitors identified to date are, you guessed it, stress and glucocorticoids—as little as a few hours of either in a rat.

Two key questions arise. First, when the stress stops, does neurogenesis recover and, if so, how fast? No one knows yet. Second, what does it matter that stress inhibits adult neurogenesis? Intrinsic in this question is the larger question of what adult neurogenesis is good for. This is incredibly controversial, an issue that has adversaries practically wrestling each other on the podium during scientific conferences. At one extreme are studies that suggest that under the right conditions, there are tons of neurogenesis in the adult hippocampus, that these new neurons form connections with other neurons, and that these new connections, in fact, are needed for certain types of learning. At the other extreme, every one of these findings is questioned. So the jury's out on this one.

Fourth, hippocampal neurons become endangered. As noted, within seconds of the onset of stress, glucose delivery throughout the brain increases. What if the stressor continues? By about thirty minutes into a continuous stressor, glucose delivery is no longer enhanced, and has returned to normal levels. If the stressor goes on even longer, the delivery of glucose to the brain is even inhibited, particularly in the hippocampus. Delivery is inhibited about 25 percent, and the effect is due to glucocorticoids.[†]

---

* The other region supplies new neurons to the olfactory system; for some strange reason, neurons that process odors constantly die off and have to be replaced. It turns out that there is a huge burst in the production of those new olfactory neurons early during pregnancy. They are fully on line just around the time of birth, and the scientists who discovered this speculated that these new olfactory neurons are tagged for the task of imprinting forever on the smell of your offspring (a critical event for mothers of most mammals). And what happens early in pregnancy, when those new olfactory neurons are showing up, but not quite making sense yet? I bet this has something to do with the famed nausea of pregnancy, the food aversions and olfactory sensitivities. This has nothing to do with stress, but it is too cool not to mention.

[†] An obvious question: over and over I've emphasized how important it is during stress to cut down energy delivery to unessential outposts in your body, diverting it instead to exercising muscle. In the previous section, we added your hippocampus to that list of places that are spoon-fed energy with the onset of a stressor. It seems like that would be a clever area to continue to stoke, as the stressor goes on. Why should glucose delivery eventually be inhibited there? Probably because, as time goes by, you are running more on automatic, relying more on the implicit memory outposts in the brain to do things that involve reflexive movement—the martial arts display you put on to disarm the terrorist or, at least, the coordinated swinging of the softball bat at the company

Decreasing glucose uptake to this extent in a healthy, happy neuron is no big deal. It just makes the neuron a little queasy and light-headed. But what if the neuron isn't healthy and happy, and is instead in the middle of a neurological crisis? It's now more likely to die than usual.

Glucocorticoids will compromise the ability of hippocampal neurons to survive an array of insults. Take a rat, give it a major epileptic seizure, and the higher the glucocorticoid levels at the time of the seizure, the more hippocampal neurons will die. Same thing for cardiac arrest, where oxygen and glucose delivery to the brain is cut off, or for a stroke, in which a single blood vessel in the brain shuts down. Same for concussive head trauma, or drugs that generate oxygen radicals. Disturbingly, same thing for the closest there is to a rat neuron's equivalent of being damaged by Alzheimer's disease (exposing the neuron to fragments of an Alzheimer's-related toxin called *beta-amyloid*). Same for a rat hippocampus's equivalent of having AIDS-related dementia (induced by exposing the neuron to a damaging constituent of the AIDS virus called *gp120*).*

My lab and others have shown that the relatively mild energy problem caused by that inhibition of glucose storage by glucocorticoids or stress makes it harder for a neuron to contain the eleventy things that go wrong during one of these neurological insults. All of these neurological diseases are ultimately energy crises for a neuron: cut off the glucose to a neuron (hypoglycemia), or cut off both the glucose and oxygen (hypoxia-ischemia), or make a neuron work like mad (a seizure) and energy stores drop precipitously. Damaging tidal waves of neurotransmitters and ions flood into the wrong places, oxygen radicals are generated. If you throw in glucocorticoids on top of that, the neuron is even less able to afford to clean up the mess. Thanks to that stroke or seizure, today's the worst day of that neuron's life, and it goes into the crisis with 25 percent less energy in the bank than usual.

Finally, there is now evidence that truly prolonged exposure to stress or glucocorticoids can actually kill hippocampal neurons. The

---

picnic that you've been nervous about. And thus, the decreased glucose delivery to highfalutin brain regions like the hippocampus and cortex may be a means to divert energy to those more reflexive brain regions.

* Chapter 3 described how stress can indirectly give rise to a stroke or cardiac arrest. But for the other neurological problems noted—seizure, head trauma, AIDS-related dementia, and most important, Alzheimer's disease—there is no evidence that stress or glucocorticoids *cause* these maladies. Instead, the possibility is that they worsen pre-existing cases.

first hints of this came in the late 1960s. Two researchers showed that if guinea pigs are exposed to pharmacological levels of glucocorticoids (that is, higher levels than the body ever normally generates on its own), the brain is damaged. Oddly, damage was mainly limited to the hippocampus. This was right around the time that Bruce McEwen was first reporting that the hippocampus is loaded with receptors for glucocorticoids and no one really appreciated yet how much the hippocampus was the center in the brain for glucocorticoid actions.

Beginning in the early 1980s, various researchers, including myself, showed that this "glucocorticoid neurotoxicity" was not just a pharmacological effect, but was relevant to normal brain aging in the rat. Collectively, the studies showed that lots of glucocorticoid exposure (in the range seen during stress) or lots of stress itself would accelerate the degeneration of the aging hippocampus. Conversely, diminishing glucocorticoid levels (by removing the adrenals of the rat) would delay hippocampal aging. And as one might expect by now, the extent of glucocorticoid exposure over the rat's lifetime not only determined how much hippocampal degeneration there would be in old age, but how much memory loss as well.

Where do glucocorticoids and stress get off killing your brain cells? Sure, stress hormones can make you sick in lots of ways, but isn't neurotoxicity going a bit beyond the bounds of good taste? A dozen years into studying the phenomenon, we're not yet sure.

 ## WHAT ABOUT DAMAGE TO THE HUMAN HIPPOCAMPUS?

We know from earlier in this chapter that an excess of stress and/or glucocorticoids can disrupt functioning of the hippocampus. Is there any evidence that this can include the sort of overt damage to the hippocampus that we've been discussing? That is, can it disconnect neural networks by the atrophying of processes, inhibit the birth of new neurons, worsen the neuron death caused by other neurological insults, or overtly kill neurons?

To date, six sets of findings in humans should raise some worries:

1. Cushing's syndrome. As discussed above, Cushing's involves any of a number of types of tumors that produce a vast, damaging excess of glucocorticoids, where the consequences include impairment of hippocampal-dependent memory. Monica Starkman at the University of Michigan has used brain imaging techniques on

Cushing's patients to look at the overall size of the brain, and the sizes of various subsections. She reports that there is a selective decrease in the volume of the hippocampus in these individuals. Moreover, the more severe the glucocorticoid excess, the greater the loss of hippocampal volume and the greater the memory problems.

2. Post-traumatic stress disorder (PTSD). As will be discussed in more detail in chapter 15, this anxiety disorder can arise from a variety of types of traumatic stressors. Work pioneered by Douglas Bremner of Emory University, replicated by others, shows that people with PTSD from repeated trauma (as opposed to a single trauma)—soldiers exposed to severe and repeated carnage in combat, individuals repeatedly abused as children—have smaller hippocampi. Again, the volume loss appears to be only in the hippocampus, and in at least one of those studies, the more severe the history of trauma, the more extreme the volume loss.

3. Major depression. As will be detailed in chapter 14, major depression is utterly intertwined with prolonged stress, and this connection includes elevated glucocorticoid levels in about half the people with major depression. Yvette Sheline of Washington University and others have shown that prolonged major depression is, once again, associated with a smaller hippocampus. The more prolonged the history of depression, the more volume loss. Furthermore, it is in patients with the subtype of depression that is most associated with elevated glucocorticoid levels where you see the smaller hippocampus.

4. Repeated jet lag. Chapter 11 will consider a single but intriguing study examining airline flight attendants with long careers of shifting time zones on intercontinental flights. The shorter the average time allowed to recover from each large bout of jet lag over a career, the smaller the hippocampus and the more memory problems.

5. Normative aging. Work by Sonia Lupien of McGill University, and replicated by others, has examined healthy elderly people. Check out what their resting glucocorticoid levels are, the size of their hippocampus, and the quality of their hippocampal-dependent memory. Then come back some years later and retest them. As will be discussed in chapter 12, on aging, there is somewhat of a rise in resting glucocorticoid levels with age in humans, although there is a lot of variability in this. What is seen is that those whose glucocorticoid levels have been rising over the years since the study began are the ones who have had the most severe loss of hippocampal volume and the greatest decline in memory.

6. Interactions between glucocorticoids and neurological insults. A handful of studies report that for the same severity of a stroke, the higher the glucocorticoid levels in a person at the time they come into an emergency room, the more ultimate neurological impairment.

So these studies collectively demonstrate that glucocorticoids damage the human hippocampus. Well, let's hold on a second. There are some problems and complications:

First, there have been some studies suggesting that PTSD involves *lower* than normal levels of glucocorticoids. Thus it can't be the case that an excess of the hormones is damaging the hippocampus. However, it looks as if in those PTSD patients with the low levels, there is excessive *sensitivity* to the glucocorticoids. So the hormones are still plausible culprits.

As a next issue, it isn't clear whether the loss of hippocampal volume in PTSD is caused by the trauma itself, or by the post-traumatic period; amid that uncertainty, there has been at least one excellent study upending both of those ideas. It suggested instead that having a small hippocampus comes *before* the PTSD and, in fact, makes you more likely to develop PTSD when exposed to trauma.

Finally, it should be remembered that the aging studies present a relationship that is merely correlative. In other words, yes, it could be that increasing glucocorticoid levels with age lead to hippocampal atrophy. But there are at least as good reasons to think that it is the other way around, that progressive hippocampal atrophy leads to the rising glucocorticoid levels (as will be explained more fully in chapter 12, this is because the hippocampus also helps to inhibit glucocorticoid release, such that an atrophied hippocampus isn't very good at that task).

In other words, no one is quite sure yet what is going on. One of the biggest problems is a lack of studies of brains like these *after* people have died. Phenomenally obsessive research could be carried out that would tell us whether the hippocampus is smaller because there are fewer of the millions of hippocampal neurons or because neurons have fewer and shorter cables connectiong them to other neurons. Or both. If it turned out that there were fewer neurons, you might even be able to tell whether it is because more of them have died than usual, or because fewer of them were born. Or, again, both.

Actually, even without the postmortem studies, there are a few hints about the sources of the volume loss. Intriguingly, when the tumor that gave rise to the Cushing's syndrome is removed and glucocorticoid levels revert to normal, the hippocampus slowly comes back to normal size. As noted before, when glucocorticoids cause the cables connecting neurons to shrivel up, it is not a permanent process—stop the glucocorticoid excess and the processes can slowly regrow. Thus, the best guess is that the volume loss in Cushing's is based on the retraction of processes. In contrast, the volume losses in PTSD and major depression appear to be something approaching permanent, in that the loss persists in the former case decades after the trauma, and, in the latter, years to decades after the depression has been gotten under control with medication. So in those cases, the volume loss in the hippocampus probably can't be due to shriveling processes of neurons, given that the shriveling can reverse.

Beyond that, no one knows at this point why the hippocampus winds up being smaller in these disorders and situations. It is the knee-jerk reflex of all scientists to say, "More research is needed," but more research really is needed in this case. For the moment, I think it is fair to say that there is decent but not definitive evidence that stress and/or prolonged exposure to glucocorticoids can cause structural, as well as functional, changes in the hippocampus, that these are changes that you probably wouldn't want to have happen to your hippocampus, and that these changes can be long-lasting.

What are some of the disturbing implications of these findings? The first concerns the use by neurologists of synthetic versions of glucocorticoids (such as hydrocortisone, dexamethasone, or prednisone) after someone has had a stroke. As we know from our introduction to glands and hormones in chapter 2, glucocorticoids are classic anti-inflammatory compounds and are used to reduce the edema, the damaging brain swelling that often occurs after a stroke. Glucocorticoids do wonders to block the edema that occurs after something like a brain tumor, but it turns out that they don't do much for post-stroke edema. Worse, there's increasing evidence that those famously anti-inflammatory compounds can actually be pro-inflammatory, worsening inflammation in the injured brain. Yet tons of neurologists still prescribe the stuff, despite decades-old warnings by the best people in the field and findings that the glucocorticoids tend to worsen the neurological outcome. So these recent findings add a voice to that caution—clinical use of glucocorticoids tends to be bad news for neurological diseases that involve a precarious hippocampus. (As a caveat, however, it turns out that huge doses of glucocorticoids can occasionally help reduce damage after a spinal cord injury, for reasons having nothing to do with stress or with much of this book.)

Related to this is the concern that physicians may use synthetic glucocorticoids to treat problems outside the nervous system and, in the process, might endanger the hippocampus. A scenario that particularly disturbs me concerns the ability of these hormones to worsen gp120 damage to neurons and its relevance to AIDS-related dementia. (Remember?—the gp120 protein is found in the AIDS virus and appears to play a central role in damaging neurons and causing the dementia.) If, many experiments down the line, it turns out that glucocorticoids can worsen the cognitive consequences of HIV infection, this will be worrisome. That isn't just because people with AIDS are under stress. It's also because people with AIDS are often treated with extremely high doses of synthetic glucocorticoids to combat other aspects of the disease.

This same logic extends to the use of glucocorticoids in other realms of clinical medicine. About 16 million prescriptions are written annually in the United States for glucocorticoids. Much of the use is benign—a little hydrocortisone cream for some poison ivy, a hydrocortisone injection for a swollen knee, maybe even use of steroid inhalants for asthma (which is probably not a worrisome route for glucocorticoids to get into the brain). But there are still hundreds of thousands of people taking high-dose glucocorticoids to suppress the inappropriate immune responses in autoimmune diseases (such as lupus, multiple sclerosis, or rheumatoid arthritis). As discussed earlier, prolonged glucocorticoid exposure in these individuals is associated with problems with hippocampal-dependent memory. So should you avoid taking glucocorticoids for your autoimmune disease in order to avoid the possibility of accelerated hippocampal aging somewhere down the line? Almost certainly not—these are often devastating diseases and glucocorticoids are often highly effective treatments. Potentially, the memory problems are a particularly grim and unavoidable side effect.

An even more disturbing implication of these findings is that if glucocorticoids turn out to endanger the human hippocampus (making it harder for neurons to survive an insult), you're still in trouble, even if your neurologist doesn't administer synthetic glucocorticoids to you. This is because your body secretes boatloads of the stuff during many neurological crises—humans coming into ERs after neurological insults have immensely high levels of glucocorticoids in their bloodstreams. And what we know from rats is that the massive outpouring of glucocorticoids at that time adds to the damage—remove the adrenals of a rat right after a stroke or seizure, or use a drug that will transiently shut down adrenal secretion of glucocorticoids, and less hippocampal damage will result. In other words, what we think of as typical amounts of brain damage after a stroke or seizure is damage being worsened by the craziness of our bodies having stress-responses at the time.

Consider how bizarre and maladaptive this is. Lion chases you; you secrete glucocorticoids in order to divert energy to your thigh muscles—great move. Go on a blind date, secrete glucocorticoids in order to divert energy to your thigh muscles—probably irrelevant. Have a grand mal seizure, secrete glucocorticoids in order to divert energy to your thigh muscles—and make the brain damage worse. This is as stark a demonstration as you can ask for that a stress-response is not always what you want your body to be having.

How did such maladaptive responses evolve? The most likely explanation is that the body simply has not evolved the tendency *not* to secrete glucocorticoids during a neurological crisis. Stress-induced glucocorticoid secretion works roughly the same in all the mammals, birds, and fish . . . and it has only been in the last half-century or so that westernized versions of just one of those species had much of a chance of surviving something like a stroke. There simply has not been much evolutionary pressure yet to make the body's response to massive neurological injury more logical.

We are now fifty, sixty years into thinking about ulcers, blood pressure, and aspects of our sex lives as being sensitive to stress. Most of us recognize the ways in which stress can also disrupt how we learn and remember. This chapter raises the possibility that the effects of stress in the nervous system might extend even to damaging our neurons, and the next chapter continues this theme, in considering how stress might well accelerate the aging of our brains. The noted neuroscientist Woody Allen once said, "My brain is my second-favorite organ." My guess is that most of us would rank our brains even higher up on a list.

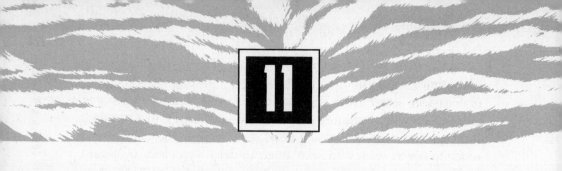

11

STRESS AND A GOOD NIGHT'S SLEEP

Then there was the day when my son was about two weeks old. He was our first born, and we had been plenty nervous about how demanding parenting was going to be. It had been a great day—he'd slept well through the night, waking up a few times to nurse, and took some long naps during the day that allowed us to do the same. We'd settled into a schedule. My wife did the nursing, and I fetched the tureens of cranberry juice that she had become obsessed with since giving birth. Our son filled his diapers on cue, and his every gesture was confirming how wondrous he was. Things were calm.

In the evening, as he slept and we settled into our old routines, like doing dishes (the first time in days), I indulged myself in some editorializing about the human condition. "You know, this newborn business is really quite manageable if you just stay on top of things. You need to work as a team, be organized, roll with the punches." I went on fatuously like this for a while.

That night, our son woke up to nurse right after we fell asleep. He was fussy, wouldn't go back to sleep unless I patted him repeatedly, protested each time I tried to stop by waking up. This went on for an insane hour and then he needed to nurse again. Then, after patting him some more, he responded by blowing out his diaper, making a mess of his onesie and me. Then he screamed bloody murder when I washed him off. Finally, he then slept contentedly without patting, for about twenty minutes, before needing to nurse again, another blowout soiling of his fresh onesie, followed by our discovery that we had no clean ones, having neglected to do the laundry.

Rather than doing something useful, I orated in a half-psychotic state, "We can't do this, we're going to die, I'm serious, people DIE from lack of sleep, it's not possible to do this, it's physiologically proven, we're all going to DIE." I swung my arms with emphasis, knocking over and loudly breaking a glass of cranberry juice. This woke up our, by then, happily sleeping son, causing all three of us to burst into tears. He eventually settled down and slept like a baby for the rest of the night, while I tossed anxiously, waiting for him to wake up again.

Contained in this are the two central features of this chapter. Not getting enough sleep is a stressor; being stressed makes it harder to sleep. Yup, we've got a dread vicious cycle on our hands.

 ## THE BASICS OF SLEEP

All things considered, sleeping is pretty creepy. For a third of your life, you're just not there, floating in this suspended state, everything slowed down. Except, at points, your brain is more active than when you're awake, making your eyelids all twitchy, and it's consolidating memories from the day and solving problems for you. Except when it's dreaming, when it's making no sense. And then you sometimes walk or talk in your sleep. Or drool. And then there's those mysterious penile or clitoral erections that occur intermittently during the night.*

Weird. What's going on here? To start, sleep is not a monolithic process, a uniform phenomenon. Instead, there are different types of sleep—shallow (also known as stages 1 and 2) sleep, where you are easily awakened. Deep sleep (also known as stages 3 and 4, or "slow wave sleep"). Rapid Eye Movement (REM) sleep, where the puppy's paws flutter and our eyes dart around and dreams happen. There are not only these different stages, but a structure, an architecture to them. You start off shallow, gradually sleep your way down to slow wave sleep, followed by REM, then back up again, and then repeat the

---

* And this isn't even going into the subject of species that sleep with only half of their brain at a time, in order to keep one eye and half the brain open to look out for predators. Mallards, for example, that are stuck on the edge of their group at night keep their outward facing eye, and the half of the brain that responds to it, preferentially awake. As more oddities, dolphins can swim while sleeping and some birds can fly.

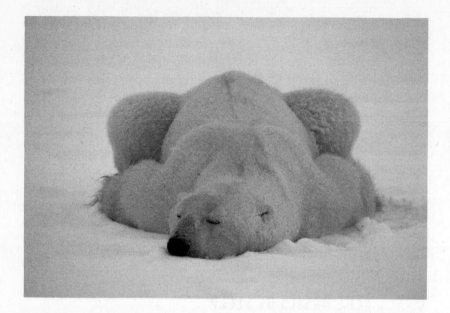

whole cycle about every ninety minutes (and as we'll see in chapter 14, something goes wrong with the architecture of sleep during a major depression).

Not surprisingly, the brain works differently in different stages of sleep. This can be studied by having people sleep in a brain scanner, while you measure the levels of activity of different brain regions. Take some volunteers, sleep-deprive them for some godawful length of time, stick them in one of these imaging machines, poke them awake a little more while you get a measure of their brains' activity when they're awake, and then, snug as a bug in a scanner, let them go to sleep with the scanner running.

The picture during slow wave sleep makes lots of sense. Parts of the brain associated with arousal activity slow down. Ditto for brain regions involved in controlling muscle movement. Interestingly, regions involved in the consolidation and retrieval of memories don't have much of a decrease in metabolism. However, the pathways that bring information to and from those regions shut down dramatically, isolating them. The parts of the brain that first respond to sensory information have somewhat of a metabolic shutdown, but the more dramatic changes are in downstream brain areas that integrate, associate those bytes of sensory information, and give them meaning. What you've got is a metabolically quiescent, sleeping brain. This makes sense, as deep slow wave sleep is when energy restoration occurs. This is shown by the fact that the extent of sleep deprivation is not a great predictor of the total amount you will ultimately sleep, but it is a good predictor of how much slow wave sleep there'll be—a very active brain or a sleep-deprived brain tends to consume a lot of a particular form of energy; the breakdown product of that depleted form of energy is the signal that biases toward slow wave sleep.

A very different picture emerges during REM sleep. Overall, there's an increase in activity. Some brain regions become even more metabolically active than when you're awake. Parts of the brain that regulate muscle movement, brain stem regions that control breathing and heart rate—all increase their metabolic rate. In a part of the brain called the limbic system, which is involved in emotion, there is an increase as well. The same for areas involved in memory and sensory processing, especially those involved in vision and hearing.

Something particularly subtle goes on in the visual processing regions. The part of the cortex that processes the first bits of visual information does not show much of an increase in metabolism, whereas there is a big jump in the downstream regions that integrate simple visual information.* How can this be, when, on top of it, your eyes are closed? This is dreaming.

That tells us something about how dream imagery arises. But something else that happens in the brain tells us something about the *content* of dreams. There's a part of the brain, briefly mentioned in the last chapter, called the frontal cortex. It's the most recently evolved part of the human brain, is disproportionately huge in primates, and is the last part of our brain to fully mature. The frontal cortex is the nearest thing we have to a superego. Starting from toilet training, it helps you to do the harder, rather than easier thing—for example, thinking in a logical, sequential manner, rather than bouncing all over the place cognitively. It keeps you from murdering someone just because you feel like it, stops you from telling someone exactly what you think of their hideous outfit and instead finds something complimentary. The frontal cortex does all this disciplining of you by inhibiting that frothy, emotional limbic system.† If you damage the frontal cortex, someone gets "frontally disinhibited"—doing and saying the things we may think about but would never act upon. During REM sleep, metabolism in the frontal cortex goes way down, disinhibiting the limbic system to come up with

---

* Harking back to chapter 10, this is the Hubel and Weisel part of the visual cortex that responds to simple stuff like dots and lines.

† Amazingly, the frontal cortex is the last part of the brain to fully mature, typically not going completely online until you are well into your *twenties*. Doesn't that begin to explain a lot of the imprudent things you did back when?

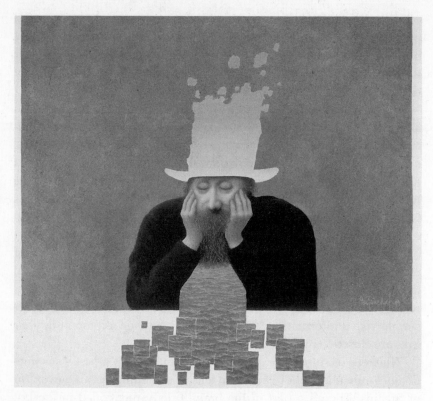

Alfredo Castañeda, Our Dream *(detail), 1999.*

the most outlandish ideas. That's why dreams are dreamlike—illogical, nonsequential, hyperemotional. You breathe underwater, fly in the air, communicate telepathically; you announce your love to strangers, invent languages, rule kingdoms, star in Busby Berkeley musicals.

So those are the nuts and bolts of sleep. But what is sleep for? You die without it. Even fruit flies do. The most obvious answer is to have a stretch where your brain is going at half speed, in order to build up supplies of energy. Your brain consumes phenomenal amounts of energy to pull off all that calculus and symphony writing that you do—the brain constitutes something like 3 percent of your body weight but needs nearly a quarter of the energy. So stores tend to decline during the day and some solid slow wave sleep is needed to restock those stores (mostly of a molecule called glycogen, which is also an energy store in liver and muscle).*

---

* Despite this, your brain is actually pretty lousy at storing energy, given the magnitude of its energy demands. This comes back to haunt your neurons big-time during a number of neurological disasters involving a shortage of energy.

Others speculate that sleep is for decreasing brain temperature, letting it cool off from all that daytime brainstorming, or for detoxifying the brain. Weirdly, another major reason to sleep is to dream. If you skip a night's sleep, when you finally get to sleep the next night, you have more REM sleep than normal, suggesting that you've built up a real deficit of dreaming. Some extremely difficult studies that make me queasy just to contemplate deprive people or animals of REM sleep preferentially, and the study subjects go to pieces much faster than they do for the equivalent amount of deprivation of other types of sleep.

Thus, this begs the question of what dreaming is for. To work out unresolved issues about your mother? To provide a living for surrealists and dadaists? So you can have a sex dream about some unlikely person in your waking life and then act all weird around that person the next morning by the water cooler? Well, maybe. The marked increase in metabolic activity during REM sleep, and in some of the most inhibited areas of the brain during waking, have suggested to some a sort of "use it or lose it" scenario in which dreaming gives some aerobic exercise to otherwise underutilized brain pathways (that is, the oft-neglected Busby Berkeley musical brain circuit).

What has become clear is that sleep plays a role in cognition. For example, sleep can facilitate problem solving. This is the realm of "sleeping on a problem," and then suddenly discovering a solution the next morning while you're cleaning crud out of the corners of your eyes. The neurobiologist Robert Stickgold of Harvard has emphasized that this type of problem solving is the kind where a morass of unhelpful facts are broken through to get to feelings. As he says, you don't forget a phone number and then "sleep on it" to remember it. You do it for some complex, ambiguous problem.

Both slow wave and REM sleep also seem to play roles in the formation of new memories, the consolidation of information from the previous day, even information that became less accessible to you while awake over the course of the day. One type of evidence supporting this is the fact that if you teach an animal some task and disrupt its sleep that night, the new information isn't consolidated. While this has been shown in many different ways, the interpretation remains controversial. As we saw in the last chapter, stress can disrupt memory consolidation. As we're about to see in great detail, sleep deprivation is stressful. Maybe sleep deprivation disrupts memory consolidation merely because of the stress, which wouldn't prove that sleep normally helps memory consolidation. But the pattern of memory disruption caused by sleep deprivation is different from that caused by stress.

Another type of evidence is correlative. Being exposed to lots of new information during the day is associated with more REM sleep that night. Moreover, the amount of certain subtypes of sleep at night predicts how well new information is recalled the next day. For example, lots of REM sleep during the night predicts better consolidation of emotional information from the day before, while lots of stage 2 sleep predicts better consolidation of a motor task, and a combination of lots of REM and slow wave sleep predicts better retention of perceptual information. Others have taken this further, reporting that it's not just the amount of some subtype of sleep that predicts some subtype of learning, but whether it occurs early or late in the night.

Another style of evidence for the "sleep helps you consolidate memories" story was first obtained by Bruce McNaughton of the University of Arizona. As we saw in chapter 10, the hippocampus has a central role in explicit learning. McNaughton recorded the activity of single hippocampal neurons in rats, identifying ones that became particularly busy while the rat was learning some new explicit information. That night, during slow wave sleep, it would be those same neurons that would be particularly busy. Taking that one step further, he showed that *patterns* of activation of hippocampal neurons that occur during learning are then repeated when the animal is sleeping. Brain-imaging studies with humans have shown something similar. There's even evidence that when consolidation is going on during REM, genes are activated that help form new connections between neurons. During slow wave sleep, metabolism remains surprisingly high in areas like the hippocampus. It's as if sleep is the time when the brain practices those new memory patterns over and over, cementing them into place.

Weirdly, amid this general picture of sleep deprivation disrupting cognition, at least one type of learning is facilitated by sleep deprivation, as shown in some recent work by a graduate student of mine, Ilana Hairston. Suppose you have some unlikely task where you have to learn to recite the months of the year backward as rapidly as possible. Why is this going to be hard? Because there will repeatedly be the pull to recite the months in the way that you've done your whole life, which is forward; the previous, overlearned version of the task interferes with this new reversal task. Who would excel at this task? Someone who has never learned to do January, February, March, etc., automatically in that direction. If you sleep deprive some rats and give them a rat's equivalent of a reversal task, they do better than do control animals. Why? Because they can't remember the prior overlearned version of the task well enough for it to intrude now.

So now we have the basics of sleep and what it might be good for. *Entrez* stress.

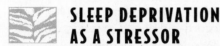

SLEEP DEPRIVATION AS A STRESSOR

As we glide down into slow wave sleep, some obvious things occur to facets of the stress-response system. For starters, the sympathetic nervous system shuts down, in favor of that calm, vegetative parasympathetic nervous system. In addition, glucocorticoid levels go down. As introduced back in chapter 2, CRH is the hypothalamic hormone that gets the pituitary to release ACTH in order to trigger adrenal release of glucocorticoids. Some of the hypothalamic control of pituitary hormone release consists of an accelerator and a brake—a releasing factor and an inhibiting factor. For years, there's been evidence floating around for a hypothalamic "corticotropin *inhibiting* factor" (CIF) that would inhibit the release of ACTH, counteracting the effects of CRH. No one's sure what CIF is, or if it really exists, but there's some decent evidence that CIF is a brain chemical that helps bring on slow wave sleep (called "delta sleep-inducing factor"). Thus, sleep deeply, and you turn off glucocorticoid secretion.

In contrast, during REM, as you're mobilizing all that energy to generate that outlandish dream imagery and to move your eyes rapidly, glucocorticoid secretion and the sympathetic nervous system rev up again. But given that most of what counts as a good night's sleep consists of slow wave sleep, sleep is predominately a time when the stress-response is turned off. This is seen in species whether they're nocturnal or diurnal (that is, sleeping during the dark hours, like us). About an hour before you wake up, levels of CRH, ACTH, and glucocorticoids begin to rise. This is not just because merely rousing from slumber is a mini-stressor, requiring mobilization of some energy, but because those rising stress hormone levels play a role in terminating sleep.

So deprive yourself of sleep, and the sleep-induced decline in the levels of those stress hormones doesn't occur. And, no surprise, they rise instead. Glucocorticoid levels increase and the sympathetic nervous system is activated; commensurate with everything that's been reviewed in previous chapters, down go levels of growth hormone and of various sex hormones. Sleep deprivation definitely stimulates glucocorticoid secretion, although not to a massive extent in most studies (unless the sleep deprivation is really prolonged; however, "it is postulated that these increases [in response to severe sleep deprivation] are due to the stress of dying rather than to sleep loss," dryly noted one journal article).

The elevated glucocorticoid levels during sleep deprivation play a role in breaking down some of the stored forms of energy in the brain. This, along with many of the glucocorticoid effects on memory, could have something to do with why learning and memory are so lousy when you're sleep-deprived. That's something we all learned when doing an all-nighter and discovering the next morning during the final exam that we can barely recall what month it was, let alone any of the factoids crammed in our heads the previous night. A recent study beautifully demonstrated one way in which our brains become impaired when we try to think hard on no sleep. Take a normally rested subject, stick her in a brain imager, and ask her to solve some "working memory" problems (holding on to some facts and manipulating them—like adding sequences of three-digit numbers). As a result, her frontal cortex lights up metabolically. Now, take someone who is sleep deprived and he's awful at the working memory task. And what's going on in his brain? What you might have guessed is that frontal metabolism would be inhibited, too groggy to get activated in response to the task. Instead, the opposite occurs—the frontal cortex is activated, but so are large parts of the rest of the cortex. It's as if sleep deprivation has reduced this gleaming computer of a frontal cortex to a bunch of unshaven gibbering neurons counting on their toes, having to ask the rest of their cortical buddies to help out with this tough math problem.

So why care if sleep deprivation is a stressor? It's obvious. We're accustomed to all sorts of amenities in our modern lives: overnight deliveries of packages, advice nurses who can be called at two in the morning, round-the-clock technical support staff. Therefore, people are required to work under conditions of sleep deprivation. We're not a nocturnal species and if a person works at night or works swing shifts, regardless of how many total hours of sleep she's getting, it's going against her biological nature. People who work those sorts of hours tend to overactivate the stress-response, and there's little habituation that goes on. Given that an overactive stress-response makes every page of this book relevant, it is not surprising that night work or shift work increases the risk of cardiovascular disease, gastrointestinal disorders, immune suppression, and fertility problems.

A widely reported study a few years back really brought this into focus. Recall how prolonged stress and glucocorticoids can damage the hippocampus and impair hippocampal-dependent explicit memory. Kei Cho of the University of Bristol studied flight attendants working for two different airlines. On one airline, after you worked a transcontinental flight with major jet lag, you'd have a 15-day break until being scheduled for the next transcontinental flight. In contrast, on Airline #2, presumably with a weaker union, you got a 5-day break before the next transcontinental flight.* Cho controlled for total amount of flying time and total number of time zones shifted in the course of flying. Thus, Airline #2's crews didn't experience more total jet lag, just less time to recover. Finally, Cho considered only employees who had been doing this for more than five years. He found that Airline #2's attendants had, on average, impaired explicit memory, higher glucocorticoid levels, and a smaller temporal lobe (the part of the brain that contains the hippocampus). (This study was briefly alluded to in chapter 10). This is obviously not a good thing for the employees working under these conditions. And this may make it less likely that the flight attendant will remember that 17C requested a mixture of ginger ale and skim milk with ice. But it kind of makes one wonder whether the back-to-the-grind-after-5-days *pilot* is having trouble remembering whether or not this little ol' switch turns the engine on or off.

These worries about sleep deprivation are relevant to even those whose 9-to-5 job is 9-to-5 during daylight hours. We have an unprecedented number of ways to make us sleep deprived, beginning with something as simple as indoor lighting. In 1910, the average American slept nine hours a night, disturbed only by the occasional Model T backfiring. We now average 7.5 and declining. When there's the lure of 24-hour-a-day fun, activities, and entertainment or, for the workaholic, the knowledge that somewhere, in some time zone, someone else is working while you indulge yourself in sleep, that pull of "just a few more minutes," of pushing yourself, becomes irresistible. And damaging.†

---

* Either out of good manners or fear of getting his keister sued, Cho did not identify the airlines.

† Just to be perfectly up front, I'm being a complete hypocrite here and it's scandalous that I even have the nerve to spout off about this. For the most part I'm without vices— I don't smoke, have never had a drink or illicit drug in my life, don't eat meat or drink tea or coffee. But I'm incredibly bad at getting enough sleep; I've needed a nap since the Carter administration. I've got this colleague, William Dement, who is considered the dean of sleep research, absolutely evangelical about the health risks of sleep deprivation, and on days when I'm really a mess from lack of sleep, I live in dread of running into him. So on this one, do as I say, not as I do.

AND STRESS AS A DISRUPTOR OF SLEEP

What should happen to sleep during stress? This one's simple, given a zebra-o-centric view of the world: lion coming, don't nap (or, as the old joke goes, "The lion and the lamb shall lie down together. But the lamb won't get much sleep."). The hormone CRH seems to be most responsible for this effect. As you'll recall, the hormone not only starts the glucocorticoid cascade by stimulating ACTH release from the pituitary, but it is also the neurotransmitter that activates all sorts of fear, anxiety, and arousal pathways in the brain. Infuse CRH into a sleeping rat's brain and you suppress sleep—it's like throwing ice water onto those happily dozing neurons. Part of this is due to the direct effects of CRH in the brain, but part is probably due to CRH activating the sympathetic nervous system. If you go up to high altitude without acclimating, your heart is going to be racing, even when you're not exerting yourself. This is not because you are stressed or anxious, but simply because your heart has to beat more often to deliver sufficient oxygen. Suddenly you discover that it's awfully hard to fall asleep with your eyeballs throbbing rhythmically 110 times a minute. So the bodily consequences of sympathetic activation make sleeping hard.

Not surprisingly, about 75 percent of cases of insomnia are triggered by some major stressor. Moreover, many (but not all) studies show that poor sleepers tend to have higher levels of sympathetic arousal or of glucocorticoids in their bloodstream.

So, lots of stress and, potentially, little sleep. But stress not only can decrease the total amount of sleep but can compromise the *quality* of whatever sleep you do manage. For example, when CRH infusion decreases the total amount of sleep, it's predominantly due to a decrease in slow wave sleep, exactly the type of sleep you need for energy restoration. Instead, your sleep is dominated by more shallow sleep stages, meaning you wake up more easily—fragmented sleep. Moreover, when you do manage to get some slow wave sleep, you don't even get the normal benefits from it. When slow wave sleep is ideal, really restoring those energy stores, there's a characteristic pattern in what is called the delta power range that can be detected on an EEG (electroencephalogram) recording. When people are stressed presleep, or are infused with glucocorticoids during sleep, you get less of that helpful sleep pattern during slow wave sleep.

Glucocorticoids compromise something else that occurs during good quality sleep. Jan Born of the University of Lubeck in Germany has shown that if you infuse glucocorticoids into someone while

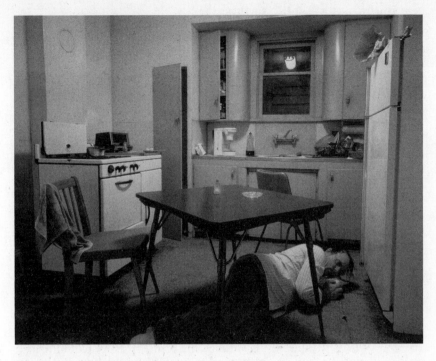

Jeff Wall, Insomnia, *transparency in lightbox, 1994.*

they're sleeping, you impair the memory consolidation that would normally be occurring during slow wave sleep.

 ## A CAUSES *B* CAUSES *A* CAUSES *B* CAUSES . . .

We have the potential for some real problems here, insofar as lack of sleep or poor-quality sleep activates the stress-response, and an activated stress-response makes for less sleep or lower-quality sleep. Each feeds on the other. Does that mean that experiencing even a smidgen of stress, or staying up late once to see Ted Koppel interview Britney Spears about the evidence for and against global warming, and—that's it, you're finished—downward spiral of stress and sleep deprivation?

Obviously not. For one thing, as mentioned, sleep deprivation doesn't cause all that massive of a stress-response. Moreover, the need to sleep will eventually overcome the most stressful of stressors.

Nonetheless, a fascinating study suggests how the two halves might interact, along the lines that the expectation that you're going to sleep poorly makes you stressed enough to get poor-quality sleep. In the study, one group of volunteers was allowed to sleep for as long as they wanted, which turned out to be until around nine in the morning. As would be expected, their stress hormone levels began to rise around eight. How might you interpret that? These folks had enough sleep, happily restored and reenergized, and by about eight in the morning, their brains knew it. Start secreting those stress hormones to prepare to end the sleep.

But the second group of volunteers went to sleep at the same time but were told that they would be woken up at six in the morning. And what happened with them? At five in the morning, their stress hormone levels began to rise.

This is important. Did their stress hormone levels rise three hours earlier than the other group because they needed three hours less sleep? Obviously not. The rise wasn't about them feeling rejuvenated. It was about the stressfulness of anticipating being woken up earlier than desirable. Their brains were feeling that anticipatory stress while sleeping, demonstrating that a sleeping brain is still a working brain.

What might be happening, then, if you go to sleep thinking that not only will you be woken up earlier than you would like, but at an *unpredictable* time? Where any minute could be your last minute of sleep for the night? It's quite possible that stress hormone levels will be elevated throughout the night, in nervous anticipation of that wake-up call. As we've seen, with an elevated stress-response during sleep, the quality of the sleep is going to be compromised.

Thus, there is a hierarchy as to what counts as miserable sleep. Continuous, uninterrupted sleep, but too little of it—deadline looming, go to sleep late, get up early, not good. Even worse is too little sleep that is fragmented. As an example, I once did an experiment where every three hours for days I had to take blood samples from some animals. Even though I did next to nothing on these nights and days other than sleep, in fact I got more total sleep per day than was usual for me, I was a wreck. But worst of all is too little sleep that is *unpredictably* fragmented. You finally get back to sleep, but with the corrosive knowledge that five hours or five minutes from now, another patient will come into the emergency room, or the alarms will go off and it's back to the fire truck, or someone's diaper will slowly but surely fill up.

This teaches us a lot about what counts as good sleep and how stress can prevent it. But as we'll see in a couple of chapters, this generalizes beyond sleep. When it comes to what makes for psychological stress, a lack of predictability and control are at the top of the list of things you want to avoid.

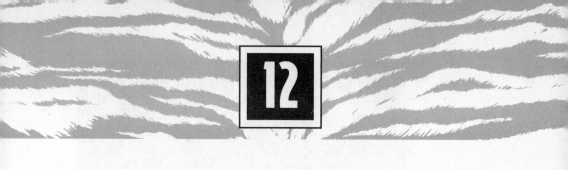

12

AGING AND DEATH

Predictably, it comes at the most unpredictable times. I'll be lecturing, bored, telling the same story about neurons I did last year, daydreaming, looking at the ocean of irritatingly young undergraduates, and then it hits, producing almost a sense of wonderment. "How can you just sit there? Am I the only one who realizes that we're all going to die someday?" Or I'll be at a scientific conference, this time barely understanding someone else's lecture, and amid the roomful of savants, the wave of bitterness will sweep over me. "All of you damned medical experts, and not one of you can make me live forever."

It first really dawns on us emotionally sometime around puberty. Woody Allen, once our untarnished high priest of death and love, captures its roundabout assault perfectly in *Annie Hall*. The protagonist is shown, in flashback, as a young adolescent. He is sufficiently depressed for the worried mother to drag him to the family doctor—"Listen to what he keeps saying, what's wrong with him, does he have the flu?" The Allenesque adolescent, glazed with despair and panic, announces in a monotone: "The universe is expanding." It's all there—the universe is expanding; look how big infinity is and how finite we are—and he has been initiated into the great secret of our species: we will die and we know it. With that rite of passage, he has found the mother lode of psychic energy that fuels our most irrational and violent moments, our most selfish and our most altruistic ones, our neurotic dialectic of simultaneously mourning and denying, our diets and exercising, our myths of paradise and resurrection. It's as if we were trapped in a mine, shouting out for rescuers, Save us, we're alive but we're getting old and we're going to die.

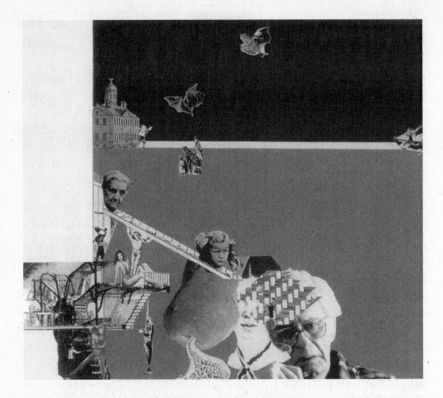

Morris Zlapo, Gepetto's Dementia, *collage, 1987.*

And, of course, before dying, most of us will become old, a process aptly described as not for sissies: wracking pain. Dementia so severe we can't recognize our children. Cat food for dinner. Forced retirement. Colostomy bags. Muscles that no longer listen to our commands, organs that betray us, children who ignore us. Mostly that aching sense that just when we finally grow up and learn to like ourselves and to love and play, the shadows lengthen. There is so little time.

Oh, it doesn't have to be that bad. For many years I have spent part of each year doing stress research on wild baboons in East Africa. The people living there, like many people in the nonwesternized world, clearly think differently about these issues than we do. No one seems to find getting old depressing. How could they?—they wait their whole lives to become powerful elders. My nearest neighbors are of the Masai tribe, nomadic pastoralists. I often patch up their various minor injuries and ills. One day, one of the extremely old men of the village (perhaps sixty years old) tottered into our camp. Ancient, wrinkled beyond measure, tips missing from a few fingers, frayed ear-lobes, long-forgotten battle scars. He spoke only Masai and not Swahili, the lingua franca of East Africa, so he was accompanied by

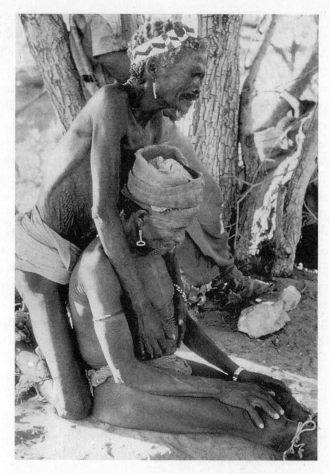

An elderly hunter-gatherer shaman in the Kalahari Desert.

his more worldly, middle-aged neighbor, who translated for him. He had an infected sore on his leg, which I washed and treated with antibiotic ointment. He also had trouble seeing—"cataracts" was my barely educated guess—and I explained that they were beyond my meager curative powers. He seemed resigned, but not particularly disappointed, and as he sat there cross-legged, naked except for the blanket wrapped around him, basking in the sun, the woman stood behind him and stroked his head. In a voice as if describing last year's weather she said, "Oh, when he was younger, he was beautiful and strong. Soon he will die." That night in my tent, sleepless and jealous of the Masai, I thought, "I'll take your malaria and parasites, I'll take your appalling infant mortality rates, I'll take the chances of being attacked by buffalo and lions. Just let me be as unafraid of dying as you are."

Maybe we will luck out and wind up as respected village elders. Perhaps we will grow old with grace and wisdom. Perhaps we will be honored, surrounded by strong, happy children whose health and fecundity will feel like immortality to us. Gerontologists studying the aging process find increasing evidence that most of us will age with a fair degree of success. There's far less institutionalization and disability than one might have guessed. While the size of social networks shrink with age, the quality of the relationships improves. There are types of cognitive skills that improve in old age (these are related to social intelligence and to making good strategic use of facts, rather than merely remembering them easily). The average elderly individual thinks his or her health is above average, and takes pleasure from that. And most important, the average level of happiness increases in old age; fewer negative emotions occur and, when they do, they don't persist as long. Connected to this, brain-imaging studies show that negative images have less of an impact, and positive images have more of an impact on brain metabolism in older people, as compared to young.

So maybe old age is not so bad. The final chapter of this book reviews some of the patterns seen in aged people who are particularly

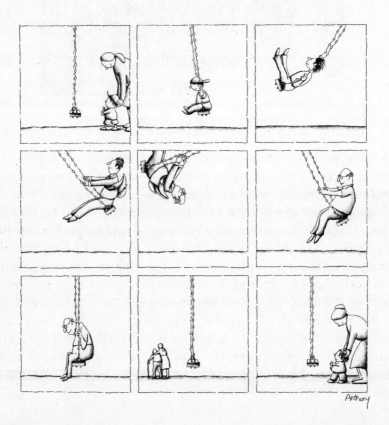

Anthony

successful in their aging. The purpose of this chapter is to review what stress has to do with the aging process and whether we wind up with the honored village elder model of aging, or the cat food variant.

 ## AGED ORGANISMS AND STRESS

How do aged organisms deal with stress? Not very well, it turns out. In many ways, aging can be defined as the progressive loss of the ability to deal with stress, and that certainly fits our perception of aged individuals as fragile and vulnerable. This can be stated more rigorously by saying that many aspects of the bodies and minds of old organisms work fine, just as they do in young ones, so long as they aren't pushed. Throw in an exercise challenge, an injury or illness, time pressure, novelty—any of a variety of physical, cognitive, or psychological stressors—and aged organisms don't do so well.

"Not doing so well" in the stress-response department can take at least two forms that should be familiar by now. The first is failing to activate a sufficient stress-response when it is needed. This occurs at many levels during aging. For example, individual cells have a variety of defenses they can mobilize in response to a challenge that can be viewed as a cellular stress-response. Heat a cell to an unhealthy extent and "heat shock proteins" are synthesized to help stabilize cellular function during a crisis. Damage DNA and DNA repair enzymes are activated. Generate oxygen radicals and antioxidant enzymes are made in response. And all of these cellular stress-responses become less responsive to challenge during aging.

A similar theme comes through at the level of how whole organ systems respond to stress. For example, after you eliminate from your study elderly people who have heart disease and look only at healthy subjects of different ages (so as to study aging, instead of inadvertently studying disease), many aspects of cardiac function are unchanged by age. But challenge the system with exercise, for example, and old hearts do not respond as adequately as do young ones, in that the maximal work capacity and the maximal heart rate that can be achieved are nowhere near as great as in a young person.* Similarly, in

---

* The problem here is not that elderly individuals fail to secrete sufficient epinephrine or norepinephrine during exercise. They secrete plenty, more than young individuals, in fact. But the heart and various blood vessels in an aged organism do not respond as vigorously to the epinephrine and norepinephrine.

the absence of stress, old and young rat brains contain roughly the same amount of energy. But when you stress the system by cutting off the flow of oxygen and nutrients, energy levels decline faster in the old brains. Or, as a classic example, normal body temperature, 98.6 degrees, does not change with age. Nevertheless, aged bodies are impaired in mounting a thermoregulatory stress-response, and thus it takes the bodies of the elderly longer to restore a normal temperature after being warmed or chilled.

The idea also applies to measures of cognition. What happens to IQ test scores as people get older? (You'll notice that I didn't say "intelligence." What that has to do with IQ test scores is a controversy I don't want to touch.) The dogma in the field was once that IQ declined with age. Then it was that it did not decline. It depends on how you test it. If you test young and old people and give them lots of time to complete the test, there is little difference. As you stress the system—in this case, by making the subjects race against a time limit—scores fall for all ages, but much further among older people.

So sometimes the problem in aging is not enough of a stress-response. Predictably, in some realms, the problem is too much of a stress-response—either one turned on all the time, or one that takes too long to turn off at the end of a stressor.

As an example, older individuals are impaired at turning off epinephrine, norepinephrine, or glucocorticoid secretion after a stressor has finished; it takes longer for levels of these substances to return to baseline. Moreover, even in the absence of the stressor, epinephrine, norepinephrine, and glucocorticoid levels are typically elevated in aged rats, nonhuman primates, and humans as well.*

Do aged organisms pay a price for having these components of the stress-response turned on too often? This seems to be the case. As one example, which was discussed in the chapter on memory, stress and glucocorticoids inhibit the birth of new neurons in the adult hippocampus and inhibit the growth of new processes in preexisting neurons. Is the birth of new neurons and the elaboration of neuronal processes preferentially inhibited in old rats? Yes, and if their gluco-

---

* The literature used to show that resting glucocorticoid levels did not rise with age in humans. However, those studies came from a time when someone age sixty would be classified as "elderly." Modern gerontologists do not consider someone aged until the late seventies or eighties, and more recent studies show a big jump in resting glucocorticoid levels in that age group.

corticoid levels are lowered, neurogenesis and process growth increase to levels seen in young animals.

We know by now that, ideally, the hormones of the stress-response should be nice and quiet when nothing bad is happening, secreted in tiny amounts. When a stressful emergency hits, your body needs a huge and fast stress-response. At the end of the stressor, everything should shut off immediately. And these traits are precisely what old organisms typically lack.*

 ## WHY YOU SELDOM SEE REALLY OLD SALMON

We shift over to the other half of the aging-stress relationship—not whether aged organisms can deal well with stress, but whether stress can accelerate aspects of aging. There is some decent evidence that an excess of stress can increase the risk of some of the diseases of aging. Remarkably, it turns out that in more than a dozen species, glucocorticoid excess is *the* cause of death during aging.

Pictures of heroic wild animals, à la Marlin Perkins: penguins who stand all winter amid the Antarctic cold, keeping their eggs warm at their feet. Leopards dragging massive kills up trees with their teeth, in order to eat them free of harassment by lions. Desiccated camels marching scores of miles. And then there's salmon, leaping over dams and waterfalls to return to the freshwater stream of their birth. Where they spawn a zillion eggs. After which most of them die over the next few weeks.

Why do salmon die so soon after spawning? No one is quite sure, but evolutionary biologists are rife with theories about why this and the rare other cases of "programmed die-offs" in the animal kingdom may make some evolutionary sense. What is known, however, is the proximal mechanism underlying the sudden die-off (not "How come they die, in terms of evolutionary patterns over the millennia?" but "How come they die, in the sense of which parts of the body's functioning suddenly go crazy?"). It is glucocorticoid secretion.

---

* Aging also brings about a dramatic decline in the levels of a hormone called DHEA, which has gotten tons of attention. There is some evidence that DHEA serves as an "anti-stress" hormone, blocking the actions of glucocorticoids, and that it can have some beneficial effects in aged populations. I've buried DHEA in this footnote, however, because the subject is quite controversial and in need of some more convincing studies, in my view.

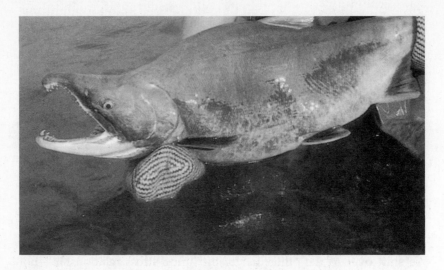

A male sockeye salmon, after the onset of programmed aging.

If you catch salmon right after they spawn, just when they are look-ing a little green around the gills, you find they have huge adrenal glands, peptic ulcers, and kidney lesions; their immune systems have collapsed, and they are teeming with parasites and infections. Aha, kind of sounds like Selye's rats way back when.* Moreover, the salmon have stupendously high glucocorticoid concentrations in their blood-streams. When salmon spawn, regulation of their glucocorticoid secre-tion breaks down. Basically, the brain loses its ability to measure accurately the quantities of circulating hormones and keeps sending a signal to the adrenals to secrete more of them. Lots of glucocorticoids can certainly bring about all those diseases with which the salmon are festering. But is the glucocorticoid excess really responsible for their death? Yup. Take a salmon right after spawning, remove its adrenals, and it will live for a year afterward.

The bizarre thing is that this sequence of events not only occurs in five species of salmon, but also among a dozen species of Australian marsupial mice. All the male mice of these species die shortly after sea-sonal mating; cut out their adrenal glands, however, and they too keep living. Pacific salmon and marsupial mice are not close relatives. At least twice in evolutionary history, completely independently, two

---

* As a very weird and provocative observation, these salmon even have deposits in their brains of the "beta-amyloid" protein that is found in the brains of people with Alzheimer's disease. No one is quite sure what to make of that.

very different sets of species have come up with the identical trick: if you want to degenerate very fast, secrete a ton of glucocorticoids.

 ## CHRONIC STRESS AND THE AGING PROCESS IN THE MAINSTREAM

That is all fine for the salmon looking for the fountain of youth, but we and most other mammals age gradually over time, not in catastrophic die-offs over the course of days. Does stress influence the rate of gradual mammalian aging?

Intuitively, the idea that stress accelerates the aging process makes sense. We recognize that there is a connection between how we live and how we die. Around 1900, a madly inspired German physiologist, Max Rubner, tried to define this connection scientifically. He looked at all sorts of different domestic species and calculated things like lifetime number of heartbeats and lifetime metabolic rate (not the sort of study that many scientists have tried to replicate). He concluded that there is only so long a body can go on—only so many breaths, so many heartbeats, so much metabolism that each pound of flesh can carry out before the mechanisms of life wear out. A rat, with approximately 400 heartbeats a minute, uses up its heartbeat allotment faster (after approximately two years) than an elephant (with approximately 35 beats per minute and a sixty-year life span). Such calculations lay behind ideas about why some species lived far longer than others. Soon the same sort of thinking was applied to how long different individuals within a species live—if you squander a lot of your heartbeats being nervous about blind dates when you're sixteen, there would be that much less metabolic reserve available to you at eighty.

In general, Rubner's ideas about life spans among different species have not held up well in their strictest versions, while the "rate of living" hypotheses about individuals within a species that his ideas inspired have been even less tenable. Nevertheless, they led many people in the field to suggest that a lot of environmental perturbations can wear out the system prematurely. Such "wear and tear" thinking fit in naturally with the stress concept. As we have seen, excessive stress increases the risks of adult-onset diabetes, hypertension, cardiovascular disease, osteoporosis, reproductive decline, and immune suppression. All of these conditions become more common as we age. Moreover, in chapter 4 it was shown that if you have a lot of the indices of allostatic load, it increases your risk of Metabolic syndrome; that same study showed that it increased your mortality risk as well.

We return to the tendency of very old rats, humans, and primates to have elevated resting levels of glucocorticoids in the bloodstream. Some aspect of the regulation of normal glucocorticoid secretion is disrupted during aging. To get a sense of why this happens, we must return to chapter 1's interest about why the water tank on your toilet does not overflow when it's refilling. Once again, the process of refilling can trigger a sensor—the flotation device—to decrease the amount of water flowing into the tank. Engineers who study this sort of thing term that process *negative feedback inhibition* or *end-product inhibition*: increasing amounts of water accumulating in the tank decrease the likelihood of further release of water.

Most hormonal systems, including the CRH/ACTH/glucocorticoid axis, work by this feedback-inhibition process. The brain triggers glucocorticoid release indirectly via CRH and pituitary release of ACTH. The brain needs to know whether to keep secreting more CRH. It does this by sensing the levels of glucocorticoids in the circulation (sampling the hormone from the bloodstream coursing through the brain) to see if levels are at, below, or above a "set point." If levels are low, the brain keeps secreting CRH—just as when water levels in the toilet tank are still low. Once glucocorticoid levels reach or exceed that set point, there is a negative feedback signal and the brain stops secreting CRH. As a fascinating complication, the set point can shift. In the absence of stress, the brain wants different levels of glucocorticoids in the bloodstream from those required when something stressful is happening. (This implies that the quantity of glucocorticoids in the bloodstream necessary to turn off CRH secretion by the brain should vary with different situations, which turns out to be the case.)

This is how the system works normally, as can be shown experimentally by injecting a person with a massive dose of a synthetic glucocorticoid (dexamethasone). The brain senses the sudden increase and says, in effect, "My God, I don't know what is going on with those idiots in the adrenal, but they just secreted *way* too many glucocorticoids." The dexamethasone exerts a negative feedback signal, and soon the person has stopped secreting CRH, ACTH, and her own glucocorticoids. This person would be characterized as "dexamethasone-responsive." If negative feedback regulation is not working very well, however, the person is "dexamethasone-resistant"—she keeps secreting the various hormones, despite the whopping glucocorticoid signal in the bloodstream. And that is precisely what happens in old people, old nonhuman primates, and old rats. Glucocorticoid feedback regulation no longer works very well.

This may explain why very old organisms secrete excessive gluco-corticoids (in the absence of stress and during the recovery period after the end of a stressor). Why the failure of feedback regulation? There is a fair amount of evidence that it is due to the degeneration during aging of one part of the brain. The entire brain does not serve as a "glu-cocorticoid sensor"; instead, that role is served by only a few areas with very high numbers of receptors for glucocorticoids and the means to tell the hypothalamus whether or not to secrete CRH. In chapter 10, I described how the hippocampus is famed for its role in learning and memory. As it turns out, it is also one of the important negative feedback sites in the brain for controlling glucocorticoid secretion. It also turns out that during aging, hippocampal neurons may become dysfunctional. When this occurs, some of the deleterious consequences include a tendency to secrete an excessive amount of glucocorticoids—this could be the reason aged people may have ele-vated resting levels of the hormone, may have trouble turning off secretion after the end of stress, or may be dexamethasone-resistant. It is as if one of the brakes on the system has been damaged, and hor-mone secretion rushes forward, a little out of control.

The elevated glucocorticoid levels of old age, therefore, arise because of a problem with feedback regulation in the damaged hip-pocampus. Why are neurons damaged in the aging hippocampus? It's glucocorticoid exposure, as was discussed in chapter 10.

If you've read carefully, you will begin to note something truly insidious embedded in these findings. When the hippocampus is dam-aged, the rat secretes more glucocorticoids. Which should damage the hippocampus further. Which should cause even more glucocorticoid secretion. . . . Each makes the other worse, causing a degenerative cas-cade that appears to occur in many aging rats, and whose potential pathological consequences have been detailed throughout virtually every page of this book.

Does this degenerative cascade occur in humans? As noted, gluco-corticoid levels rise with extreme old age in the human, and chapter 10 outlines the first evidence that these hormones might have some bad effects on the human hippocampus. The primate and human hip-pocampus appear to be negative feedback regulators of glucocorticoid release, such that hippocampal damage is associated with glucocorti-coid excess, just as in the rodent. So the pieces of the cascade appear to be there in the human, raising the possibilities that histories of severe stress, or of heavy use of synthetic glucocorticoids to treat some dis-ease, might accelerate aspects of this cascade.

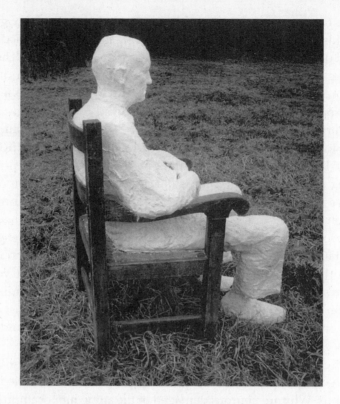

George Segal, Man in a Chair, *wood and plaster, 1969.*

Does that mean that all is lost, that this sort of dysfunction is an obligatory part of aging? Certainly not. It was not by chance that two paragraphs above, I described this cascade as occurring in "many" aging rats, rather than in "all." Some rats age successfully in a way that spares them this cascade, as do many humans—these pleasing stories are part of the final chapter of this book.

It is thus not yet clear whether the "glucocorticoid neurotoxicity" story applies to how our brains age. Unfortunately, the answer is not likely to be available for years; the subject is difficult to study in humans. Nevertheless, from what we know about this process in the rat and monkey, glucocorticoid toxicity stands as a striking example of ways in which stress can accelerate aging. Should it turn out to apply to us as well, it will be an aspect of our aging that will harbor a special threat. If we are crippled by an accident, if we lose our sight or hearing, if we are so weakened by heart disease as to be bed-bound, we cease having so many of the things that make our lives worth living. But when it is our brains that are damaged, when it is our ability to recall old memories or to form new ones that is destroyed, we fear we'll cease to exist as sentient, unique individuals—the version of aging that haunts us most.

Even the most stoic of readers should be pretty frazzled by now, given the detailing in the twelve chapters so far about the sheer number of things that can go wrong with stress. It is time to shift to the second half of the book, which examines stress management, coping, and individual differences in the stress-response. It is time to begin to get some good news.

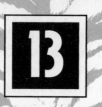

13

WHY IS PSYCHOLOGICAL
STRESS STRESSFUL?

Some people are born to biology. You can spot them instantly as kids—they're the ones comfortably lugging around the toy microscopes, dissecting some dead animal on the dining room table, being ostracized at school for their obsession with geckos.* But all sorts of folks migrate to biology from other fields—chemists, psychologists, physicists, mathematicians.

Several decades after stress physiology began, the discipline was inundated by people who had spent their formative years as engineers. Like physiologists, they thought there was a ferocious logic to how the body worked, but for bioengineers, that tended to mean viewing the body a bit like the circuitry diagram that you get with a radio: input-output ratios, impedance, feedback loops, servomechanisms. I shudder even to write such words, as I barely understand them; but the bioengineers did wonders for the field, adding a tremendous vigor.

Suppose you wonder how the brain knows when to stop glucocorticoid secretion—when enough is enough. In a vague sort of way,

---

* I used to collect the leftover chicken bones from everyone at the Friday-night dinner table, clean them with my knife, and proudly display an articulated skeleton by the end of dessert. In retrospect, I think this was more to irritate my sister than to begin an anatomical quest. A biography of Teddy Roosevelt, however, recently helped me to appreciate that the world lost one of its great potential zoologists when he lapsed into politics. At age eighteen, he had already published professionally in ornithology; when he was half that age, he reacted to the news that his mother had thrown out his collection of field mice, stored in the family icebox, by moping around the house, proclaiming, "The loss to science! The loss to science!"

everyone knew that somehow the brain must be able to measure the amount of glucocorticoids in the circulation, compare that to some desired set point, and then decide whether to continue secreting CRH or turn off the faucet (returning to the toilet tank model). The bioengineers came in and showed that the process was vastly more interesting and complicated than anyone had imagined. There are "multiple feedback domains"; some of the time the brain measures the *quantity* of glucocorticoids in the bloodstream, and sometimes the *rate* at which the level is changing. The bioengineers solved another critical issue: Is the stress-response linear or all-or-nothing? Epinephrine, glucocorticoids, prolactin, and other substances are all secreted during stress; but are they secreted to the same extent regardless of the intensity of the stressor (all-or-nothing responsiveness)? The system turns out to be incredibly sensitive to the size of the stressor, demonstrating a linear relationship between, for example, the extent of the drop in blood pressure and the extent of epinephrine secretion, between the degree of hypoglycemia (drop in blood sugar) and glucagon release. The body not only can sense something stressful, but it also is amazingly accurate at measuring just how far and how fast that stressor is throwing the body out of allostatic balance.

Beautiful stuff, and important. Hans Selye loved the bioengineers, which makes perfect sense, since in his time the whole stress field must have still seemed a bit soft-headed to some mainstream physiologists. Those physiologists knew that the body does one set of things when it is too cold, and a diametrically opposite set when it is too hot, but here were Selye and his crew insisting that there were physiological mechanisms that respond equally to cold *and* hot? *And* to injury *and* hypoglycemia *and* hypotension? The beleaguered stress experts welcomed the bioengineers with open arms. "You see, it's for real; you can do math about stress, construct flow charts, feedback loops, formulas. . . ." Golden days for the business. If the system was turning out to be far more complicated than ever anticipated, it was complicated in a way that was precise, logical, mechanistic. Soon it would be possible to model the body as one big input-output relationship: you tell me exactly to what degree a stressor impinges on an organism (how much it disrupts the allostasis of blood sugar, fluid volume, optimal temperature, and so on), and I'll tell you exactly how much of a stress-response will occur.

This approach, fine for most of the ground that we've covered up until now, will probably allow us to estimate quite accurately what the pancreas of that zebra is doing when the organism is sprinting from a lion. But the approach is not going to tell us which of us will get an ulcer when the factory closes down. Starting in the late 1950s, a new style of experiments in stress physiology began to be conducted that burst that lucid, mechanistic bioengineering bubble. A single example will suffice. An organism is subjected to a painful stimulus, and you are interested in how great a stress-response will be triggered. The bioengineers had been all over that one, mapping the relationship between the intensity and duration of the stimulus and the response. But this time, when the painful stimulus occurs, the organism under study can reach out for its mommy and cry in her arms. Under these circumstances, this organism shows less of a stress-response.

Nothing in that clean, mechanistic world of the bioengineers could explain this phenomenon. The input was still the same; the same number of pain receptors should have been firing while the child underwent some painful procedure. Yet the output was completely different. A critical realization roared through the research community: the physiological stress-response can be modulated by psychological factors. Two identical stressors with the same extent of allostatic disruption can be *perceived*, can be *appraised* differently, and the whole show changes from there.

Suddenly the stress-response could be made bigger or smaller, depending on psychological factors. In other words, psychological variables could *modulate* the stress-response. Inevitably, the next step was demonstrated: in the absence of any change in physiological reality—any actual disruption of allostasis—psychological variables alone could *trigger* the stress-response. Flushed with excitement, Yale physiologist John Mason, one of the leaders in this approach, even went so far as to proclaim that all stress-responses were psychological stress-responses.

The old guard was not amused. Just when the conception of stress was becoming systematized, rigorous, credible, along came this rabble of psychologists muddying up the picture. In a series of published exchanges in which they first praised each other's achievements and ancestors, Selye and Mason attempted to shred each other's work. Mason smugly pointed to the growing literature on psychological initiation and modulation of the stress-response. Selye, facing defeat, insisted that all stress-responses couldn't be psychological and perceptual: if an organism is anesthetized, it still gets a stress-response when a surgical incision is made.

The psychologists succeeded in getting a place at the table, and as they have acquired some table manners and a few gray hairs, they have been treated less like barbarians. We now have to consider which psychological variables are critical. Why is psychological stress stressful?

THE BUILDING BLOCKS OF
PSYCHOLOGICAL STRESSORS

Outlets for frustration You would expect key psychological variables to be mushy concepts to uncover, but in a series of elegant experiments, the physiologist Jay Weiss, then at Rockefeller University, demonstrated exactly what is involved. The subject of one experiment is a rat that receives mild electric shocks (roughly equivalent to the static shock you might get from scuffing your foot on a carpet). Over a series of these, the rat develops a prolonged stress-response: its heart rate and glucocorticoid secretion rate go up, for example. For convenience, we can express the long-term consequences by how likely the rat is to get an ulcer, and in this situation, the probability soars. In the next room, a different rat gets the same series of shocks—identical pattern and intensity; its allostatic balance is challenged to exactly the same extent. But this time, whenever the rat gets a shock, it can run over to a bar of wood and gnaw on it. The rat in this situation is far less likely to get an ulcer. You have given it an *outlet for frustration*. Other types of outlets work as well—let the stressed rat eat something, drink water, or sprint on a running wheel, and it is less likely to develop an ulcer.

We humans also deal better with stressors when we have outlets for frustration—punch a wall, take a run, find solace in a hobby. We are even cerebral enough to *imagine* those outlets and derive some relief: consider the prisoner of war who spends hours imagining a golf game in tremendous detail. I have a friend who passed a prolonged and very stressful illness lying in bed with a mechanical pencil and a notepad, drawing topographic maps of imaginary mountain ranges and taking hikes through them.

A central feature of an outlet being effective is if it distracts from the stressor. But, obviously, more important is that it also be something positive for you—a reminder that there is more to life than whatever is making you crazed and stressed at the time. The frustration-reducing effects of exercise provide an additional layer of benefit, one harking back to my dichotomy, repeated ad nauseam, between the zebra running for its life and the psychologically stressed human. The stress-response is about preparing your body for an explosive burst of energy consumption *right now*; psychological stress is about doing all the same things to your body for no physical reason whatsoever. Exercise finally provides your body for the outlet that it was preparing for.

A variant of Weiss's experiment uncovers a special feature of the outlet-for-frustration reaction. This time, when the rat gets the identical series of electric shocks and is upset, it can run across the cage, sit next to another rat and ... bite the hell out of it. Stress-induced displacement of aggression: the practice works wonders at minimizing the stressfulness of a stressor. It's a real primate specialty as well. A male baboon loses a fight. Frustrated, he spins around and attacks a subordinate male who was minding his own business. An extremely high percentage of primate aggression represents frustration displaced onto innocent bystanders. Humans are pretty good at it, too, and we have a technical way of describing the phenomenon in the context of stress-related disease: "He's one of those guys who doesn't get ulcers, he gives them." Taking it out on someone else—how well it works at minimizing the impact of a stressor.

Social support An additional way we can interact with another organism to minimize the impact of a stressor on us is considerably more encouraging for the future of our planet than is displacement aggression. Rats only occasionally use it, but primates are great at it. Put a primate through something unpleasant: it gets a stress-response. Put it through the same stressor while in a room full of other primates and ... it depends. If those primates are strangers, the stress-response gets worse. But if they are friends, the stress-response is decreased. Social support networks—it helps to have a shoulder to cry on, a hand to hold, an ear to listen to you, someone to cradle you and to tell you it will be okay.

The same is seen with primates in the wild. While I mostly do laboratory research on how stress and glucocorticoids affect the brain, I spend my summers in Kenya studying patterns of stress-related physiology and disease among wild baboons living in a national park. The social life of a male baboon can be pretty stressful—you get beaten up as a victim of displaced aggression; you carefully search for some tuber to eat and clean it off, only to have it stolen by someone of higher rank; and so on. Glucocorticoid levels are elevated among low-ranking baboons and among the entire group if the dominance hierarchy is unstable, or if a new aggressive male has just joined the troop. But if you are a male baboon with a lot of friends, you are likely to have lower glucocorticoid concentrations than males of the same general rank who lack these outlets. And what counts as friends? You play with kids, have frequent nonsexual grooming bouts with females (and social grooming in nonhuman primates lowers blood pressure).

Social support is certainly protective for humans as well. This can be demonstrated even in transient instances of support. In a number of subtle studies, subjects were exposed to a stressor such as having to give a public speech or perform a mental arithmetic task, or having

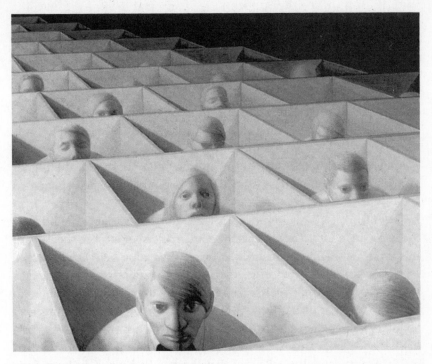

George Tooker, Landscape with Figures, *egg tempera on gesso, 1966.*

two strangers argue with them, with or without a supportive friend present. In each case, social support translated into less of a cardiovascular stress-response. Profound and persistent differences in degrees of social support can influence human physiology as well: within the same family, there are significantly higher glucocorticoid levels among stepchildren than among biological children. Or, as another example, among women with metastatic breast cancer, the more social support, the lower the resting cortisol levels.

As noted in chapter 8, people with spouses or close friends have longer life expectancies. When the spouse dies, the risk of dying rises. Recall also from that chapter the study of parents of Israeli soldiers killed in the Lebanon war: in the aftermath of this stressor, there was no notable increase in risk of diseases or mortality, except among those who were already divorced or widowed. Some additional examples concern the cardiovascular system. People who are socially isolated have overly active sympathetic nervous systems. Given the likelihood that this will lead to higher blood pressure and more platelet aggregation in their blood vessels (remember that from chapter 3?), they are more likely to have heart disease—two to five times as likely, as it turns out. And once they have the heart disease, they are more likely to die at a younger age. In a study of patients with severe coronary heart disease, Redford Williams of Duke University and colleagues found that half of those lacking social support were dead within five years— a rate three times higher than was seen in patients who had a spouse or close friend, after controlling for the severity of the heart disease.*

Finally, support can exist at the broad community level (stay tuned for chapter 17). If you are a member of an ethnic minority, the fewer members there are of your group in your neighborhood, the higher your risks of mental illness, psychiatric hospitalization, and suicide.

Predictability Weiss's rat studies uncovered another variable modulating the stress-response. The rat gets the same pattern of electric shocks, but this time, just before each shock, it hears a warning bell. Fewer ulcers. *Predictability* makes stressors less stressful. The rat with the warning gets two pieces of information. It learns when something dreadful is about to happen. The rest of the time, it learns that something dreadful is *not* about to happen. It can relax. The rat without a warning can always be a half-second away from the next shock. In effect, information that increases predictability tells you that there is bad news, but comforts you that it's not going to be worse—you are going to get shocked soon, but it's never going to be sprung on you without warning.

We all know a human equivalent of this principle: you're in the dentist's chair, no novocaine, the dentist drilling away. Ten seconds of

---

* Recently, I learned about the protective effects of social support in an unexpected way. A local TV station was doing a piece on how stressful rush-hour traffic was, and I wound up giving them advice—turning this chapter into a 15-second sound bite. Somewhere along the way we stumbled onto the great idea of getting a certified Type-A individual (we eventually found one through a local Type-A cardiology clinic) who did the commute each day and measuring his stress hormone levels before and during a commute. The film crew would take some saliva samples from which glucocorticoid levels would be measured. Great. Get to the guy's house just before his commute, collect some spit in a test tube. Then into traffic—with the film crew increasingly stressed by the worry that there wouldn't be any tie-ups. But soon the snarls began, bumper to bumper. Then the second saliva sample was taken. Laboratory analysis, anxious TV producers awaiting results. Baseline sample at home: highly elevated glucocorticoid levels. Rush-hour level: *way down*. Oh no. I'm convinced that the explanation for the outcome of that unscientific experiment was the social support. For this guy, who Type-A's his way through rush hour each day, this was fabulous. A chance to be on television, a bunch of people there with him to document what a stressful commute he endures, getting to feel he's the chosen representative of all Type A's, their anointed. He apparently spent the entire ride cheerfully pointing out how horrible it was, how much worse he's seen ("You think this is bad?! This isn't bad. You should have been in Troy in '47."). He had a fabulous time. The punch line? Everyone should have a friendly film crew in tow when they're stuck in traffic.

nerve-curling pain, some rinsing, five seconds of drilling, a pause while the dentist fumbles a bit, fifteen seconds of drilling, and so on. In one of the pauses, frazzled and trying not to whimper, you gasp, "Almost done?"

"Hard to say," the dentist mumbles, returning to the intermittent drilling. Think how grateful we are for the dentist who, instead, says, "Two more and we're done." The instant the second burst of drilling ends, down goes blood pressure. By being given news about the stressor to come, you are also implicitly being comforted by now knowing what stressors are not coming.

As another variant on the helpfulness of predictability, organisms will eventually habituate to a stressor if it is applied over and over; it may knock physiological allostasis equally out of balance the umpteenth time that it happens, but it is a familiar, predictable stressor by then, and a smaller stress-response is triggered. One classic demonstration involved men in the Norwegian military going through parachute training—as the process went from being hair-raisingly novel to something they could do in their sleep, their anticipatory stress-response went from being gargantuan to nonexistent.

The power of loss of predictability as a psychological stressor is shown in an elegant, subtle study. A rat is going about its business in its cage, and at measured intervals the experimenter delivers a piece of food down a chute into the cage; rat eats happily. This is called an intermittent reinforcement schedule. Now, change the pattern of food delivery so that the rat gets *exactly* the same total amount of food over the course of an hour, but at a random rate. The rat receives just as much reward, but less predictably, and up go glucocorticoid levels. There is not a single physically stressful thing going on in the rat's world. It's not hungry, pained, running for its life—nothing is out of allostatic balance. In the absence of any stressor, loss of predictability triggers a stress-response.

There are even circumstances in which a stress-response can be *more* likely to occur in someone despite the reality that the outside world is *less* stressful. Work by the zoologist John Wingfield of the University of Washington has shown an example of this with wild birds. Consider some species that migrates between the Arctic and the tropics. Bird #1 is in the Arctic, where the temperature averages 5 degrees and where it is, indeed, 5 degrees outside that day. In contrast, Bird #2 is in the tropics, where the average temperature is 80 degrees, but today it has dropped down to 60. Who has the bigger stress-response? Amazingly, Bird #2. The point isn't that the temperature in the tropics is 55 degrees warmer than in the Arctic (what kind of stressor would that be?). It's that the temperature in the tropics is 20 degrees colder than anticipated.

A human version of the same idea has been documented. During the onset of the Nazi blitzkrieg bombings of England, London was hit every night like clockwork. Lots of stress. In the suburbs the bombings were far more sporadic, occurring perhaps once a week. Fewer stressors, but much less predictability. There was a significant increase in the incidence of ulcers during that time. Who developed more ulcers? The suburban population. (As another measure of the importance of unpredictability, by the third month of the bombing, ulcer rates in all the hospitals had dropped back to normal.)

Despite the similarity between the responses of humans and of other animals to a lack of predictability, I suspect that there they are not identical, and in an important way. The warning of impending shocks to a rat has little effect on the size of the stress-response *during* the shocks; instead, allowing the rat to feel more confident about when it *doesn't* have to worry reduces the rat's anticipatory stress-response the rest of the time. Analogously, when the dentist says, "Only two more times and then we're done," it allows us to relax *at the end* of the second burst of drilling. But I suggest, although I cannot prove it, that unlike the case for the rat, proper information will also lower our stress-response *during* the pain. If you were told "only two times more" versus "only ten times more," wouldn't you use different mental strategies to try to cope? With either scenario, you would pull out the comforting thought of "only one more and then it's the last one" at different times; you would save your most distracting fantasy for a different point; you would try counting to zero from different numbers. Predictive information lets us know what internal coping strategy is likely to work best during a stressor.

We often wish for information about the course of some medical problem because it aids our strategizing about how we will cope. A simple example: you have some minor surgery, and you're given predictive information—the first post-surgical day, there is going to be a lot of pain, pretty constant, whereas by the second day, you'll just feel a bit achy. Armed with that information, you are more likely to plan on watching the eight distracting videos on day one and to devote day two to writing delicate haikus than the other way around. Among other reasons, we wish to optimize our coping strategies when we request the most devastating piece of medical information any of us will ever face: "How much time do I have left?"

Control Rat studies also demonstrate a related facet of psychological stress. Give the rat the same series of shocks. This time, however, you study a rat that has been trained to press a lever to avoid electric shocks. Take away the lever, shock it, and the rat develops a massive stress-response. It's as if the rat were thinking, "I can't believe this. I know what to do about electric shocks; give me a damned lever and I could handle this. This isn't fair." Ulceration city (as well as higher glucocorticoid levels, poorer immune function, and faster tumor growth). Give the trained rat a lever to press; even if it is disconnected from the shock mechanism, it still helps: down goes the stress-response. So long as the rat has been exposed to a higher rate of shocks previously, it will think that the lower rate now is due to its having control over the situation. This is an extraordinarily powerful variable in modulating the stress-response.

The identical style of experiment with humans yields similar results. Place two people in adjoining rooms, and expose both to intermittent noxious, loud noises; the person who has a button and believes that pressing it decreases the likelihood of more noise is less hypertensive. In one variant on this experiment, subjects with the button who did not bother to press it did just as well as those who actually pressed the button. Thus, the *exercise* of control is not critical; rather, it is the *belief* that you have it. An everyday example: airplanes are safer than cars, yet more of us are phobic about flying. Why? Because your average driver believes that he is a better-than-average driver, thus more in control. In an airplane, we have no control at all. My wife and I tease each other on plane flights, exchanging control: "Okay, you rest for a while, I'll take over concentrating on keeping the pilot from having a stroke."

The issue of control runs through the literature on the psychology of stress. As will be discussed in the final chapter on coping, exercise can be a great stress reducer, but only so long as it is something that seems even remotely desirable. Amazingly, the same is seen in a rat—let a rat run voluntarily in a running wheel, and it makes it feel great. *Force* a rat to do the same amount of exercise and it gets a massive stress-response.

The issue of control runs through the extensive literature on occupational stress. Sure, there are some jobs where stress comes in the form of someone having too much control and responsibility—that rare occupation where, over the course of an average workday, you might find yourself having to direct the landing pattern of an array of circling jumbo jets at the local airport, personally excise someone's cerebral aneurysm, and make the final decision as to whether taffeta is going to be in at the fall runway show in Milan. For most, though, occupational stress is built more around lack of control, work life spent as a piece of the machine. Endless studies have shown that the link between occupational stress and increased risk of cardiovascular and metabolic diseases is anchored in the killer combination of high demand and low control—you have to work hard, a lot is expected of you, and you have minimal control over the process. This is the epitome of the assembly line, the combination of stressors that makes for Marx's alienation of the workers. The control element is more powerful than the demand one—low demand and low control is more damaging to one's health than high demand and high control.

The stressfulness of lack of control on the job applies in only certain domains, however. For example, there is the issue of what product is made, and lack of control in this realm tends not to be all that stressful—few people are ulcerating because of their deep conviction that all of their capable and motivated fellow workers should be cranking vast numbers of stuffed Snoopys out of this factory instead of ball bearings. Instead, it is stress about lack of control over the process—what work rate is expected and how much flexibility there is about it, what amenities there are and how much control you have over them, how authoritarian the authorities are.

These issues can apply just as readily to some less expected workplaces, ones that can be highly prestigious and desirable. For example, professional musicians in orchestras generally have lower job satisfaction and more stress than those in small chamber groups (such as a string quartet). Why? One pair of researchers suggest that this is because of the lack of autonomy in an orchestra, where centuries of tradition hold that orchestras are subservient to the dictatorial whims of the maestro conducting them. For example, it was only in recent years that orchestra unions won the right for regularly scheduled bathroom breaks during rehearsals, instead of having to wait until the conductor cared to note how squirmy the reed players had become.*

So the variable of control is extremely important; controlling the rewards that you get can be more desirable than getting them for nothing. As an extraordinary example, both pigeons and rats prefer to press a lever in order to obtain food (so long as the task is not too difficult) over having the food delivered freely—a theme found in the activities and statements of many scions of great fortunes, who regret the contingency-free nature of their lives, without purpose or striving.

---

* Interestingly, the paper was written by Seymour Levine, one of the giants in this field, and his son, Robert, a professional orchestra musician.

Loss of control and lack of predictive information are closely related. Some researchers have emphasized this, pointing out that the common theme is that the organism is subjected to novelty. You thought you knew how to manage things, you thought you knew what would happen next, and it turns out you are wrong in this novel situation. The potency of this is demonstrated in primate studies in which merely placing the animal into a novel cage suppresses its immune system. Others have emphasized that these types of stressors cause arousal and vigilance, as you search for the new rules of control and prediction. Both views are different aspects of the same issue.

A perception of things worsening Yet another critical psychological variable in the stress-response has been uncovered. A hypothetical example: two rats get a series of electric shocks. On the first day, one gets ten shocks an hour; the other, fifty. Next day, both get twenty-five shocks an hour. Who becomes hypertensive? Obviously, the one going from ten to twenty-five. The other rat is thinking, "Twenty-five? Piece of cheese, no problem; I can handle that." Given the same degree of disruption of allostasis, a perception that events are improving helps tremendously.

The principle often pops up in the realm of human illness. Recall in chapter 9 the scenario where pain is less stressful, can even be welcome, when it means, for example, that the drugs are working, the tumor is shrinking. One classic study demonstrated that in examining parents of children who had a 25 percent chance of dying of cancer. Astonishingly, these parents showed only a moderate rise in glucocorticoid levels in the bloodstream. How could that be? Because the children were all in remission after a period in which the odds of death had been far higher. Twenty-five percent must have seemed like a miracle. Twenty-five shocks an hour, a certain degree of social instability, a one-in-four chance of your child dying—each can imply either good news or bad, and only the latter seems to stimulate a stress-response. It's not just the external reality; it's the meaning you attach to it.

A version of this can be observed among the baboons I study in Kenya. In general, when dominance hierarchies are unstable, resting glucocorticoid levels rise. This makes sense, because such instabilities make for stressful times. Looking at individual baboons, however, shows a more subtle pattern: given the same degree of instability, males whose ranks are *dropping* have elevated glucocorticoid levels, while males whose ranks are *rising* amid the tumult don't show this endocrine trait.

NOT SO FAST

Thus, some powerful psychological factors can trigger a stress-response on their own or make another stressor seem more stressful: loss of control or predictability, loss of outlets for frustration or sources of support, a perception that things are getting worse. There are obviously some overlaps in the meaning of these different factors. As we saw, control and predictability are closely aligned; combine them with a perception of things worsening, and you have the situation of bad things happening, out of your control, and utterly unpredictable. The primatologist Joan Silk of UCLA has emphasized how, among primates, a great way to maintain dominance is for the alpha individual to mete out aggression in a randomly brutal way. This is our primate essence of terrorism.

Sometimes these different variables conflict and it becomes a question as to which is more powerful. This often involves a dichotomy between control/predictability issues and the perception of whether things are improving or worsening. For example, someone unexpectedly wins the lottery big-time. Is this a stressor? It depends on what is more powerful, the beneficial "perception of things getting better" part or the stressful "lack of predictability" part. Not surprisingly, if the lottery win is big enough, most people's psyches can handle some unpredictability. Nonetheless, some nonhuman primate studies in which rank was manipulated by the experimenters show that it can go in the other way, that if the change is sufficiently unexpected, it can be stressful, even if it is good change (and psychotherapy often must delve into the reasons why people sometimes find change for the good to be less desirable than persisting with a known misery). Conversely, if a situation is sufficiently awful, the fact that it may have been predictable offers little comfort.

These factors play a major role in explaining how we all go through lives full of stressors, yet differ so dramatically in our vulnerability to them. The final chapter of this book examines the bases of these individual differences in greater detail. This will serve as a blueprint for analyzing how to learn to exploit these psychological variables—how, in effect, to manage stress better.

The ways in which these different psychological variables can interact brings up a key point, one that will dominate the final chapter. This is that stress management cannot consist merely of the simple-minded solution of "Maximize control. Maximize predictability. Maximize outlets for frustration." As we will now see, it is considerably

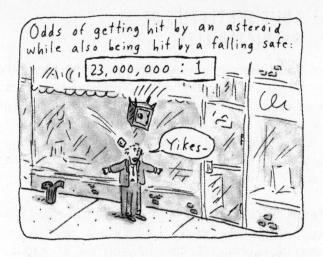

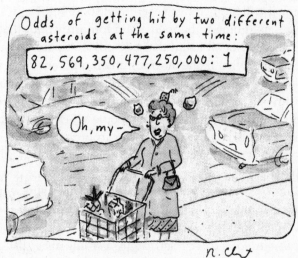

more complicated than that. As the most obvious first pass at this, some lack of control and predictability can be a great thing—a good roller-coaster ride, a superbly terrifying movie, a mystery novel with a great surprise ending, winning a lottery, being subject to a random act of kindness. And sometimes, an overabundance of predictability is a disaster—boredom on the job. The right amounts of loss of control and predictability are what we call stimulation. In chapter 16, we will look at the biology of why stimulation makes us happy, rather than stressed. The goal is never to generate lives in which there is never a challenge to allostasis. And the remainder of this chapter considers when increasing a sense of control and predictability reduces stress.

SOME SUBTLETIES OF PREDICTABILITY

We have already seen how predictability can ameliorate the consequences of stress: one rat gets a series of shocks and develops a higher risk for an ulcer than the rat who gets warnings beforehand. Predictability doesn't always help, however. The experimental literature on this is pretty dense; some human examples of this point make it more accessible. (Remember, in these scenarios, the stressor is inevitable; the warning cannot change the stressor, just the perception of it.)

How predictable is the stressor, in the absence of a warning? What if, one morning, an omnipotent voice says, "There is no way out of it; a meteor is going to crush your car while you're at work today (but it's the only time it will happen this year)." Not soothing. There's the good news that it's not going to happen again tomorrow, but that's hardly comforting; this is not an event that you anxiously fret over often. At the other extreme, what if one morning an omnipotent voice whispers, "Today it's going to be stressful on the freeway—lots of traffic, stops and go's. Tomorrow, too. In fact, every day this year, except November 9, when there'll hardly be any traffic, people will wave to each other, and a highway patrol cop will stop you in order to share his coffee cake with you." Who needs predictive information about the obvious fact that driving to work is going to be stressful? Thus, warnings are less effective for very rare stressors (you don't usually worry much about meteors) and very frequent ones (they approach being predictable even without the warning).

How far in advance of the stressor does the warning come? Each day, you go for a mysterious appointment: you are led into a room with your eyes closed and are seated in a deep, comfortable chair. Then, with roughly even probabilities but no warning, either a rich, avuncular voice reads you to sleep with your favorite childhood stories, or a bucket of ice water is sloshed over your head. Not a pleasing prospect, I would bet. Would the whole thing be any less unsettling if you were told which treatment you were going to get five seconds before the event? Probably not—there is not enough time to derive any psychological benefits from the information. At the other extreme, how about predictive information long in the future? Would you wish for an omnipotent voice to tell you, "Eleven years and twenty-seven days from now your ice-water bath will last ten full minutes"? Information either just before or long before the stressor does little good to alleviate the psychological anticipation.

Some types of predictive information can even increase the cumulative anticipatory stressor. For example, if the stressor is truly terrible. Would you be comforted by the omnipotent message: "Tomorrow an unavoidable accident will mangle your left leg, although your right leg will remain in great shape"?

Likewise, predictive information can make things worse if the information is vague. As I write this section, we continue to be stressed by the maddening vagueness of predictive information in our post-9/11 world, when we are given warnings that read like horoscopes from hell: "Orange Alert: We don't know what the threat is, but be extra alert about everything for the next few days."*

Collectively, these scenarios tell us that predictability does not always work to protect us from stress. The much more systematic studies with animals suggest that it works only in a midrange of frequencies and intensities of stressors, and with certain lag times and levels of accurate information.

 ## SUBTLETIES OF CONTROL

To understand some important subtleties of the effects of control on stress, we need to return to the paradigm of the rat being shocked. It had been previously trained to press a lever to avoid shocks, and now it's pounding away like crazy on a lever. The lever does nothing; the rat is still getting shocked, but with less chance of an ulcer because the rat thinks it has control. To introduce a sense of control into the experimental design decreases the stress-response because, in effect, the rat is thinking, "Ten shocks an hour. Not bad; just imagine how bad it would be if I wasn't on top of it with my lever here." But what if things backfire, and adding a sense of control makes the rat think, "Ten shocks an hour, what's wrong with me? I have a lever here, I should have avoided the shocks, it's my fault." If you believe you have control over stressors that are, in fact, beyond your control, you may consider it somehow to be your fault that the inevitable occurred.

---

* The satirical newspaper *The Onion* mocked the imprecision of this information with a facetious article in which Tom Ridge, secretary of Homeland Security, supposedly announces new levels of alert. "The newly added levels are Orange-Red Alert, Red-Orange Alert, Maroon Alert, Burnt Sienna Alert, and Ochre Alert," Ridge said. "They indicate, in ascending order of fear: concern, deep dread, severe apprehension, near-crippling fright, and pants-shitting terror. Please make a note of this." (*The Onion* 39, no. 7, 26 February 2003)

An inappropriate sense of control in the face of awful events can make us feel terrible. Some of our most compassionate words to people experiencing tragedy involve minimizing their perceived sense of control. "It's not your fault, no one could have stopped in time; she just darted out from between the cars." "It's not something you could have done anything about; you tried your best, the economy's just lousy now." "Honey, getting him the best doctor in the world couldn't have cured him." And some of the most brutally callous of society's attempts to shift blame attribute more personal control during a stressor than exists. "She was asking for it if she was going to dress that way" (rape victims have the control to prevent the rape). "Your child's schizophrenia was caused by your mothering style" (this was a destructive belief that dominated psychiatry for decades before the disease was recognized to be neurochemical). "If they'd only made the effort to assimilate, they wouldn't have these problems" (minorities have the power to prevent their persecution).

The effects of the sense of control on stress are highly dependent on context. In general, if the stressor is of a sort where it is easy to imagine how much worse it could have been, inserting an artificial sense of control helps. "That was awful, but think of how bad it would have been if I hadn't done X." But when the stressor is truly awful, an artificial sense of control is damaging—it is difficult to conceive a yet-worse scenario that you managed to avoid, but easy to be appalled by the disaster you didn't prevent. You don't want to feel as if you could have controlled the uncontrollable when the outcome is awful. People with a strong internal locus of control (in other words, people who think they are the masters of their own ship—that what goes on around them reflects their actions) have far greater stress-responses than do those with external loci when confronted with something uncontrollable. This is a particular risk for the elderly (especially elderly men) as life generates more and more things beyond their control. As we will see in the final chapter, there is even a personality type whose tendency to internalize control in the face of bad, uncontrollable things greatly increases the risk of a particular disease.

These subtleties about control and predictability help to explain a confusing feature about the studies of stress. In general, the less control or predictability, the more at risk you are for a stress-induced disease. Yet an experiment conducted by Joseph Brady in 1958 with monkeys gave rise to the view that more control and more predictability cause ulcers. Half the animals could press a bar to delay shocks ("executive" monkeys); the other half were passively yoked to one of the "executives" such that they received a shock whenever the first one did. In this widely reported study, the executive monkeys were more likely to develop ulcers. Out of these studies came the popular concept of the "executive stress syndrome" and associated images of executive humans weighed down with the stressful burdens of control, leadership, and responsibility. Ben Natelson, of the VA Medical Center in East Orange, New Jersey, along with Jay Weiss, noted some problems with that study. First, it was conducted with parameters where control and predictability are bad news. Second, the "executive" and "nonexecutive" monkeys were not chosen randomly; instead, the monkeys that tended to press the bar first in pilot studies were selected to be executives. Monkeys that press sooner have since been shown to be more emotionally reactive animals, so Brady was inadvertently stacking the executive side with the more reactive, ulcer-prone monkeys. In general, executives of all species are more likely to be giving ulcers than to be getting them, as we will see in chapter 17.

To summarize, stress-responses can be modulated or even caused by psychological factors, including loss of outlets for frustration and of social support, a perception of things worsening, and under some circumstances, a loss of control and of predictability. These ideas have vastly expanded our ability to answer the question: Why do only some of us get stress-related diseases? Obviously we differ as to the number of stressors that befall us. After all the chapters on physiology, you can guess that we differ in how fast our adrenals make glucocorticoids, how many insulin receptors we have in our fat cells, the thickness of our stomach walls, and so on. But in addition to those physiological differences, we can now add another dimension. We differ in the psychological filters through which we perceive the stressors in our world. Two people participating in the same event—a long wait at the supermarket checkout, public speaking, parachuting out of an airplane—may differ dramatically in their psychological perception of the event. "Oh, I'll just read a magazine while I wait" (outlet for frustration); "I'm nervous as hell, but by giving this after-dinner talk, I'm a shoo-in for that promotion" (things are getting better); "This is great—I've always wanted to try sky-diving" (this is something I'm in control of).

In the next two chapters we will consider psychiatric disorders such as depression and anxiety, and personality disorders, in which there's a bad match between how stressful the real world is and how stressful the person perceives it to be. As we'll see, the mismatch between the two can take a variety of forms, but the thing in common is the fact that a potentially considerable price is paid by the sufferer. Following that, in chapter 16, we consider what psychological stress has to do with the process of addiction. Following that is a chapter examining how your place in society, and the type of society it is, can have profound effects on stress physiology and patterns of disease. In the final chapter we will examine how stress-management techniques can aid us by teaching how to exploit these psychological defenses.

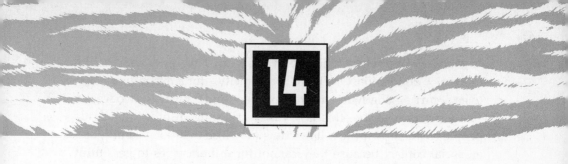

14

STRESS AND DEPRESSION

We are morbidly fascinated with the exotica of disease. They fill our made-for-television movies, our tabloids, and the book reports of adolescents hoping to become doctors someday. Victorians with Elephant Man's disease, murderers with multiple personality disorders, ten-year-olds with progeria, idiot savants with autism, cannibals with kuru. Who could resist? But when it comes to the bread and butter of human misery, try a major depression. It can be life-threatening, it can destroy lives, demolish the families of sufferers. And it is dizzyingly common—the psychologist Martin Seligman has called it the common cold of psychopathology. Best estimates are that from 5 to 20 percent of us will suffer a major, incapacitating depression at some point in our lives, causing us to be hospitalized or medicated or nonfunctional for a significant length of time. Its incidence has been steadily increasing for decades—by the year 2020, depression is projected to be the second leading cause of medical disability on earth.

This chapter differs a bit from those that preceded it in which the concept of "stress" was at the forefront. Initially, that may not seem to be the case in our focus on depression. The two appear to be inextricably linked, however, and the concept of stress will run through every page of this chapter. It is impossible to understand either the biology or psychology of major depressions without recognizing the critical role played in the disease by stress.

To begin to understand this connection, it is necessary to get some sense of the disorder's characteristics. We have first to wrestle with a semantic problem. *Depression* is a term that we all use in an everyday sense. Something mildly or fairly upsetting happens to us, and we get "the blues" for a while, followed by recovery. This is not what occurs in a major depression. One issue is chronicity—for a major depression to be occurring, the symptoms to have persisted for at least two weeks. The other is severity—this is a vastly crippling disorder that leads people to attempt suicide; its victims may lose their jobs, family, and all social contact because they cannot force themselves to get out of bed, or refuse to go to a psychiatrist because they feel they don't deserve to get better. It is a horrific disease, and throughout this chapter I will be referring to this major, devastating form of depression, rather than the transient blues that we may casually signify with the term "feeling depressed."

 ## THE SYMPTOMS

The defining feature of a major depression is loss of pleasure. If I had to define a major depression in a single sentence, I would describe it as a "genetic/neurochemical disorder requiring a strong environmental trigger whose characteristic manifestation is an inability to appreciate sunsets." Depression can be as tragic as cancer or a spinal cord injury. Think about what our lives are about. None of us will live forever, and on occasion we actually believe it; our days are filled with disappointments, failures, unrequited loves. Despite this, almost inconceivably, we not only cope but even feel vast pleasures. I, for example, am resoundingly mediocre at soccer, but nothing keeps me from my twice-weekly game. Invariably there comes a moment when I manage to gum up someone more adept than I; I'm panting and heaving and pleased, and there's still plenty more time to play and a breeze blows and I suddenly feel dizzy with gratitude for my animal existence. What could be more tragic than a disease that, as its defining symptom, robs us of that capacity?

This trait is called anhedonia: hedonism is "the pursuit of pleasure," anhedonia is "the inability to feel pleasure" (also often called dysphoria—I'll be using the terms interchangeably). Anhedonia is consistent among depressives. A woman has just received the long-sought promotion; a man has just become engaged to the woman of his dreams—and, amid their depression, they will tell you how they feel nothing, how it really doesn't count, how they don't deserve it. Friendship, achievement, sex, food, humor—none can bring any pleasure.

This is the classic picture of depression, and some recent research, much of it built around work of the psychologist Alex Zautra of the

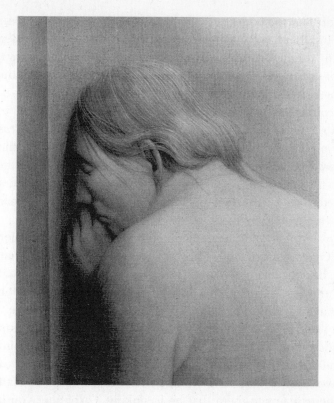

George Tooker, Woman at the Wall, *egg tempera on gesso, 1974.*

University of Arizona, shows that the story is more complex. Specifically, positive and negative emotions are not mere opposites. If you take subjects and, at random times throughout the day, have them record how they are feeling at that moment, the frequencies of feeling good and feeling bad are not inversely correlated. There's normally not much of a connection between how much your life is filled with strongly positive emotions and how much with strongly negative ones. Depression represents a state where those two independent axes tend toward collapsing into one inverse relationship—too few positive emotions and too many negative ones. Naturally, the inverse correlation isn't perfect, and a lot of current research focuses on questions like: Are different subtypes of depression characterized more by the absence of positive emotions or the overabundance of negatives?

Accompanying major depression are great grief and great guilt. We often feel grief and guilt in the everyday sadnesses that we refer to as "depression." But in a major depression, they can be incapacitating, as the person is overwhelmed with the despair. There can be complex layers of these feelings: not just obsessive guilt, for example, about something that has contributed to the depression, but obsessive guilt about the depression itself—what it has done to the sufferer's family, the guilt of not being able to overcome depression, a life lived but once and wasted amid this disease. Small wonder that, worldwide, depression accounts for 800,000 suicides per year.*

In a subset of such patients, the sense of grief and guilt can take on the quality of a delusion. By this, I do not mean the thought-disordered delusions of schizophrenics; instead, delusional thinking in depressives is of the sort where facts are distorted, over- or underinterpreted to the point where one must conclude that things are terrible and getting worse, hopeless.

An example: a middle-aged man, out of the blue, has a major heart attack. Overwhelmed by his implied mortality, the transformation of his life, he slips into a major depression. Despite this, he is recovering from the attack reasonably well, and there is every chance that he will resume a normal life. But each day he's sure he's getting worse.

The hospital in which he is staying is circular in construction, with a corridor that forms a loop. One day, the nurses walk him once around the hospital before he collapses back in bed. The next day, he does two laps; he is getting stronger. That evening, when his family visits, he explains to them that he is sinking. "What are you talking about? The nurses said that you did two loops today; yesterday you only did one." No, no, he shakes his head sadly, you don't understand. He explains that the hospital is being renovated and, um, well, last night they closed off the old corridor and opened a newer, smaller one. And, you see, the distance around the new loop is less than half the distance of the old one, so two laps today is still less than I could do yesterday.

This particular incident occurred with the father of a friend, an engineer who lucidly described radii and circumferences, expecting his family to believe that the hospital had opened up a new corridor through the core of the building in one day. This is delusional thinking; the emotional energies behind the analysis and evaluation are disordered so that the everyday world is interpreted in a way that leads to depressive conclusions—it's awful, getting worse, and this is what I deserve.

---

* Some suicide statistics: women are more likely to attempt suicide when depressed than are men; men are more likely to be successful. The group most at risk are single white males over sixty-five years of age with, naturally, access to guns.

Cognitive therapists, like Aaron Beck of the University of Pennsylvania, even consider depression to be primarily a disorder of thought, rather than emotion, in that sufferers tend to see the world in a distorted, negative way. Beck and colleagues have conducted striking studies that provide evidence for this. For example, they might show a subject two pictures. In the first, a group of people are gathered happily around a dinner table, feasting. In the second, the same people are gathered around a coffin. Show the two pictures rapidly or simultaneously; which one is remembered? Depressives see the funeral scene at rates higher than chance. They are not only depressed about something, but see the goings-on around them in a distorted way that always reinforces that feeling. Their glasses are always half empty.

Another frequent feature of a major depression is called psychomotor retardation. The person moves and speaks slowly. Everything requires tremendous effort and concentration. She finds the act of merely arranging a doctor's appointment exhausting. Soon it is too much even to get out of bed and get dressed. (It should be noted that not all depressives show psychomotor retardation; some may show the opposite pattern, termed psychomotor agitation.) The psychomotor retardation accounts for one of the important clinical features of depression, which is that severely, profoundly depressed people rarely attempt suicide. It's not until they begin to feel a bit better. If the psychomotor aspects make it too much for this person to get out of bed, they sure aren't going to find the often considerable energy needed to kill themselves.

A key point: many of us tend to think of depressives as people who get the same everyday blahs as you and I, but that for them it just spirals out of control. We may also have the sense, whispered out of earshot, that these are people who just can't handle normal ups and downs, who are indulging themselves. (Why can't they just get themselves together?) A major depression, however, is as real a disease as diabetes. Another set of depressive symptoms supports that view. Basically, many things in the bodies of depressives work peculiarly; these are called vegetative symptoms. You and I get an everyday depression. What do we do? Typically, we sleep more than usual, probably eat more than usual, convinced in some way that such comforts will make us feel better. These traits are just the opposite of the vegetative symptoms seen in most people with major depressions. Eating declines. Sleeping does as well, and in a distinctive manner. While depressives don't necessarily have trouble falling asleep, they have the problem of "early morning wakening," spending months on end sleepless and exhausted from three-thirty or so each morning. Not only is sleep shortened but, as mentioned in chapter 11, the "architecture" of sleep is different as well—the normal pattern of shifting between deep and shallow sleep, the rhythm of the onset of dream states, are disturbed.

An additional vegetative symptom is extremely relevant to this chapter, namely that major depressives often experience elevated levels of glucocorticoids. This is critical for a number of reasons that will be returned to, and helps to clarify what the disease is actually about. When looking at a depressive sitting on the edge of the bed, barely able to move, it is easy to think of the person as energy-less, enervated. A more accurate picture is of the depressive as a tightly coiled spool of wire, tense, straining, active—but all inside. As we will see, a psychodynamic view of depression shows the person fighting an enormous, aggressive mental battle—no wonder they have elevated levels of stress hormones.

Chapter 10 reviewed how glucocorticoids can impair aspects of memory that depend on the hippocampus, and the frequently elevated glucocorticoid levels in depression may help explain another feature of the disease, which is problems with hippocampal-dependent memory. The memory problems may reflect, in part, a lack of motivation on the part of the depressed person (why work hard on some shrink's memory test when everything, everything, is hopeless and pointless?), or an anhedonic inability to respond to the rewards of remembering something in a task. Nonetheless, amid those additional factors, the pure process of storing and retrieving memories via the hippocampus is often impaired. As we'll see shortly, this fits extraordinarily well with recent findings showing that the hippocampus is smaller than average in many depressives.

Another feature of depression also confirms that it is a real disease, rather than merely the situation of someone who simply cannot handle everyday ups and downs. There are multiple types of depressions, and they can look quite different. In one variant, unipolar depression, the sufferer fluctuates from feeling extremely depressed to feeling reasonably normal. In another form, the person fluctuates between deep depression and wild, disorganized hyperactivity. This is called bipolar depression or, more familiarly, manic depression. Here we run into another complication because, just as we use depression in an everyday sense that is different from the medical sense, mania has an everyday connotation as well. We may use the term to refer to madness, as in made-for-television homicidal maniacs. Or we could describe someone as being in a manic state when he is buoyed by some unexpected good news—talking quickly, laughing, gesticulating. But the mania found in manic depression is of a completely different magnitude. Let me give an example of the disorder: a woman comes into the emergency room; she's bipolar, completely manic, hasn't been taking her medication. She's on welfare, doesn't have a cent to her name, and in the last week she's bought three Cadillacs with money from loan sharks. And, get this, she doesn't even know how to drive. People in manic states will go for days on three hours of sleep a night and feel rested, will talk nonstop for hours at a time, will be vastly distractible, unable to concentrate amid their racing thoughts. In outbursts of irrational grandiosity, they will behave in ways that are foolhardy or dangerous to themselves and others—at the extreme, poisoning themselves in attempting to prove their immortality, burning down their homes, giving away their life savings to strangers. It is a profoundly destructive disease.

The strikingly different subtypes of depression and their variability suggest not just a single disease, but a heterogeneity of diseases that have different underlying biologies. Another feature of the disorder also indicates a biological abnormality. Suppose a patient comes to a doctor in the tropics. The patient is running a high fever that abates, only to come back a day or two later, abate again, return again, and so on every 48 to 72 hours. The doctor will recognize this instantly as malaria, because of the rhythmicity of the disorder. It has to do with the life cycle of the malarial parasite as it moves from red blood cells to the liver and spleen. The rhythmicity screams biology. In the same way, certain subtypes of depression have a rhythm. A manic-depressive may be manic for five days, severely depressed for the following week, then mildly depressed for half a week or so, and, finally, symptom-free for a few weeks. Then the pattern starts up again, and may have been doing so for a decade. Good things and bad things happen, but the same cyclic rhythm continues, which suggests just as much deterministic biology as in the life cycle of the malarial parasite. In another subset of depression the rhythm is annual, where sufferers get depressed during the winter. These are called seasonal affective disorders (SADs; "affective" is the psychiatric term for emotional responses), and are thought to be related to patterns of exposure to light; recent work has uncovered a class of retinal cells that respond to light intensity and, surprisingly, send their information directly into the limbic system, the emotional part of the brain. Again, the rhythmicity appears independent of external life events; a biological clock is ticking away in there that has something to do with mood, and something is seriously wrong with its ticking.

THE BIOLOGY OF DEPRESSION

Neurochemistry and Depression

Considerable evidence exists that something is awry with the chemistry of the brains of depressives. In order to appreciate that, it is necessary to learn a bit about how brain cells communicate with one another. The illustration on page 279 shows a schematic version of two neurons, the principal type of brain cell. If a neuron has become excited with some thought or memory (metaphorically speaking), its excitement is electrical—a wave of electricity sweeps from the dendrites over the cell body, down the axon to the axon terminals. When the wave of electrical excitation reaches the axon terminal, it releases chemical messengers that float across the synapse. These messengers—neurotransmitters—bind to specialized receptors on the adjacent dendrite, causing the second neuron to become electrically excited.

A minor piece of housekeeping, however: What happens to the neurotransmitter molecule after it has done its job and floats off the receptor? In some cases, it is recycled—taken back up by the axon terminal of the first neuron and repackaged for future use. Or it can be degraded in the synapse and the debris flushed out to sea (the cerebrospinal fluid, then to the blood, and then the urine). If these processes of clearing neurotransmitters out of the way fail (reuptake ceases or degradation stops or both), suddenly a lot more neurotransmitter remains in the synapse, giving a stronger signal to the second neuron than usual. Thus, the proper disposal of these powerful messengers is integral to normal neuronal communication.

There are trillions of synapses in the brain. Do we need trillions of chemically unique neurotransmitters? Certainly not. You can generate a seemingly infinite number of messages with a finite number of messengers; consider how many words we can form with the mere twenty-six letters in our alphabet. All you need are rules that allow for the same messenger to convey different meanings, metaphorically speaking, in different contexts. At one synapse, neurotransmitter A sends a message relevant to pancreatic regulation, while at another synapse the same neurotransmitter substance may pertain to adolescent crushes. There are many neurotransmitters, probably on the order of a few hundred, but certainly not trillions.

So that's a primer on how neurons talk to each other with neurotransmitters. The best evidence suggests that depression involves abnormal levels of the neurotransmitters norepinephrine, serotonin,

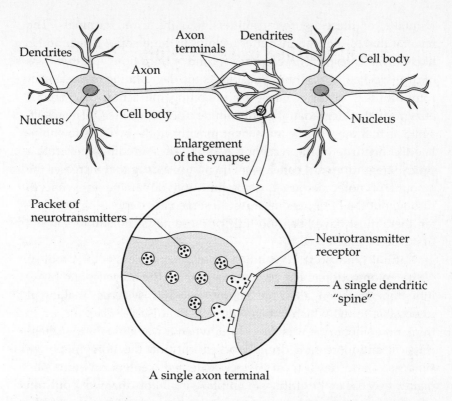

Packet of neurotransmitters

Neurotransmitter receptor

A single dendritic "spine"

A single axon terminal

A neuron that has been excited conveys information to other neurons by means of chemical signals at synapses, the contact points between neurons. When the impulse reaches the axon terminal of the signaling neuron, it induces the release of neurotransmitter molecules. Transmitters diffuse across a narrow cleft and bind to receptors in the adjacent neuron's dendritic spine.

and dopamine. Before reviewing the evidence, it's important to clear up a point. You are no doubt thinking, "Wasn't there something about norepinephrine and the sympathetic nervous system many chapters ago?" Absolutely, and that proves the point about the varied roles played by any given neurotransmitter. In one part of the body (the heart, for example), norepinephrine is a messenger concerning arousal and the Four F's, while in a different part of the nervous system, norepinephrine seems to have something to do with the symptoms of depression.

Why is it likely that there is something wrong with norepinephrine, serotonin, or dopamine in depression? The best evidence is that most of the drugs that lessen depression increase the amount of signaling by these neurotransmitters. One class of antidepressants, called tricyclics (a reference to their biochemical structure), stops the recycling, or reuptake, of these neurotransmitters into the axon terminals. The result is that the neurotransmitter remains in the synapse longer and is likely to hit its respective receptor a second or third time. Another class of drugs, called MAO inhibitors, blocks the degradation of these neurotransmitters in the synapse by inhibiting the action of a crucial enzyme in that degradation, monoamine oxidase, or MAO. The result, again, is that more of the messenger remains in the synapse to stimulate the dendrite of the receiving neuron. These findings generate a pretty straightforward conclusion: if you use a drug that increases the amount of norepinephrine, serotonin, and dopamine in synapses throughout the brain, and as a result, someone's depression gets better, there must have been too little of those neurotransmitters in the first place. Case closed.

Naturally, not so fast. As a first issue of confusion, is the problem with serotonin, dopamine, or norepinephrine? The tricyclics and MAO inhibitors work on all three neurotransmitter systems, making it impossible to tell which one is critical to the disease. People used to think norepinephrine was the culprit, when it was thought that those classical antidepressant drugs worked only on the norepinephrine synapse. These days, most of the excitement centers on serotonin, mainly because of the efficacy of reuptake inhibitors that work only on serotonin synapses (selective serotonin reuptake inhibitors, or SSRIs, of which Prozac is the most famous). However, there still remains some reason to think that the other two neurotransmitters remain part of the story, since some of the newest antidepressants appear to work on them more than on serotonin.*

A second piece of confusion is actually quite major. Is the defect in depression with these neurotransmitters really one of too little neurotransmitter in the synapse? You would think this was settled—the effective antidepressant drugs increase the amounts of these neurotransmitters in the synapse and alleviate depression; thus, the problem had to be too little of the stuff to begin with. However, some clinical data suggest that this might not be so simple.

The stumbling block has to do with timing. Expose the brain to some tricyclic antidepressant, and the amount of signaling with these

---

* The current herbal rage, St. John's wort, has been gaining some credibility in traditional scientific circles. It inhibits the uptake of serotonin, dopamine, and norepinephrine, and seems to be roughly as effective an antidepressant as Prozac. Moreover, in people who are not taking any additional medication, it appears to have somewhat fewer side effects than do the SSRIs. However, there is increasing evidence that it can seriously disrupt the effectiveness of a wide variety of other medications.

neurotransmitters in the synapses changes within hours. However, give that same drug to a depressed person, and it takes weeks for the person to feel better. Something doesn't quite fit. Two theories have arisen in recent years that might reconcile this problem with timing, and they are both extremely complicated.

Revisionist theory 1, the "it's not too little neurotransmitter, it's actually too much" hypothesis. First, some orientation. If somebody constantly yells at you, you stop listening. Analogously, if you inundate a cell with lots of a neurotransmitter, the cell will not "listen" as carefully—it will "down-regulate" (decrease) the number of receptors for that neurotransmitter, in order to decrease its sensitivity to that messenger. If, for example, you double the amount of serotonin reaching the dendrites of a cell and that cell down-regulates its serotonin receptors by 50 percent, the changes roughly cancel out. If the cell down-regulates less than 50 percent, the net result is more serotonin signaling in the synapse; if more than 50 percent, the result is actually less signaling in the synapse. In other words, how strong the signal is in a synapse is a function both of how loudly the first neuron yells (the amount of neurotransmitter released) and of how sensitively the second neuron listens (how many receptors it has for the neurotransmitter).

Okay, ready. This revisionist theory states that the original problem is that there is actually too much norepinephrine, serotonin, and/or dopamine in parts of the brains of depressives. What happens when you prescribe antidepressants that increase signaling of these neurotransmitters even further? At first, that should make the depressive symptoms worse. (Some psychiatrists argue that this actually does occur.) Over the course of a few weeks, however, the dendrites say, "This is intolerable, all this neurotransmitter; let's down-regulate our receptors a whole lot." If this occurs and, critical to the theory, more than compensates for the increased neurotransmitter signal, the depressive problem of excessive neurotransmitter signaling goes away: the person feels better.

Revisionist theory 2, "It really is too little norepinephrine, serotonin, and/or dopamine after all." This theory is even more complicated than the first, and also requires orientation. Not only do dendrites contain receptors for neurotransmitters, but it turns out that on the axon terminals of the "sending" neuron as well there are receptors for the very neurotransmitters being released by that neuron. What possible purpose could these so-called autoreceptors serve? Neurotransmitters are released, float into the synapse, bind to the standard receptors on the second neuron. Some neurotransmitter molecules, however, will float back and wind up binding to the autoreceptors. They serve as some sort of feedback signal; if, say, 5 percent of the released neurotransmitter reaches the autoreceptors, the first neuron can count its toes, multiply by 20, and figure out how much neurotransmitter it has released. Then it can make some decisions—should I release more neurotransmitter or stop now? Should I start synthesizing more? and so on. If this process lets the first neuron do its bookkeeping on neurotransmitter expenditures, what happens if the neuron down-regulates a lot of these autoreceptors? Underestimating the amount of neurotransmitter it has released, the neuron will inadvertently start increasing the amount it synthesizes and discharges.

With this as background, here's the reasoning behind the second theory (that there really is too little norepinephrine, serotonin, or dopamine in a part of the brain of depressives). Give the antidepressant drugs that increase signaling of these neurotransmitters. Because of the increased signaling, over the course of weeks there will be down-regulation of norepinephrine, serotonin, and dopamine receptors. Critical to this theory is the idea that the autoreceptors on the first neuron will down-regulate to a greater extent than the receptors on the second neuron. If that happens, the second neuron may not be listening as well, but the first one will be releasing sufficient extra neurotransmitter to more than overcome that. The net result is enhanced neurotransmitter signaling, and depressive symptoms abate. (This mechanism may explain the efficacy of electroconvulsive therapy, ECT, or "shock therapy." For decades psychiatrists have used this technique to alleviate major depressions, and no one has quite known why it works. It turns out that among its many effects ECT decreases the number of norepinephrine autoreceptors, at least in experimental animal models.)

If you are confused by now, you are in some good company, as the entire field is extremely unsettled. Norepinephrine, serotonin, or dopamine? Too much or too little signaling? If it is, for example, too little serotonin signaling, is it because too little serotonin is being released into synapses, or because there is some defect blunting the sensitivity of serotonin receptors? (To give you a sense of how big a can of worms that one is, there are currently recognized more than a dozen different types of serotonin receptors, with differing functions, efficacies, and distributions in the brain.) Maybe there are a variety of different neurochemical routes for getting to a depression, and different pathways are associated with different subtypes of depression (unipolar versus manic depression, or one that is triggered by outside events versus one that runs with its own internal clockwork, or one dominated by psychomotor retardation versus one dominated by sui-cidalism). This is a very reasonable idea, but the evidence for it is still scant.

Amid all those questions, another good one—why does having too much or too little of these neurotransmitters cause a depression? There are a lot of links between these neurotransmitters and function. For example, serotonin is thought to have something to do with incessant ideation in depression, the uncontrollable wallowing in those dark thoughts. Connected with this, SSRIs are often effective on people with obsessive-compulsive disorder. There is a commonality here: in the depressive case, it is the obsessive sense of failure, of doom, of despair, while in the latter case, it can be obsessive worries that you left the gas on at home when you left, that your hands are dirty and need to be washed, and so on. Trapped in a mind that just circles and circles around the same thoughts or feelings.

Norepinephrine is thought to play a different role in the symptoms of depression. The major pathway that utilizes norepinephrine is an array of projections from a brain region called the locus ceruleus. That projection extends diffusely throughout the brain and seems to play a role in alerting other brain regions—increasing their baseline level of activation, lowering their threshold for responding to outside signals. Thus, a shortage of norepinephrine in this pathway might begin to explain the psychomotor retardation.

Dopamine, meanwhile, has something to do with pleasure, a con-nection that will be reviewed at length in chapter 16. Several decades ago, some neuroscientists made a fundamental discovery. They had implanted electrodes into the brains of rats and stimulated areas here and there, seeing what would happen. By doing so, they found an extraordinary area of the brain. Whenever this area was stimulated, the rat became unbelievably happy. So how can one tell when a rat is unbelievably happy? You ask the rat to tell you, by charting how-many times it is willing to press a lever in order to be rewarded with stimulation in that part of the brain. It turns out that rats will work themselves to death on that lever to get stimulation. They would rather be stimulated there than get food when they are starv-ing, or have sex, or receive drugs even when they're addicted and going through withdrawal. The region of the brain targeted in these studies was promptly called the "pleasure pathway" and has been famous since.

That humans have a pleasure pathway was discovered shortly afterward by stimulating a similar part of the human brain during neurosurgery.* The results are pretty amazing. Something along the lines of "Aaaaah, boy, that feels good. It's kind of like getting your back rubbed but also sort of like sex or playing in the backyard in the leaves when you're a kid and Mom calling you in for hot chocolate and then you get into your pajamas with the feet. . . ." Where can we sign up?

This pleasure pathway seems to make heavy use of dopamine as a neurotransmitter (and in chapter 16, we'll see how dopamine signals the anticipation of reward more than it signals reward itself). The strongest evidence for this is the ability of drugs that mimic dopamine, such as cocaine, to act as euphoriants. Suddenly, it seems plausible to hypothesize that depression, which is characterized above all by dysphoria, might involve too little dopamine and, thus, dysfunction of those pleasure pathways.

Thus, these are the big three when it comes to the neurotransmitters implicated in depression, with attention these days probably being the most for serotonin and the least for dopamine. All of the leading antidepressant drugs—the SSRIs, and older classes such as tricyclics or MAO inhibitors—work by altering the levels of one or more of these three neurotransmitters. At this point, there is nothing close to resembling a science as to which sort of person will respond best to which type of antidepressants.

Naturally, there's a spate of other neurotransmitters that may be involved. One particularly interesting one is called Substance P. Decades of work have shown that Substance P plays a role in pain perception, with a major role in activating the spinal cord pathways discussed in chapter 9. Remarkably, some recent studies indicate that drugs that block the action of Substance P can work as antidepressants in some individuals. What's this about? Perhaps the sense of depression as a disease of "psychic pain" may be more than just a metaphor.

Neuroanatomy and Depression

I introduce an illustration here of what the brain looks like, to consider a second way in which brain function might be abnormal in

---

* Because the brain is not sensitive to pain, a lot of such surgery is done on patients who are awake (with their scalps anesthetized, of course). This is helpful, because prior to modern imaging techniques, surgeons often had to have the patient awake to guide what they were doing. Place an electrode in the brain, stimulate, the patient flops her arm. Go a little deeper with the electrode, stimulate, and the patient flops her leg. Quick, consult your brain road map, figure out where you are, go an inch deeper, hang a left past the third neuron, and there's the tumor. That sort of thing.

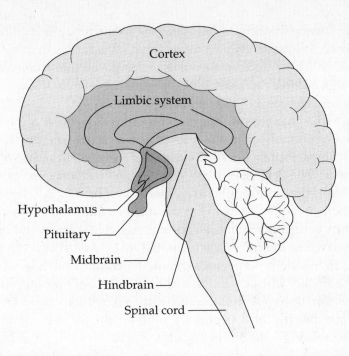

Cortex

Limbic system

Hypothalamus —

Pituitary —

Midbrain —

Hindbrain —

Spinal cord —

The triune brain.

depressives, in addition to the neurochemistry discussed. One region regulates processes like your breathing and heart rate. It includes the hypothalamus, which is busy releasing hormones and instructing the autonomic nervous system. If your blood pressure drops drastically, causing a compensatory stress-response, it is the hypothalamus, midbrain, and hindbrain that kick into gear. All sorts of vertebrates have roughly the same connections here.

Layered on top of that is a region called the limbic system, the functioning of which is related to emotion. As mammals, we have large limbic systems; lizards have relatively tiny limbic systems—they are not noted for the complexity of their emotional lives. If you get a stress-response from smelling the odor of a threatening rival, it's your limbic system that is involved.

Above that is the cortex. Everyone in the animal kingdom has some, but it is a real primate specialty. The cortex does abstract cognition, invents philosophy, remembers where your car keys are. The stuff of the previous chapter.

Now think for a second. Suppose you are gored by an elephant. You may feel a certain absence of pleasure afterward, maybe a sense of grief. Throw in a little psychomotor retardation—you're not as eager for your calisthenics as usual. Sleeping and feeding may be disrupted, glucocorticoid levels may be a bit on the high side. Sex may lose its appeal for a while. Hobbies are not as enticing; you don't jump up to go out with friends; you pass up that all-you-can-eat buffet. Sound like some of the symptoms of a depression?

Now, what happens during a depression? You think a thought about your mortality or that of a loved one; you imagine children in refugee camps, the rain forests disappearing and endless species of life evaporating, late Beethoven string quartets, and suddenly you experience some of the same symptoms as after being gored by the elephant. On an incredibly simplistic level, you can think of depression as occurring when your cortex thinks an abstract negative thought and manages to convince the rest of the brain that this is as real as a physical stressor. In this view, people with chronic depressions are those whose cortex habitually whispers sad thoughts to the rest of the brain. Thus, an astonishingly crude prediction: cut the connections between the cortex and the rest of a depressive's brain, and the cortex will no longer be able to get the rest of the brain depressed.

Remarkably, it actually works sometimes. Neurosurgeons may perform this procedure on people with vastly crippling depressions that are resistant to drugs, ECT, or other forms of therapy. Afterward, depressive symptoms seem to abate.*

Obviously, this is a simplified picture—no one actually disconnects the entire cortex from the rest of the brain. After all, the cortex does more than mope around feeling bad about the final chapter of *Of Mice and Men*. The surgical procedure, called a cingulotomy, or a cingulum bundle cut, actually disconnects just one area toward the front of the cortex, called the anterior cingulate cortex (ACC). The ACC is turning out to have all the characteristics of a brain region you'd want to take offline in a major depression. It's a part of the brain that is very concerned with emotions. Show people arrays of pictures: in one case, ask them to pay attention to the emotions being expressed by people in the pictures; in another case, ask them to pay attention to details like whether these are indoor or outdoor photographs. In only the former case do you get activation of the ACC.

---

* What else changes after this surgical procedure? If the cortex can no longer send abstract thoughts to the rest of the brain, the person should not only lose the capacity for abstract misery but for abstract pleasure as well, and this is what happens; but surgery such as this is a therapy employed only in patients completely incapacitated by their illness, who spend decades on the back ward of some state hospital, rocking and clutching themselves and feebly attempting suicide with some regularity.

And the emotions that the ACC is involved in seem to be negative ones. Induce a positive state in someone by showing something amusing, and ACC metabolism decreases. In contrast, if you electrically stimulate the ACC in people, they feel a shapeless sense of fear and foreboding. Moreover, neurons in the ACC, including in humans, respond to pain of all sorts. But the ACC response isn't really about the pain; it more concerns feelings about the pain. As was discussed in chapter 9, give someone a hypnotic suggestion that they will not feel the pain of dipping their hand into ice water. The primary parts of the brain that get pain projections from the spinal cord get just as active as if there were no hypnotic suggestion. But this time, the ACC doesn't activate.

In addition, the ACC and adjacent brain regions activate when you show widows pictures of their lost loved ones (versus pictures of strangers). As another example of this, put a volunteer in a brain-imaging machine and, from inside, ask them to play some game with two other people, via a computer console. Rig up the flow of the game so that, over time, the other two (actually, a computer program) gradually begin just playing with each other, excluding the test subject. Neuronal activity in the ACC lights up, and the more left out the person feels, the more intensely the ACC activates. How do you know this has something to do with that dread junior high school feeling of being picked last for the team? Because of a clever control in the study: set the person up to play with the supposed other two players. Once again, it winds up that the other two only play against each other. The difference, this time, though, is that early on the subject is told there's been a technical glitch and that their computer console isn't working. Excluded because of a snafu in the technology, there's no ACC activation.

Given these functions of the ACC, it is not surprising that its resting level of activity tends to be elevated in people with a depression—this is the fear and pain and foreboding churning away at those neurons. Interestingly, another part of the brain, called the amygdala, seems to be hyperactive in depressives as well. We will hear lots about the role of the amygdala in fear and anxiety in the next chapter. However, in depressives, the amygdala seems to have been recruited into a different role. Show a depressed person a fearful human face and his amygdala doesn't activate all that much (in contrast to the response you'd see in the amygdala of a control subject). But show him a sad face and the amygdala gets a highly exaggerated activation.

Sitting just in front of the ACC is the frontal cortex which, as we saw in chapter 11, is one of the most distinctly human parts of the brain. Work by Richard Davidson of the University of Wisconsin has shown that one subregion called the prefrontal cortex (PFC) seems highly responsive to mood, and in a lateralized way. Specifically, activation of the left PFC is associated with positive moods, and activation of the right PFC, with negative. For example, induce a positive state in someone (by asking him to describe the happiest day of his life), and the left PFC lights up, in proportion to the person's subjective assessment of his pleasure. Ask him to remember a sad event, and the right PFC dominates. Similarly, separate an infant monkey from its mother and right PFC metabolism rises while left PFC decreases. Thus, not surprisingly, in depressives, there is decreased left PFC activity and elevated activity in the right PFC.

There are a few other anatomical changes in the brain in depression, but to make sense of those, we have to consider what hormones have to do with the disease.

Genetics and Depression

It is hard to look at the biology of anything these days without genes coming into the picture, and depression is no exception. Depression has a genetic component. As a first observation, depression runs in families. For a long time, that would have been sufficient evidence for some folks that there is a genetic link, but this conclusion is undone by the obvious fact that not only do genes run in families, environment does as well. Growing up in a poor family, an abusive family, a persecuted family, can all increase the risk of depression running through that family without genes having anything to do with it.

So we look for a tighter relationship. The more closely related two individuals are, the more genes they share in common and, as it turns out, the more likely they are to share a depressive trait. As one of the most telling examples of this, take any two siblings (who are not identical twins). They share something like 50 percent of their genes. If one of them has a history of depression, the other has about a 25 percent likelihood, considerably higher than would be expected by chance. Now, compare two identical twins, who share all of their genes in common. And if one of them is depressive, the other has a 50 percent chance. This is quite impressive—the more genes in common, the more likelihood of sharing the disease. But there remains a confound: the more genes people share within a family, the more environment they share as well (starting with the fact that identical twins grow up treated more similarly than are non-identical twins).

Tighten the relationship further. Look at children who were adopted at an early age. Consider those whose biological mother had a history of depression, but whose adoptive mother did not. They have an increased risk of depression, suggesting a genetic legacy shared with their biological mother. But the confound there, as we saw in chapter 6, is that "environment" does not begin at birth, but begins much earlier, with the circulatory environment shared in utero with one's biological mother.

For any card-carrying molecular biologist in the twenty-first century, if you want to prove that genes have something to do with depression, you're going to have to identify the specific genes, the specific stretches of DNA that code for specific proteins that increase the risk for depression. As we'll see shortly, precisely that has occurred in recent years.

Immunology and Depression

This subsection did not exist in previous editions of this book. Immunity is about fighting off pathogens, depression is about feeling sad—unrelated subjects. Well, they can be related, but in an idiotically obvious way—like, duh, being sick can be depressing.

But it's more complicated than that. Chronic illness that involves overactivation of the immune system (for example, chronic infections, or an autoimmune disease where the immune system has accidentally activated and is attacking some part of your body) is more likely to cause depression than other equally severe and prolonged illnesses that don't involve the immune system. Some more threads of interconnection involve the cytokines that act as messengers between immune cells. As you'll recall from chapter 8, cytokines can also get into the brain, where they can stimulate CRH release. More recently, it's becoming clear that they also interact with norepinephrine, dopamine, and serotonin systems. Critically, cytokines can cause depression. This is shown in animal models of depression. Furthermore, certain types of cancers are sometimes treated with cytokines (to enhance immune function), and this typically results in depression. So this represents a new branch of study for biological psychiatry—the interactions between immune function and mood.

Endocrinology and Depression

Abnormal levels of a number of different hormones often go hand in hand with depression. To begin, people who secrete too little thyroid hormone can develop major depressions and, when depressed, can be atypically resistant to antidepressant drugs working. This is particularly important because many people, seemingly with depressions of a purely psychiatric nature, turn out to have thyroid disease.

There is another aspect of depression in which hormones may play a role. The incidence of major, unipolar depression differs greatly, with women suffering far more than men. Even when you consider manic depression, where there is no sex difference in its incidence, bipolar women have more depressive episodes than do bipolar men.

Why this female bias? It has nothing to do with the obvious first guess, which is that women are more likely to see a health professional for depression than are men. The difference holds up even when such reporting biases are controlled for. One theory, from the school of cognitive therapy, concentrates on the ways in which women and men tend to think differently. When something upsetting happens, women are more likely to ruminate over it—think about it or want to talk about it with someone else. And men, terrible communicators that they so often are, are more likely to want to think about anything but the problem, or even better, go and do something—exercise, use power tools, get drunk, start a war. A ruminative tendency, the cognitive psychologists argue, makes you more likely to become depressed.

Another theory about the sex difference is psychosocial in nature. As we will see, much theorizing about the psychology of depression suggests that it is a disorder of lack of power and control, and some scientists have speculated that because women in so many societies traditionally have less control over the circumstances of their lives than do men, they are at greater risk for depression. In support of this idea, some psychiatrists have produced data suggesting that the elevated rates of depression in women decline to the levels seen in men in some traditional societies in which women don't have a subordinate role. Yet another theory suggests that men really do have as high a rate of depression as do women, but they are simply more likely to mask it with substance abuse.

All of these ideas are reasonable, although they run into trouble when one considers that women and men, as noted, have the same rate of bipolar depression; it is only unipolar depression that is more common among women. These theories seem particularly weak in their failure to explain a major feature of female depressions, namely, that women are particularly at risk for depressions at certain reproductive points: menstruation, menopause, and most of all, the weeks immediately after giving birth. A number of researchers believe such increased risks are tied to the great fluctuations that occur during menstruation, menopause, and parturition in two main hormones: estrogen and progesterone. As evidence, they cite the fact that women can get depressed when they artificially change their estrogen or progesterone levels (for example, when taking birth-control pills). Critically, both of these hormones can regulate neurochemical events in the brain, including the metabolism of neurotransmitters such as norepinephrine and serotonin. With massive changes in hormone levels (a thousandfold for progesterone at the time of giving birth, for example), current speculation centers on the possibility that the ratio of estrogen to progesterone can change radically enough to trigger a major depression. This is a new area of research with some seemingly contradictory findings, but there is more and more confidence among scientists that there is a hormonal contribution to the preponderance of female depressions.

Obviously, the next subject in a section on hormones and depression will have to look at glucocorticoids. But given how central this is to the whole venture of this book, the subject requires expansion.

 ## HOW DOES STRESS INTERACT WITH THE BIOLOGY OF DEPRESSION?

Stress, Glucocorticoids, and the Onset of Depression

The first stress-depression link is an obvious one, in that stress and depression tend to go together. This can run in two directions. First, studies of what is called "stress generation" among depressives look at the fact that people who are prone to depression tend to experience stressors at a higher than expected rate. This is even seen when comparing them to individuals with other psychiatric disorders or health problems. Much of this appears to be stressors built around lack of social support. This raises the potential for a vicious cycle to emerge. This is because if you interpret the ambiguous social interactions around you as signs of rejection, and respond as if you have been rejected, it can increase the chances of winding up socially isolated, thereby confirming your sense that you have been rejected. . . .

But the major way in which people think about a link between stress and depression, and the one that concerns us here, has causality running in the other direction. Specifically, people who are undergoing a lot of life stressors are more likely than average to succumb to a major depression, and people sunk in their first major depression are more likely than average to have undergone recent and significant stress. Obviously, not everyone who undergoes major stressors sinks into depression, and what those individual differences are about should be clearer as we proceed through this chapter.

As noted, some people have the grave misfortune of suffering from repeated depressive episodes, ones that can take on a rhythmic pattern stretching over years. When considering the case histories of those people, stressors emerge as triggers for only the first few depressions. In other words, have two, three major bouts of depression and, statistically, you are no more at risk for subsequent major depression than anyone else. But somewhere around the fourth depression or so, a mad clockwork takes over, and the depressive waves crash, regardless of whether the outside world pummels you with stressors. What that transition is about will be considered below.

Laboratory studies also link stress and the symptoms of depression. Stress a lab rat, and it becomes anhedonic. Specifically, it takes a stronger electrical current than normal in the rat's pleasure pathways to activate a sense of pleasure. The threshold for perceiving pleasure has been raised, just as in a depressive.

Critically, glucocorticoids can do the same. A key point in chapter 10 was how glucocorticoids and stress could disrupt memory. Part of the evidence for that came from people with Cushing's syndrome (as a reminder, that is a condition in which any of a number of different types of tumors wind up causing vast excesses of glucocorticoids in the bloodstream), as well as from people prescribed high doses of glucocorticoids to treat a number of ailments. It has also been known for decades that a significant subset of Cushingoid patients and patients prescribed synthetic glucocorticoids become clinically depressed, independent of memory problems. This has been a bit tricky to demonstrate. First, when someone is initially treated with synthetic glucocorticoids, the tendency is to get, if anything, euphoric and even manic, perhaps for a week or so before the depression kicks in. You can immediately guess that we are dealing with one of our dichotomies between short- and long-term stress physiology; chapter 16 will explore in even more detail where that transient euphoria comes from. As a second complication, does someone with Cushing's syndrome or someone taking high pharmacological doses of synthetic glucocorticoids get depressed because glucocorticoids cause that state, or is it because they recognize they have a depressing disease? You show it is the glucocorticoids that are the culprits by demonstrating higher depression rates in this population than among people with, for example, the same disease and the same severity but not receiving glucocorticoids. At this stage, there's also not much of a predictive science to this phenomenon. For example, no clinician can reliably predict beforehand which patient is going to get depressed when put on high-dose glucocorticoids, let alone at what dose, and whether it is when the dose is raised or lowered to that level. Nonetheless, have lots of glucocorticoids in the bloodstream and the risk of a depression increases.

Stress and glucocorticoids tangle up with biology in predisposing a person toward depression in an additional, critical way. Back to that business about there being a genetic component to depression. Does this mean that if you have "the gene" (or genes) "for" depression, that's it, you're up the creek, it's inevitable? Obviously not, and the best evidence for this is that factoid about identical twins. One has depression and the other, sharing all the same genes, has about a 50 percent chance of having the disease as well, a much higher rate than in the general population. There, pretty solid evidence for genes being involved. But flip this the other way. Share every single gene with someone who is depressive and you still have a 50 percent chance of *not* having the disease.

Genes are rarely about inevitability, especially when it comes to humans, the brain, or behavior. They're about vulnerability, propensities, tendencies. In this case, genes increase the risk of depression only in certain environments: you guessed it, only in stressful environments. This is shown in a number of ways, but most dramatically in a recent study by Avshalom Caspi at King's College, London. Scientists identified a certain gene in humans that increases the risk of depression. More specifically, it is a gene that comes in a few different "allelic versions"—a few different types or flavors that differ slightly in function; have one of those versions, and you're at increased risk. What that gene is I'm not telling yet; I'm saving it for the end of this chapter, as it is a doozy. But the key thing is that having version X of this gene Z doesn't guarantee you get depression, it just increases your risk. And, in fact, knowing nothing more about someone than which version of gene Z she has doesn't increase your odds of predicting whether she gets depressed. Version X increases depression risk only when coupled with a history of repeated major stressors. Amazingly, the same has been shown with studies of some nonhuman primate species, who carry a close equivalent of that gene Z. It's not the gene that causes it. It's that the gene interacts with a certain environment. More specifically, a gene that makes you vulnerable in a stressful environment.

Glucocorticoid profiles once a depression has been established

Not surprisingly, glucocorticoid levels are typically abnormal in people who are clinically depressed. A relatively infrequent subtype of depression, called "atypical depression," is dominated by the psychomotor features of the disease—an incapacitating physical and psychological exhaustion. Just as is the case with chronic fatigue syndrome, atypical depression is characterized by lower than normal glucocorticoid levels. However, the far more common feature of depression is one of an overactive stress-response—somewhat of an overly activated sympathetic nervous system and, even more dramatically, elevated levels of glucocorticoids. This adds to the picture that depressed people, sitting on the edge of their beds without the energy to get up, are actually vigilant and aroused, with a hormonal profile to match—but the battle is inside them.

Research stretching back some forty years has explored why, on a nuts-and-bolts level, glucocorticoid levels are often elevated in depression. The elevated levels appear to be due to too much of a stress signal from the brain (back to chapter 2—remember that the adrenals typically secrete glucocorticoids only when they are commanded to by the brain, via the pituitary), rather than the adrenals just getting some depressive glucocorticoid hiccup all on their own now and then. Moreover, the excessive secretion of glucocorticoids is due to what is called feedback resistance—in other words, the brain is less effective than it should be at shutting down glucocorticoid secretion. Normally, the levels of this hormone are tightly regulated—the brain senses circulating glucocorticoid levels, and if they get higher than desired (the "desired" level shifts depending on whether events are calm or stressful), the brain stops secreting CRH. Just like the regulation of water in a toilet bowl tank. In depressives, this feedback regulation fails—concentrations of circulating glucocorticoids that should shut down the system fail to do so, as the brain does not sense the feedback signal.*

---

* Careful readers will recall a discussion on page 248 of the use of the dexamethasone suppression test to show that many aged organisms have trouble turning off glucocorticoid secretion. The same test is used here. The truly obsessively careful reader will recall that during aging, the problem of shutting off glucocorticoid secretion—the "dexamethasone resistance"—probably arises from damage to a part of the brain that helps to terminate the glucocorticoid stress-response. Does similar damage occur in depression? As we'll see, this might occur in some long-term depressives. However, the elevated glucocorticoid levels occur in depressives with no evidence of damage. Most likely, sustained stress decreases the number of glucocorticoid receptors in that part of the brain, making the neurons less effective at sensing the hormone in the bloodstream.

What are the consequences of elevated glucocorticoid levels before and during a depression?

The first most critical question to ask is, how does an excess of glucocorticoids increase the risk of depression? A preceding section detailed, at great length, the considerable confusion about whether depression is about serotonin or norepinephrine or dopamine. To the extent that this is the case, the glucocorticoid angle fits well, in that the hormones can alter features of all three neurotransmitter systems—the amount of neurotransmitter synthesized, how fast it is broken down, how many receptors there are for each neurotransmitter, how well the receptors work, and so on. Moreover, stress has been shown to cause many of the same changes as well. Sustained stress will deplete dopamine from those "pleasure" pathways, and norepinephrine from that alerting locus ceruleus part of the brain. Moreover, stress alters all sorts of aspects of the synthesis, release, efficacy, and breakdown of serotonin. It is not clear which of those stress effects are most important, simply because it is not clear which neurotransmitter or neurotransmitters are most important. However, it is probably safe to say that whatever neurochemical abnormalities wind up being shown definitively to underlie depression, there is precedent for stress and glucocorticoids causing those same abnormalities.

Those elevated glucocorticoid levels appear to have some other consequences as well. They may play a role, for example, in the fact that depressive patients often are at least mildly immunosuppressed, and are more prone to osteoporosis. Moreover, prolonged major depression increases the risk of heart disease about three- to fourfold, even after controlling for smoking and alcohol consumption, and the glucocorticoid excess is likely to contribute to that as well.

And there may be more consequences. Think back to chapter 10 and its discussion of the many ways in which glucocorticoids can damage the hippocampus. As that literature emerged in the 1980s, it immediately suggested that there may be problems with the hippocampus in people with major depression. This speculation was reinforced by the fact that the type of memory most often impaired in depression—declarative memory—is mediated by the hippocampus. As was discussed in chapter 10, there is atrophy of the hippocampus in long-term depression. The atrophy emerges as a result of the depression (rather than precedes it), and the longer the depressive history, the more atrophy and the more memory problems. While no one has explicitly shown yet that the atrophy occurs only in those depressives with the elevated glucocorticoid levels, the atrophy is most common in the subtypes of depression in which the glucocorticoid excess is most common. Chronic depression has also been associated in some studies with decreased volume in the frontal cortex. This was initially puzzling for those of us who view the world through glucocorticoid-tinted glasses, but has recently been resolved. In the rat, the hippocampus is overwhelmingly *the* target in the brain for glucocorticoid action, as measured by the density of receptors for the hormone; however, in the primate brain, the hippocampus and frontal cortex seem to be equally and markedly sensitive to glucocorticoids.

So some pretty decent circumstantial evidence suggests that the glucocorticoid excess of depression may have something to do with the decreased volume of the hippocampus and frontal cortex. Chapter 10 noted an array of bad things that glucocorticoids could do to neurons. Some obsessively careful studies have shown loss of cells in the frontal cortex accompanying the volume loss in depression—as one point of confusion, it is those supportive glial cells rather than neurons that are lost. But in the hippocampus, no one has a clue yet; it could be the killing or atrophying of neurons, the inhibition of the birth of new neurons, or all the above.* Whatever the explanation is at the cellular level, it appears to be permanent; years to decades after these major depressions have been gotten under control (typically with medication), the volume loss is still there.

Anti-glucocorticoids as antidepressants

The glucocorticoid-depression link has some important implications. When I first introduced that link at the beginning of the chapter, it was

---

* Chapter 10 detailed the revolutionary finding that the adult brain, particularly the hippocampus, can make new neurons. It also showed that stress and glucocorticoids are the strongest inhibitors of such neurogenesis. The finding also noted that it is not clear yet what these new neurons are good for, although it wouldn't be crazy to think that new neurons in the hippocampus might have something good to do for memory. Thus, it doesn't seem crazy, either, to speculate that an inhibition of neurogenesis in the hippocampus before and during depression might contribute to the memory problems that have been reviewed. This seems plausible to me. But there is also the additional idea floating around in the field that the inhibition of neurogenesis gives rise to the *emotional* symptoms as well (that is to say, the anhedonia and grief that define a depression), and that antidepressants work by jump-starting hippocampal neurogenesis. This theory has garnered a lot of attention, and there have been some highly visible studies supporting it. Nonetheless, I don't find those studies or the basic idea to be too convincing—I can come up with a route that links the functions of the hippocampus to the emotional features of a depression, but it feels way too convoluted to be at the core of what causes this disease. (You'll note that I bury this in a footnote, in the hope that some colleagues whom I like and respect on the other side of this question won't come and stab me.)

meant to give some insight into the flavor of what a depression is like—a person looks like an enervated sea sponge, sitting there motionless on the edge of his bed, but he's actually boiling, in the middle of an internal battle. Tacit in that description was the idea that undergoing a depression is actually immensely stressful, and, therefore, among other things, stimulates glucocorticoid secretion. The data just reviewed suggest the opposite scenario—stress and glucocorticoid excess can be a cause of depression, rather than merely a consequence.

If that is really the case, then a novel clinical intervention should work: take one of those depressives with high glucocorticoid levels, find some drug that works on the adrenals to lower glucocorticoid secretion, and the depression should lessen. And, very exciting, that has been shown. The approach, though, is filled with problems. You don't want to suppress glucocorticoid levels too much because, umpteen pages into this book, it should be apparent by now that those hormones are pretty important. Moreover, the "adrenal steroidogenesis inhibitors," as those drugs are called, can have some nasty side effects. Nonetheless, some solid reports have shown them to have antidepressant effects in people with high-glucocorticoid depressions.

Another version of the same approach is to use a drug that blocks glucocorticoid receptors in the brain. These exist and are relatively safe, and there's now decent evidence that they work as well.* A relatively obscure hormone called DHEA, which has some ability to block glucocorticoid access to its receptor, has been reported to have some antidepressant qualities as well. Thus, these recent studies not only teach us something about the bases of depression, but may open the way for a whole new generation of medications for the disease.

Some investigators have built on these observations with a fairly radical suggestion. For those biological psychiatrists concerned with the hormonal aspects of depression, the traditional glucocorticoid scenario is outlined above. In it, depressions are stressful and raise glucocorticoid levels; when someone is treated with antidepressants, the abnormal neurochemistry (related to serotonin, norepinephrine, etc.) is normalized, lessening the depression and, by the way, making life feel less stressful, with glucocorticoid levels returning to normal as a by-product. The new scenario is the logical extension of the inverted causality also just discussed. In this version, for any of a number of

---

* Interestingly, the best glucocorticoid receptor out there is a drug already famous—notorious to some—namely, RU486, the "abortion drug." Not only does it block receptors in the uterus for progesterone, another steroid hormone, but it blocks glucocorticoid receptors effectively.

reasons, glucocorticoid levels rise in someone (because the person is under a lot of stress, because something about the regulatory control of glucocorticoids is awry in that person), causing changes in the chemistry of serotonin (or norepinephrine, etc.) and a depression. In this scenario, antidepressants work by normalizing glucocorticoid levels, thereby normalizing the brain chemistry and alleviating the depression.

For this view to be supported, it has to be shown that the primary mechanism of action of the different classes of antidepressants is to work on the glucocorticoid system, and that changes in glucocorticoid levels precede the changes in brain chemistry or depressive symptoms. A few researchers have presented evidence that antidepressants work to rapidly alter numbers of glucocorticoid receptors in the brain, altering regulatory control of the system and lowering glucocorticoid levels, and these changes precede changes in the traditional symptoms of depression; other researchers have not observed this. As usual, more research is needed. But even if it turns out that, in some patients, depression is driven by elevated glucocorticoid levels (and recovery from depression thus mediated by reduction of those levels), that can't be the general mechanism of the disease in all cases: only about half of depressives actually have elevated glucocorticoid levels. In the other half, the glucocorticoid system seems to work perfectly normally. Perhaps this particular stress/depression link is relevant only during the first few rounds of someone's depression (before the endogenous rhythmicity kicks in), or only in a subset of individuals.

We have now seen ways in which stress and glucocorticoids are intertwined with the biology of depression. That intertwining is made even tighter when considering the psychological picture of the disease.

 ## STRESS AND THE PSYCHODYNAMICS OF MAJOR DEPRESSIONS

I have to begin with Freud. I know it is obligatory to dump on Freud, and some of it is deserved, but there is much that he still has to offer. I can think of few other scientists who, nearly a century after their major contributions, are still considered important and correct enough for anyone to want to bother pointing out their errors instead of just consigning them to the library archives.

Freud was fascinated with depression and focused on the issue that we began with—why is it that most of us can have occasional terrible experiences, feel depressed, and then recover, while a few of us collapse into major depression (melancholia)? In his classic essay

"Mourning and Melancholia" (1917), Freud began with what the two have in common. In both cases, he felt, there is the loss of a love object. (In Freudian terms, such an "object" is usually a person, but can also be a goal or an ideal.) In Freud's formulation, in every loving relationship there is ambivalence, mixed feelings—elements of hatred as well as love. In the case of a small, reactive depression—mourning—you are able to deal with those mixed feelings in a healthy manner: you lose, you grieve, and then you recover. In the case of a major melancholic depression, you have become obsessed with the ambivalence—the simultaneity, the irreconcilable nature of the intense love alongside the intense hatred. Melancholia—a major depression—Freud theorized, is the internal conflict generated by this ambivalence.

This can begin to explain the intensity of grief experienced in a major depression. If you are obsessed with the intensely mixed feelings, you grieve doubly after a loss—for your loss of the loved individual and for the loss of any chance now to ever resolve the difficulties. "If only I had said the things I needed to, if only we could have worked things out"—for all of time, you have lost the chance to purge yourself of the ambivalence. For the rest of your life, you will be reaching for the door to let you into a place of pure, unsullied love, and you can never reach that door.

It also explains the intensity of the guilt often experienced in major depression. If you truly harbored intense anger toward the person along with love, in the aftermath of your loss there must be some facet of you that is celebrating, alongside the grieving. "He's gone; that's terrible but . . . thank god, I can finally live, I can finally grow up, no more of this or that." Inevitably, a metaphorical instant later, there must come a paralyzing belief that you have become a horrible monster to feel any sense of relief or pleasure at a time like this. Incapacitating guilt.

This theory also explains the tendency of major depressives in such circumstances to, oddly, begin to take on some of the traits of the lost loved/hated one—and not just any traits, but invariably the ones that the survivor found most irritating. Psychodynamically, this is wonderfully logical. By taking on a trait, you are being loyal to your lost, beloved opponent. By picking an irritating trait, you are still trying to convince the world you were right to be irritated—you see how you hate it when I do it; can you imagine what it was like to have to put up with that for years? And by picking a trait that, most of all, you find irritating, you are not only still trying to score points in your argument with the departed, but you are punishing yourself for arguing as well.

Out of the Freudian school of thought has come one of the more apt descriptions of depression—"aggression turned inward." Suddenly the loss of pleasure, the psychomotor retardation, the impulse to suicide all make sense. As do the elevated glucocorticoid levels. This does not describe someone too lethargic to function; it is more like the actual state of a patient in depression, exhausted from the most draining emotional conflict of his or her life—one going on entirely within. If that doesn't count as psychologically stressful, I don't know what does.

Like other good parts of Freud, these ideas are empathic and fit many clinical traits; they just feel "right." But they are hard to assimilate into modern science, especially biologically oriented psychiatry. There is no way to study the correlation between serotonin receptor density and internalization of aggression, for example, or the effects of estrogen-progesterone ratios on love-hate ratios. The branch of psychological theorizing about depression that seems most useful to me, and is most tightly linked to stress, comes from experimental psychology. Work in this field has generated an extraordinarily informative model of depression.

 ## STRESS, LEARNED HELPLESSNESS, AND DEPRESSION

In order to appreciate the experimental studies underlying this model, recall that in the preceding chapter on psychological stress, we saw that certain features dominated as psychologically stressful: a loss of control and of predictability within certain contexts, a loss of outlets for frustration, a loss of sources of support, a perception of life worsening. In one style of experiment, pioneered by the psychologists Martin Seligman and Steven Maier, animals are exposed to pathological amounts of these psychological stressors. The result is a condition strikingly similar to a human depression.

Although the actual stressors may differ, the general approach in these studies always emphasizes repeated stressors with a complete absence of control on the part of the animal. For example, a rat may be subjected to a long series of frequent, uncontrollable, and unpredictable shocks or noises, with no outlets.

After awhile, something extraordinary happens to that rat. This can be shown with a test. Take a fresh, unstressed rat, and give it something easy to learn. Put it in a room, for example, with the floor divided into two halves. Occasionally, electricity that will cause a mild shock is delivered to one half, and just beforehand, there is a signal indicating which half of the floor is about to be electrified. Your run-of-the-mill rat can learn this "active avoidance task" easily, and within a short time it readily and calmly shifts the side of the room it sits in according to the signal. Simple. Except for a rat who has recently been exposed to repeated uncontrollable stressors. That rat cannot learn the task. It does not learn to cope. On the contrary, it has learned to be helpless.

This phenomenon, called learned helplessness, is quite generalized; the animal has trouble coping with all sorts of varied tasks after its exposure to uncontrollable stressors. Such helplessness extends to tasks having to do with its ordinary life, like competing with another animal for food, or avoiding social aggression. One might wonder whether the helplessness is induced by the physical stress of receiving the shocks or, instead, the psychological stressor of having no control over or capacity to predict the shocks. It is the latter. The clearest way to demonstrate this is to "yoke" pairs of rats—one gets shocked under conditions marked by predictability and a certain degree of control, the other rat gets the identical pattern of shocks, but without the control or predictability. Only the latter rat becomes helpless.

Seligman argues persuasively that animals suffering from learned helplessness share many psychological features with depressed humans. Such animals have a motivational problem—one of the reasons that they are helpless is that they often do not even attempt a coping response when they are in a new situation. This is quite similar to the depressed person who doesn't even try the simplest task that would improve her life. "I'm too tired, it seems overwhelming to take on something like that, it's not going to work anyway. . . ."

Animals with learned helplessness also have a cognitive problem, something awry with how they perceive the world and think about it. When they do make the rare coping response, they can't tell whether it works or not. For example, if you tighten the association between a coping response and a reward, a normal rat's response rate increases (in other words, if the coping response works for the rat, it persists in that response). In contrast, linking rewards more closely to the rare coping responses of a helpless rat has little effect on its response rate. Seligman believes that this is not a consequence of helpless animals somehow missing the rules of the task; instead, he thinks, they have actually learned not to bother paying attention. By all logic, that rat should have learned, "When I am getting shocked, there is absolutely nothing I can do, and that feels terrible, but it isn't the whole world; it isn't true for everything." Instead, it has learned, "There is nothing I can do. Ever." Even when control and mastery are potentially made available to it, the rat cannot perceive them. This is very similar to the depressed human who always sees glasses half empty. As Beck and other cognitive therapists have emphasized, much of what constitutes a depression is centered around responding to one awful thing and overgeneralizing from it—cognitively distorting how the world works.

The learned helplessness paradigm produces animals with other features strikingly similar to those in humans with major depressions. There is a rat's equivalent of dysphoria—the rat stops grooming itself and loses interest in sex and food. The rat's failure even to attempt coping responses suggests that it experiences an animal equivalent of psychomotor retardation.* In some models of learned helplessness, animals mutilate themselves, biting at themselves. Many of the vegetative symptoms appear as well—sleep loss and disorganization of sleep architecture, elevated glucocorticoid levels. Most critically, these animals tend to be depleted of norepinephrine in certain parts of the brain, while antidepressant drugs and ECT speed up their recovery from the learned helplessness state.

Learned helplessness has been induced in rodents, cats, dogs, birds, fish, insects, and primates, including humans. It takes surprisingly little in terms of uncontrollable unpleasantness to make humans give up and become helpless in a generalized way. In one study by Donald Hiroto, student volunteers were exposed to either escapable or inescapable loud noises (as in all such studies, the two groups were paired so that they were exposed to the same amount of noise). Afterward, they were given a learning task in which a correct response turned off a loud noise; the "inescapable" group was significantly less capable of learning the task. Helplessness can even be generalized to

---

* One might wonder if the entire learned helplessness phenomenon is really just about psychomotor retardation. Perhaps the rat is so wiped out after the uncontrollable shocks that it simply doesn't have the energy to perform active avoidance coping tasks. This would shift the emphasis away from learned helplessness as a cognitive state ("there is nothing I can do about this") or an anhedonic emotional state ("nothing feels pleasurable") to one of psychomotor inhibition ("everything seems so exhausting that I'm just going to sit here"). Seligman and Maier strongly object to this interpretation and present data showing that rats with learned helplessness are not only as active as control rats but, more important, are also impaired in "passive avoidance tasks"— learning situations where the coping response involves remaining still, rather than actually *doing* something (in other words, situations where a little psychomotor retardation should *help*). Championing the psychomotor retardation view is another major figure in this field, Jay Weiss, who presents an equal amount of data showing that "helpless" rats perform normally on passive avoidance tasks, indicating that the helplessness is a motor phenomenon and not a cognitive or emotional one. This debate has been going on for decades and I sure don't know how to resolve the conflicting views.

nonaversive learning situations. Hiroto and Seligman did a follow-up study in which, again, there was either controllable or uncontrollable noise. Afterward the latter group was less capable of solving simple word puzzles. Giving up can also be induced by stressors far more subtle than uncontrollable loud noises. In another study, Hiroto and Seligman gave volunteers a learning task in which they had to pick a card of a certain color according to rules that they had to discern along the way. In one group, these rules were learnable; in the other group, the rules were not (the card color was randomized). Afterward, the latter group was less capable of coping with a simple and easily solved task. Seligman and colleagues have also demonstrated that unsolvable tasks induced helplessness afterward in social coping situations.

Thus humans can be provoked into at least transient cases of learned helplessness, and with surprising ease. Naturally, there is tremendous individual variation in how readily this happens—some of us are more vulnerable than others (and you can bet that this is going to be important in considering stress management in the final chapter). In the experiment involving inescapable noise, Hiroto had given the students a personality inventory beforehand. Based on that, he was able to identify the students who came into the experiment with a strongly "internalized locus of control"—a belief that they were the masters of their own destiny and had a great deal of control in their lives—and, in contrast, the markedly "externalized" volunteers, who tended to attribute outcomes to chance and luck. In the aftermath of the uncontrollable stressor, the externalized students were far more vulnerable to learned helplessness. Transferring that to the real world, with the same external stressors, the more that someone has an internal locus of control, the less the likelihood of a depression.

Collectively, these studies strike me as extremely important in forming links among stress, personality, and depression. Our lives are replete with incidents in which we become irrationally helpless. Some are silly and inconsequential. Once in the African camp that I shared with Laurence Frank, the zoologist whose hyenas figured in chapter 7, we managed to make a disaster of preparing macaroni and cheese over the campfire. Inspecting the mess, we ruefully admitted that it might have helped if we had bothered to read the instructions on the box. Yet we had both avoided doing that; in fact, we both felt a formless dread about trying to make sense of such instructions. Frank summed it up: "Face it. We suffer from learned cooking helplessness."

But life is full of more significant examples. If a teacher at a critical point of our education, or a loved one at a critical point of our emotional development, frequently exposes us to his or her own specialized uncontrollable stressors, we may grow up with distorted beliefs about what we cannot learn or ways in which we are unlikely to be loved. In one chilling demonstration of this, some psychologists studied inner-city school kids with severe reading problems. Were they intellectually incapable of reading? Apparently not. The psychologists circumvented the students' resistance to learning to read by, instead, teaching them Chinese characters. Within hours they were capable of reading more complex symbolic sentences than they could in English. The children had apparently been previously taught all too well that reading English was beyond their ability.

A major depression, these findings suggest, can be the outcome of particularly severe lessons in uncontrollability for those of us who are already vulnerable. This may explain an array of findings that show that if a child is stressed in certain ways—loss of a parent to death, divorce of parents, being a victim of abusive parenting—the child is more at risk for depression years later. What could be a more severe lesson that awful things can happen that are beyond our control than a lesson at an age when we are first forming our impressions about the nature of the world? As an underpinning of this, Paul Plotsky and Charles Nemeroff of Emory University have shown that rats or monkeys exposed to stressors early in life have a lifelong increase in CRH levels in their brain.

"According to our model," writes Seligman, "depression is not generalized pessimism, but pessimism specific to the effects of one's own skilled actions." Subjected to enough uncontrollable stress, we learn to be helpless—we lack the motivation to try to live because we assume the worst; we lack the cognitive clarity to perceive when things are actually going fine, and we feel an aching lack of pleasure in everything.*

---

* Before we leave the issue of learned helplessness, let me acknowledge that these are brutal experiments to subject an animal to. Is there no alternative? Painfully, I think not. You can study cancer in a petri dish—grow a tumor and then see if some drug slows the tumor's growth, and with what other toxicity; you can experiment with atherosclerotic plaque formation in a dish—grow blood-vessel cells and see if your drug removes cholesterol from their sides, and at what dosage. But you can't mimic depression in a petri dish, or with a computer. Millions of us are going to succumb to this nightmarish disorder, the treatments are still not very good, and animal models remain the best methods for seeking improvement. If you are of the school that believes that animal research, while sad, is acceptable, your goal is to do only good science on the smallest number of animals with the least pain.

ATTEMPTING AN INTEGRATION

Psychological approaches to depression give us some insight into the nature of the disease. According to one school, it is a state brought about by pathological overexposure to loss of control and outlets for frustration. In another psychological view, the Freudian one, it is the internalized battle of ambivalences, aggression turned inward. These views contrast with the more biological ones—that depression is a disorder of abnormal neurotransmitter levels, abnormal communication between certain parts of the brain, abnormal hormone ratios, genetic vulnerability.

There are extremely different ways of looking at the world, and researchers and clinicians from different orientations often don't have a word to say to one another about their mutual interest in depression. Sometimes they seem to be talking radically different languages— psychodynamic ambivalence versus neurotransmitter autoreceptors, cognitive overgeneralization versus allelic variants of genes.

What I view as the main point of this chapter is that stress is the unifying theme that pulls together these disparate threads of biology and psychology.

We have now seen some important links between stress and depression: extremes of psychological stress can cause something in a laboratory animal that looks pretty close to a depression. Moreover, stress is a predisposing factor in human depression as well, and brings about some of the typical endocrine changes of depression. In addition, genes that predispose to depression only do so in a stressful environment. Tightening the link further, glucocorticoids, as a central hormone of the stress-response, can bring about depression-like states in an animal, and can cause depression in humans. And finally, both stress and glucocorticoids can bring about neurochemical changes that have been implicated in depression.

With these findings in hand, the pieces begin to fit together. Stress, particularly in the form of extremes of lack of control and outlets, causes an array of deleterious changes in a person. Cognitively, this involves a distortive belief that there is no control or outlets in any circumstance-learned helplessness. On the affective level, there is anhedonia; behaviorally, there is psychomotor retardation. On the neurochemical level, there are likely disruptions of serotonin, norepinephrine, and dopamine signaling—as will be shown in chapter 16, prolonged stress can deplete dopamine in the pleasure pathways.

Physiologically, there are alterations in, among other things, appetite, sleep patterns, and sensitivity of the glucocorticoid system to feedback regulation. We call this array of changes, collectively, a major depression.

This is terrific. I believe we have a stress-related disease on our hands. But some critical questions remain to be asked. One concerns why it is that after three or so bouts of major depression the stress-depression link uncouples. This is the business about depressive episodes taking on an internal rhythm of their own, independent of whether the outside world is actually pummeling you with stressors. Why should such a transition occur? At present, there's a lot of theorizing but very little in the way of actual data.

But the most basic question remains, why do only some of us get depressed? An obvious answer is because some of us are exposed to a lot more stressors than others. And, when factoring in development, that can be stated in a way that also includes history—not only are some of us exposed to more stressors than others, but if we are exposed to some awful stressors early in life, forever after we will be more vulnerable to whatever subsequent stressors are thrown at us. This is the essence of allostatic load, of wear and tear, where exposure to severe stress produces rents of vulnerability.

So differential incidences of depression can be explained by differences in the amount of stress, and/or in stress histories. But even for the same stressors and the same history of stress, some of us are more vulnerable than others. Why should some of us succumb more readily?

To begin to make sense of this, we have to invert that question, to state it in a more world-weary way. How is it that any of us manage to *avoid* getting depressed? All things considered, this can be an awful world, and at times it must seem miraculous that any of us resist despair.

The answer is that we have built into us a biology of recovering from the effects of stress that provoke depression. As we've seen, stress and glucocorticoids can bring about many of the same alterations in neurotransmitter systems that have been implicated in depression. One of the best documented links is that stress depletes norepinephrine. No one is sure exactly why the depletion occurs, although it probably has something to do with norepinephrine being consumed faster than usual (rather than its being made more slowly than usual).

Critically, not only does stress deplete norepinephrine, but it simultaneously initiates the gradual synthesis of *more* norepinephrine. At the same time that norepinephrine content is plummeting, shortly after the onset of stress, the brain is starting to make more of the key enzyme tyrosine hydroxylase, which synthesizes norepinephrine. Both glucocorticoids and, indirectly, the autonomic nervous system play a role in inducing the new tyrosine hydroxylase. The main point is that, in most of us, stress may cause depletion of norepinephrine, but only transiently. We're about to see there are similar mechanisms related to serotonin. Thus, while everyday stressors bring about some of the neurochemical changes linked to depression along with some of the symptoms—we feel "blue"—at the same time, we are already building in the mechanisms of recovery. We get over it, we put things behind us, we get things in perspective, we move on with our lives . . . we heal and we recover.

So, given the same stressors and stress histories, why do only some of us get depressed? There is increasing evidence for a reasonable answer, which is that the biology of vulnerability to depression is that you don't recover from stressors very well. Back to that finding of the different versions of "gene Z," where one version increases your risk for depression, but only when coupled with a history of major stressors. The gene turns out to code for a protein called the serotonin transporter (also known as 5-HTT, derived from the fact that the chemical abbreviation for serotonin is "5-HT"). In other words, the pump that causes the reuptake of serotonin from the synapse. Whose actions are inhibited by drugs like Prozac, which are SSRIs—selective serotonin reuptake inhibitors. Aha. A whole bunch of pieces here are teetering on the edge of falling into place. The different allelic versions of the 5-HTT gene differ as to how good they are at removing serotonin from the synapse. And where does stress fit in? Glucocorticoids help regulate how much 5-HTT is made from the gene. And, critically, glucocorticoids differ in how good they are at doing that, depending on which allelic version of the 5-HTT gene you have. This allows us to come up with a working model of depression risk. It is a simplistic one, and a more realistic version must incorporate the likelihood of scads more examples of interactions among genes and stressors than simply this stress/glucocorticoids/5-HTT story.* Nonetheless, maybe what occurs is something like this: a major stressor comes along and produces some of the neurochemical changes of depression. The more prior history of stress you have, especially early in life, the less of a stressor it takes to produce those neurochemical changes. But the same stress signal, namely glucocorticoids, alters norepinephrine synthesis, serotonin

---

* For example, there is probably an equivalent story concerning stress, glucocorticoids, and the genetics of tyrosine hydroxylase.

trafficking, and so on, starting you on the road toward recovery. Unless your genetic makeup means that those recovery steps don't work very well.

This is the essence of the interaction between biology and experience. Take a sufficiently severe stressor and, as studies suggest, virtually all of us will fall into despair. No degree of neurochemical recovery mechanisms can maintain your equilibrium in the face of some of the nightmares that life can produce. Conversely, have a life sufficiently free of stress, and even with a genetic predisposition, you may be safe—a car whose brakes are faulty presents no danger if it is never driven. But in between those two extremes, it is the interaction between the ambiguous experiences that life throws at us and the biology of our vulnerabilities and resiliencies that determines which of us fall prey to this awful disease.

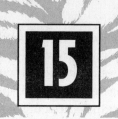

PERSONALITY, TEMPERAMENT, AND THEIR STRESS-RELATED CONSEQUENCES

The main point of chapter 13 was that psychological factors can modulate stress-responses. Perceive yourself in a given situation to have expressive outlets, control, and predictive information, for example, and you are less likely to have a stress-response. What this chapter explores is the fact that people habitually differ in how they modulate their stress-responses with psychological variables. Your style, your temperament, your personality have much to do with whether you regularly perceive opportunities for control or safety signals when they are there, whether you consistently interpret ambiguous circumstances as implying good news or bad, whether you typically seek out and take advantage of social support. Some folks are good at modulating stress in these ways, and others are terrible. These fall within the larger category of what Richard Davidson has called "affective style." And this turns out to be a very important factor in understanding why some people are more prone toward stress-related diseases than others.

We start with a study in contrasts. Consider Gary. In the prime of his life, he is, by most estimates, a success. He's done okay for himself materially, and he's never come close to going hungry. He's also had more than his share of sexual partners. And he has done extremely well in the hierarchical world that dominates most of his waking hours. He's good at what he does, and what he does is compete—he's already Number 2 and breathing down the neck of Number 1, who's grown complacent and a bit slack. Things are good and likely to get better.

But you wouldn't call Gary satisfied. In fact, he never really has been. Everything is a battle to him. The mere appearance of a rival rockets him into a tensely agitated state, and he views every interaction with a potential competitor as an in-your-face personal provocation. He views virtually every interaction with a distrustful vigilance. Not surprisingly, Gary has no friends to speak of. His subordinates give him a wide, fearful berth because of his tendency to take any frustration out on them. He behaves the same toward Kathleen, and barely knows their daughter Caitland—this is the sort of guy who is completely indifferent to the cutest of infants. And when he looks at all he's accomplished, all he can think of is that he is still not Number 1.

Gary's profile comes with some physiological correlates. Elevated basal glucocorticoid levels—a constant low-grade stress-response because life is one big stressor for him. An immune system that you wouldn't wish on your worst enemy. Elevated resting blood pressure, an unhealthy ratio of "good" to "bad" cholesterol, and already the early stages of serious atherosclerosis. And, looking ahead a bit, a premature death in late middle-age.

Contrast that with Kenneth. He's also prime-aged and Number 2 in his world, but he got there through a different route, one reflecting the different approach to life that he's had ever since he was a kid. Someone caustic or jaded might dismiss him as merely being a politician, but he's basically a good guy—works well with others, comes to their aid, and they in turn to his. Consensus builder, team player, and if he's ever frustrated about anything, and it isn't all that certain he ever is, he certainly doesn't take it out on those around him.

A few years ago, Kenneth was poised for a move to the Number 1 spot, but he did something extraordinary—he walked away from it all. Times were good enough that he wasn't going to starve, and he had reached the realization that there were things in life more important than fighting your way up the hierarchy. So he's spending time with his kids, Sam and Allan, making sure they grow up safe and healthy. He has a best friend in their mother, Barbara, and never gives a thought to what he's turned his back on.

Not surprisingly, Kenneth has a physiological profile quite different from Gary's, basically the opposite on every stress-related measure, and enjoys a robust good health. He is destined to live to a ripe old age, surrounded by kids, grandkids, and Barbara.

Normally, with these sorts of profiles, you try to protect the privacy of the individuals involved, but I'm going to violate that by including pictures of Gary and Kenneth on the next page. Check them out.

Isn't that something? Some baboons are driven sharks, avoid ulcers by giving them, see the world as full of water holes that are half empty.

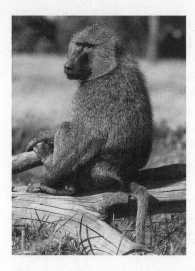

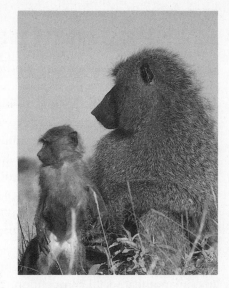

"Gary."

"Kenneth" (with infant).

And some baboons are the opposite in every way. Talk to any pet owner, and they will give ardent testimonials as to the indelible personality of their parakeet, turtle, or bunny. And they'd usually be at least somewhat right—people have published papers on animal personality. Some have concerned lab rats. Some rats have an aggressive proactive style for dealing with stressors—put a new object in their cage and they bury it in the bedding. These animals don't have much in the way of a glucocorticoid stress response. In contrast, there are reactive animals who respond to a menacing by avoiding it. They have a more marked glucocorticoid stress-response. And then there are studies about stress-related personality differences in geese. There's even been a great study published about sunfish personalities (some of whom are shy, and some of whom are outgoing social butterflies). Animals are strongly individualistic, and when it comes to primates, there are astonishing differences in their personalities, temperaments, and coping styles. These differences carry some distinctive physiological consequences and disease risks related to stress. This is not the study of what external stressors have to do with health. This is, instead, the study of the impact on health of how an individual perceives, responds to, and copes with those external stressors. The lessons learned from some of these animals can be strikingly relevant to humans.

STRESS AND THE SUCCESSFUL PRIMATE

If you are interested in understanding the stressors in our everyday lives and how some folks cope with them better than others, study a troop of baboons in the Serengeti—big, smart, long-lived, highly social animals who live in groups of from 50 to 150. The Serengeti is a great place for them to live, offering minimal problems with predators, low infant-mortality rates, easy access to food. Baboons there work per-haps four hours a day, foraging through the fields and trees for fruits, tubers, and edible grasses. This has a critical implication for me, which has made them the perfect study subjects when I've snuck away from my laboratory to the Serengeti during the summers of the past two decades. If baboons are spending only four hours a day filling their stomachs, that leaves them with eight hours a day of sunlight to be vile to one another. Social competition, coalitions forming to gang up on other animals, big males in bad moods beating up on someone smaller, snide gestures behind someone's back—just like us.

I am not being facetious. Think about some of the themes of the first chapter—how few of us are getting our ulcers because we have to walk ten miles a day looking for grubs to eat, how few of us become hypertensive because we are about to punch it out with someone over the last gulp from the water hole. We are ecologically buffered and privileged enough to be stressed mainly over social and psychological matters. Because the ecosystem of the Serengeti is so ideal for savanna baboons, they have the same luxury to make each other sick with social and psychological stressors. Of course, like ours, theirs is a world filled with affiliation, friendships, relatives who support each other; but it is a viciously competitive society as well. If a baboon in the Serengeti is miserable, it is almost always because another baboon has worked hard and long to bring about that state. Individual styles of coping with the social stress appear to be critical. Thus, one of the things I set out to test was whether such styles predicted differences in stress-related physiology and disease. I watched the baboons, col-lected detailed behavioral data, and then would anesthetize the ani-mals under controlled conditions, using a blowgun. Once they were unconscious, I could measure their glucocorticoid levels, their ability to make antibodies, their cholesterol profiles, and so on, under basal conditions and a range of stressed conditions.*

---

* The controls are daunting. You have to find an anesthetic that does not distort the lev-els of hormones that you are measuring. You have to dart every animal at the same time

The cases of Gary and Kenneth already give us a sense of how different male baboons can be. Two males of similar ranks may differ dramatically as to how readily they form coalitional partnerships with other males, how much they like to groom females, whether they play with kids, whether they sulk after losing a fight or go beat up on someone smaller. Two students, Justina Ray and Charles Virgin, and I analyzed years of behavioral data to try to formalize different elements of style and personality among these animals. We found some fascinating correlations between personality styles and physiology.

Among males who were in the higher-ranking half of the hierarchy, we observed a cluster of behavioral traits associated with low resting glucocorticoid levels independent of their specific ranks. Some of these traits were related to how males competed with one another. The first trait was whether a male could tell the difference between a threatening and a neutral interaction with a rival. How does one spot this in a baboon? Look at a particular male and two different scenarios. First scenario: along comes his worst rival, sits down next to him, and makes a threatening gesture. What does our male subject do next? Alternative scenario: our guy is sitting there, his worst rival comes along and . . . wanders off to the next field to fall asleep. What does our guy do in this situation?

Some males can tell the difference between these situations. Threatened from a foot away, they get agitated, vigilant, prepared; when they instead see their rival is taking a nap, they keep doing whatever they were doing. They can tell that one situation is bad news, the other is meaningless. But some males get agitated even when their rival is taking a nap across the field—the sort of situation that happens five times a day. If a male baboon can't tell the difference between the two

---

of day to control for daily fluctuations in hormone levels. If you want to get a first blood sample in which hormone levels reflect basal, nonstressed conditions, you can't dart someone who is sick or injured or who has had a fight or intercourse that day. For some of the cholesterol studies, I could not dart anyone who had eaten in the preceding twelve hours. If you are trying to measure resting hormone levels, you can't spend all morning making the same animal nervous as you repeatedly try to dart him; instead you get one shot, and you can't let him see it coming. Finally, once you dart him, you have to obtain the first blood sample rapidly, before hormone levels change in response to the dart. Quite a thing to do with your college education.

Why are these studies exclusively about males? Because of the difficulties inherent in trying to dart and anesthetize females. At any given time in this baboon population, approximately 80 percent of the adult females are either pregnant or nursing their young. You don't want to dart a female who is pregnant, as there is a good chance that the anesthesia will endanger the pregnancy. And you don't want to dart a female who has a youngster holding on to her in a panic as she goes down, or spends a day badly endangered for lack of milk while Mom is anesthetized.

situations, on the average his resting glucocorticoid levels are twice as high as those of the guy who can tell the difference—after correcting for rank as a variable. If a rival napping across the field throws a male into turmoil, the latter's going to be in a constant state of stress. No wonder his glucocorticoid levels are elevated. These stressed baboons are similar to the hyperreactive macaque monkeys that Jay Kaplan has studied. As you will recall from chapter 3, these are individuals who respond to every social provocation with an overactivation of their stress-response (the sympathetic nervous system) and carry the greater cardiovascular risk.

Next variable: if the situation really is threatening (the rival's a foot away and making menacing moves), does our male sit there passively and wait for the fight, or does he take control of the situation and strike first? Males who sit there passively, abdicating control, have much higher glucocorticoid levels than the take-charge types, after rank is eliminated as a factor in the analysis. We see the same pattern in low-ranking as well as high-ranking males.

A third variable: after a fight, can the baboon tell whether he won or lost? Some guys are great at it; they win a fight, and they groom their best friend. They lose a fight, and they beat up someone smaller. Other baboons react the same way regardless of outcome; they can't tell if life is improving or worsening. The baboon who can't tell the difference between winning and losing has much higher glucocorticoid levels, on average, than the guys who can, independent of rank.

Final variable: if a male has lost a fight, what does he do next? Does he sulk by himself, groom someone, or beat someone up? Discouragingly, it turns out that the males who are most likely to go beat on someone—thus displaying displaced aggression—have lower glucocorticoid levels, again after rank is eliminated as a variable. This is true for both subordinate baboons and the high-ranking ones.

Thus, after factoring out rank, lower basal glucocorticoid levels are found in males who are best at telling the difference between threatening and neutral interactions; who take the initiative if the situation clearly is threatening; who are best at telling whether they won or lost; and, in the latter case, who are most likely to make someone else pay for the defeat. This echoes some of the themes from the chapter on psychological stress. The males who were coping best (at least by this endocrine measure) had high degrees of social control (initiating the fights), predictability (they can accurately assess whether a situation is threatening, whether an outcome is good news), and outlets for frustration (a tendency to give rather than get ulcers). Remarkably, this style is stable over the years of these individuals' lives, and carries a big payoff—males with this cluster of low-glucocorticoid traits remain high ranking significantly longer than average.

Our subsequent studies have shown another set of traits that also predict low basal glucocorticoid levels. These traits have nothing to do with how males compete with one another. Instead, they are related to patterns of social affiliation. Males who spent the most time grooming females not in heat (not of immediate sexual interest—just good old platonic friends), who are groomed by them the most frequently, who spend the most time playing with the young—these are the low-glucocorticoid guys. Put most basically (and not at all anthropomor-phically), these are male baboons who are most capable of developing friendships. This finding is remarkably similar to those discussed in previous chapters regarding the protective effects of social affiliation against stress-related disease in humans. And as will be discussed in the final chapter of this book, this cluster of personality traits is also stable over time and comes with a distinctive payoff as well—a male baboon's equivalent of a successful old age.

Thus, among some male baboons, there are at least two routes for winding up with elevated basal glucocorticoid levels, independent of social rank—an inability to keep competition in perspective and social isolation. Stephen Suomi at the National Institutes of Health has stud-ied rhesus monkeys and identified another personality style that should seem familiar, which carries some physiological correlates. About 20 percent of rhesus are what he calls "high-reactors." Just like the baboons who find a rival napping to be an arousing threat, these individual monkeys see challenges everywhere. But in their case, the response to the perceived threat is a shrinking timidity. Put them into a novel environment that other rhesus monkeys would find to be a stimulating place to explore, and they react with fear, pouring out glucocorticoids. Place them with new peers, and they freeze with anxiety—shy and withdrawn, and again releasing vast amounts of glucocorticoids. Separate them from a loved one, and they are atypi-cally likely to collapse into a depression, complete with excessive glu-cocorticoids, overactivation of the sympathetic nervous system, and immunosuppression. These appear to be lifelong styles of dealing with the world, beginning early in infancy.

From where do these various primate personalities arise? When it comes to the baboons, I'll never know. Male baboons change troops at puberty, often moving dozens of miles before finding an adult troop to join. It is virtually impossible to track the same individuals from birth to adulthood, so I have no idea what their childhoods were like, whether their mothers were permissive or stern, whether they were forced to take piano lessons, and so on. But Suomi has done elegant work that indicates both genetic and environmental components to these personality differences. For example, he has shown that an infant monkey has a significant chance of sharing a personality trait with its father, despite the formation of social groups in which the father is not present—a sure hint at a heritable, genetic component. In contrast, the high-reactivity personality in these monkeys can be completely prevented by fostering such animals early in life to atypically nurturing mothers—a powerful vote for environmental factors built around mothering style.

Broadly, these various studies suggest two ways that a primate's personality style might lead down the path to stress-related disease. In the first way, there's a mismatch between the magnitude of the stressors they are confronted with and the magnitude of their stress-response—the most neutral of circumstances is perceived as a threat, demanding either a hostile, confrontational response (as with some of my baboons and Kaplan's macaques) or an anxious withdrawal (as with some of Suomi's monkeys). At the most extreme they even react to a situation that most certainly does not constitute a stressor (for example, winning a fight) the same way as if it were a stressful misery (losing one). In their second style of dysfunction, the animal does not take advantage of the coping responses that might make a stressor more manageable—they don't grab the minimal control available in a tough situation, they don't make use of effective outlets when the going gets tough, and they lack social support.

It would seem relatively straightforward to pull together some sound psychotherapeutic advice for these unhappy beasts. But in reality, it's hopeless. Baboons and macaques get distracted during therapy sessions, habitually pulling books off the shelves, for example; they don't know the days of the week and thus constantly miss appointments; they eat the plants in the waiting room, and so on. Thus, it might be more useful to apply those same insights to making sense of some humans who are prone toward an overactive stress-response and increased risk of stress-related disease.

 ## THE HUMAN REALM: A CAUTIONARY NOTE

There are, by now, some fairly impressive and convincing studies linking human personality types with stress-related diseases. Probably the best place to start, however, is with a bit of caution about some reported links that, I suspect, should be taken with a grain of salt.

I've already noted some skepticism about early psychoanalytic theorizing that linked certain personality types with colitis (see chapter 5). Another example concerns miscarriages and abortions. Chapter 7 reviewed the mechanisms by which stress can cause the loss of a pregnancy, and one hardly needs to have experienced that personally to have an inkling of the trauma involved. Thus, you can imagine the particular agony for women who miscarry repeatedly, and the special state of misery for those who never get a medical explanation for the problem—no expert has a clue what's wrong. Into that breach have charged people who have attempted to uncover personality traits common to women labeled as "psychogenic aborters."

Some researchers have identified one subgroup of women with repeated "psychogenic" abortions (accounting for about half the cases) as being "retarded in their psychological development." They are characterized as emotionally immature women, highly dependent on their husbands, who on some unconscious level view the impending arrival of the child as a threat to their own childlike relationship with their spouse. Another personality type identified, at the opposite extreme, are women who are characterized as being assertive and independent, who really don't want to have a child. Thus, a common theme in the two supposed profiles is an unconscious desire not to have the child—either because of competition for the spouse's attention or because of reluctance to cramp their independent lifestyles.

Many experts are skeptical about the studies behind these characterizations, however. The first reason harks back to a caveat I aired early in the book: a diagnosis of "psychogenic" anything (impotency, amenorrhea, abortion, and so on) is usually a diagnosis by exclusion. In other words, the physician can't find any disease or organic cause, and until one is discovered, the disorder gets tossed into the psychogenic bucket. This may mean that, legitimately, it is heavily explained by psychological variables, or it may simply mean that the relevant hormone, neurotransmitter, or genetic abnormality has not yet been discovered. Once it is discovered, the psychogenic disease is magically transformed into an organic problem—"Oh, it wasn't your personality after all." The area of repeated aborting seems to be one that is rife with recent biological insights—in other words, if so many of last decade's psychogenic aborters now have an organic explanation for their malady, that trend is likely to continue. So be skeptical of any current "psychogenic" label.

Another difficulty is that these studies are all retrospective in design: the researchers examine the personalities of women after they have had repeated abortions. A study may thus cite the case of a woman who has had three miscarriages in a row, noting that she is emotionally withdrawn and dependent on her husband. But because of the nature of the research design, one can't tell whether these traits are a cause of the miscarriages or a response to them—three successive miscarriages could well exact a heavy emotional price, perhaps making the subject withdrawn and more dependent on her husband. In order to study the phenomenon properly, one would need to look at personality profiles of women before they become pregnant, to see if these traits predict who is going to have repeated miscarriages. To my knowledge, this kind of study has not yet been carried out.

As a final problem, none of the studies provides any reasonable speculation as to how a particular personality type may lead to a tendency not to carry fetuses to term. What are the mediating physiological mechanisms? What hormones and organ functions are disrupted? The absence of any science in that area makes me pretty suspicious of the claims. Psychological stressors can increase the risk of a miscarriage, but although there is precedent in the medical literature for thinking that having a certain type of personality is associated with an increased risk for miscarriages, scientists are far from being able to agree on what personality is associated, let alone whether the personality is a cause or consequence of the miscarriages.

PSYCHIATRIC DISORDERS AND ABNORMAL STRESS-RESPONSES

A number of psychiatric disorders involve personalities, roles, and temperaments that are associated with distinctive stress-responses. We have seen an example of this in the previous chapter on depression—about half of depressives have resting glucocorticoid levels that are dramatically higher than in other people, often sufficiently elevated to cause problems with metabolism or immunity. Or in some cases, depressives are unable to turn off glucocorticoid secretion, their brains being less sensitive to a shut-off signal.

A theme in the previous section on some troubled nonhuman primates is that there is a discrepancy between the sorts of stressors they are exposed to and the coping responses they come up with. Learned helplessness, which we saw to be an underpinning of depression, appears to be another example of such discrepancy. A challenge occurs, and what is the response of a depressive individual? "I can't, it's too much, why bother doing anything, it isn't going to work anyway, nothing I do ever works. . . ." The discrepancy here is that in the face of stressful challenges, depressives don't even attempt to mount a coping response. A different type of discrepancy is seen with people who are anxiety-prone.

Anxiety Disorders

What is anxiety? A sense of disquiet, of disease, of the sands constantly shifting menacingly beneath your feet—where constant vigilance is the only hope of effectively protecting yourself.

Anxiety disorders come in a number of flavors. To name just a few: generalized anxiety disorder is just that—generalized—whereas phobias focus on specific things. In people with panic attacks, the anxiety boils over with a paralyzing, hyperventilating sense of crisis that causes massive activation of the sympathetic nervous system. In obsessive-compulsive disorder, the anxiety buries and busies itself in endless patterns of calming, distracting ritual. In post-traumatic stress disorder, the anxiety can be traced to a specific trauma.

In none of these cases is the anxiety about fear. Fear is the vigilance and the need to escape from something real. Anxiety is about dread and foreboding and your imagination running away with you. Much as with depression, anxiety is rooted in a cognitive distortion. In this case, people prone toward anxiety overestimate risks and the likelihood of a bad outcome.

Unlike depressives, the anxiety-prone person is still attempting to mobilize coping responses. But the discrepancy is the distorted belief that stressors are everywhere and perpetual, and that the only hope for safety is constant mobilization of coping responses. Life consists of the concrete, agitated present of solving a problem that someone else might not even consider to exist.*

Awful. And immensely stressful. Not surprisingly, anxiety disorders are associated with chronically overactive stress-responses, and with increased risk of many of the diseases that fill the pages of this book (anxiety-prone rats, for example, have a shortened life span). However, glucocorticoid excess is not the usual response. Instead, it's too much sympathetic activation, an overabundance of circulating catecholamines (epinephrine and norepinephrine).

We have now seen some interesting contrasts between glucocorticoids and the catecholamines (epinephrine and norepinephrine). Chapter 2 emphasized how the former defend you against stressors by

---

* Emphasizing the concrete nature of anxiety, the psychoanalyst Anna Aragno has written, "Anxiety wipes out the space wherein the symbol is born."

handing out guns from the gun locker within seconds, in contrast to glucocorticoids, which defend you by constructing new weapons over the course of minutes to hours. Or there can be an elaboration of this time course, in which catecholamines mediate the response to a current stressor while glucocorticoids mediate preparation for the next stressor. When it comes to psychiatric disorders, it seems that increases in the catecholamines have something to do with still trying to cope and the effort that involves, where overabundance of glucocorticoids seems more of a signal of having given up on attempting to cope. You can show this with a lab rat. Rats, being nocturnal creatures, don't like bright lights, are made anxious by them. Put a rat in a cage whose edges are dark, just the place a rat likes to hunker down. But the rat is really hungry and there's some wonderful food in the middle of the cage, under a bright light. Massive anxiety—the rat starts toward the food, pulls back, again and again, frantically tries to figure ways to the food that avoid the light. This is anxiety, a disorganized attempt to cope, and this phase is dominated by catecholamines. If it goes on for too long, the animal gives up, just lies there, in the shaded perimeter. And that is depression, and it is dominated by glucocorticoids.

The Biology of Anxiety

The main point of this chapter is to explore how different psychiatric disorders and personality styles involve dealing poorly with stress, and we've just seen how anxiety fits the bill. But it is worth looking at the biology of the disease a bit.

There are some things that mammals get anxious about that are innate. Bright lights for a rat. Being dangled up in the air if you are a terrestrial creature. Having your breathing obstructed for most any animal. But most things that make us anxious are learned. Maybe because they are associated with some trauma, or maybe because we've generalized them based on their similarity to something associated with a trauma. Organisms are predisposed to learn some of those associations more readily than others—humans and spiders, for example, or monkeys and snakes. But we can learn to be anxious about utterly novel things—as we speed up to get across a suspension bridge quickly, wondering if the guy in that panel truck is from Al-Qaeda.

This is a different type of learning than what we focused on in chapter 10, which concerned the hippocampus and declarative learning. This is implicit learning, where a certain autonomic response in your body has been conditioned. Thus, consider a woman who has suffered a traumatic assault, where her brain has become conditioned

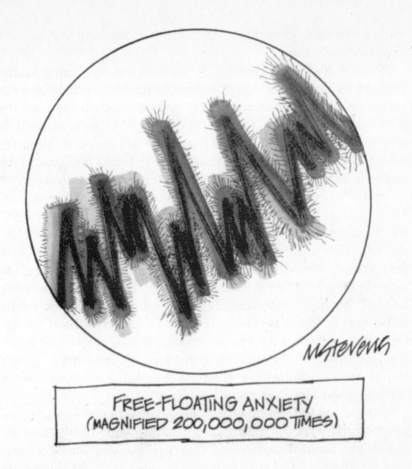

FREE-FLOATING ANXIETY
(MAGNIFIED 200,000,000 TIMES)

to speed up her heart every time she sees a similar-looking man. Pavlovian learning—ring the bell associated with food, and the brain has learned to activate salivary glands; see a certain type of face, and the brain has learned to activate the sympathetic nervous system. The conditioned memory can be elicited without you even being conscious of it. That woman finds herself in a crowded party, having a fine time, when suddenly the anxiety is there, she's gasping, heart racing, and she hasn't a clue why. It is not until a few seconds later that she realizes that the man talking just behind her has an accent just like *the* man. The body responds before there is consciousness of the similarity.

As we saw in chapter 10, while mild transient stress enhances declarative learning, prolonged or severe stress disrupts it. But in the case of this pre-conscious, implicit, autonomic learning, any type of stress enhances it. For example, make a loud sound and a lab rat will have a startle response—in a few milliseconds, its muscles tense. Stress the rat beforehand with any type of stressor and the startle response is exaggerated and more likely to become a habitual, conditioned response. Same in us.

As mentioned, this is outside the realm of the hippocampus, that wonderfully rational conduit of declarative memory, helping us recall someone's birthday. Instead, anxiety and fear conditioning are the province of a related structure, the amygdala.* To begin to make sense of its function, you have to look at brain areas that project to the amygdala, and where the amygdala projects to, in turn. One route to the amygdala is from pain pathways. Which brings us back to chapter 9 and how there's pain and then there's subjective pain interpretation. The amygdala is about the latter. The structure also gets sensory information. Remarkably, the amygdala gets sensory information before that information reaches the cortex and causes conscious awareness of the sensation—the woman's heart races before she is even aware of the accent of the man. The amygdala gets information from the autonomic nervous system. What's the significance of this? Suppose some ambiguous information is filtering in, and your amygdala is "deciding" whether this is a time to get anxious. If your heart is pounding and your stomach is in your throat, that input will bias the amygdala to vote for anxiety.† And, to complete the picture, the amygdala is immensely sensitive to glucocorticoid signals.

The outputs from the amygdala make perfect sense—mostly projections to the hypothalamus and related outposts, which initiate the cascade of glucocorticoid release and activate the sympathetic nervous system.‡ And how does the amygdala communicate?—by using CRH as a neurotransmitter.

Some of the most convincing work implicating the amygdala in anxiety comes from brain-imaging studies. Put people in a scanner, flash various pictures, see what parts of the brain are activated in response to each. Show a scary face, and the amygdala lights up. Make

---

* The amygdala is also all about aggression. It is hard to understand why organisms are aggressive outside of the context of understanding that they are anxious or fearful.

† An exciting clinical implication of this can be found in the recent work of Larry Cahill and Roger Pitman of Harvard. They report that if you block the sympathetic nervous system in someone who has just suffered a major trauma (with a drug from chapter 3 called a beta-blocker), you decrease the odds of the person developing post-traumatic stress disorder. What's the rationale? Decrease the sympathetic signal to the amygdala, and the amygdala is less likely to decide that this is an event that should provoke wild arousal forever after.

‡ So an aroused amygdala activates the sympathetic nervous system and, as we saw in the previous paragraph, an aroused sympathetic nervous system increases the odds of the amygdala activating. Anxiety can feed on itself.

the pictures subliminal—flash them for thousandths of a second, too fast to be consciously seen (and too fast to activate the visual cortex), and the amygdala lights up.*

How does the functioning of the amygdala relate to anxiety? People with anxiety disorders have exaggerated startle responses, see menace that others don't. Give people some reading task, where they are flashed a series of nonsense words and have to quickly detect the real ones. Everyone slows down slightly for a menacing word, but people with anxiety disorders slow down even more. Commensurate with these findings, the amygdala in such a person shows the same hyperreactivity. A picture that is sort of frightening, that doesn't quite activate the amygdala in a control subject, does so in an anxious person. A frightening picture that is flashed up too briefly to be even noted subliminally in a control subject does the trick to the amygdala in someone who is anxious. No wonder the sympathetic nervous system then races—alarms are always going off in the amygdala.

Why does the amygdala work differently in someone who is anxious? Some amazing research in recent years shows how this might work. As we saw in chapter 10, major stressors and glucocorticoids disrupt hippocampal function—the synapses aren't able to do that long-term potentiation business, and the dendritic processes in neurons shrink. Remarkably, stress and glucocorticoids do just the opposite in the amygdala—synapses become more excitable, neurons grow more of the cables that connect the cells to each other. And if you artificially make the amygdala of a rat more excitable, the animal shows an anxiety-like disorder afterward.

Joseph LeDoux of New York University, who pretty much put the amygdala on the map when it comes to anxiety, has constructed a remarkable model out of these findings. Suppose a major traumatic stressor occurs, of a sufficient magnitude to disrupt hippocampal function while enhancing amygdaloid function. At some later point, in a similar setting, you have an anxious, autonomic state, agitated and fearful, and you haven't a clue why—this is because you never consolidated memories of the event via your hippocampus while your amygdala-mediated autonomic pathways sure as hell remember. This is a version of free-floating anxiety.

---

* Some recent studies that I find truly unsettling show that if you flash a picture of a face of someone from a different race, the amygdala tends to light up. Endless studies need to be done looking at what sort of face is flashed and what sort of person is observing it. But in the meantime, just think about the implications of that finding.

TYPE A AND THE ROLE OF UPHOLSTERY IN CARDIOVASCULAR PHYSIOLOGY

A number of proposed links between personality and cardiovascular disease have been reported. Amid these, there is one proposed connection between personality and heart disease that has become so well-known that it has suffered the ultimate accolade—namely, being distorted beyond recognition in many people's minds (usually winding up being ascribed to the most irritating behavioral trait that you want to complain about in someone else, or indirectly brag about in yourself). I'm talking being "Type A."

Two cardiologists, Meyer Friedman and Ray Rosenman, coined the term *Type A* in the early 1960s to describe a collection of traits that they found in some individuals. They didn't describe these traits in terms related to stress (for example, defining Type-A people as those who responded to neutral or ambiguous situations as if they were stressful), although I will attempt to do that reframing below. Instead, they characterized Type-A people as immensely competitive, overachieving, time-pressured, impatient, and hostile. People with that profile, they reported, had an increased risk of cardiovascular disease.

This was met with enormous skepticism in the field. You're some 1950s Ozzie-and-Harriet cardiologist and you think about heart valves and circulating lipids, not about how someone deals with a slow line at the supermarket. Thus, there was an initial tendency among many in the field to view the link between the behavior and the disease as the reverse of what Friedman and Rosenman proposed—getting heart disease might make some people act in a more Type-A manner. But Friedman and Rosenman did prospective studies that showed that the Type A-ness preceded the heart disease. This finding made a splash, and by the 1980s, some of the biggest guns in cardiology convened, checked the evidence, and concluded that being Type A carries at least as much cardiac risk as does smoking or having high cholesterol levels.

Everyone was delighted, and "Type A" entered common parlance. The trouble was, soon thereafter some careful studies failed to replicate the basic findings of Friedman and Rosenman. Suddenly, Type A wasn't looking good after all. Then, to add insult to injury, two studies showed that once you had coronary heart disease, being Type A was associated with better survival rates (in the notes at the end of the book, I discuss subtle ways to explain this finding).

By the late 1980s, the Type-A concept underwent some major modifications. One was the recognition that personality factors are more predictive of heart disease when considering people who get their first heart attack at an early age—by later years, the occurrence of a first heart attack is more about fats and smoking. Moreover, work by Redford Williams of Duke University convinced most in the field that the key factor in the list of Type A–ish symptoms is the hostility. For example, when scientists reanalyzed some of the original Type-A studies and broke the constellation of traits into individual ones, hostility popped out as the only significant predictor of heart disease. The same result was found in studies of middle-aged doctors who had taken personality inventory tests twenty-five years earlier as an exercise in medical school. And the same thing was found when looking at American lawyers, Finnish twins, Western Electric employees—a range of populations. As another example, there is a correlation between how hostile people are in ten American cities and the mortality rates due to cardiovascular disease.* These various studies have suggested that a high degree of hostility predicts coronary heart disease, atherosclerosis, hemorrhagic stroke, and higher rates of mortality with these diseases. Many of these studies, moreover, controlled for important variables like age, weight, blood pressure, cholesterol levels, and smoking. Thus, it is unlikely that the hostility–heart disease connection could be due to some other factor (for example, that hostile people are more likely to smoke, and the heart disease arises from the smoking, not the hostility). More recent studies have shown that hostility is associated with a significant overall increase in mortality across all diseases, not just those of the heart.[†]

Friedman and colleagues stuck with an alternative view. They suggested that at the core of the hostility is a sense of "time-pressuredness"—"Can you believe that teller, how slowly he's working. I'm going to be here all day. I can't waste my life on some bank line. How did that kid know I was in a rush? I could kill him"—and that the core of being time-pressured is rampant insecurity. There's no time to savor anything you've accomplished, let alone enjoy anything that anyone else has done, because you must rush off to prove yourself all over again, and try to hide from the world for another day what a fraud you are. Their work suggested that a persistent sense of insecurity is, in fact, a better predictor of cardiovascular profiles

---

* The hostility measures were self-rated in a Gallup poll. What was the rank order of the cities in terms of hostility? From highest to lowest: Philadelphia, New York, Cleveland, Des Moines, Chicago, Detroit, Denver, Minneapolis, Seattle, Honolulu. This mostly makes sense to me, except what's up with Des Moines?

[†] Perhaps modifying a wonderful aphorism to "I will let no man degrade my soul *or my health* by making me hate him."

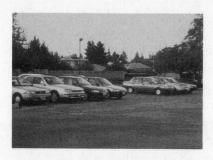 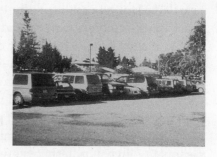

Type A's in action. The photo on the left shows the early-morning parking pattern of a patient support group for Type-A individuals with cardiovascular disease—everyone positioned for that quick getaway that doesn't waste a second. On the right, the same scene later in the day.

than is hostility, although theirs appears to be a minority view in the field.

Insofar as hostility has something to do with your heart (whether as a primary factor or as a surrogate variable), it remains unclear which aspects of hostility are bad news. For example, the study of lawyers suggested that overt aggressiveness and cynical mistrust were critical—in other words, frequent open expression of the anger you feel predicts heart disease. In support of that, experimental studies show that the full expression of anger is a powerful stimulant of the cardiovascular system. By contrast, in the reanalysis of the original Type-A data a particularly powerful predictor of heart disease was not only high degrees of hostility, but also the tendency not to express it when angry. This latter view is supported by some fascinating work by James Gross of Stanford University. Show volunteers a film clip that evokes some strong emotion. Disgust, for example (thanks to a gory view of someone's leg being amputated). They writhe in discomfort and distaste and, no surprise, show the physiological markers of having turned on their sympathetic nervous systems. Now, show some other volunteers the same film clip but, beforehand, instruct them to try not to express their emotions ("so that if someone were watching, they'd have no idea what you were feeling"). Run them through the blood and guts, and, with them gripping the arms of their chairs and trying to remain stoic, and still, the sympathetic activation becomes even greater. Repressing the expression of strong emotions appears to exaggerate the intensity of the physiology that goes along with them.

Why would great hostility (of whatever variant) be bad for your heart? Some of it is likely to be that roundabout realm of risk factors, in that hostile individuals are more likely to smoke, eat poorly, drink to excess. Moreover, there are psychosocial variables, in that hostile people lack social support because they tend to drive people away. But there are direct biological consequences to hostility as well. Subjectively, we can describe hostile persons as those who get all worked up and angry over incidents that the rest of us would find only mildly provocative, if provocative at all. Similarly, their stress-responses switch into high gear in circumstances that fail to perturb everyone else's. Give both hostile and non-hostile people a nonsocial stressor (like some math problems) and nothing exciting happens; everyone has roughly the same degree of mild cardiovascular activation. But if you generate a situation with a social provocation, the hostile people dump more epinephrine, norepinephrine, and glucocorticoids into their bloodstreams and wind up with higher blood pressures and a host of other undesirable features of their cardiovascular systems. All sorts of social provocations have been used in studies: the subjects may be requested to take a test and, during it, be repeatedly interrupted; or they may play a video game in which the opponent not only is rigged to win but acts like a disparaging smart aleck. In these and other cases, the cardiovascular stress-responses of the non-hostile are relatively mild. But blood pressure goes through the roof in the hostile people. (Isn't it remarkable how similar these folks are to Jay Kaplan's hyperreactive monkeys, with their exaggerated sympathetic responses to stressors and their increased risk of cardiovascular disease? Or to my baboons, the ones who can't differentiate between threatening and nonthreatening events in their world? There are card-carrying Type-A individuals out there with tails.) Here is that discrepancy again. For anxious people, life is full of menacing stressors that demand vigilant coping responses. For the Type A, life is full of menacing stressors that demand vigilant coping responses of a particularly hostile nature. This is probably representative of the rest of their lives. If each day is filled with cardiovascular provocations that everyone else responds to as no big deal, life will slowly hammer away at the hearts of the hostile. An increased risk of cardiovascular disease is no surprise.

A pleasing thing is that Type A-ness is not forever. If you reduce the hostility component in Type-A people through therapy (using some of the approaches that will be outlined in the final chapter), you reduce the risk for further heart disease. This is great news. I've noticed that many health professionals who treat Type-A people are mostly trying to reform these folks. Basically, many Type-A people are abusive pains in the keister to lots of folks around them. When you talk to some of the Type-A experts, there is an odd tone between the lines that Type A-ness (of which many of them are admittedly perfect examples) is a kind of ethical failing, and that the term is a fancied-up medical way of describing people who just aren't nice to others. Added to this is a tendency I've noticed for a lot of the Type-A experts to be lay preachers, or descendants of clergy. That religious linkage will even sneak in the back door. I once talked with two leaders in the field, one an atheist and the other agnostic, and when they tried to give me a sense of how they try to get through to Type-A subjects about their bad ways, they made use of a religious sermon.* I finally asked these two M.D.s an obvious question—were they in the business of blood vessels or souls? Was the work that they do about heart disease or about ethics? And without a beat they both chose ethics. Heart disease was just a wedge for getting at the bigger issues. I thought this was wonderful. If it takes turning our coronary vessels into our ledgers of sin and reducing circulating lipids as an act of redemption in order to get people to be more decent to each other, more power to them.

Interior Decorating as Scientific Method

A final question about this field: How was Type-A behavior discovered? We all know how scientists make their discoveries. There are the discoveries in the bathtub (Archimedes and his discernment of the displacement of water), discoveries in one's sleep (Kekule and his dream of carbons dancing in a ring to form benzene), discoveries at the symphony (our scientist, strained by overwork, is forced to the concert by a significant other; during a quiet woodwind section, there's the sud-

---

* I listened to a tape of this sermon, called "Back in the Box," by the Reverend John Ortberg. It concerns an incident from his youth. His grandmother, saintly, kind, nurturant, also happened to be a viciously competitive and skillful Monopoly player, and his summer visits to her were littered with his defeats at the game. He described one year where he practiced like mad, honed his Machiavellian instinct, developed a ruthless jugular-gripping style, and finally mopped up the board with her. After which, his grandmother rose and calmly put the pieces away.

"You know," she said offhandedly, "this is a great game, but when it is all over with, the pieces just go back in the box." Amass your property, your hotels . . . [the sermon takes off from there] . . . your wealth, your accomplishments, your awards, your whatevers, and eventually it will all be over with and those pieces go back in the box. And all you are left with is how you lived your life.

I listened to this tape while racing to beat red lights on my way to a 5:00 A.M. commuter train, Powerbook ready so as not to miss a moment of work on the train, eating breakfast one-handed while driving, using the time to listen to this sermon on tape as research for this chapter. And this sermon, whose trajectory was obvious from the first sentence and was filled with Jesus and other things I do not subscribe to, reduced me to tears.

den realization, the scribbled equation on the program notes, the rushed "Darling, I must leave this instant for the laboratory [accent on second syllable, like in *Masterpiece Theater*]," with the rest being history). But every now and then someone else makes the discovery and comes and tells the scientist about it. And who is that someone? Very often someone whose role in the process could be summed up by an imaginary proverb that will probably never end up embroidered on someone's pot holder: "If you want to know if the elephant at the zoo has a stomachache, don't ask the veterinarian, ask the cage cleaner." People who clean up messes become attuned to circumstances that change the amount of mess there is. Back in the 1950s that fact caused a guy to just miss changing the course of medical history.

I had the privilege of hearing the story from the horse's mouth, Dr. Meyer Friedman. It was the mid-1950s, Friedman and Rosenman had their successful cardiology practice, and they were having an unexpected problem. They were spending a fortune having to reupholster the chairs in their waiting rooms. This is not the sort of issue that would demand a cardiologist's attention. Nonetheless, there seemed to be no end of chairs that had to be fixed. One day, a new upholsterer came in to see to the problem, took one look at the chairs, and discovered the Type A–cardiovascular disease link. "What the hell is wrong with your patients? People don't wear out chairs this way." It was only the front-most few inches of the seat cushion and of the padded armrests that were torn to shreds, as if some very short beavers spent each night in the office craning their necks to savage the fronts of the chairs. The patients in the waiting rooms all habitually sat on the edges of their seats, fidgeting, clawing away at the armrests.

The rest should have been history: up-swelling of music as the upholsterer is seized by the arms and held in a penetrating gaze—"Good heavens, man, do you realize what you've just said?" Hurried conferences between the upholsterer and other cardiologists. Frenzied sleepless nights as teams of idealistic young upholsterers spread across the land, carrying the news of their discovery back to Upholstery/Cardiology Headquarters—"Nope, you don't see that wear pattern in the waiting-room chairs of the urologists, or the neurologists, or the oncologists, or the podiatrists, just the cardiologists. There's something different about people who wind up with heart disease"—and the field of Type-A therapy takes off.

Instead, none of that happened. Dr. Friedman sighs. A confession. "I didn't pay any attention to the man. I was too busy; it went in one ear and out the other." It wasn't until four or five years later that

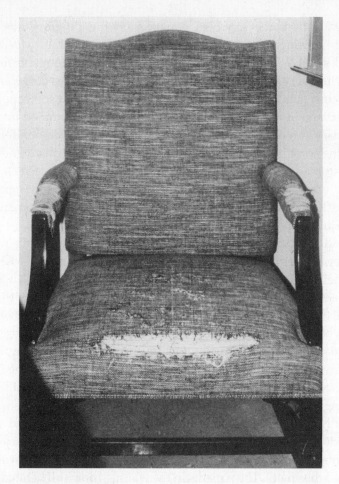

How it all began . . . almost.

Dr. Friedman's formal research with his patients began to yield some hints, at which point there was the thunderclap of memory—Oh, my god, the upholsterer, remember that guy going on about the wear pattern? And to this day, no one remembers his name.*

---

* Since the last edition, it has been necessary to edit this section into the past tense. Friedman, who was somewhat of a father figure to me, passed away recently at age ninety-one. He was a man who, statistically, had so little time left, yet he had somehow beaten that ticking toxic clock, and he had all the time in the world. But he hadn't turned into a contentless geezer—up until his last days, he was seeing patients, running an institute at UCSF Medical Center, cranky about delays in his work, anticipating his next data, arguing with competitors with a different take on the subject. Full of appetites, but with an appetite being its own reward and no rancor at the idea that it might not be fulfilled. And

There have been a host of other studies concerning personality, temperament, and stress-related physiology. Scientists have reported differences in stress-related immune function between optimists and pessimists. Others have shown higher glucocorticoid levels in shyer individuals in social settings. Others have considered neurosis as a factor. But let's consider one more subject, one that is particularly interesting because it concerns the last people on earth who you'd think were stressed.

 ## WHEN LIFE CONSISTS OF NOTHING BUT SQUEEZING TIGHTLY

This chapter has discussed personality types associated with overactive stress-responses, and argued that a common theme among them is a discrepancy between what sort of stressors life throws at these folks and what sort of coping responses they come up with. This final section is about a newly recognized version of an overactive stress-response. And it's puzzling.

These are not people who are dealing with their stressors too passively, too persistently, too vigilantly, or with too much hostility. They don't appear to have all that many stressors. They claim they're not depressed or anxious, and the psychological tests they are given show they're right. In fact, they describe themselves as pretty happy, successful, and accomplished (and, according to personality tests, they really are). Yet, these people (comprising approximately 5 percent of the population) have chronically activated stress-responses. What's their problem?

Their problem, I think, is one that offers insight into an unexpected vulnerability of our human psyche. The people in question are said to

---

deeply engaged with the idea that the world would be a more decent place if something was done about those Type-A people—Friedman was one of the two people I described a few paragraphs back (along with his medical director, Bart Sparagon) who said he was in the business of ethics. Friedman would do something very interesting and confessional with this. He was a gentle, courtly man who had been a driven, steamrolling son of a bitch before a heart attack in his fifties. He'd stand up in front of a group of his patients, ruthless CEO Type-A barracudas with their first heart attacks at age forty-two, and say, "Look at me—not look at me, I used to be so Type A that I developed a bad heart, but look at me, I used to be so Type A that I was a bad person," and then he'd prove it—tales of people he was curt to, whose efforts he never noticed, whose accomplishments he envied. And here he was at age ninety, metaphorically the ex-alcoholic preacher who has been there. Cardiology as redemption. It would be hard to make a choice between making the world a healthier place or a kinder place. Here was a man who did both. I miss him.

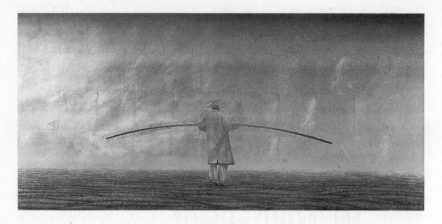

Clifford Goodenough, Figure Walking in a Landscape, *goldleaf, tempera, oil on masonite, 1991.*

have "repressive" personalities, and we all have met someone like them. In fact, we usually regard these folks with a tinge of envy—"I wish I had their discipline; everything seems to come so easily to them. How do they do it?"

These are the archetypal people who cross all their *t*'s and dot all their *i*'s. They describe themselves as planners who don't like surprises, who live structured, rule-bound lives—walking to work the same way each day, always wearing the same style of clothes—the sort of people who can tell you what they're having for lunch two weeks from Wednesday. Not surprisingly, they don't like ambiguity and strive to set up their world in black and white, filled with good or bad people, behaviors that are permitted or strictly forbidden. They keep a tight lid on their emotions. Stoic, regimented, hardworking, productive, solid folks who never stand out in a crowd (unless you begin to wonder at the unconventional nature of their extreme conventionality).

Some personality tests, pioneered by Richard Davidson, identify repressive individuals. For starters, as noted, the personality tests show that these people aren't depressed or anxious. Instead, the tests reveal their need for social conformity, their dread of social disapproval, and their discomfort with ambiguity, as shown by the extremely high rates at which they agree with statements framed as absolutes, statements filled with "never" and "always." No gray tones here.

Intertwined with those characteristics is a peculiar lack of emotional expression. The tests reveal how repressive people "inhibit negative affect"—no expressing of those messy, complicated emotions for them, and little recognition of those complications in others. For example, ask repressors and non-repressors to recall an experience associated with a specific strong emotion. Both groups report that particular emotion with equal intensity. However, when asked what else they were feeling, non-repressors typically report an array of additional, nondominant feelings: "Well, it mostly made me angry, but also a little sad, and a little disgusted too. . . ." Repressors steadfastly report no secondary emotions. Black-and-white feelings, with little tolerance for subtle blends.

Are these people for real? Maybe not. Maybe beneath their tranquil exteriors, they're actually anxious messes who won't admit to their frailties. Careful study indicates that some repressors are indeed mostly concerned about keeping up appearances. (One clue is that they tend to give less "repressed" answers on personality questionnaires when they can be anonymous.) And so their physiological symptoms of stress are easy to explain. We can cross those folks off the list.

What about the rest of the repressors? Could they be deceiving themselves—roiling with anxiety, but not even aware of it? Even careful questionnaires cannot detect that sort of self-deception; to ferret it out, psychologists traditionally rely on less structured, more open-ended tests (of the "What do you see in this picture?" variety). Those tests show that, yes, some repressors are far more anxious than they realize; their physiological stress is also readily explained.

Yet even after you cross the anxious self-deceivers off the list, there remains a group of people with tight, constrained personalities who are truly just fine: mentally healthy, happy, productive, socially interactive. But they have overactive stress-responses. The levels of glucocorticoids in their bloodstream are as elevated as among highly depressed people, and they have elevated sympathetic tone as well. When exposed to a cognitive challenge, repressors show unusually large increases in heart rate, blood pressure, sweating, and muscle tension. And these overaroused stress-responses exact a price. For example, repressive individuals have relatively poor immune function. Furthermore, coronary disease patients who have repressive personalities are more vulnerable to cardiac complications than are non-repressors.

Overactive, endangering stress-responses—yet the people harboring them are not stressed, depressed, or anxious. Back to our envious thought—"I wish I had their discipline. How do they do it?" The way they do it, I suspect, is by working like maniacs to generate their structured, repressed world with no ambiguity or surprises. And this comes with a physiological bill.

Davidson and Andrew Tomarken of Vanderbilt University have used electroencephalographic (EEG) techniques to show unusually enhanced activity in a portion of the frontal cortex of repressors. As will be covered at length in the next chapter, this is a region of the brain involved in inhibiting impulsive emotion and cognition (for example, metabolic activity in this area has been reported to be decreased in violent sociopaths). It's the nearest anatomical equivalent we have to a superego; makes you say you love the appalling dinner, compliment the new hairdo, keeps you toilet trained. It keeps those emotions tightly under control, and as Gross's work showed with emotional repression, it takes a lot of work to keep an especially tight squeeze on those emotional sphincters.

It can be a frightening world out there, and the body may well reflect the effort of threading our way through those dark, menacing forests. How much better it would be to be able to sit, relaxed, on the sun-drenched porch of a villa, far, far from the wild things baying. Yet, what looks like relaxation could well be exhaustion—exhaustion from the labor of having built a wall around that villa, the effort of keeping out that unsettling, challenging, vibrant world. A lesson of repressive personality types and their invisible burdens is that, sometimes, it can be enormously stressful to construct a world without stressors.

16

JUNKIES, ADRENALINE JUNKIES, AND PLEASURE

Okay, it's great that we're trying to understand how stress works and how to live healthier lives and make the world a better place and all that, but it's time we devoted a little space to a really important issue—why can't we tickle ourselves?

Before tackling this profound question, we first need to consider why not all people can make you feel ticklish. It probably requires that it be a person that you feel positive about. Thus, you're five and there's no one who can evoke ticklish feelings in you like your nutty uncle who chases you around the room first. Or you're twelve and it's the person in junior high school who's making your stomach feel like it's full of butterflies and making other parts of your body feel all mysterious and weird. It's why most of us probably wouldn't get the giggles if we were tickled by, say, Slobodan Milosovic.

Most of us feel fairly positive about ourselves. So why can't we tickle ourselves? Philosophers have ruminated on this one through the ages, and have come up with some speculations. But theories about self-tickling are a dime a dozen. Finally, a scientist has tackled this mystery by doing an experiment.

Sarah-Jayne Blackmore of the University College of London first theorized that you can't tickle yourself because you *know* exactly when and where you're going to be tickled. There's no element of surprise. So she set out to test this by inventing a tickling machine. It consists of a lever attached to a foam pad where, thanks to various pulleys and fulcrums run by a computer, when you move the lever with one hand, the foam pad almost instantaneously strokes the palm of the other hand, moving in the same direction as the movement of the lever.

Being a hard-nosed scientist, Blackmore quantified the whole thing, coming up with a Tickle Index. Then reinvent the wheel—if someone else operates the lever, it tickles you; if you do, nope. No element of surprise. You can't tickle yourself, even with a tickle machine.

Then Blackmore tested her theory by removing the sense of predictability from the self-tickling process. First, remove the sense of predictability about *when* the tickling occurs—the person moves the lever and, unexpectedly, there's a time lag until the foam pad moves. Anything more than three-tenths of a second delay and it scores as high of a Tickle Index as if someone else had done it. Now, remove the sense of predictability about *where* the tickling occurs—the person moves the lever, say, forward and back, and, unexpectedly, the foam pad moves in a different direction. Anything more than a 90-degree deviation from where you expected the pad to move, and it feels as ticklish as if someone else had done it.*

Now we've gotten somewhere. Being tickled doesn't feel ticklish until there is an element of surprise. Of unpredictability. Of lack of control. And suddenly, our beautiful world of tickle science is shattered around us. We spent a whole bunch of time some pages back learning about how the cornerstones of psychological stress are built around a lack of control and predictability. Those were *bad* things, yet most of us *like* being tickled by the right person.†

Hey, wait a second—more pieces of our grand edifice begin to crumble—we stand in long lines to see movies that surprise and terrify us, we bungee jump and go on roller coasters that most definitely deprive us of a sense of control and predictability. We pay good money

---

* An experiment this elegant and clever and eccentric makes me proud to be a scientist.

† A brief digression into tickling political correctness. I once read some weird screed about how no one actually likes being tickled, that it is all about power and control on the part of the tickler, particularly when children are involved, and how the laughing isn't really pleasurable but is reflexive, and the requesting to be tickled is some sign of their acquiescence to their subordinance and loving of their chains, and soon terms like "phallocentric" and "dead white male" and fake quotes from Chief Seattle were being bandied about. As a biologist, one of the first things you do when confronting a puzzle like this is to go for the Phylogenetic Precedent to gain insight into a human phenomenon—do other species do this? Because if other, closely related species do the same thing, that weakens arguments about how the whole phenomenon is embedded in human culture. I can report here that chimps love to be tickled. All those chimps who get trained in American Sign Language—one of the first words they master is "tickle" and one of the first sentences is "tickle me." In college, I worked with one of those chimps. He'd do the "tickle me" sequence correctly, and you'd tickle him like mad—chimps curl up and cover their ribs and make this fast, soundless, breathy giggle when they're being tickled. Stop, he sits up, catches his breath, mops his brow because of how it's all just too much. Then he gets a gleamy look in his eye and it's, "Tickle me," all over again.

to be stressed sometimes. And, as long as we're at it, as we've seen already, we turn on the sympathetic nervous system and secrete ample amounts of glucocorticoids during sex, what's up with that? Chapter 9 oriented us to the role of stress-induced analgesia in making us feel less awful during stress. But, as the starting point of this chapter, if you get the right amount of stress, if you get allostatically challenged just right, it doesn't just feel less awful; it can feel *great*.

So how does that work? And why do some people find stress and risk-taking to feel so great that they get addicted? And how does stress interact with the pleasures and addictive qualities of various substances of abuse?

 ## THE NEUROCHEMISTRY OF PLEASURE

As we saw in chapter 14, the brain contains a pleasure pathway that makes heavy use of the neurotransmitter dopamine. As we also saw in that chapter, if that pathway becomes depleted of dopamine, anhedonia or dysphoria can be an outcome. This "dopaminergic" projection begins in a region deep in the brain called the ventral tegmentum. It then projects to something called the nucleus accumbens and then, in turn, goes on to all sorts of other places. These include the frontal cortex which, as we saw in chapters 10 and 12, plays a key role in executive function, decision making, and impulse control. There are also projections to the anterior cingulate cortex which, as we saw in chapter 14, seems to play a role in having a sense of sadness (leading to the idea that the dopaminergic projection normally inhibits the cingulate). There's also a heavy projection into the amygdala which, as we saw in the last chapter, plays a key role in anxiety and fear.

The relationship between dopamine and pleasure is subtle and critical. On first pass, one might predict that the neurotransmitter is about pleasure, about reward. For example, take a monkey who has been trained in a task: a distinctive bell sounds, which means that the monkey now presses a lever ten times; this leads, ten seconds later, to a desirable food reward. You might initially guess that activation of the dopamine pathway causes neurons in the frontal cortex to become their most active in response to the reward. Some brilliant studies by Wolfram Schultz of the University in Fribourg in Switzerland showed something more interesting. Yes, frontal neurons become excited in response to reward. But the biggest response comes earlier, around the time of the bell sounding and the task commencing. This isn't a signal

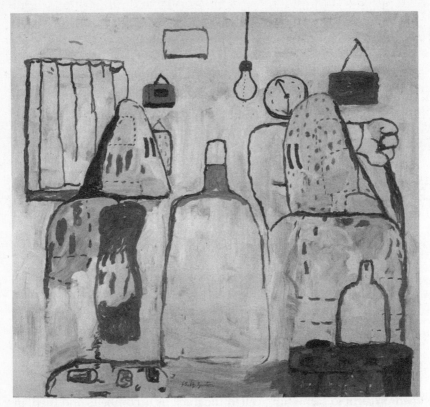

Philip Guston, Bad Habits, *oil on canvas, 1970.*

of, "This feels great." It's about mastery and expectation and confidence. It's "I know what that light means. I know the rules: IF I press the lever, THEN I'm going to get some food. I'm all over this. This is going to be great." The pleasure is in the *anticipation* of a reward; from the standpoint of dopamine, the reward is almost an afterthought.

Psychologists refer to the period of anticipation, of expectation, of working for reward as the "appetitive" stage, one filled with appetite, and call the stage that commences with reward the "consummatory" stage. What Schultz's findings show is that if you know your appetite is going to be sated, pleasure is more about the appetite than about the sating.*

---

* A college friend, who had a seemingly endless string of disastrous relationships, summed up this concept with a cynicism that would have made George Bernard Shaw proud: "A relationship is the price you pay for the anticipation of it." (It was Shaw who once wrote, "Love is the gross exaggeration of the differences between one person and everybody else.")

The next key thing to learn is that the dopamine and its associated sense of pleasurable anticipation fuels the work needed to get that reward. Paul Phillips from the University of North Carolina has used some immensely fancy techniques to measure millisecond bursts of dopamine in rats and has showed with the best time resolution to date that the burst comes just before the behavior. Then, in the clincher, he artificially stimulated dopamine release and, suddenly, the rat would start lever pressing. The dopamine does indeed fuel the behavior.

The next critical point is that the strength of these pathways can change, just like in any other part of the brain. There's the burst of dopaminergic pleasure once that light comes on, and all that is required is to train for longer and longer intervals between light and reward, for those anticipatory bursts of dopamine to fuel ever-increasing amounts of lever pressing. This is how gratification post-ponement works—the core of goal-directed behavior is expectation. Soon we're forgoing immediate pleasure in order to get good grades in order to get into a good college in order to get a good job in order to get into the nursing home of our choice.

Recent work by Schultz adds a twist to this. Suppose in one setup, the subject gets a signal, does a task, and then gets a reward. In the second situation, there's the signal, the task, and then, rather than a certainty of reward, there's simply a high probability of it. In other words, within a generally benevolent context (that is, the outcome is still likely to be good), there's an element of surprise. Under those conditions, there is even greater release of dopamine. Right after the task is completed, dopamine release starts to rise far higher than usual, peaking right around the time that the reward, if it's going to happen, should be arriving. Introduce, "This is going to be great . . . maybe . . . probably . . ." and your neurons spritz dopamine all over the place in anticipation. This is the essence of why, as we learned in Intro Psych, intermittent reinforcement is so reinforcing. What these findings show is that if you think there's a reasonably good chance that your appetite is going to be sated, but you're not positive, pleasure becomes even *more* about the appetite than about the sating.

So dopamine plays an important role in the anticipation of pleasure and in energizing you in order to respond to incentives. However, it can't be the whole story of pleasure, reward, and anticipation. For example, rats can still respond to reward to some extent even when artificially depleted of dopamine in those pathways. Opioids probably play a role in the other pathways involved. Moreover, the dopamine pathway might be most relevant to spiky, intense versions of anticipation. A recent and fascinating study shows this. Get some college students (either gender) who are in what they believe to be their "one true love" relationship. Put them in a scanner and flash up various familiar but neutral faces. Somewhere along the way, flash up a picture of the student's beloved. For people who were in the first few months of the relationship, the dopamine pathways lit up. For people whose relationship was more on the order of years, that's not what happened. Instead, there was activation of the anterior cingulate, that part of the brain discussed in the chapter on depression. The tegmentum/accumbens dopamine system seems to be about edgy, make-you-crazy-with-anticipation passion. Two years later, it's the cingulate weighing in, mediating something akin, perhaps, to comfort and warmth . . . or maybe even a nonhyperventilating version of love.

 STRESS AND REWARD

So the really good thing about being tickled is the anticipation of being tickled. The element of surprise and lack of control. In other words, we're back to where we started—when does a lack of control and predictability fuel dopamine release and a sense of anticipatory pleasure, and when is it the core of what makes psychological stress stressful?

The key seems to be whether the uncertainty occurs in a benign or malevolent context. If it's the right person tickling you in that adolescent stage of being on the cusp of sexuality, maybe, just maybe, that tickling is going to be followed by something *really* good, like hand-holding. In contrast, if it's Slobodan Milosovic who is tickling you, maybe, just maybe, it will be followed up by his trying to ethnically cleanse you. If the context is one of you being at risk for getting shocked, the lack of predictability adds to the stress. If the context is one in which that special someone is likely to eventually say yes, her running hot and cold is all that's needed to start you off on a fifty-year courtship. Part of what makes the Las Vegas world of gambling so addictive is the brilliant ways in which people are manipulated into thinking that the environment is a benign, rather than malevolent, one—the belief that the outcome is likely to be a good one, especially for someone as lucky and special as *you* . . . so long as you keep putting in those coins and pressing that lever.

What makes for the benign sort of environment in which uncertainty is pleasurable, rather than stressful? One key element is how long the experience goes on. Pleasurable lack of control is all about transience—it's not for nothing that roller-coaster rides are three minutes rather than three weeks long. Another thing that biases toward uncertainty being pleasurable is if it comes bound within a larger package of control and predictability. No matter how real and viscerally gripping the scary movie may be, you still know that Anthony Perkins is stalking Janet Leigh, not you. No matter how wild and scary and unpredictable and exhilarating the bungee jumping is, it's still in the context of having assured yourself that these folks have a license from the Bungee Jumping Safety Police. This is the essence of play. You surrender some degree of control—think of how a dog initiates play with another dog by crouching down, making himself smaller, more vulnerable and less in control. But it has to be within a larger context of safety. You don't roll over and expose your throat in play to someone you haven't sniffed over carefully.

Time now to introduce some really unexpected neurochemistry that ties this all together. Glucocorticoids, those hormones which have been discovered at the scene of the crime for virtually all the stress-related pathology we've been learning about, those same villainous glucocorticoids . . . will trigger the release of dopamine from pleasure pathways. It's not some generic effect upon all the dopamine pathways in the brain. Just the pleasure pathway. Most remarkably, Pier Vincenzo Piazza and Michel Le Moal of the University of Bordeaux in France have shown that lab rats will even work in order to get infused with glucocorticoids, will lever-press the exact amount needed to maximize the amount of dopamine released by the hormone.

And what is the pattern of glucocorticoid exposure that maximized dopamine release? You can probably guess already. A moderate rise that doesn't go on for too long. As we've seen, experience severe and prolonged stress, and learning, synaptic plasticity, and immune defenses are impaired. As we saw, experience moderate and transient stress, and memory, synaptic plasticity, and immunity are enhanced. Same thing here. Experience severe and prolonged glucocorticoid exposure, and we've returned to chapter 14—dopamine depletion, dysphoria, and depression. But with moderate and transient glucocorticoid elevation you release dopamine. And transient activation of the amygdala releases dopamine as well. Couple the glucocorticoid rise with the accompanying activation of the sympathetic nervous system, and you're also enhancing glucose and oxygen delivery to the brain.

You feel focused, alert, alive, motivated, anticipatory. You feel great. We have a name for such transient stress. We call it "stimulation."*

 ## ADRENALINE JUNKIES

What does this tell us about the subset of people who thrive on stress and risk-taking, who are most alive under circumstances that would ulcerate anyone else?[†] These are the folks who push every envelope. They spend every last dollar in Monopoly, have furtive sex in public places, try out a new, complicated recipe on important dinner guests, answer the ad in *Soldier of Fortune*. What's up with them?

We can make some pretty informed guesses. Maybe they release atypically low amounts of dopamine. Or, as another version of the same problem, maybe they have versions of dopamine receptors that are atypically unresponsive to a dopamine signal. In that scenario, it's hard to "just say no" to some thrilling possibility when there's not a whole lot of pleasurable yes's in one's life (a point that we'll return to when considering substance abuse). Supporting this idea are some reports of atypical versions of dopamine receptors in people with addictive personalities.[‡]

As another possibility, maybe the baseline of dopamine signaling is fine, but those transients of stimulation cause whopping great rises of dopamine, bigger anticipatory pleasure signals than in most other people. That would certainly encourage one to try the stuff again.

There's yet another possibility. Experience something thrilling with the right intensity and duration, and dopamine is released in the pleasure pathway. End of experience, dopamine levels go back down to baseline. What if someone's brain happens not to be great at keeping up with dopamine reserves in the pleasure pathway? As a result, at

---

* This explains a pattern, noted in chapter 14, that is often seen when people are administered synthetic glucocorticoids to control an autoimmune or inflammatory disease. Eventually, people typically feel depressed. But the first few days, it's the opposite—energized and euphoric.

† What should be obvious is that instead of the term "adrenaline junkies" or even "epinephrine junkies," more proper would be "transiently and moderately increased levels of glucocorticoids junkies."

‡ Many in the field of addiction research believe that there are personalities that are addictive across the board in a wide range of areas—with drugs of abuse, with alcohol, with gambling, with being financially or sexually imprudent. This is controversial, however.

the end of a stimulating increase in dopamine release, dopamine levels not only drop back to baseline, but to a smidgen *below* baseline. In other words, a little lower than where you started. What's the only solution then to counteract this mild dysphoria, this mild inability to anticipate pleasure? Find something else that's thrilling and, of necessity, a bit riskier, in order to achieve the same dopamine peak of the prior time. Afterward, your baseline drops a bit lower. Necessitating another, and another stimulant, each one having to be bigger, in the search for the giddy heights of dopamine that you reached that first time.

This is the essence of the downward ratcheting of addiction. Once, a long time ago, the sixteen-year-old Evel Knievel, behind the steering wheel with his brand-new driver's permit, sped up to beat a red light, and got a bit of a buzz from this. He then discovered, the next time doing it, that it didn't feel quite as exciting.

 ADDICTION

There's an astonishing number of substances that different cultures have come up with that can cause you to be ruinously addicted, to compulsively take the substance despite negative consequences. The field of addiction research has long had to grapple with the sheer variety of these compounds, from the standpoint of understanding their effects on brain chemistry. Alcohol is very different from tobacco or cocaine. Let alone trying to make sense of how things like gambling or shopping wind up being addictive.

Amid this variety, though, there's a critical commonality, which is that these compounds all cause the release of dopamine in the ventral tegmentum–nucleus accumbens pathway. Not all to the same extent. Cocaine, which directly causes the release of dopamine from those neurons, is extremely good at doing it. Other drugs which do so through intervening steps are much less potent—alcohol, for example. But they all do to at least some extent, and in brain-imaging studies of humans taking addictive drugs, the more subjectively pleasurable a person finds a particular exposure to a drug to have been, the more activation of that pathway. This certainly makes sense and defines an addictive substance—you anticipate how pleasurable it will be and thus come back for more.

But addictive substances are not only addictive, but also typically have the property of causing tolerance, or habituation. In other words,

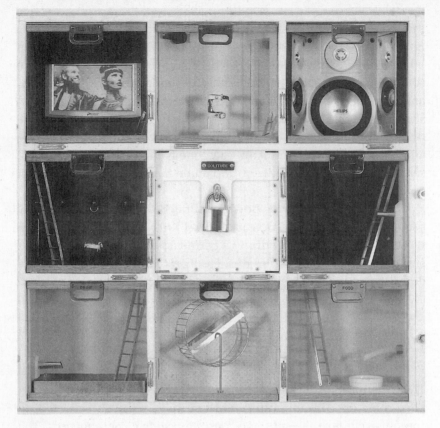

Toland Grinnell, Rodent Addiction System (White), *detail, mixed media,*
2003.

you need increasing amounts of the stuff to get the same anticipatory
oomph as before. The explanation lies, in part, with the magnitude of
dopamine released by these compounds. Consider some of the sources
of pleasure we have—promotion at work, beautiful sunset, great sex,
getting a parking spot where there's still time on the meter. They all
release dopamine for most people. Same thing for a rat. Food for a
hungry rat, sex for a horny one, and dopamine levels rise 50 to 100 percent in this pathway. But give the rat some cocaine and there is a
THOUSAND-FOLD increase in dopamine release.

What's the neurochemical consequence of this tidal wave of
dopamine? We considered a related version in chapter 14. If someone
always yells at you, you stop listening. If you flood a synapse with a
gazillion times more of a neurotransmitter than is usually the case, the
recipient neuron has to compensate by becoming less sensitive. No
one is sure what the mechanism is for what's termed an "opponent

process" that counteracts the dopamine blast. Maybe fewer dopamine receptors, maybe fewer of whatever the dopamine receptors connect to. But regardless of the mechanism, the next time, it is going to take even more dopamine release to have the same impact on that neuron. This is the addictive cycle of escalating drug use.

Around this point, there is a transition in the process of addiction. Early on, addiction is about "wanting" the drug, anticipating its effects, and about how high those dopamine levels are when they're pouring out in a drug-induced state (in addition, the release of endogenous opiates around this time fuels that sense of "wanting"). It's about the motivation to get the reward of a drug. With time there's the transition to "needing" the drug, which is about how low the dopamine lows are without the drug. The stranglehold of addiction is when it is no longer the issue of how good the drug feels, but how bad its absence feels. It's about the motivation to avoid the punishment of not having the drug. George Koob of the Scripps Research Institute has shown that when rats are deprived of a drug they are addicted to, there is a tenfold increase in levels of CRH in the brain, particularly in pathways mediating fear and anxiety, such as in the amygdala. No wonder you feel so awful. Brain-imaging studies of drug users at that stage show that viewing a film of actors pretending to use drugs activates dopamine pathways in the brain more than does watching porn films.

This process emerges in the context of the uncertainty and intermittent reinforcement that we discussed earlier. You're pretty sure you've scraped together enough money, you're pretty sure you can find a dealer, you're pretty sure you won't get caught, you're pretty sure it will be good stuff—but still, there's that element of uncertainty amid the anticipation, and that stokes the addictiveness like crazy.

So this tells us something about the acquisition of addiction, the downward spiral of tolerance to the drug, and the psychological contexts in which those processes can occur. There's a last basic feature of addiction that needs to be discussed. Consider the rare individual who has beaten his addiction, left his demons behind, rebooted and started a new life. It's been months, years, even decades since he's gone near the drug. But uncontrollable circumstances put him back where he always used the drug back when—back on that same street corner, in that same music studio, back in the same overstuffed armchair near the bar in the country club—and the craving comes roaring back like it was yesterday. The capacity to induce that craving doesn't necessarily decline with time; as many drug abusers in that situation will say, it is as if they had never stopped using.

This is the phenomenon of context-dependent relapse—the itch is stronger in some places than others, specifically in places that you associate with prior drug use. You can show the identical phenomenon in a lab rat. Get them addicted to some substance, where they are willing to lever-press like mad to get infused with the stuff. Stick them in a novel cage with a lever and you may get some lever pressing out of them. But put them back in the cage that they associate with the drug exposure, and they lever-press like mad. And, as with humans, the potential for relapse doesn't necessarily decrease over time.

This process of associating drug use with a particular setting is a type of learning, and a lot of current addiction research explores the neurobiology of such learning. This work focuses not so much on those dopamine neurons, but on the neurons that project to them. Many of them come from cortical and hippocampal regions that carry information about setting. If you repeatedly use a drug in the same setting, those projections onto those dopamine neurons are repeatedly activated and eventually become potentiated, strengthened, in the same ways as the hippocampal synapses we learned about in chapter 10. When those projections get strong enough, if you return to that setting, the dopamine anticipation of the drug gets triggered merely by the context. In a lab rat in this situation, you don't even need to place the animal back into the same setting. Just electrically stimulate those pathways that project onto the dopamine neurons, and you reinstate the drug craving. As goes one of the clichés of addiction, there's really no such thing as an *ex*-addict—it is simply an addict who is not in the context that triggers use.

 ## STRESS AND SUBSTANCE ABUSE

We are finally in a position to consider the interactions between stress and drug abuse. We begin by considering what taking any of various psychostimulant drugs does to the stress-response. And everyone knows the answer to that one—"I'm not feeling any pain." Drugs of abuse make you feel less stressed.

In general, the evidence is pretty decent for this, given a few provisos. People do generally report themselves as feeling less stressed, less anxious, if a stressor occurs after some psychoactive drug's effects have kicked in. Alcohol is best known for this, and is formally termed an *anxiolytic,* a drug that "lyses," or disintegrates anxiety. You can show this with a lab rat. As discussed in the last chapter, rats hug the dark corners when put into a brightly lit cage. Put a hungry rat in a cage with some food in the brightly lit center, and how long does it take to overcome its anxious conflict and go for the food? Alcohol decreases the time to do this, as do many other addictive compounds.

How does this work? Many drugs, including alcohol, raise gluco-corticoid levels when they are first taken. But with more sustained use, various drugs can blunt the nuts and bolts of the stress-response. Alcohol, for example, has been reported in some cases to decrease the extent of sympathetic nervous system arousal and to dampen CRH-mediated anxiety. In addition, drugs may change the cognitive appraisal of the stressor. What does that jargon mean? Basically, if you're in such a mess of an altered state that you can barely remember what species you are, you may not pick up on the subtle fact that something stressful has occurred.

Intrinsic in that explanation is the downside of the anxiety-reducing consequences of getting wasted. As the blood levels of the drug drop, as the effects wear off, the cognition and reality sneak back in and, if anything, the drugs become just the opposite, become anxiety-generating. The dynamics of many of these drugs in the body is such that the amount of time that blood levels are rising, with their stress-reducing effects, is shorter than the amount of time that they are dropping. So what's the solution? Drink, ingest, inhale, shoot up, snort all over again.

So various psychostimulants can decrease stress-responses, secondary to blunting the machinery of the stress-response, plus making you such a disoriented mess that you don't even notice that there's been a stressor. How about the flip side of this relationship: What does stress have to do with the likelihood of taking (and abusing) drugs? The clear punch line is that stress pushes you toward more drug use and a greater chance of relapse, although it's not completely clear how stress does this.

The first issue is the effect of stress on initially becoming addicted. Set up a rat in a situation where if it presses a lever X number of times, it gets infused with some potentially addictive drug—alcohol, amphetamines, cocaine. Remarkably, only some rats get into this "self-administration" paradigm enough to get addicted (and we'll see shortly which rats are more likely). If you stress a rat just before the start of this session of drug exposure, it is now more likely to self-administer to the point of addiction. And just as you'd expect from chapter 13, unpredictable stress drives a rat toward addiction more effectively than does predictable stress. Similarly, put a rat or a monkey in a position of being socially subordinate, and the same increased risk occurs. And, no surprise, stress clearly increases alcohol consumption in humans as well.

Importantly, stress increases the addictive potential of a drug only if the stressor comes right before the drug exposure. In other words, short-term stress. The type that boosts dopamine levels transiently. Why does stress have this effect? Imagine that you go into a bout of exposure to a novel, potentially addictive drug, and you just happen to be the type of rat or human for whom the drug doesn't do a whole lot—you're not releasing much dopamine or the other neurotransmitters involved, you're not getting this anticipatory sense afterward of wanting to do it again. But couple that same ho-hum dopamine rise with a rise due to stress and, whoa, you erroneously decide that something cosmic has just happened—where can you get some more? Thus, acute stress increases the reinforcing potential of a drug.

All that makes sense. But, naturally, things get more complicated. Stress increases the likelihood of self-administering a drug to an addictive extent, but this time we're talking about stress during childhood. Or even as a fetus. Stress a pregnant rat and her offspring will have an increased propensity for drug self-administration as adults. Give a rat an experimentally induced birth complication by briefly depriving it of oxygen at birth, and you produce the same. Ditto if stressing a rat in its infancy. The same works in nonhuman primates—separate a monkey from its mother during development, and that animal is more likely to self-administer drugs as an adult. The same has been shown in humans.

In these instances, the stressor during development can't be working merely by causing a transient rise in dopamine release. Something long term has to be occurring. We're back in chapter 6 and perinatal experiences causing lifelong "programming" of the brain and body. It's not clear how this works in terms of addictive substances, other than that there obviously has to be a permanent change in the sensitivity of the reward pathways.

What about once the addiction has occurred—what does ongoing stress do to the extent of abuse? No surprise, it increases it. How does this work? Maybe because of transient stressors briefly boosting dopamine levels and giving the drug more oomph. But by now, the main point for the addict may not be about wanting the high as much as needing to avoid the low of drug withdrawal. As noted, during this time, levels of anxiety-mediating CRH are way up in the amygdala. Moreover, glucocorticoid secretion is consistently elevated during withdrawal, into the range where it depletes dopamine. And what happens if you add additional stress on top of that? All that the extra glucocorticoids can do in this scenario is make the dopamine depletion even worse. Thus increasing the craving for that drug-induced boost of dopamine.

What about that rare individual who manages to stop abusing whatever drug she's addicted to and successfully goes on the wagon? Stress increases the odds of her relapsing into drug use. As usual, the same is true in rats. Get a rat who is self-administering a drug by lever pressing to the point of addiction. Now, switch the rat to being infused with saline instead of with the drug. Soon the lever pressing "extinguishes"—the rat gives up on it, won't bother with the lever anymore. Some time later, return the rat to that cage with the drug-associated lever and there's an increased likelihood that the rat will try lever pressing for the drug again. Infuse the rat with a bit of the drug just before returning it to that familiar locale and it's even more likely to start self-administering again—you've reawakened the taste for that drug. If you stress the rat right before you return it to the cage, it's even more likely to restart the drug use. As usual, unpredictable and uncontrollable stressors are the ones that really revive the drug use. And, as usual, the human studies show basically the same thing.

How does stress do this? It's not entirely clear. The effects of glucocorticoids on dopamine release may be relevant, but I have not seen a clear model built around their interaction. Maybe it's the stress-induced increase in sympathetic arousal, mediated by CRH in the amygdala. There's also some evidence suggesting that stress will increase the strength of those associative projections into the pleasure pathway. Perhaps it has something to do with stress impairing the functioning of the frontal cortex, which normally has that sensible, restraining role of gratification postponement and decision making—shut down your frontal cortex and suddenly you have what seems like an irresistibly clever idea: "I know, why don't I start taking that drug again which nearly destroyed my life."

So stress can increase the odds of abusing a drug to the point of addiction in the first place, make withdrawal harder, and make relapse more likely. Why do all the above happen more readily to some people than others? Immensely interesting work by Piazza and Le Moal has started to answer this.

Remember those apples and pears in chapter 5? Who are the individuals who are more prone toward putting on fat around their gut, becoming apples, the less healthy version of fat deposition? We saw that they are likely to be people with more of a tendency to secrete glucocorticoids in response to stressors, and to have a slower recovery from such a stress-response. Same thing here. Which rats are most likely to self-administer when given a chance and, once self-administering, to do so to the point of escalating addiction? The ones who are "high reactors," who are most behaviorally disrupted by being placed in a novel environment, who are more reactive to stress. They secrete glucocorticoids longer than the other rats in response to a stressor, causing them to pour out more dopamine when they are first exposed to the drug. So if you're the kind of rat who is particularly thrown out of kilter by stress, you're atypically likely to try something that temporarily promises to make things right.

 ## THE REALM OF SYNTHETIC PLEASURE

Chapter 13 raised the important point that positive and negative affect are not mere opposites of each other, and that they can independently influence one's risk of depression. Addiction maps onto this point well, in that an addiction can broadly serve two dissociable functions. One involves positive affect—drugs can generate pleasure (albeit with an ultimate cost that offsets the transient rewards). The other function concerns negative affect—drugs can be used to try to self-medicate away pain, depression, fear, anxiety, and stress. This dual purpose transitions us to the next chapter with its theme that society does not evenly distribute healthy opportunities for pleasure, or sources of fear and anxiety. It is hard to "just say no" when life demands a constant vigilance and when there are few other things to which to say "yes."

The premise of this book is that we humans, especially we westernized humans, have come up with some pretty strange sources of negative emotions—worrying about and being saddened by purely psychological events that are displaced over space and time. But we westernized humans have also come up with some strange sources of positive emotions.

Once, during a concert of cathedral organ music, as I sat there amid that tsunami of sound getting gooseflesh, I was struck with a thought—way back when, for a medieval peasant, this must have been the loudest human-made sound they would ever experience, something that would be awe-inspiring in ways we can no longer imagine. No wonder they signed up for the religion being proffered. And now

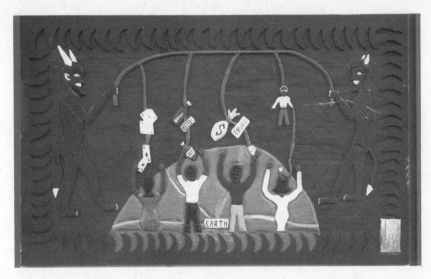

Leroy Almon, Mr. and Mrs. Satan Fishing, *1994.*

we are constantly pummeled with sounds that dwarf quaint cathedral organs. Once, hunter-gatherers might chance upon a gold mine—honey from a wild bee hive—and thus would briefly satisfy one of our most hard-wired food cravings. Now we have hundreds of carefully engineered, designed, and marketed commercial foods filled with rapidly absorbed processed sugars that cause a burst of sensation that can't be matched by some lowly natural food. Once, we had lives that, amid considerable privation and negatives, also offered a huge array of subtle and often hard-won pleasures. And now we have drugs that cause spasms of pleasure and dopamine a thousand-fold higher than anything stimulated in our drug-free world.

Peter Sterling, of allostasis fame, has written brilliantly about how our sources of pleasure have become so narrowed and artificially strong. His thinking centers around the fact that our anticipatory pleasure pathway is stimulated by many different things. For this to work, the pathway must rapidly habituate, must desensitize to any given source that has stimulated it, so that it is prepared to respond to the next stimulant. But unnaturally strong explosions of synthetic experience and sensation and pleasure evoke unnaturally strong degrees of habituation. This has two consequences. As the first, soon we hardly notice anymore the fleeting whispers of pleasure caused by leaves in autumn, or by the lingering glance of the right person, or by the promise of reward that will come after a long, difficult, and worthy task. The other consequence is that, after awhile, we even habituate to those artificial deluges of intensity and moment-ness. If we were nothing but machines of local homeostatic regulation, as we consume more, we would desire less. But instead, our tragedy is that we just become hungrier. More and faster and stronger. "Now" isn't as good as it used to be, and won't suffice tomorrow.

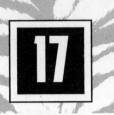

17

THE VIEW FROM THE BOTTOM

Toward the end of the first chapter, I voiced a caveat—when I discuss a way in which stress can make you sick, that is merely shorthand for discussing how stress can make you more likely to get diseases that make you sick. That was basically a first pass at a reconciliation between two very different camps that think about poor health. At one extreme, you have the mainstream medical crowd that is concerned with reductive biology. For them, poor health revolves around issues of bacteria, viruses, genetic mutations, and so on. At the other extreme are the folks anchored in mind-body issues, for whom poor health is about psychological stress, lack of control and efficacy, and so on. A lot of this book has, as one of its goals, tried to develop further links between those two viewpoints. This has come in the form of showing how sensitive reductive biology can be to some of those psychological factors, and exploring the mechanisms that account for this. And it has come in the form of criticizing the extremes of both camps: on the one hand, trying to make clear how limiting it is to believe that humans can ever be reduced to a DNA sequence, and on the other, trying to indicate the damaging idiocy of denying the realities of human physiology and disease. The ideal resolution harks back to the wisdom of Herbert Weiner, as discussed in chapter 8, that disease, even the most reductive of diseases, cannot be appreciated without considering the person who is ill.

Terrific; we're finally getting somewhere. But this analysis, and most pages of this book up until now, have left out a third leg in this stool—the idea that poor health also has something to do with poor jobs in a shrinking economy, or a diet funded by food stamps with too many meals consisting of Coke and Cheetos, or living in a crummy overcrowded apartment close to a toxic waste dump or without enough heat in winter. Let alone living on the streets or in a refugee camp or a war zone. If we can't consider disease outside the context of the person who is ill, we also can't consider it outside the context of the society in which that person has gotten ill, and that person's place in that society.

I recently found support for this view in an unexpected corner. Neuroanatomy is the study of the connections between different areas of the nervous system, and it can sometimes seem like a mind-numbing form of stamp collecting—some multisyllabically named part of the brain sends its axons in a projection with another multisyllabic name to eighteen multisyllabic target sites, whereas in the next county over in the brain. . . . During a period of my errant youth I took particular pleasure in knowing as much neuroanatomy as possible, the more obscure, the better. One of my favorite names was that given to a tiny space that exists between two layers of the meninges, the tough fibrous wrapping found around the brain. It was called the "Virchow-Robin space," and my ability to toss off that name won me the esteem of my fellow neuroanatomy dorks. I never figured out who Robin was, but Virchow was Rudolph Virchow, a nineteenth-century German pathologist and anatomist. Man, to be honored by having your name attached to some microscopic space between two layers of Saran brain wrap—this guy must have been the king of reductive nuts-and-bolts science to merit that. I'd bet he even wore a monocle, which he'd remove before peering down a microscope.

And then I found out a bit about Rudolph Virchow. As a young physician, he came of age with two shattering events—a massive typhus outbreak in 1847 that he attempted to combat firsthand and the doomed European revolutions of 1848. The first was the perfect case for teaching that disease can be as much about appalling living conditions as it is about microorganisms. The second taught just how effectively the machinery of power can subjugate those in appalling living conditions. In its aftermath, he emerged not just as someone who was a scientist plus a physician plus a public health pioneer plus a progressive politician—that would be plenty unique. But in addition, through a creative synthesis, he saw all those roles as manifestations of a single whole. "Medicine is a social science, and politics nothing but medicine on a large scale," he wrote. And, "Physicians are the natural attorneys of the poor." This is an extraordinarily large vision for a man getting microscopic spaces named for him. And unless one happens to be a very atypical physician these days, this vision must also seem extraordinarily quaint, as sadly quaint as Picasso thinking he could throw some paint on a canvas, call it *Guernica,* and do something to halt Fascism.

The history of status thymicolymphaticus, the imaginary disease of a supposedly enlarged thymus gland in infants, detailed at the end of chapter 8, taught us that your place in society can leave its imprint on the corpse you eventually become. The purpose of this chapter is to show how your place in society, and the sort of society it is, can leave an imprint on patterns of disease while you are alive, and to show that part of understanding this imprint incorporates the notion of stress. This will be preparatory for an important notion to be discussed in the final chapter on stress management—that certain techniques for reducing stress work differently depending on where you dwell in your society's hierarchy.

A strategy that I've employed in a number of chapters is to introduce some phenomenon in the context of animals, often social primates. This has been in order to show some principle in a simplified form before turning to the complexity of humans. I do the same in this chapter, beginning with a discussion of what social rank has to do with health and stress-related diseases among animals. But this time, there is a paradoxical twist that, by the end of this chapter, should seem depressing as hell—this time, it is we humans who provide a brutally simple version and our nonhuman primate cousins the nuance and subtlety.

 ## PECKING ORDERS AMONG BEASTS WITH TAILS

While pecking orders—dominance hierarchies—might have first been discerned among hens, they exist in all sorts of species. Resources, no matter how plentiful, are rarely divvied up evenly. Instead of every contested item being fought for with bloodied tooth and claw, dominance hierarchies emerge. As formalized systems of inequities, these are great substitutes for continual aggression between animals smart enough to know their place.

Hierarchical competition has been taken to heights of animal complexity by primates. Consider baboons, the kind running around savannas in big social groups of a hundred or so beasts. In some cases, the hierarchy can be fluid, with ranks changing all the time; in other cases, rank is hereditary and lifelong. In some cases, rank can depend on the situation—A outranks B when it comes to a contested food item, but the order is reversed if it is competition for someone of the opposite sex. There can be circularities in hierarchies—A defeats B defeats C defeats A. Ranking can involve coalitional support—B gets trounced by A, unless receiving some well-timed help from C, in which case A is sent packing. The actual confrontation between two animals can include anything ranging from a near fatal brawl to a highly dominant individual doing nothing more than shifting menacingly and giving subordinates the willies.

Regardless of the particulars, if you're going to be a savanna baboon, you probably don't want to be a low-ranking one. You sit there for two minutes digging some root out of the ground to eat, clean it off and . . . anyone higher ranking can rip it off from you. You spend hours sweet-talking someone into grooming you, getting rid of those bothersome thorns and nettles and parasites in your hair, and the grooming session can be broken up by someone dominant just for the sheer pleasure of hassling you. Or you could be sitting there, minding your own business, bird-watching, and some high-ranking guy having a bad day decides to make you pay for it by slashing you with his canines. (Such third-party "displacement aggression" accounts for a huge percentage of baboon violence. A middle-ranking male gets trounced in a fight, turns and chases a subadult male, who lunges at an adult female, who bites a juvenile, who slaps an infant.) For a subordinate animal, life is filled with a disproportionate share not only of physical stressors but of psychological stressors as well—lack of control, of predictability, of outlets for frustration.

It's not surprising, then, that among subordinate male baboons, resting levels of glucocorticoids are significantly higher than among dominant individuals—for a subordinate, everyday basal circumstances are stressful. And that's just the start of subordinates' problems with glucocorticoids. When a real stressor comes along, their glucocorticoid response is smaller and slower than in dominant individuals. And when it's all passed, their recovery appears to be delayed. All these are features that count as an inefficient stress-response.*

More problems for subordinate individuals: elevated resting blood pressure; sluggish cardiovascular response to real stressors; a sluggish

---

* I spent about a dozen summers with my baboons figuring out the neuroendocrine mechanisms that give rise to the inefficient glucocorticoid system in the subordinate animals. "Neuroendocrine mechanisms" means the steps linking the brain, the pituitary, and the adrenals in the regulation of glucocorticoid release. The question becomes which of the steps—brain, pituitary, adrenals—is the spot where there is a problem. There turn out to be a number of sites where things work differently in subordinate and dominant baboons. Interestingly, the mechanisms that give rise to the pattern in subordinate baboons are virtually identical with those that give rise to the elevated glucocorticoid levels that occur in many humans with major depression.

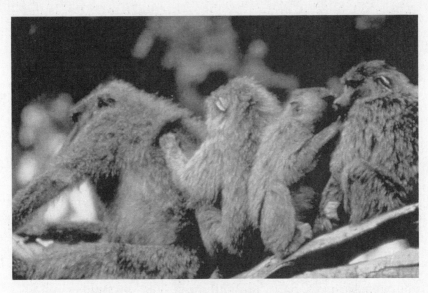

Grooming, a wonderful means of social cohesion and stress reduction, in a society where everyone's back is not scratched equally.

recovery; suppressed levels of the good HDL cholesterol; among male subordinates, testosterone levels that are more easily suppressed by stress than in dominant males; fewer circulating white blood cells; and lower circulating levels of something called *insulin-like growth factor-I*, which helps heal wounds. As should be clear umpteen pages into this book, all these are indices of bodies that are chronically stressed.

A chronically activated stress-response (elevated glucocorticoid levels, or resting blood pressure that is too high, or an enhanced risk of atherosclerosis) appears to be a marker of being low ranking in lots of other animal species as well. This occurs in primates ranging from standard-issue monkeys like rhesus to beasts called prosimians (such as mouse lemurs). Same for rats, mice, hamsters, guinea pigs, wolves, rabbits, pigs. Even fish. Even sugar gliders, whatever they might be.

A critical question: I'm writing as if being low ranking and subject to all those physical and psychological stressors chronically activates the stress-response. Could it be the other way around? Could having a second-rate stress-response set you up for being low ranking?

You can answer this question with studies of captive animals, where you can artificially form a social group. Monitor glucocorticoid levels, blood pressure, and so on when the group is first formed, and again once rankings have emerged, and the comparison will tell you in which direction the causality works—do physiological differences

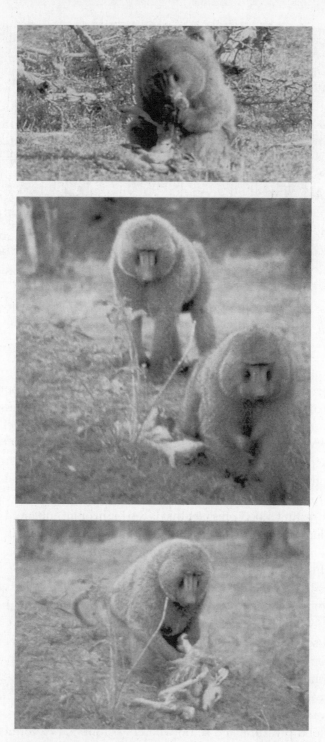

A middle-ranking baboon, who has spent all morning stalking an impala, has the kill stolen from him by a high-ranking male.

predict who is going to wind up with which rank, or is it the other way around? The answer, overwhelmingly, is that rank emerges first, and drives the distinctive stress profile.

So we've developed a pretty clear picture. Social subordination equals being chronically stressed equals an overactive stress-response equals more stress-related disease. Now it's time to see why that's simplistic and wrong.

The first hint is hardly a subtle one. When you stand up at some scientific meeting and tell about the health-related miseries of your subordinate baboons or tree shrews or sugar gliders, invariably some other endocrinologist who studies the subject in some other species gets up and says, "Well, *my* subordinate animals don't have high blood pressure or elevated glucocorticoid levels." There are lots of species in which social subordination is not associated with an overactive stress-response.

Why should that be? Why should being subordinate not be so bad in that species? The answer is that in that species, it's not so bad being subordinate, or possibly it's actually a drag being dominant.

An example of the first is seen with a South American monkey called the marmoset. Being subordinate among them does not involve the misery of physical and psychological stressors; it isn't a case of subjugation being forcibly imposed on you by big, mean, dominant animals. Instead, it is a relaxed waiting strategy—marmosets live in small social groups of related "cooperative breeders," where being subordinate typically means you are helping out your more dominant older sibling or cousin and waiting your turn to graduate into that role. Commensurate with this picture, David Abbott at the Wisconsin Regional Primate Research Center has shown that subordinate marmosets don't have overactive stress-responses.

Wild dogs and dwarf mongooses provide examples of the second situation in which subordination isn't so bad. Being dominant in those species doesn't mean a life of luxury, effortlessly getting the best of the pickings and occasionally endowing an art museum. None of that status quo stuff. Instead, being dominant requires the constant reassertion of high rank through overt aggression—one is tested again and again. As Scott and Nancy Creel at Montana State University have shown, it's not the subordinate animals among those species who have the elevated basal glucocorticoid levels, it's the dominant ones.

Recently, Abbott and I drew on the collaborative efforts of a large number of colleagues who have studied rank/stress physiology issues in nonhuman primates. We formalized what features of a primate society predict whether it is the dominant or the subordinate animals who have the elevated stress-responses. To the experts on each primate species, we posed the same questions: in the species that you study, what are the rewards of being dominant? How much of a role does aggression play in maintaining dominance? How much grief does a subordinate individual have to take? What sources of coping and support (including the presence of relatives) do subordinates of that species have available to them? What covert alternatives to competition are available? If subordinates cheat at the rules, how likely are they to get caught and how bad is the punishment? How often does the hierarchy change? Amid seventeen questions asked concerning the dozen different species for which there are decent amounts of data available, the best predictors of elevated glucocorticoid levels among subordinate animals turn out to be if they are frequently harassed by dominant individuals and if they lack the opportunities for social support.

So rank means different things in different species. It turns out that rank can also mean different things in different social groups within the same species. Primatologists these days talk about primate "culture," and this is not an anthropomorphic term. For example, chimps in one part of the rain forest can have a very different culture from the folks four valleys over—different frequencies of social behaviors, use of similar vocalizations but with different meanings (in other words, something approaching the concept of a "dialect"), different types of tool use. And intergroup differences influence the rank-stress relationship.

One example is found among female rhesus monkeys, where subordinates normally take a lot of grief and have elevated basal glucocorticoid levels—except in one social group that was studied, which, for some reason, had high rates of reconciliatory behaviors among animals after fights. The same is found in a baboon troop that just happened to be a relatively benign place to be a low-ranking individual. Another example concerns male baboons where, as noted, subordinates normally have the elevated glucocorticoid levels—except during a severe drought, when the dominant males were so busy looking for food that they didn't have the time or energy to hassle everyone else (implying, ironically, that for a subordinate animal, an environmental stressor can be a blessing, insofar as it saves you from a more severe social stressor).

A critical intergroup difference in the stress-response concerns the stability of the dominance hierarchy. Consider an animal who is, say, Number 10 in the hierarchy. In a stable system, that individual is getting trounced 95 percent of the time by Number 9 but, in turn, thrashes Number 11 95 percent of the time. In contrast, if Number 10 were winning only 51 percent of interactions with Number 11, that suggests that the two may be close to switching positions. In a stable hierarchy, 95 percent of the interactions up and down the ranks reinforce the status quo. Under those conditions, dominant individuals are stably entrenched and have all the psychological perks of their position—control, predictability, and so on. And under those conditions, among the various primate species discussed above, it is the dominant individuals who have the healthiest stress-responses.

In contrast, there are rare periods when the hierarchy becomes unstable—some key individual has died, someone influential has transferred into the group, some pivotal coalitional partnership has formed or come apart—and a revolution results, with animals changing ranks left and right. Under those conditions, it is typically the dominant individuals who are in the very center of the hurricane of instability, subject to the most fighting, the most challenges, and who are most affected by the see-sawing of coalitional politics.* During such unstable periods among those same primate species, the dominant individuals no longer have the healthiest stress-responses.

So while rank is an important predictor of individual differences in the stress-response, the meaning of that rank, the psychological baggage that accompanies it in a particular society, is at least as important. Another critical variable is an animal's personal experience of both its rank and society. For example, consider a period when an immensely aggressive male has joined a troop of baboons and is raising hell, attacking animals unprovoked left and right. One might predict stress-responses throughout the troop thanks to this destabilizing brute. But, instead, the pattern reflects the individual experience of animals—for those lucky enough never to be attacked by this character, there were no changes in immune function. In contrast, among those attacked, the more frequently that particular baboon suffered at this guy's teeth, the more immunosuppressed she was. Thus, you ask the question, "What are the effects of an aggressive, stressful individual on immune function in a social group?" The answer is, "It depends—it's not the abstract state of living in a stressful society which is immunosuppressive. Instead, it is the concrete state of how often your own nose is being rubbed in that instability."†

---

* After all, do you think it would have been restful to have been the czar of Russia in 1917?

† All you have to do to appreciate that bad times for a group as a whole do not necessarily translate into bad times for every individual is to consider all the people who have made fortunes black-marketing penicillin or hoarding critical food supplies during wartime.

As a final variable, it is not just rank that is an important predictor of the stress-response, not just the society in which the rank occurs, or how a member of the society experiences both; it's also personality—the topic of chapter 15. As we saw, some primates see glasses as half empty and life as full of provocations, and they can't take advantage of outlets or social support—those are the individuals with overactive stress-responses. For them, their rank, their society, their personal experiences might all be wonderfully salutary, but if their personality keeps them from perceiving those advantages, their hormone levels and arteries and immune systems are going to pay a price.

All things considered, this presents a pretty subtle picture of what social rank has to do with stress-related disease among primates. It's reasonable to expect the picture to be that much more complicated and subtle when considering humans. Time for a surprise.

 ## DO HUMANS HAVE RANKS?

I personally was always picked last for the whiffleball team as a kid, being short, uncoordinated, and typically preoccupied with some book I was lugging around. Thus, having been perpetually ensconced at the bottom of that pecking order, I am skeptical about the notion of ranking systems for humans.

Part of the problem is definitional, in that some supposed studies of human "dominance" are actually examining Type-A features—people defined as "dominant" are ones who, in interviews, have hostile, competitive contents to their answers, or who speak quickly and interrupt the interviewer. This is not dominance in a way that any zoologist would endorse.

Other studies have examined the physiological correlates of individual differences in humans who are competing directly against one another in a way that looks like dominance. Some have examined, for example, the hormonal responses in college wrestlers depending on whether they won or lost their match. Others have examined the endocrine correlates of rank competition in the military. One of the most fruitful areas has been to examine ranks in the corporate world. Chapter 13 showed how the "executive stress syndrome" is mostly a myth—people at the top give ulcers, rather than get them. Most studies have shown that it is middle management that succumbs to the stress-related diseases. This is thought to reflect the killer combination that these folks are often burdened with, namely, high work demands but little autonomy—responsibility without control.

Collectively, these studies have produced some experimentally reliable correlations. I'm just a bit dubious as to what they mean. For starters, I'm not sure what a couple of minutes of competitive wrestling between two highly conditioned twenty-year-olds teaches us about which sixty-year-old gets clogged arteries. At the other end, I wonder what the larger meaning is of rankings among business executives— while primate hierarchies can ultimately indicate how hard you have to work for your calories, corporate hierarchies are ultimately about how hard you have to work for, say, a plasma TV. Another reason for my skepticism is that for 99 percent of human history, societies were most probably strikingly unhierarchical. This is based on the fact that contemporary hunter-gatherer bands are remarkably egalitarian.

But my skepticism is most strongly anchored in two reasons having to do with the complexity of the human psyche. First, humans can belong to a number of different ranking systems simultaneously, and ideally are excelling in at least one of them (and thus, may be giving the greatest psychological weight to that one). So, the lowly subordinate in the mailroom of the big corporation may, after hours, be deriving tremendous prestige and self-esteem from being the deacon of his church, or the captain of her weekend softball team, or may be at the top of the class at the adult-extension school. One person's highly empowering dominance hierarchy may be a mere 9-to-5 irrelevancy to the person in the next cubicle, and this will greatly skew results.

And most important, people put all sorts of spin inside their heads about ranks. Consider a marathon being observed by a Martian scientist studying physiology and rank in humans. The obvious thing to do is keep track of the order in which people finish the race. Runner 1 dominates 5, who clearly dominates 5,000. But what if runner 5,000 is a couch potato who took up running just a few months ago, who half expected to keel over from a coronary by mile 13 and instead finished— sure, hours after the crowds wandered off—but finished, exhausted and glowing. And what if runner 5 had spent the previous week reading in the sports section that someone of their world-class quality should certainly finish in the top three, maybe even blow away the field. No Martian on earth could predict correctly who is going to feel exultantly dominant afterward.

People are as likely to race against themselves, their own previous best time, as against some external yardstick. This can be seen in the corporate world as well. An artificial example: the kid in the mailroom is doing a fabulous job and is rewarded, implausibly, with a $50,000 a year salary. A senior vice president screws up big-time and is punished, even more implausibly, with a $50,001 a year salary. By the perspective of that Martian, or even by a hierarchically minded wildebeest, it's obvious that the vice president is in better shape to acquire the nuts and berries needed for survival. But you can guess who is going to be going to work contentedly and who is going to be making angry phone calls to a headhunter from the cell phone in the BMW. Humans can play internal, rationalizing games with rank based on their knowledge of what determined their placement. Consider the following fascinating example: guys who win at some sort of competitive interaction typically show at least a small rise in their circulating testosterone levels—unless they consider the win to have come from sheer luck.

When you put all those qualifiers together, I think the net result is some pretty shaky ground when it comes to considering human rank and its relevance to the stress-response. Except in one realm. If you want to figure out the human equivalent of being a low-ranking social animal, an equivalent that carries with it atypically high rates of physical and psychological stressors, which is ecologically meaningful in that it's not just about how many hours you have to work to buy an iPod, which is likely to overwhelm most of the rationalizations and alternative hierarchies that one can muster—check out a poor human.

 ## SOCIOECONOMIC STATUS, STRESS, AND DISEASE

If you want to see an example of chronic stress, study poverty. Being poor involves lots of physical stressors. Manual labor and a greater risk of work-related accidents. Maybe even two or three exhausting jobs, complete with chronic sleep deprivation. Maybe walking to work, walking to the laundromat, walking back from the market with the heavy bag of groceries, instead of driving an air-conditioned car. Maybe too little money to afford a new mattress that might help that aching back, or some more hot water in the shower for that arthritic throb; and, of course, maybe some hunger thrown in as well. . . . The list goes on and on.

Naturally, being poor brings disproportionate amounts of psychological stressors as well. Lack of control, lack of predictability: numbing work on an assembly line, an occupational career spent taking orders or going from one temporary stint to the next. The first one laid off when economic times are bad—and studies show that the deleterious effects of unemployment on health begin not at the time the person is laid off, but when the mere threat of it first occurs. Wondering if the money will stretch to the end of the month. Wondering if the rickety car will get you to tomorrow's job interview on time. How's this for an implication of lack of control: one study of the working poor showed that they were less likely to comply with their doctors' orders to take antihypertensive diuretics (drugs that lower blood pressure by making you urinate) because they weren't allowed to go to the bathroom at work as often as they needed to when taking the drugs.

As a next factor, being poor means that you often can't cope with stressors very efficiently. Because you have no resources in reserve, you can never plan for the future, and can only respond to the present crisis. And when you do, your solutions in the present come with a whopping great price later on—metaphorically, or maybe not so metaphorically, you're always paying the rent with money from a loan shark. Everything has to be reactive, in the moment. Which increases the odds that you'll be in even worse shape to deal with the next stressor—growing strong from adversity is mostly a luxury for those who are better off.

Along with all of that stress and reduced means of coping, poverty brings with it a marked lack of outlets. Feeling a little stressed with life and considering a relaxing vacation, buying an exercycle, or taking some classical guitar lessons to get a little peace of mind? Probably not. Or how about quitting that stressful job and taking some time off at home to figure out what you're doing with your life? Not when there's an extended family counting on your paycheck and no money in the bank. Feeling like at least jogging regularly to get some exercise and let off some steam? Statistically, a poor person is far more likely to live in a crime-riddled neighborhood, and jogging may wind up being a hair-raising stressor.

Finally, along with long hours of work and kids to take care of comes a serious lack of social support—if everyone you know is working two or three jobs, you and your loved ones, despite the best of intentions, aren't going to be having much time to sit around being supportive. Thus, poverty generally equals more stressors—and though the studies are mixed as to whether or not the poor have more major catastrophic stressors, they have plenty more chronic daily stressors.

All these hardships suggest that low socioeconomic status (SES—typically measured by a combination of income, occupation, housing conditions, and education) should be associated with chronic activation of the stress-response. Only a few studies have looked at this, but they support this view. One concerned school kids in Montreal, a city with fairly stable communities and low crime. In six- and eight-year-old children, there was already a tendency for lower-SES kids to have elevated glucocorticoid levels. By age ten, there was a step-wise gradient, with low-SES kids averaging almost double the circulating glucocorticoids as the highest SES kids. Another example concerns people in Lithuania. In 1978, men in Lithuania, then part of the USSR, had the same mortality rates for coronary heart disease as did men in nearby Sweden. By 1994, following the disintegration of the Soviet Union, Lithuanians had four times the Swedish rate. In 1994 Sweden, SES was not related to glucocorticoid levels, whereas in 1994 Lithuania, it was strongly related.

Findings like these suggest that being poor is associated with more stress-related diseases. As a first pass, let's just ask whether low SES is associated with more diseases, period. And is it ever.

The health risk of poverty turns out to be a huge effect, the biggest risk factor there is in all of behavioral medicine—in other words, if you have a bunch of people of the same gender, age, and ethnicity and you want to make some predictions about who is going to live how long, the single most useful fact to know is each person's SES. If you want to increase the odds of living a long and healthy life, don't be poor. Poverty is associated with increased risks of cardiovascular disease, respiratory disease, ulcers, rheumatoid disorders, psychiatric diseases, and a number of types of cancer, just to name a few.* It is associated with higher rates of people judging themselves to be of poor health, of infant mortality, and of mortality due to all causes. Moreover, lower SES predicts lower birth weight, after controlling for body size—and we know from chapter 6 the lifelong effects of low birth weight. In other words, be born poor but hit the lottery when you're three weeks

---

* As but one example, across the countries of Europe, socioeconomic status accounts for 68 percent of the variance as to who gets a stroke. However, not all diseases are more prevalent among the poor, and, fascinatingly, some are even more common among the wealthy. Melanoma is an example, suggesting that sun exposure in a lounge chair may have different disease risks than getting your neck red from stooped physical labor (or that a huge percentage of poor people laboring away in the sun have a fair amount of melanin in their skin, if you know what I mean). Or multiple sclerosis, and a few other autoimmune diseases and, during its heyday, polio. Or "hospitalism," a pediatric disease of the 1930s in which infants would waste away in hospitals. It is now understood that it was mostly due to lack of contact and sociality—and kids who would wind up in poorer hospitals were less subject to this, since the hospitals couldn't afford state-of-the-art incubators, necessitating that staff actually hold them.

old, spend the rest of your life double-dating with Donald Trump, and you're still going to have a statistical increase in some realms of disease risk for the rest of your life.

Is the relationship between SES and health just some little statistical hiccup in the data? No—it can be a huge effect. In the case of some of those diseases sensitive to SES, if you cling to the lowest rungs of the socioeconomic ladder, it can mean ten times the prevalence compared with those perched on top.* Or stated another way, this translates into a five- to ten-year difference in life expectancy in some countries when comparing the poorest and wealthiest, and decades' worth of differences when comparing subgroups of the poorest and wealthiest.

Findings such as these go back centuries. For example, one study of men in England and Wales demonstrated a steep SES gradient in mortality in every decade of the twentieth century. This has a critical implication that has been pointed out by Robert Evans of the University of British Columbia: the diseases that people were dying of most frequently a century ago are dramatically different from the most common ones now. Different causes of death, but same SES gradient, same relationship between SES and health. Which tells you that the gradient arises less from disease than from social class. Thus, writes Evans, the "roots [of the SES health gradient] lie beyond the reach of medical therapy."

So SES and health are tightly linked. What direction is the causality? Maybe being poor sets you up for poor health. But maybe it's the other way around, where being sickly sets you up for spiraling down into poverty. The latter certainly happens, but most of the relationship is due to the former. This is demonstrated by showing that your SES at one point in life predicts important features of your health later on. For example, poverty early in life has adverse effects on health forever after—harking back to chapter 6 and the fetal origins of adult disease. One remarkable study involved a group of elderly nuns. They took their vows as young adults, and spent the rest of their lives sharing the same diet, same health care, same housing, and so on. Despite controlling for all these variables, in old age their patterns of disease, of dementia, and of longevity were still predicted by the SES status they had when they became nuns more than half a century before.

Thus, SES influences health, and the greater cumulative percentage of your life you've spent poor, the more of an adverse impact on

---

* A number of writers in the field have noted (even pre-DiCaprio) that there was a strict SES gradient as to who survived on the *Titanic*.

health.* Why should SES influence health? A century ago in the United States, or today in a developing country, the answer would be obvious. It would be about poor people getting more infectious diseases, less food, and having an astronomically higher infant mortality rate. But with our shift toward the modern prevalence of slow, degenerative diseases, the answers have shifted as well.

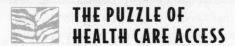

THE PUZZLE OF HEALTH CARE ACCESS

Let's start with the most plausible explanation. In the United States, poor people (with or without health insurance) don't have the same access to medical care as do the wealthy. This includes fewer preventive check-ups with doctors, a longer lag time for testing when something bothersome has been noted, and less adequate care when something has actually been discovered, especially if the medical care involves an expensive, fancy technique. As one example of this, a 1967 study showed that the poorer you are judged to be (based on the neighborhood you live in, your home, your appearance), the less likely paramedics are to try to revive you on the way to the hospital. In more recent studies, for the same severity of a stroke, SES influenced your likelihood of receiving physical, occupational, or speech therapy, and how long you waited until undergoing surgery to repair the damaged blood vessel that caused the stroke.

This sure seems like it should explain the SES gradient. Make the health care system equitable, socialize that medicine, and away would go that gradient. But it can't be only about differential health care access, or even mostly about it.

For starters, consider countries in which poverty is robustly associated with increased prevalence of disease: Australia, Belgium, Denmark, Finland, France, Italy, Japan, the Netherlands, New Zealand, the former Soviet Union, Spain, Sweden, the United Kingdom, and, of course, the U.S. of A. Socialize the medical care system, socialize the whole country, turn it into a worker's paradise, and you still get the gradient. In a place like England, the SES gradient has gotten worse over this century, despite the imposition of universal health care allowing everyone equal health care access.

---

* What that means is that you're not completely sunk if you're born poor; social mobility helps to some extent.

You could cynically and correctly point out that systems of wonderfully egalitarian health care access are probably egalitarian in theory only—even the Swedish health care system is likely to be at least a smidgen more attentive to the wealthy industrialist, sick doctor, or famous jock than to some no-account poor person cluttering up a clinic. Some people always get more of their share of equality than others. But in at least one study of people enrolled in a prepaid health plan, where medical facilities were available to all participants, poorer people had more cardiovascular disease, despite making more use of the medical resources.

A second vote against the importance of differential health care access is because the relationship forms the term I've been using, namely, a *gradient*. It's not the case that only poor people are less healthy than everyone else. Instead, for every step lower in the SES ladder, there is worse health (and the lower you get in the SES hierarchy, the bigger is each step of worsening health). This was a point made screamingly clear in the most celebrated study in the field, the Whitehall studies of Michael Marmot of University College of London. Marmot considered a system where gradations in SES status are so clear that occupational rank practically comes stamped on people's foreheads—the British civil service system, which ranges from unskilled blue-collar workers to high-powered executives. Compare the highest and lowest rungs and there's a fourfold difference in rates of cardiac disease mortality. Remember, this is in a system where everyone has roughly equal health care access, is paid a living wage, and, very important in the context of the effects of unpredictability, is highly likely to continue to be able to earn that living wage.

A final vote against the health care access argument: the gradient exists for diseases that have nothing to do with access. Take a young person and, each day, scrupulously, give her a good medical examination, check her vitals, peruse her blood, run her on a treadmill, give her a stern lecture about good health habits, and then, for good measure, centrifuge her a bit, and she is still just as much at risk for some diseases as if she hadn't gotten all that attention. Poor people are still more likely to get those access-proof diseases. Theodore Pincus of Vanderbilt University has carefully documented the existence of an SES gradient for two of those diseases, juvenile diabetes and rheumatoid arthritis.

Thus, the leading figures in this field all seem to rule out health care access as a major part of the story. This is not to rule it out completely (let alone suggest that we not bother trying to establish universal

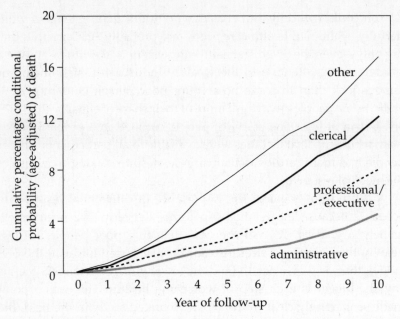

The Whitehall Study, Mortality by Professional Level of Follow-up.

health care access). As evidence, sweaty capitalist America has the worst gradient, while the socialized Scandinavian countries have the weakest. But they still have hefty gradients, despite their socialism. The main cause has to be somewhere else. Thus, we move on to the next most plausible explanation.

 RISK FACTORS AND PROTECTIVE FACTORS

Poorer people in westernized societies are more likely to drink and smoke excessively (sufficiently so that it's been remarked that smoking is soon going to be almost exclusively a low-SES activity). These excesses take us back to the last chapter and having trouble "just saying no" when there are few yes's. Moreover, the poor are more likely to have an unhealthy diet—in the developing world, being poor means having trouble affording food, while in the westernized world, it means having trouble affording *healthy* food. Thanks to industrialization, fewer jobs in our society involve physical exertion and, when combined with the costs of membership in some tony health club, the poor get less exercise. They're more likely to be obese, and in an apple-ish way. They are less likely to use a seat belt, wear a motorcycle helmet, own a car with air bags. They are more likely to live near a toxic dump, be mugged, have inadequate heat in the winter, live in crowded conditions (thereby increasing exposure to infectious diseases). The list seems endless, and they all adversely impact health.

Being poor is statistically likely to come with another risk factor—being poorly educated. Thus, maybe poor people don't understand, don't know about the risk factors they are being exposed to, or the health-promoting factors they are lacking—even if it is within their power to do something, they aren't informed. As one example that boggles me, substantial numbers of people are apparently not aware that cigarettes do bad things to you, and the studies show that these aren't folks too busy working on their doctoral dissertations to note some public health trivia. Other studies indicate that, for example, poor women are the least likely to know of the need for Pap smears, thus increasing their risk for cervical cancer.* The intertwining of poverty and poor education probably explains the high rates of poor people who, despite their poverty, could still be eating somewhat more healthfully, using seat belts or crash helmets, and so on, but don't. And it probably helps to explain why poor people are less likely to comply with some treatment regime prescribed for them that they can actually afford—they are less likely to have understood the instructions or to think that following them is important. Moreover, a high degree of education generalizes to better problem-solving skills across the board. Statistically, being better educated predicts that your community of friends and relatives is better educated as well, with those attendant advantages.

However, the SES gradient isn't much about risk factors and protective factors. To show this requires some powerful statistical techniques in which you see if an effect still exists after you control for one or more of these factors. For example, the lower your SES, the greater your risk of lung cancer. But the lower your SES, the greater the likelihood of smoking. So control for smoking—comparing only people who smoke—does the incidence of lung cancer still increase with declining SES? Take it one step further—for the same *amount* of smoking, does lung cancer incidence still increase? For the same amount of smoking *and* drinking, does . . . and so on. These types of analyses show that these risk factors matter—as Robert Evans has written, "Drinking sewage is probably unwise even for Bill Gates." They just

---

* In a subtle but striking complication to this story, education actually worsens health inequality. As medical research generates new advances in health care and preventive medicine, it is the educated who first hear about it, appreciate it, and adopt it, and thus differentially benefit from it, amplifying the health gradient even more.

don't matter that much. For example, in the Whitehall studies, smoking, cholesterol levels, blood pressure, and level of exercise explain away only about a third of the SES gradient. For the same risk factors and same lack of protective factors, throw in poverty and you're more likely to get sick.

So differential exposure to risk factors or protective factors does not explain a whole lot. This point is brought home in another way. Compare countries that differ in wealth. One can assume that being in a wealthier country gives you more opportunities to buy protective factors and to avoid risk factors. For example, you find the least pollution in very poor and very wealthy countries; the former because they are nonindustrial and the latter because they either do it cleanly or farm it out to someone else. Yet, when you consider the wealthiest quarter or so countries on earth, there is no relationship between a country's wealth and the health of its citizens.* This is a point heavily emphasized by Stephen Bezruchka of the University of Washington, in considering the United States—despite the most expensive and sophisticated health care system in the world, there's an unconscionable number of less wealthy nations whose citizens live longer, healthier lives than our own.†

So out go major roles for health care access, and risk factors. This is where things get tense at the scientific conferences. Much of this book has been about how a certain style of "mainstream" medicine, overly focused on how disease is exclusively about viruses, bacteria, and mutations, has grudgingly had to make room for the relevance of psychological factors, including stress. In a similar way, among the "social epidemiologists" who think about the SES/health gradients, the mainstream view has long focused on health care access and risk factors. And thus, they too have had to make room for psychological factors. Including stress. Big-time.

---

* This may seem like an aside, but is as central a point as any in this book. Once you get past the 25 percent poorest countries on earth, there's no relationship between the wealth of a country and the percentage of its citizens who say they are happy. (How many countries were on the list whose citizens are at least as happy, if not happier, than Americans, despite being in less wealthy countries? Ten, most with social welfare systems. And unhappiness? The dozen most unhappy are all ex-states of the Soviet Union, or of Eastern Europe.)

† In 1960, the United States was 13th in life expectancy, pretty lousy in and of itself. By 1997, it was 25th. As one example, Greeks, who have approximately half the average income of Americans, have a longer life expectancy.

STRESS AND THE SES GRADIENT

As discussed, the poor certainly have a hugely disproportionate share of both daily and major stressors. If you've gotten this far into this book and aren't wondering whether stress has something to do with the SES health gradient, you should get your money back. Does it?

In the last edition of this book, I argued for a major role for stress based on three points. First, the poor have all those chronic daily stressors. Second, when one examines the SES gradient for individual diseases, the strongest gradients occur for diseases with the greatest sensitivity to stress, such as heart disease, diabetes, Metabolic syndrome, and psychiatric disorders. Finally, once you've rounded up the usual suspects—health care access and risk factors—and ruled them out as being of prime importance, what else is there to pin the SES gradient on? Sunspots?

Kinda flimsy. With that sort of evidence, the social epidemiologists were willing to let in some of those psychologists and stress physiologists, but through the back door, and—Cook, find them something to eat in the *kitchen*, if you please.

So that was the stress argument a half decade back. But since then, striking new findings make the stress argument very solid.

BEING POOR VERSUS FEELING POOR

A central concept of this book is that stress is heavily rooted in psychology once you are dealing with organisms who aren't being chased by predators, and who have adequate shelter and sufficient calories to sustain good health. Once those basic needs are met, it is an inevitable fact that if everyone is poor, and I mean everyone, then no one is. In order to understand why stress and psychological factors have so much to do with the SES/health gradient, we have to begin with the obvious fact that it is never the case that everyone is poor thereby making no one poor. This brings us to a critical point in this field—the SES/health gradient is not really about a distribution that bottoms out at being poor. It's not about being poor. It's about *feeling* poor, which is to say, it's about feeling *poorer* than others around you.

Beautiful work regarding this has been carried out by Nancy Adler of the University of California at San Francisco. Instead of just looking at the relationship between SES and health, Adler looks at what health has to do with what someone *thinks and feels* their SES is—their "subjective SES." Show someone a ladder with ten rungs on it and ask them, "In society, where on this ladder would you rank yourself in terms of how well you're doing?" Simple.

First off, if people were purely accurate and rational, the answers across a group should average out to the middle of the ladder's rungs. But cultural distortions come in—expansive, self-congratulatory European-Americans average out at higher than the middle rung (what Adler calls her Lake Wobegon Effect, where all the children are above average); in contrast, Chinese-Americans, from a culture with less chest-thumping individualism, average out to below the middle rung. So you have to correct for those biases. In addition, given that you're asking how people feel about something, you need to control for people who have an illness of feeling, namely depression.

Once you've done that, look at what health measures have to do with one's subjective SES. Amazingly, it is at least as good a predictor of these health measures as is one's actual SES, and, in some cases, *it is even better.* Cardiovascular measures, metabolism measures, glucocorticoid levels, obesity in kids. *Feeling* poor in our socioeconomic world predicts poor health.

This really isn't all that surprising. We can be an immensely competitive, covetous, invidious species, and not particularly rational in how we make those comparisons. Here's an example from a realm unrelated to this subject—show a bunch of women volunteers a series of pictures of attractive female models and, afterward, they feel in a worse mood, with lower self-esteem, than before seeing the pictures (and even more depressingly, show those same pictures to men and afterward what declines is their stated satisfaction with their wives).

So it's not about being poor. It's about feeling poor. What's the difference? Adler shows that subjective SES is built around education, income, and occupational position (in other words, the building blocks of subjective SES), plus satisfaction with standard of living and feeling of financial security about the future. Those last two measures are critical. Income may tell you something (but certainly not everything) about SES; satisfaction with standard of living is the world of people who are poor and happy and zillionaires who are still grasping for more. All that messy stuff that dominates this book. And what is "feelings about financial security" tapping into? Anxiety. So SES reality plus your satisfaction with that SES plus your confidence about how predictable your SES is are collectively better predictors of health than SES alone.

This is not a hard and fast rule, and Adler's most recent work shows that subjective SES is not necessarily that great of a predictor in certain ethnic groups—stay tuned for more, no doubt. But overall, this strikes me as immensely impressive—when you're past the realm of worrying about having adequate shelter and food, being poor is not as bad for you as feeling poor.

POVERTY VERSUS POVERTY AMID PLENTY

In many ways, an even more accurate tag line for this whole phenomenon is, It's about being *made* to feel poor. This point is made clearer when considering the second body of research in this area, championed by Richard Wilkinson of the University of Nottingham in England. Wilkinson took a top-down approach, looking at the "How are you doing?" ladder from the societal level.

Let's consider how answers to "How are you doing?" can be distributed along the ladder. Suppose there is a business with ten employees. Each earns $5.50 an hour. Thus the company is paying out a total of $55/hour in salary, and the average income is $5.50/hour. With that distribution, the wealthiest employee is making $5.50/hour, or 10 percent of the total income ($5.50/$55).

Meanwhile, in the next business, there are also ten employees. One earns $1/hour, the next $2/hour, the next $3, and so on. Once again, the company pays a total of $55/hour in salary, and the average salary is again $5.50/hour. But now the wealthiest employee, earning $10/hour, takes home 18 percent of the total income ($10/$55).

Now, in the third company, nine of the employees earn $1/hour, and the tenth earns $46/hour. Again, the company pays a total of $55/hour, and the average salary is $5.50/hour. And here, the wealthiest employee takes home 84 percent of the total income ($46/$55).

What we have here are businesses of increasingly unequal incomes. What Wilkinson and others have shown is that poverty is not only a predictor of poor health but, independent of absolute income, so is poverty amid plenty—the more income inequality there is in a society, the worse the health and mortality rates.

This has been shown repeatedly, and at multiple levels. For example, income inequality predicts higher infant mortality rates across a bunch of European countries. Income inequality predicts mortality rates across all ages (except the elderly) in the United States, whether you consider this at the level of states or cities. In a world of science often filled with wishy-washy data, the effect is extremely reliable—income inequality across American states is a really strong predictor of mortality rates among working men. When you compare the most egalitarian state, New Hampshire, with the least egalitarian, Louisiana, the latter has about a 60 percent higher mortality rate.* Finally, Canada is both markedly more egalitarian and healthier than the United States—despite being a "poorer" country.

Amid extraordinary findings like that, the relationship between income inequality and poor health doesn't seem to be universal. Note how flat the curve is for Canada—moreover, you don't find it when considering adults throughout Western Europe, particularly in countries with well-established social welfare systems like Denmark. In other words, you probably can't pick up this effect when comparing individual parishes in Copenhagen because the overall pattern is so egalitarian in a place like that. But it's a reasonably robust relationship in the United Kingdom, while the flagship for the health/income inequality relationship is the United States, where the top 1 percent of the SES ladder controls nearly 40 percent of the wealth, and it's a huge effect (and persists even after controlling for race).

These studies of nations, states, and cities raise the issue of whom someone is comparing themselves to when they think of where they are on a how-are-you-doing ladder. Adler tries to get at this by asking her question twice. First, you're asked to place yourself on the ladder with respect to "society as a whole," and second, with respect to "your immediate community." The top-down Wilkinson types get at this by comparing the predictive power of data at the national, state, and city levels. Neither literature has given a clear answer yet, but both seem to suggest that it is one's immediate community that is most important. As Tip O'Neil, the consummate politician, used to say, "All politics is local."

This is obviously the case in traditional settings where all people know about is the immediate community of their village—look at how many chickens *he* has, I'm *such* a loser. But thanks to urbanization, mobility, and the media that makes for a global village, something absolutely unprecedented can now occur—we can now be made to feel poor, or poorly about ourselves, by people *we don't even know*. You can feel impoverished by the clothes of someone you pass in a midtown crowd, by the unseen driver of a new car on the freeway, by

---

* The most egalitarian states tend to be in New England, prairie states like the Dakotas or Iowa, and Utah; the least egalitarian are in the Deep South, plus Nevada.

Bill Gates on the evening news, even by a fictional character in a movie. Our perceived SES may arise mostly out of our local community, but our modern world makes it possible to have our noses rubbed in it by a local community that stretches around the globe.

Income inequality seems really important for making sense of the SES/health gradient. But maybe it isn't that important. Maybe the inequality business is just a red herring built around the fact that places with big inequalities tend to be poor places as well (in other words, back to the key thing being "poverty," instead of "poverty amid plenty"). But, control for absolute income, and the inequality data still stand.

There's a second potential problem (WARNING: skip this paragraph if you're math-phobic—as a synopsis of the plot, the income inequality hypothesis is menaced by math villains but is saved in a cliffhanger finish). Moving up the SES ladder is associated with better health (by whatever measure you are using) but, as noted, each incremental step gets smaller. A mathematical way of stating this is that the SES/health relationship forms an asymptote—going from very poor to lower middle class involves a steep rise in health that then tends to flatten out as you go into the upper SES range. So if you examine wealthy nations, you are examining countries where SES averages out to somewhere in the flat part of the curve. Therefore, compare two equally wealthy nations (that is to say, which have the same average SES on the flat part of the curve) that differ in income inequality. By definition, the nation with the greater inequality will have more data points coming from the steeply declining part of the curve, and thus must have a lower average level of health. In this scenario, the income inequality phenomenon doesn't really reflect some feature of society as a whole, but merely emerges, as a mathematical inevitability, from individual data points. However, some fairly fancy mathematical modeling studies show that this artifact can't explain all of the health–income inequality relationship in the United States.

But, alas, there might be a third problem. Suppose in some society the poor health of the poor was more sensitive to socioeconomic factors than the good health of the rich. Now suppose you make income distribution in that society more equitable by transferring some wealth from the wealthy to the poor.* Maybe by doing that, you make the health of the wealthy a little worse, and the health of the poor a lot

---

* Appropriately, the proportion of the society's wealth that must be transferred in order to make for completely equal income is termed the Robin Hood index.

better. A little worse in the few wealthy plus a lot better in the numerous poor and, overall, you've got a healthier society. That wouldn't be very interesting in the context of stress and psychological factors. But Wilkinson makes an extraordinary point—in societies that have more income equality, both the poor *and the wealthy* are healthier than their counterparts in a less equal society with the same average income. There is something more profound happening here.

 ## HOW DOES INCOME INEQUALITY AND FEELING POOR TRANSLATE INTO BAD HEALTH?

Income inequality and feeling poor could give rise to bad health through a number of routes. One, pioneered by Ichiro Kawachi of Harvard University, focuses on how income inequality makes for a psychologically crappier, more stressful life for everyone. He draws heavily upon a concept in sociology called "social capital." While "financial capital" says something about the depth and range of financial resources you can draw on in troubled times, social capital refers to the same in the social realm. By definition, social capital occurs at the level of a community, rather than at the level of individuals or individual social networks.

What makes for social capital? A community in which there is a lot of volunteerism and numerous organizations that people can join which make them feel like they're part of something bigger than themselves. Where people don't lock their doors. Where people in the community would stop kids from vandalizing a car even if they don't know whose car it is. Where kids don't try to vandalize cars. What Kawachi shows is that the more income inequality in a society, the lower the social capital, and the lower the social capital, the worse the health.

Obviously, "social capital" can be measured in a lot of ways and is still evolving as a hard-nosed measure, but, broadly, it incorporates elements of trust, reciprocity, lack of hostility, heavy participation in organizations for a common good (ranging from achieving fun—a bowling league—to more serious things—tenant organizations or a union) and those organizations accomplishing something. Most studies get at it with two measures: how people answer a question like, "Do you think most people would try to take advantage of you if they got a chance, or would they try to be fair?" and how many organizations people belong to. Measures like those tell you that on the levels of states, provinces, cities, and neighborhoods, low social capital tends to mean poor health, poor self-reported health, and high mortality rates.*

Findings such as these make perfect sense to Wilkinson. In his writing, he emphasizes that trust requires reciprocity, and reciprocity requires equality. In contrast, hierarchy is about domination, not symmetry and equality. By definition, you can't have a society with both dramatic income inequality and lots of social capital. These findings would also have made sense to the late Aaron Antonovsky, who was one of the first to study the SES/health gradient. He stressed how damaging it is to health and psyche to be an invisible member of society. To recognize the extent to which the poor exist without feedback, just consider the varied ways that most of us have developed for looking through homeless people as we walk past them.

So income inequality, minimal trust, lack of social cohesion all go together. Which causes which, and which is most predictive of poor health? To figure this out, you need some fancy statistical techniques called path analysis. An example we're comfortable with by now from earlier chapters: chronic stress makes for more heart disease. Stress can do this by directly increasing blood pressure. But stress also makes lots of people eat less healthfully. How much is the path from stress to heart disease directly via blood pressure, and how much by the indirect route of changing diet? That's the sort of thing that a path analysis can tell you. And Kawachi's work shows that the strongest route from income inequality (after controlling for absolute income) to poor health is via the social capital measures.

How does lots of social capital turn into better health throughout a community? Less social isolation. More rapid diffusion of health information. Potentially, social constraints on publicly unhealthy behaviors. Less psychological stress. Better organized groups demanding better public services (and, related to that, another great measure of social capital is how many people in a community bother to vote).

So it sounds like a solution to life's ills, including some stress-related ills, is to get into a community with lots of social capital. However, as will be touched on in the next chapter, this isn't always a great thing. Sometimes, communities get tremendous amounts of social capital by having all of their members goose-step to the same thoughts and beliefs and behaviors, and don't cotton much to anyone different.

---

* Even at the level of college campuses—the more social capital on a campus, by these measures, the less binge drinking.

Research by Kawachi and others shows another feature of income inequality that translates into more physical and psychological stress: the more economically unequal a society, the more crime—assault, robbery, and, particularly, homicide—and the more gun ownership. Critically, income inequality is consistently a better predictor of crime than poverty per se. This has been demonstrated on the level of states, provinces, cities, neighborhoods, even individual city blocks. And just as we saw in chapter 13 when we looked at the prevalence of displacement aggression, poverty amid plenty predicts more crime—but not against the wealthy. The have-nots turn upon the have-nots.

Meanwhile, Robert Evans (University of British Columbia), John Lynch, and George Kaplan (the latter two both of the University of Michigan) offer another route linking income inequality to poor health, once again via stress. This pathway is one that, once you grasp it, is so demoralizing that you immediately want to man the barricades and sing revolutionary songs from *Les Miz*. It goes as follows:

If you want to improve health and quality of life, and decrease the stress, for the average person in a society, you do so by spending money on public goods—better public transit, safer streets, cleaner water, better public schools, universal health care. The bigger the income inequality is in a society, the greater the financial distance between the wealthy and the average. The bigger the distance between the wealthy and the average, the less benefit the wealthy will feel from expenditures on the public good. Instead, they would derive much more benefit by spending the same (taxed) money on their private good—a better chauffeur, a gated community, bottled water, private schools, private health insurance. As Evans writes, "The more unequal are incomes in a society, the more pronounced will be the disadvantages to its better-off members from public expenditure, and the more resources will those members have [available to them] to mount effective political opposition." He notes how this "secession of the wealthy" pushes toward "private affluence and public squalor." And more public squalor means more of the daily stressors and allostatic load that drives down health for everyone. For the wealthy, this is because of the costs of walling themselves off from the rest of society, and for the rest of society, this is because they have to live in it.

So this is a route by which an unequal society makes for a more stressful reality. But this route certainly makes for more psychological stress as well—if the skew in society biases the increasingly wealthy toward wanting to avoid the public expenditures that would improve everyone else's quality of life . . . well, that might have some bad effects on trust, hostility, crime, and so on.

So we've got income inequality, low social cohesion and social capital, class tensions, and lots of crime all forming an unhealthy cluster. Let's see a grim example of how these pieces come together. By the late 1980s, life expectancy in Eastern Bloc countries was less than in every Western European country. As analyzed by Evans, these were societies in which there was a fair equity of income distribution, but a highly unequal distribution of freedoms of movement, speech, practice of beliefs, and so on. And what has happened to Russia since the dissolution of the Soviet Union? A massive increase in income inequality and crime, a decline in absolute wealth—and an overall decline in life expectancy that is unprecedented in an industrialized society.

One more grim example of how this works. America: enormous wealth, enormous income inequality, high crime, the most heavily armed nation on earth. And markedly low levels of social capital— it is virtually the constitutional right of an American to be mobile and anonymous. Show your independence. Move across the country for any job opportunity. (He lives across the street from his parents? Isn't that a little, er, stunted?) Get a new accent, get a new culture, get a new name, unlist your phone number, reboot your life. All of which are the antitheses of developing social capital. This helps to explain something subtle about the health–income inequality relationship. Compare the United States and Canada. As shown, the former has more income inequality and worse health. But restrict your analysis to a subset of atypical American systems chosen to match the low inequality of Canada—and those U.S. cities *still* have worse health and a steeper SES/health gradient. Some detailed analyses show what this is about: it's not just that America is a markedly unequal society when it comes to income. It's that even for the same degree of worsening income inequality, social capital is driven down further in the United States.

Our American credo is that people are willing to tolerate a society with miserably low levels of social capital, so long as there can be massive income inequality . . . with the hope that they will soon be sitting at the top of this steep pyramid. Over the last quarter-century, poverty and income inequality have steadily risen, and every social capital measure of trust, community participation, and voter participation has declined.* And what about American health? We have disparity

---

* The political scientist Robert Putnam of Harvard coined his famous metaphor for this spreading American anomie: "bowling alone." In recent decades, an increasing number of Americans bowl, but there are fewer people participating in that quintessential American social phenomenon, bowling leagues.

between the wealth of our nation and the health of our citizens that is also unprecedented. And getting worse.

This is pretty depressing stuff, given its implications. Adler, writing around the time when universal health insurance first became a front-page issue (as was the question of whether Hillary's hairstyle made her a more or less effective advocate for it), concluded that such universal coverage would "have a minor impact on SES-related inequalities in health." Her conclusion is anything but reactionary. Instead, it says that if you want to change the SES gradient, it's going to take something a whole lot bigger than rigging up insurance so that everyone can drop in regularly on a friendly small-town doc out of Norman Rockwell. Poverty, and the poor health of the poor, is about much more than simply not having enough money.* It's about the stressors caused in a society that tolerates leaving so many of its members so far behind.

This is relevant to an even larger depressing thought. I initially reviewed what social rank has to do with health in nonhuman primates. Do low-ranking monkeys have a disproportionate share of disease, more stress-related disease? And the answer was, "Well, it's actually not that simple." It depends on the sort of society the animal lives in, its personal experience of that society, its coping skills, its personality, the availability of social support. Change some of those variables and the rank/health gradient can shift in the exact opposite direction. This is the sort of finding that primatologists revel in—look how complicated and subtle my animals are.

The second half of this chapter looked at humans. Do poor humans have a disproportionate share of disease? The answer was "Yes, yes, over and over." Regardless of gender or age or race. In societies with universal health care and those without. In societies that are ethnically homogenous and those rife with ethnic tensions. In societies in which illiteracy is widespread and those in which it has been virtually banished. In those in which infant mortality has been plummeting and in some wealthy, industrialized societies in which rates have inexcusably been climbing. And in societies in which the central mythology is a capitalist credo of "Living well is the best revenge" and those in which it is a socialist anthem of "From each according to his ability, to each according to his needs."

What does this dichotomy between our animal cousins and us signify? The primate relationship is nuanced and filled with qualifiers;

---

* Evans makes this point by noting, "Most graduate students have had the experience of having very little money, but not of poverty. They are very different things."

the human relationship is a sledgehammer that obliterates every societal difference. Are we humans actually less complicated and sophisticated than nonhuman primates? Not even the most chauvinistic primatologists holding out for their beasts would vote for that conclusion. I think it suggests something else. Agriculture is a fairly recent human invention, and in many ways it was one of the great stupid moves of all time. Hunter-gatherers have thousands of wild sources of food to subsist on. Agriculture changed all that, generating an overwhelming reliance on a few dozen domesticated food sources, making you extremely vulnerable to the next famine, the next locust infestation, the next potato blight. Agriculture allowed for the stockpiling of surplus resources and thus, inevitably, the unequal stockpiling of them—stratification of society and the invention of classes. Thus, it allowed for the invention of poverty. I think that the punch line of the primate-human difference is that when humans invented poverty, they came up with a way of subjugating the low-ranking like nothing ever before seen in the primate world.

18

MANAGING STRESS

By now, if you are not depressed by all the bad news in the preceding chapters, you probably have only been skimming. Stress can wreak havoc with your metabolism, raise your blood pressure, burst your white blood cells, make you flatulent, ruin your sex life, and if that's not enough, possibly damage your brain.* Why don't we throw in the towel right now?

There is hope. Although it may sneak onto the scene in a quiet, subtle way, it is there. This frequently hits me at gerontology conferences. I'm sitting there, listening to the umpteenth lecture with the same general tone—the kidney expert speaking about how that organ disintegrates with age, the immunology expert on how immunity declines, and so on. There is always a bar graph set to 100 percent of Something Or Other for young subjects, with a bar showing that the elderly have only 75 percent of the kidney-related Something Or Other of young subjects, 63 percent of the muscle-related Something Or Other, and so on.

Now, there's a critical feature to those bar graphs. Research typically involves the study of populations, rather than single individuals one at a time. All those individuals never have the exact same level of Something Or Other—instead, the bars in a graph represent the average for each age (see the graph on page 386). Suppose one group of

---

* An additional pathology, for those who are really trivia fans when it comes to stress-related disease, is "stress-related alopecia areata." This is the technical term for that extraordinary state of getting so stressed and terrified by something that your hair turns white or gray over the course of days. This really does occur. The annotated notes at the end of the book detail the surprisingly frequent intersection of alopecia areata with law, history, and geopolitics.

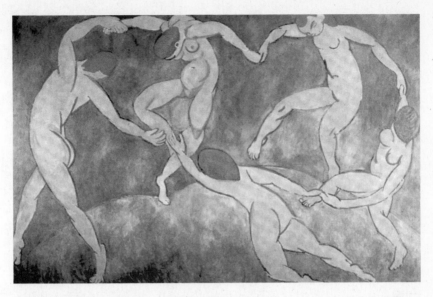

Henri Matisse, The Dance, *oil on canvas, 1910.*

three subjects has scores of 19, 20, and 21, for an average of 20. Another group may have scores of 10, 20, and 30. They also have an average score of 20, but the variability of those scores would be much larger. By the convention of science, the bars also contain a measure of how much variability there is within each age group: the size of the "T" above the bar indicates what percentage of the subjects in the group had scores within X distance of the average.

One thing that is utterly reliable is that the amount of variability increases with age—the conditions of the elderly are always much more variable than those of the young subjects. What a drag, you say as a researcher, because with that variance your statistics are not as neat and you have to include more subjects in your aged population to get a reliable average. But really *think* about that fact for a minute. Look at the size of the bars for the young and old subjects, look at the size of the T-shaped variance symbols, do some quick calculations, and suddenly the extraordinary realization hits you—to generate a bar with that large of a variance term, amid the population of, say, fifty subjects, there have to be six subjects where Something Or Other is *improving* with age. Their kidney filtration rates have gotten *better,* their blood pressures have *decreased,* they do *better* on memory tests. Suddenly you're not sitting there semi-bored in the conference, waiting for the break to grab some of those unhealthy cinnamon buns. You're on the edge of your seat. Who *are* those six? What are they

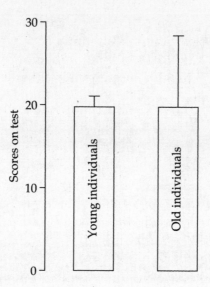

Schematic presentation of the fact that a group of young and old individuals may receive the same average score on a given test, yet the variability in the scores is typically greater among the older populations.

doing right? And with all scientific detachment abandoned, how can I do that, too?

This pattern used to be a statistical irritant to gerontologists. Now it's the trendiest subject in the field: "successful aging." Not everyone falls apart miserably with age, not every organ system poops out, not everything is bad news.

The same pattern occurs in many other realms in which life tests us. Ten men are released from years spent as political hostages. Nine come out troubled, estranged from friends and family, with nightmares, difficulties readapting to everyday life; some of those nine will never function well again. Yet invariably there is one guy who comes out saying, "Yeah, the beatings were awful, the times they put a gun to my head and cocked the trigger were the worst in my life, of course I would never want to do it again, but it wasn't until I was in captivity that I realized what is really important, that I decided to devote the rest of my life to X. I'm almost grateful." How did he do it? What explains the extraordinarily rare Holocaust survivor who came out nearly as mentally healthy as when she went in?

Consider the physiological studies of people carrying out dangerous, stressful tasks—parachuting, learning to land on an aircraft carrier in choppy seas, carrying out underwater demolition. The studies show the same pattern: most people have massive stress-responses and a subset are physiologically unflustered.

And then there's that hair-raising, push the envelope, unpredictable world of supermarket lines. You've picked the slow one, and your simmering irritation is made worse by the person behind you who looks perfectly happy standing there, daydreaming.

Despite the endless ways in which stress can disrupt, we do not all collapse into puddles of stress-related disease and psychiatric dysfunction. Of course, we are not all exposed to identical external stressors; but given the same stressors, even the same major stressors, we vary tremendously in how our bodies and psyches cope. This final chapter asks the questions born of hope. Who makes up that subset that can cope? How do they do it? And how can we? Chapter 15 suggested that some personalities and temperaments aren't well suited to dealing with stress, and it is easy to imagine the opposite case that some are. That's true, but this chapter shows that having the "right" personality doesn't explain all successful coping—there's even hope for the rest of us.

We begin by more systematically examining cases of individuals who just happen to be fabulous at dealing with stress.

 ## TALES FROM THE TRENCHES: SOME FOLKS WHO ARE AMAZING AT DEALING WITH STRESS

Successful Aging

Probably the best place to start is with successful aging, a subject that was covered at length in chapter 12. Amid a lot of good news in that chapter, one particularly bleak set of findings had to do with glucocorticoids. Old rats, recall, secrete too much of these hormones—they have elevated levels during basal, non-stressful situations and difficulty shutting off secretion at the end of stress. I discussed the evidence that this could arise from damage to the hippocampus, the part of the brain that (in addition to playing a role in learning and memory) helps inhibit glucocorticoid secretion. Then, to complete the distressing story, it was revealed that glucocorticoids could hasten the death of hippocampal neurons. Furthermore, the tendency of glucocorticoids to damage the hippocampus increases the oversecretion of glucocorticoids, which in turn leads to more hippocampal damage, more glucocorticoids, spiraling downward.

I proposed that "feed forward cascade" model around twenty years ago. It seemed to describe a basic and inevitable feature of aging in the rat, one that seemed important (at least from my provincial perspective, having just spent eighty hours a week studying it in graduate school). I was pretty proud of myself. Then an old friend, Michael Meaney of McGill University, did an experiment that deflated that grandiosity.

Meaney and colleagues studied that cascade in old rats. But they did something clever first. Before starting the studies, they tested the memory capacity of the rats. As is usual, on the average these old rats had memory problems, compared with young controls. But as usual, a subset were doing just fine, with no memory impairment whatsoever. Meaney and crew split the group of old rats into the impaired and the unimpaired. The latter turned out to show no evidence at all of that degenerative feed forward cascade. They had normal glucocorticoid levels basally and after stress. Their hippocampi had not lost neurons or lost receptors for glucocorticoids. All those awful degenerative features turned out not to be an inevitable part of the aging process. All those rats had to do was age successfully.

What was this subset of rats doing right? Oddly, it might have had something to do with their childhoods. If a rat is handled during the first few weeks of its life, it secretes less glucocorticoids as an adult. This generated a syllogism: if neonatal handling decreases the amount of glucocorticoids secreted as an adult, and such secretion in an adult influences the rate of hippocampal degeneration in old age, then handling a rat in the first few weeks of its life should alter the way it ages years later. Meaney's lab and I teamed up to test this and found exactly that. Do nothing more dramatic than pick a rat up and handle it fifteen minutes a day for the first few weeks of its life, put it back in its cage with the unhandled controls, come back two years later . . . and the handled rat is spared the entire feed forward cascade of hippocampal damage, memory loss, and elevated glucocorticoid levels.

Real rats in the real world don't get handled by graduate students. Is there a natural world equivalent of "neonatal handling" in the laboratory? Meaney went on to show that rat mothers who spend more time licking and grooming their pups in those critical first few weeks induce the same handling phenomenon. It seems particularly pleasing that this grim cascade of stress-related degeneration in old age can be derailed by subtle mothering years earlier. No doubt there are other genetic and experiential factors that bias a rat toward successful or unsuccessful aging, a subject that Meaney still pursues. Of greatest importance for our purposes now, however, is simply that this degeneration is not inevitable.

If the fates of inbred laboratory rats are this variable, how humans fare is likely to be even more diverse. Which humans age successfully? To review some of the material in chapter 12, plain old aging itself is more successful than many would guess. Levels of self-assessed contentment do not decline with age. While social networks decrease in size, they don't decline in quality. In the United States, the average eighty-five-year-old spends little time in an institution (a year and a half for women; half a year for men). The average person in that age range, taking three to eight medications a day, nevertheless typically categorizes herself as healthy. And another very good thing: despite the inherent mathematical impossibility, the average aged person considers herself to be healthier and better off than the average aged person.

Amid that good news, who are the people who age particularly successfully? As we saw in the last chapter, one factor is making sure you pick parents who were not poor. But there are other factors as well. The psychiatrist George Vaillant has been looking at this for years, beginning with his famous Harvard aging study. In 1941, a Harvard dean picked out a couple of hundred undergraduates (all male back then, naturally), who would be studied for the rest of their lives. For starters, at age sixty-five, these men had half the mortality rate of the rest of their Harvard peers, already a successfully aging crowd. Who were the students picked by that dean? Students whom he considered to be "sound." Oh hell, you're thinking—I'm a fifty-year-old woman trying to figure out how to age successfully and the prescription is to act in a way so that a 1940s Boston Brahmin with a pipe and tweed jacket would consider me to be a sound twenty-year-old fellow?

Fortunately, Vaillant's research gives us more to work with than that. Among this population, which subset has had the greatest health, contentment, and longevity in old age? A subset with an array of traits, apparent before age fifty: no smoking, minimal alcohol use, lots of exercise, normal body weight, absence of depression, a warm, stable marriage, and a mature, resilient coping style (which seems built around extroversion, social connectiveness, and low neuroticism). Of course, none of this tells you where someone gets the capacity for a mature resilient coping style, or the social means to have a stable marriage. Nor does it control for the possibility that men who, for example, have been drinking excessively have done so because they've had to deal with more than their share of miserable stressors. Despite those confounds, findings like these have emerged from other studies, and with more representative populations than Harvard graduates.

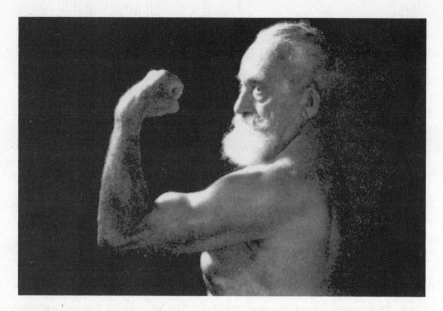

Joseph Greenstein, "The Mighty Atom," in old age. An idol of my youth, Greenstein was still performing his feats of strength in Madison Square Garden as an octogenarian. He attributed it to clean, vegetarian living.

Another literature shows the tremendous gerontological benefits of being respected and needed in old age. This has been shown in many settings, but is best appreciated with our society's equivalents of village elders—the dramatically successful aging of Supreme Court justices and conductors. It certainly fits with everything we learned about in chapter 13—you're eighty-five, and you get to influence your nation's laws for a century to come, or spend your days aerobically exercising by waving your baton about and determining whether a whole orchestra full of adults gets a potty break before or after another run through Wagner's Ring Cycle.*

The study of successful aging is a young field, and some mammoth longitudinal studies are under way that will produce a treasure trove of data, not only about what traits predict successful aging, but where those traits come from. In the meantime, though, the point for this chapter is to see that there are lots of folks out there who successfully navigate one of the most stressful passages of life.

---

* The issue of respect may help explain the highly publicized finding that winning an Oscar at any point in your life extends your life expectancy about four years, relative to actors who were nominated but didn't win.

Coping with Catastrophic Illness

In the early 1960s, when scientists were just beginning to investigate whether psychological stress triggers the same hormonal changes that physical stressors do, a group of psychiatrists conducted what has become a classic study. It concerned the parents of children dying of cancer and the high glucocorticoid levels that those parents secreted. There was great variance in this measure—some of the parents secreted immense quantities of glucocorticoids; others were in the normal range. The investigators, in in-depth psychiatric interviews, explored which parents were holding up best to this horrible stressor, and identified a number of coping styles associated with lower glucocorticoid levels.

One important variable was the ability of parents to displace a major worry onto something less threatening. A father has been standing vigil by his sick child for weeks. It's clear to everyone that he needs to get away for a few days, to gain some distance, as he is near a breaking point. Plans are made for him to leave, and just before he does, he is feeling great anxiety. Why? At one extreme is the parent who says, "I've seen how rapidly medical crises can develop at this stage. What if my daughter suddenly gets very sick and dies while I am away? What if she dies without me?" At the other extreme is the parent who can repackage the anxiety into something more manageable—"Well, I'm just worried that she'll be lonely without me, that the nurses won't have time to read her favorite stories." The latter style was associated with lower glucocorticoid levels.

A second variable had to do with denial. When a child went into remission, which frequently happened, did the parent look at him and say to the doctor, "It's over with, there's nothing to worry about, we don't even want to hear the word 'remission,' he's going to be fine"? Or did she peer anxiously at the child, wondering if every cough, every pain, every instant of fatigue was a sign that the disease had returned? During periods of remission, parents who denied that relapse and death were likely and instead focused on the seemingly healthy moment had lower glucocorticoid levels (as we will see shortly, this facet of the study had a very different postscript).

A final variable was whether the parent had a structure of religious rationalization to explain the illness. At one extreme was the parent who, while obviously profoundly distressed by her child's cancer, was deeply religious and perceived the cancer to be God's test of her family. She even reported something resembling an increase in her self-esteem: "God does not choose just anyone for a task like this; He chose us because He knew we were special and could handle this." At the other extreme was the parent who said, in effect, "Don't tell me that God works in mysterious ways. In fact, I don't want to hear about God." The researchers found that if you can look at your child having cancer and decide that God is choosing you for this special task, you are likely to have less of a stress-response (the larger issue of religious belief and health will be considered shortly).

Differences in Vulnerability to Learned Helplessness

In chapter 14, I described the learned helplessness model and its relevance to depression. I emphasized how generalized the model appears to be: animals of many different species show some version of giving up on life in the face of something aversive and out of their control.

Yet when you look at research papers about learned helplessness, there is the usual—bar graphs with T-shaped variance bars indicating large differences in response. For example, of the laboratory dogs put through one learned helplessness paradigm, about one-third wind up being resistant to the phenomenon. This is the same idea as the one out of ten hostages who comes out of captivity a mentally healthier person than when he went in. Some folks and some animals are much more resistant to learned helplessness than average. Who are the lucky ones?

Why are some dogs relatively resistant to learned helplessness? An important clue: dogs born and raised in laboratories, bred only for research purposes, are more likely to succumb to learned helplessness than those who have come to the lab by way of the pound. Martin Seligman offers this explanation: if a dog has been out in the real world, experiencing life and fending for itself (as the dogs who wind up in a pound are likely to have done), it has learned about how many controllable things there are in life. When the experience with an uncontrollable stressor occurs, the dog, in effect, is more likely to conclude that "this is awful, but it isn't the entire world." It resists globalizing the stressor into learned helplessness. In a similar vein, humans with more of an internalized locus of control—the perception that they are the masters of their own destiny—are more resistant in experimental models of learned helplessness.

More Stress Management Lessons from the Baboons

Chapters 15 and 17 introduced social primates, and some critical variables that shaped social success for them: dominance rank, the society in which rank occurs, the personal experience of both, and perhaps most important, the role played by personality. In their Machiavellian world, we saw there is more to social success and health for a male than just a lot of muscle or some big sharp canines. Just as important are social and political skills, the ability to build coalitions, and the ability to walk away from provocations. The personality traits associated with low glucocorticoid levels certainly made sense in the context of effective handling of psychological stressors—the abilities to differentiate threatening from neutral interactions with rivals, to exert some control over social conflicts, to differentiate good news from bad, to displace frustration. And, above all else, the ability to make social connections—grooming, being groomed, playing with infants. So how do these variables play out over time, as these animals age?

Baboons are long-lived animals, sticking around the savanna for anywhere from fifteen to twenty-five years. Which means you don't get to follow an animal from its first awkward bloom of puberty into old age very readily. Twenty-five years into this project, I'm just beginning to get a sense of the life histories of some of these animals, and the development of their individual differences.

As a first finding, males with the "low glucocorticoid" personalities were likely to remain in the high-ranking cohort significantly longer than rank-matched males with high glucocorticoid profiles. About three times longer. Among other things, that probably means that the low-glucocorticoid guys are outreproducing the other team. From the standpoint of evolution—passing on copies of your genes, all that jazz—this is a big difference. It suggests that if you were to go away for a couple of zillion millennia, allow that differential selection to play out, and then return to finish your doctoral dissertation, your average baboon would be a descendent of these low-glucocorticoid guys, and the baboon social world would involve a lot of impulse control and gratification postponement. Maybe even toilet training.

And what about the old ages of these individual baboons that are alive today? The most dramatic difference I've uncovered concerns the variable of social affiliation. Your average male baboon has a pretty lousy old age, once he's gotten a paunch and some worn canines and dropped down to the cellar of the hierarchy. Look at the typical pattern of dominance interactions among the males. Usually, Number 3 in the hierarchy is having most of his interactions with Numbers 2 and 4, while Number 15 is mostly concerned with 14 and 16 (except, of course, when 3 is having a bad day and needs to displace aggression on someone way down). Most interactions then usually occur between animals of adjacent ranks. However, amid that pattern, you'll note that the top-ranking half-dozen or so animals, nevertheless, are spending a lot of time subjecting poor Number 17 to a lot of humiliating dominance displays, displacing him from whatever he is eating, making him get up whenever he settles into a nice shady spot, just generally giving him a hard time. What's that about? Number 17 turns out to have been very high-ranking back when the current dominant animals were terrified adolescents. They remember, and can't believe they can make this decrepit ex-king grovel anytime they feel like it.

So as he ages, your average male baboon gets a lot of grief from the current generation of thugs, and this often leads to a particularly painful way of passing your golden years—the treatment gets so bad that the male picks up and transfers to a different troop. That's a stressful, hazardous journey, with an extremely high mortality rate for even a prime-aged animal—moving across novel terrain, chancing predators on your own. All that to wind up in a new troop, subject to an extreme version of that too-frequently-true truism about primate old age; namely, aging is a time of life spent among strangers. Clearly, for a baboon in that position, being low-ranking, aged, and ignored among strangers is better than being low-ranking, aged, and remembered by a vengeful generation.

But what about males who, in their prime, had a low-glucocorticoid personality, spending lots of time affiliated with females, grooming, sitting in contact, playing with kids? They just keep doing the same thing. They get hassled by the current rulers, but it doesn't seem to count as much as the social connectedness to these baboons. They don't transfer troops, and continue the same pattern of grooming and socialization for the rest of their lives. That seems like a pretty good definition of successful aging for any primate.

 ## APPLYING PRINCIPLES OF DEALING WITH PSYCHOLOGICAL STRESS: SOME SUCCESS STORIES

Parents somehow shouldering the burden of their child's fatal illness, a low-ranking baboon who has a network of friends, a dog resisting learned helplessness—these are striking examples of individuals who, faced with a less than ideal situation, nevertheless excel at coping. That's great, but what if you don't already happen to be that sort of individual? When it comes to rats that wish to age successfully, the useful bit of advice a previous section generates is to make sure you pick the right sort of infancy. When it comes to humans who wish to cope with stress and achieve successful aging, you should be sure to pick the right parents' genes, and the right parents' socioeconomic status as well. The other cases of successfully coping with stress may not be any more encouraging to the rest of us. What if we happen not to be the sort of baboon who looks at the bright side, the person who holds on to hope when others become hopeless, the parent of the child with cancer who somehow psychologically manages the unmanageable? There are many stories of individuals who have supreme gifts of coping. For us ungifted ones, are there ways to change the world around us and to alter our perceptions of it so that psychological stress becomes at least a bit less stressful?

The rest of the chapter is devoted to ways in which to change our coping styles. But a first thing to emphasize is that we *can* change the way we cope, both physiologically and psychologically. As the most obvious example, physical conditioning brought about by regular exercise will lower blood pressure and resting heart rate and increase lung capacity, just to mention a few of its effects. Among Type-A people, psychotherapy can change not only behaviors but also cholesterol profiles, risk of heart attack, and risk of dying, independent of changes in diet or other physiological regulators of cholesterol. As another example, the pain and stressfulness of childbirth can be modulated by relaxation techniques such as Lamaze.*

Sheer repetition of certain activities can change the connection between your behavior and activation of your stress-response. In one classic study discussed earlier, Norwegian soldiers learning to parachute were examined over the course of months of training. At the time of their first jump, they were all terrified; they felt like vats of Jell-O, and their bodies reflected it. Glucocorticoids and epinephrine levels were elevated, testosterone levels were suppressed—all for hours before and after the jump. As they repeated the experience, mastered it, stopped being terrified, their hormone secretion patterns changed. By the end of training they were no longer turning on their stress-response hours before and after the jump, only at the actual time. They were able to confine their stress-response to an appropriate moment, when there was a physical stressor; the entire psychological component of the stress-response had been habituated away.

All of these examples show that the workings of the stress-response can change over time. We grow, learn, adapt, get bored, develop an

---

* Well, I'm not so sure about that one. I've now watched my wife go through two deliveries, and Lamaze worked wonders for, like, three minutes, after which it didn't do squat, other than occupy me with pointlessly reviewing Lamaze class notes.

interest, drift apart, mature, harden, forget. We are malleable beasts. What are the buttons we can use to manipulate the system in a way that will benefit us?

The issues raised in the chapter on the psychology of stress are obviously critical: control, predictability, social support, outlets for frustration. Seligman and colleagues, for example, have reported some laboratory success in buffering people from learned helplessness when confronted with an unsolvable task—if subjects are first given "empowering" exercises (various tasks that they can readily master and control). But this is a fairly artificial setting. Some classic studies have manipulated similar psychological variables in the real world, even some of the grimmest parts of the real world. Here are two examples with startling results.

 ## SELF-MEDICATION AND CHRONIC PAIN SYNDROMES

Whenever something painful happens to me, amid all the distress I am surprised at being reminded of how painful pain is. That thought is always followed by another, "What if I hurt like this all the time?" Chronic pain syndromes are extraordinarily debilitating. Diabetic neuropathies, crushed spinal nerve roots, severe burns, recovery after surgery can all be immensely painful. This poses a medical problem, insofar as it is often difficult to give enough drugs to control the pain without causing addiction or putting the person in danger of an overdose. As any nurse will attest, this also poses a management problem, as the chronic pain patient spends half the day hitting the call button, wanting to know when his next painkiller is coming, and the nurse has to spend half the day explaining that it is not yet time. A memory that will always make me shudder: at one point, my father was hospitalized for something. In the room next door was an elderly man who, seemingly around the clock, every thirty seconds, would plaintively shout in a heavy Yiddish accent, "Nurse. Nurse! It hurts. It hurts! Nurse!" The first day it was horrifying. The second day it was irritating. By the third day, it had all the impact of the rhythmic chirping of crickets.

Awhile back some researchers got an utterly mad idea, the thought of frothing lunatics. Why not give the painkillers to the patients and let them decide when they need medication? You can just imagine the apoplexy that mainstream medicine had over that one—patients will overdose, become addicts, you can't let patients do that. It was tried with cancer patients and postsurgical patients, and it turned out that the patients did just fine when they self-medicated. In fact, the total amount of painkillers consumed *decreased*.

Why should consumption go down? Because when you are lying there in bed, in pain, uncertain of the time, uncertain if the nurse has heard your call or will have time to respond, uncertain of everything, you are asking for painkillers not only to stop the pain but also to stop the uncertainty. Reinstitute control and predictability, give the patient the knowledge that the medication is there for the instant that the pain becomes too severe, and the pain often becomes far more manageable.

INCREASING CONTROL IN NURSING HOMES

I can imagine few settings that better reveal the nature of psychological stress than a nursing home. Under the best of circumstances, the elderly tend to have a less active, less assertive coping style than young people. When confronted by stressors, the latter are more likely to try to confront and solve the problem, while the former are more likely to distance themselves from the stressor or adjust their attitude toward it. The nursing home setting worsens these tendencies toward withdrawal and passivity: it's a world in which you are often isolated from the social support network of a lifetime and in which you have little control over your daily activities, your finances, often your own body. A world of few outlets for frustration, in which you are often treated like a child—"infantilized." Your easiest prediction is "life will get worse."

A number of psychologists have ventured into this world to try to apply some of the ideas about control and self-efficacy outlined in chapter 13. In one study, for example, residents of a nursing home were given more responsibility for everyday decision making. They were made responsible for choosing their meals for the next day, signing up in advance for social activities, picking out and caring for a plant for their room, instead of having one placed there and cared for by the nurses ("Oh, here, I'll water that, dear; why don't you just get back into bed?"). People became more active—initiating more social interactions—and described themselves in questionnaires as happier. Their health improved, as rated by doctors unaware of whether they were in the increased-responsibility group or the control group. Most remarkable of all, the death rate in the former group was half that of the latter.

In other studies, different variables of control were manipulated. Almost unanimously, these studies show that a moderate increase in control produces all the salutary effects just described; in a few studies, physiological measures were even taken, showing changes like reductions in glucocorticoid levels or improved immune function. The forms that increased control could take were many. In one study, the baseline group was left alone, while the experimental group was organized into a residents' council that made decisions about life in the nursing home. In the latter group, health improved and individuals showed more voluntary participation in social activities. In another study, residents in a nursing home were being involuntarily moved to a different residence because of the financial collapse of the first institution. The baseline group was moved in the normal manner, while the experimental group was given extensive lectures on the new home and given control of a wide variety of issues connected with the move (the day of the move, the decor of the room they would live in, and so on). When the move occurred, there were far fewer medical complications for the latter group. The infantilizing effects of loss of control were shown explicitly in another study in which residents were given a variety of tasks to do. When the staff present *encouraged* them, performance improved; when the staff present *helped* them, performance declined.

Another example of these principles: this study concerned visits by college students to people in nursing homes. One nursing-home group, the baseline group, received no student visitors. In a second group, students would arrive at unpredictable times to chat. There were various improvements in functioning and health in this group, testifying to the positive effects of increased social contact. In the third and fourth groups, control and predictability were introduced—in the third group, the residents could decide when the visit occurred, whereas in the fourth they could not control it, but at least were told when the visit would take place. Functioning and health improved even more in both of those groups, compared with the second. Control and predictability help, even in settings where you think it won't make a dent in someone's unhappiness.

 ## STRESS MANAGEMENT: READING THE LABEL CAREFULLY

These studies generate some simple answers to coping with stress that are far from simple to implement in everyday life. They emphasize the importance of manipulating feelings of control, predictability, outlets for frustration, social connectedness, and the perception of whether things are worsening or improving. In effect, the nursing home and pain studies are encouraging dispatches from the front lines in this war of coping. Their simple, empowering, liberating message: if manipulating such psychological variables can work in these trying circumstances, it certainly should for the more trivial psychological stressors that fill our daily lives.

This is the message that fills stress management seminars, therapy sessions, and the many books on the topic. Uniformly, they emphasize finding means to gain at least some degree of control in difficult situations, viewing bad situations as discrete events rather than permanent or pervasive ones, finding appropriate outlets for frustration and means of social support and solace in difficult times.

That's great. But it is vital to realize that the story is not that simple. It is critical that one not walk away with the conclusion that in order to manage and minimize psychological stressors, the solution is always to have more of a sense of control, more predictability, more outlets, more social affiliation. These principles of stress management work only in certain circumstances. And only for certain types of people with certain types of problems.

I was reminded of this awhile back. Thanks to this book's having transformed me from being a supposed expert about rats' neurons to being a supposed one about human stress, I was talking to a magazine writer about the subject. She wrote for a women's magazine, the type with articles about how to maintain that full satisfying sex life while being the CEO of a Fortune 500 company. We were talking about stress and stress management, and I was giving an outline of some of the ideas in the chapter on psychological stress. All was going well, and toward the end, the writer asked me a personal question to include in the article—what are my outlets for dealing with stress. I made the mistake of answering honestly—I love my work, I try to exercise daily, and I have a fabulous marriage. Suddenly, this hard-nosed New York writer blew up at me—"I can't write about your wonderful marriage! Don't tell me about your wonderful marriage! Do you know who my readers are? They're forty-five-year-old professionals who are unlikely to ever get married and want to be told how great that is!" It struck me that she was, perhaps, in this category as well. It also struck me, as I slunk back to my rats and test tubes afterward, what an idiot I had been. You don't counsel war refugees to watch out about too much cholesterol or saturated fats in their diet. You don't tell an overwhelmed single mother living in some inner-city hellhole about the stress-reducing effects of a daily hobby. And you sure don't tell the readership of a magazine like this how swell it is to have a soul mate for life. "More control, more predictability, more outlets, more social support" is not some sort of mantra to be handed out indiscriminately, along with a smile button.

This lesson is taught with enormous power by two studies that we have already heard about, which seem superficially to be success stories in stress management but turned out not to be. Back to the parents of children with cancer who were in remission. Eventually, all the children came out of remission and died. When that occurred, how did the parents fare? There were those who all along had accepted the possibility, even probability, of a relapse, and there were those who staunchly denied the possibility. As noted, during the period of remission the latter parents tended to be the low glucocorticoid secretors. But when their illusions were shattered and the disease returned, they had the largest increases in glucocorticoid concentrations.

An equally poignant version of this unfortunate ending comes from a nursing home study. Recall the one in which residents were visited once a week by students—either unannounced, at an appointed time predetermined by the student, or at a time of the resident's choice. As noted, the sociality did everyone some good, but the people in the last two groups, with the increased predictability and control, did even better. Wonderful, end of study, celebration, everyone delighted with the clear-cut and positive results, papers to be published, lectures to be given. Student participants visit the people in the nursing home for a last time, offer an awkward, "You know that the study is over now, I, er, won't be coming back again, but, um, it's been great getting to know you." What happens then? Do the people whose functioning, happiness, and health improved now decline back to pre-experiment levels? No. They drop even further, winding up worse than before the study.

This makes perfect sense. Think of how it is to get twenty-five shocks an hour when yesterday you got ten. Think of what it feels like to have your child come out of remission after you spent the last year denying the possibility that it could ever happen. And think about those nursing home residents: it is one thing to be in a nursing home, lonely, isolated, visited once a month by your bored children. It is even worse to be in that situation and, having had a chance to spend time with bright, eager young people who seemed interested in you, to find now they aren't coming anymore. All but the most heroically strong among us would slip another step lower in the face of this loss. It is true that hope, no matter how irrational, can sustain us in the darkest of times. But nothing can break us more effectively than hope given and then taken away capriciously. Manipulating these psychological variables is a powerful but double-edged sword.

When do these principles of injecting a sense of control, of predictability, of outlets, of sociality, work and when are they disastrous to apply? There are some rules. Let's look at some specific stress management approaches and when they work, keeping those rules in mind.

 ## EXERCISE

I start with exercise because this is the stress reduction approach I rely on frequently, and I'm deeply hoping that putting it first will mean that I'll live to be very old and healthy.

Exercise is great to counter stress for a number of reasons. First, it decreases your risk of various metabolic and cardiovascular diseases, and therefore decreases the opportunity for stress to worsen those diseases.

Next, exercise generally makes you feel good. There's a confound in this, in that most people who do a lot of exercise, particularly in the form of competitive athletics, have unneurotic, extroverted, optimistic personalities to begin with (marathon runners are exceptions to this). However, do a properly controlled study, even with neurotic introverts, and exercise improves mood. This probably has something to do with exercise causing the secretion of beta-endorphin. In addition, there's the sense of self-efficacy and achievement, that good stuff you try to recall when your thigh muscles are killing you in the middle of the aerobics class. And most of all, the stress-response is about preparing your body for a sudden explosion of muscular activity. You reduce tension if you actually turn on the stress-response for that purpose, instead of merely stewing in the middle of some time-wasting meeting.

Finally, there's some evidence that exercise makes for a smaller stress-response to various psychological stressors.

That's great. Now for some qualifiers:

- Exercise enhances mood and blunts the stress-response only for a few hours to a day after the exercise session.

- Exercise is stress reducing so long as it is something you actually want to do. Let rats voluntarily run in a running wheel and their health improves in all sorts of ways. *Force* them to, even while playing great dance music, and their health worsens.

- The studies are quite clear that aerobic exercise is better than anaerobic exercise for health (aerobic exercise is the sustained type that, while you're doing it, doesn't leave you so out of breath that you can't talk).

- Exercise needs to occur on a regular basis and for a sustained period. While whole careers are consumed figuring out exactly what schedule of aerobic exercise works best (how often, for how long), it's pretty clear that you need to exercise a minimum of twenty or thirty minutes at a time, a few times a week, to really get the health benefits.

- Don't overdo it. Remember the lessons of chapter 7—too much can be at least as bad as too little.

 MEDITATION

When done on a regular, sustained basis (that is to say, something close to daily, for fifteen, thirty minutes at a time), meditation seems to be pretty good for your health, decreasing glucocorticoid levels, sympathetic tone, and all the bad stuff that too much of either can cause. Now the caveats:

First, the studies are clear in showing physiological benefits *while* someone is meditating. It's less clear that those good effects (for example, lowering blood pressure) persist for long afterward.

Next, when the good effects of meditation do persist, there may be a subject bias going. Suppose you want to study the effects of meditation on blood pressure. What do you do? You *randomly* assign some people to the control group, making sure they never meditate, and some to the group that now meditate an hour a day. But in most studies, there isn't random assignment. In other words, you study blood pressure in people who have already *chosen* to be regular meditators, and compare them to non-meditators. It's not random who chooses to meditate—maybe the physiological traits were there before they started meditating. Maybe those traits even had something to do with their choosing to meditate. Some good studies have avoided this confound, but most have not.

Finally, there are lots of different types of meditation. Don't trust anyone who says that their special brand has been proven scientifically to be better for your health than the other flavors. Watch your wallet.

GET MORE CONTROL, MORE PREDICTABILITY IN YOUR LIFE . . . MAYBE

More predictive information about impending stressors can be very stress-reducing. But not always. As noted in chapter 13, it does little good to get predictive information about common events (because these are basically inevitable) or ones we know to be rare (because you weren't anxious about them in the first place). It does little good to get predictive information a few seconds before something bad happens (because there isn't time to derive the psychological advantages of being able to relax a bit) or way in advance of the event (because who's worrying anyway?).

In some situations, predictive information can even make things worse—for example, when the information tells you little. This turfs us back to our post-9/11 world of "Go about your normal business but be extra careful"—Orange Alerts.

An overabundance of information can be stressful as well. One of the places I dreaded most in graduate school was the "new journal desk" in the library, where all the science journals received the previous week were displayed, thousands of pages of them. Everyone would circle around it, teetering on the edge of panic attacks. All that available information seemed to taunt us with how out of control we felt—stupid, left behind, out of touch, and overwhelmed.

Manipulating a sense of control is playing with the variable in psychological stress that is most likely to be double-edged. Too much of a sense of control can be crippling, whether the sense is accurate or not. An example:

When he was a medical student, a friend embarked on his surgery rotation. That first day, nervous, with no idea what to expect, he went to his assigned operating room and stood at the back of a crowd of doctors and nurses doing a kidney transplant. Hours into it, the chief surgeon suddenly turned to him: "Ah, you're the new medical student; good, come here, grab this retractor, hold it right here, steady, good boy." Surgery continued; my friend was ignored as he precariously maintained the uncomfortable position the surgeon had put him in, leaning forward at an angle, one arm thrust amid the crowd, holding the instrument, unable to see what was going on. Hours passed. He grew woozy, faint from the tension of holding still. He found himself teetering, eyes beginning to close—when the surgeon loomed before him. "Don't move a muscle because you're going to screw up *EVERYTHING*!" Galvanized, panicked, half-ill, he barely held on . . . only to discover that the "you're going to screw up everything" scenario was a stupid hazing trick done to every new med student. He had been holding an instrument over some irrelevant part of the body the entire time, fooled into feeling utterly responsible for the survival of the patient. (P.S.: He chose another medical specialty.)

As another example, recall the discussion in chapter 8 on how tenuous a link there is between stress and cancer. It is clearly a travesty to lead cancer patients or their families to believe, misinterpreting the power of the few positive studies in this field, that there is more possibility for control over the causes and courses of cancers than actually exists. Doing so is simply teaching the victims of cancer and their families that the disease is their own fault, which is neither true nor conducive to reducing stress in an already stressful situation.

So control is not always a good thing psychologically, and a principle of good stress management cannot be simply to increase the perceived amount of control in one's life. It depends on what that perception implies, as we saw in chapter 13. Is it stress-reducing to feel a sense of control when something bad happens? If you think, "Whew, that was bad, but imagine how much worse it would have been if I hadn't been in charge," a sense of control is clearly working to buffer you from feeling more stressed. However, if you think, "What a disaster and it's all my fault, I should have prevented it," a sense of control is working to your detriment. This dichotomy can be roughly translated into the following rule for when something stressful occurs: the more disastrous a stressor is, the worse it is to believe you had some control over the outcome, because you are inevitably led to think about how much better things would have turned out if only you had done something more. A sense of control works best for milder stressors. (Remember, this advice concerns the sense of control you perceive yourself as having, as opposed to how much control you actually have.)

Having an illusory sense of control in a bad setting can be so pathogenic that one version of it gets a special name in the health psychology literature. It could have been included in chapter 15, but I saved it until now. As described by Sherman James of Duke University, it is called John Henryism. The name refers to the American folk hero who, hammering a six-foot-long steel drill, tried to outrace a steam drill tunneling through a mountain. John Henry beat the machine, only to fall dead from the superhuman effort. As James defines it, John Henryism involves the belief that any and all demands can be vanquished, so long as you work hard enough. On questionnaires, John Henry individuals strongly agree with statements such as "When things don't go the way I want them, it just makes me work even harder," or "Once I make up my mind to do something, I stay with it until the job is completely done." This is the epitome of individuals with an internal locus of control—they believe that, with enough effort and determination, they can regulate all outcomes.

What's so wrong with that? Nothing, if you have the good fortune to live in the privileged, meritocratic world in which one's efforts truly do have something to do with the rewards one gets, and in a comfortable, middle-class world, an internal locus of control does wonders. For example, always attributing events in life to your own efforts (an internal locus of control) is highly predictive of lifelong health among that population of individuals who are the epitome of the privileged stratum of society—Vaillant's cohort of Harvard graduates. However, in a world of people born into poverty, of limited educational or occupational opportunities, of prejudice and racism, it can be a disaster to be a John Henry, to decide that those insurmountable odds could have been surmounted, if only, if only, you worked *even* harder—John Henryism is associated with a marked risk of hypertension and cardiovascular disease. Strikingly, James's pioneering work has shown that the dangers of John Henryism occur predominantly among the very people who most resemble the mythic John Henry himself, working-class African Americans—a personality type that leads you to believe you can control the aversively uncontrollable.

There's an old parable about the difference between heaven and hell. Heaven, we are told, consists of spending all of eternity in the study of the holy books. In contrast, hell consists of spending all of eternity in the study of the holy books. To a certain extent, our perceptions and interpretations of events can determine whether the same external circumstances constitute heaven or hell, and the second half of this book has explored the means to convert the latter to the former. But the key is, "to a certain extent." The realm of stress management is mostly about techniques to help deal with challenges that are less than disastrous. It is pretty effective in that sphere. But it just won't work to generate a cult of subjectivity in which these techniques are blithely offered as a solution to the hell of a homeless street person, a refugee, someone prejudged to be one of society's Untouchables, or a terminal cancer patient. Occasionally, there is the person in a situation like that with coping powers to make one gasp in wonder, who does indeed benefit from these techniques. Celebrate them, but that's never grounds for turning to the person next to them in the same boat and offering that as a feel-good incentive just to get with the program. Bad science, bad clinical practice, and, ultimately, bad ethics. If any hell really could be converted into a heaven, then you could make the world a better place merely by rousing yourself from your lounge chair to inform a victim of some horror whose fault it is if they are unhappy.

 ## SOCIAL SUPPORT

This far into this book, this one should be a no brainer—social support makes stressors less stressful, so go get some. Unfortunately, it's not so simple.

To begin, social affiliation is not always the solution to stressful psychological turmoil. We can easily think of people who would be the last ones on earth we would want to be stuck with when we are troubled. We can easily think of troubled circumstances where being with *anyone* would make us feel worse. Physiological studies have demonstrated this as well. Take a rodent or a primate that has been housed alone and put it into a social group. The typical result is a massive stress-response. In the case of monkeys, this can go on for weeks or months while they tensely go about figuring out who dominates whom in the group's social hierarchy.*

In another demonstration of this principle, infant monkeys were separated from their mothers. Predictably, they had pretty sizable stress-responses, with elevations in glucocorticoid levels. The elevation could be prevented if the infant was placed in a group of monkeys— but only if the infant already knew those animals. There is little to be derived in the way of comfort from strangers.

Even once animals are no longer strangers, on average half of those in any group will be socially dominant to any given individual, and having more dominant animals around is not necessarily a comfort during trouble. Even intimate social affiliation is not always helpful. We saw in psychoimmunity chapter 8 that being married is associated with all sorts of better health outcomes. Some of it is due to the old reverse causality trick—unhealthy people are less likely to get married. Some is due to the fact that marriage often increases the material well-being of people and gives you someone to remind and cajole you

---

* Some time back, the U.S. government proposed new guidelines to improve the psychological well-being of primates used for research; one well-intentioned but uninformed feature was that monkeys housed individually during a study should, at least once a week, spend time in a group of other monkeys. That precise social situation had been studied for years as a model of chronic social stress, and it was clear that the regulations would do nothing but increase the psychological well-being of these animals. Fortunately, the proposed rules were changed after some expert testimony.

into cutting back on some lifestyle risk factors. After controlling for those factors, marriage, on average, is associated with improved health. But that chapter also noted an obvious but important exception to this general rule: for women, being in a *bad* marriage is associated with immune suppression. So a close, intimate relationship with the wrong person can be anything but stress-reducing.

Expanding outward, it is also healthful to have a strong network of friends and, as we saw in the last chapter, to be in a community teeming with social capital. What's the potential downside of that? Something I alluded to. Amid all that nice, utopian social capital business lurks the inconvenient fact that a tightly cohesive, cooperative community with shared values may be all about homogeneity, conformity, and xenophobia. Maybe even brownshirts and jackboots. So social capital isn't always warm and fuzzy.

Throughout this section I have been emphasizing *getting* social support from the right person, the right network of friends, the right community. Often, one of the strongest stress-reducing qualities of social support is the act of *giving* social support, to be needed. The twelfth-century philosopher Maimonides constructed a hierarchy of the best ways to do charitable acts, and at the top was when the charitable person gives anonymously to an anonymous recipient. That's a great abstract goal, but often there is a staggering power in seeing the face that you have helped. In a world of stressful lack of control, an amazing source of control we all have is the ability to make the world a better place, one act at a time.

 ## RELIGION AND SPIRITUALITY

The idea that religiosity or spirituality protects against disease, particularly against stress-related disease, is immensely controversial. I've encountered some of the key researchers in this field, and have noticed that their read of the literature often coincides with their personal religious views. For that reason, I think it would be helpful to put my cards on the table before tackling this subject. I had a highly orthodox religious upbringing and believed devoutly. Except that now I am an atheist, have no room in my life for spirituality of any kind, and believe that religion is phenomenally damaging. Except that I wish I could be religious. Except that it makes no sense to me and I'm baffled by people who believe. Except that I'm also moved by them. So I'm confused. On to the science.

A huge literature shows that religious belief, religious practice, spirituality, and being prayed for can maintain good health—that is to say, decreases the incidence of disease, decreases the mortality rates caused by disease (put those two effects together and you have extended life span), and accelerates recovery from disease. So what's the controversy?

First, some definitional issues. What's religiosity versus spirituality? The former is about an institutionalized system with a historical precedent and a lot of adherents; the latter is more personal. As pointed out by Ken Pargament of Bowling Green University, the former has also come to mean formal, outward-oriented, doctrinal, authoritarian, and inhibiting of expression, while the latter often implies subjective, emotional, inward-oriented, and freely expressive. When comparing religious people with people who define themselves as spiritual but without a religious affiliation, the former tend to be older, less educated, and lower in socioeconomic status, with a higher percentage of men. So religiosity and spirituality can be very different things. But despite that, the health literature says roughly similar things about both, so I'm going to use them interchangeably here.

What's the controversy? Amid all those studies showing health benefits, it's whether there really *are* any benefits. Why so much uncertainty? For starters, because many of the studies are loony, or involve mistakes that should have been sorted out in the middle school science fair. But even among the serious studies, it is very hard to carry out research in this area with approaches that would count as the gold standard in the science business. For starters, most studies are retrospective. Moreover, people are usually assessing their own level of religiosity (including objective measures like how often they attend religious services), and folks are notoriously inaccurate at this sort of recall.

Another problem is one that should easily be avoided but rarely is. This is a subtle issue of statistics, and goes something like this—measure a ZILLION things related to religiosity (most of them overlapping), and measure a ZILLION things related to health (ditto), then see if anything in the first category predicts anything in the second. Even if there is no relationship at all between religiosity and health, with enough correlations, something pops up as significant by sheer chance and, *voila*, stop the presses, you've just proved that religion makes you healthy. Finally and most important in this area of science, you can't randomly assign people to different study groups ("You folks become atheists, and you guys start deeply believing in God, and we'll meet back here in ten years to check everyone's blood pressure").

So religiosity is a tough subject to do real science on, something the best people readily point out. Consider two leading thinkers in this field, Richard Sloan of Columbia University and Carl Thoresen of Stanford University. I'll be citing them a lot because each is an enormously rigorous scientist, and one is a strong advocate of the health benefits of religiosity, while the other is as strong a critic. Read their reviews of the subject and both devote half the space to savaging the, er, heck out of the literature, pointing out that the vast majority of studies in the field are plain awful and should be ignored.

Once you've separated the wheat from the voluminous chaff, what's there? Interestingly, Sloan and Thoresen agree on the next point. That is, when you consider objective medical measures, like number of days of hospitalization for an illness, there's not a shred of evidence that praying for someone improves her health (independent of her knowing that she has the social support of someone rooting for her to the higher powers). This was something already concluded by the nineteenth-century scientist, Francis Galton, who pointed out that despite having their health prayed for by overflowing churchfuls of loyal peasants each Sunday, European royals lived no longer than anyone else.

Another thing that folks like Sloan and Thoresen agree upon is that when you do see a legitimate link between religiosity and good health, you don't know which came first. Being religious may make you healthy, and being healthy may make you religious. They also agree that when you do see a link, even one in which religiosity gives rise to good health, you still don't know if it has anything to do with the religiosity. This is because being religious typically gets you a religious community, and thus social support, meaningful social roles, good role models, social capital, all that good stuff. And because in a large percentage of religions, religiosity usually means fewer of those drinking and smoking and carousing risk factors. So those need to be controlled for.

And once you've done that, remarkably, Thoresen and Sloan are still mostly in agreement, which is that religiosity does predict good health to some extent in a few areas of medicine.

Thoresen has done the most detailed analysis of this, in some hardnosed reviews of the field. He finds that regular attendance at religious services is reasonably predictive of a decreased mortality rate and of a decreased risk of cardiovascular disease and depression. However, he also finds that religiosity doesn't predict much of anything about cancer progression, cancer mortality rates, medical disability, and speed of recovery from an illness. Moreover, deeply religious people (by their own assessment) derive no more of what health benefits there are than the less deeply religious. His conclusion is that there's suggestive but not definitive evidence that religiosity, in and of itself, improves health, but the effects are pretty limited, and they're more about healthy people staying healthy than sick people staying alive and recovering faster.

Here is where Sloan becomes a strong critic. He reaches pretty much the same conclusion, but is most impressed by how small these effects are and feels that the whole subject doesn't remotely deserve the attention it has gotten. In contrast, advocates respond by saying, "These aren't much smaller effects than in other, more mainstream areas of medicine, and they're big factors in some subsets of people." And thus everyone argues back and forth until the conference session is over with and it's time for all the scientists to go to lunch.

To the extent that religiosity is good for health, once you control for social support and decreased risk factors, why is it healthful? For lots of reasons that have everything to do with stress, and with the type of deity(ies) you believe in.

To start, you can have a deity whose rules are mysterious. This is the original Judeo-Christian Yahweh, a point emphasized by Thomas Cahill in his book, *The Gift of the Jews*. Prior to the monotheistic Yahweh, the gods made sense, in that they had familiar, if supra-human appetites—they didn't just want a lamb shank, they wanted *the* best lamb shank, wanted to seduce *all* the wood nymphs, and so on. But the early Jews invented a god with none of those desires, who was so utterly unfathomable, unknowable, as to be pants-wettingly terrifying.* So even if His actions are mysterious, when He intervenes you at least get the stress-reducing advantages of attribution—it may not be clear what the deity is up to, but you at least know who is responsible for the locust swarm or the winning lottery ticket. There is Purpose lurking, as an antidote to the existential void.

Next, if it is an intervening deity with discernible rules, the deity provides the comfort of both attribution and predictive information—carry out ritual X, or Y is going to happen. And thus, when things go wrong, there is an explanation.† If it happens that things have really

---

* Tapping into this notion, the satirical newspaper *The Onion* (25 October 2001) once began an article as follows: "NEW HAVEN, CT: In a diagnosis that helps explain the confusing and contradictory aspects of the cosmos that have baffled philosophers, theologians, and other students of the human condition for millennia, God, creator of the universe and longtime deity to billions of followers, was found Monday to suffer from bipolar disorder."

† When I was young, I was taught that the Holocaust was a logical response on God's part to the affront of German Jewry inventing the Reform movement. At the time, that caused me considerable comfort and, once that whole edifice had crumbled, caused immeasurable rage.

gone wrong just to you, there is the opportunity to reframe the event, in the extraordinary way achieved by some of the parents of children with cancer—God has entrusted you with a burden that he can't entrust to just anyone.

If it is a deity who does all the above, and will respond to your personal and specific entreaties (especially if the deity *preferentially* responds to people who look/talk/eat/dress/pray like you), there is an added layer of control introduced. And if on top of all that, the deity is viewed as benign, the stress-reducing advantages must be extraordinary. If you can view cancer and Alzheimer's disease, the Holocaust and ethnic cleansing, if you can view the inevitable cessation of the beating of the hearts of all your loved ones, all in the context of a loving plan, that must constitute the greatest source of support imaginable.

Two additional areas of agreement: both Sloan and Thoresen are made very nervous by the idea that findings in this field will lead to physicians advising their patients to become religious. Both note that amid this very measured good news, religiosity can make health, mental or otherwise, a lot worse. As noted by Sharon Packer of the New School for Social Research, religion can be very good at reducing stressors, but is often the inventor of those stressors in the first place.

 ## PICKING THE RIGHT STRATEGY AT THE RIGHT TIME: COGNITIVE FLEXIBILITY

In the face of some stressor, "coping" can take a variety of forms. You can problem-solve, tackling the cognitive task of figuring out if it makes more sense to try to alter the stressor or alter your perception of it. Or you can focus on emotions—it can be stress-reducing to merely admit that you're hurting emotionally from this stressor. You can focus on relationships and social support as a means of feeling less stressed.

People obviously vary as to which style they gravitate toward. For example, an endless source of tension in heterosexual relationships is that women, on average, tend toward emotion- or relationship-based coping styles, whereas men tend toward problem-solving approaches.*

But regardless of which is your most natural coping style, a key point is that different styles tend to work better in different circumstances. As an idiotic example, suppose there's a big exam looming. One version of coping with it is to study; another is to reframe the

---

* This point is made brilliantly in a book called *You Just Don't Understand* by the linguist Deborah Tannen; this book should be required reading for newlyweds.

meaning of a bad grade ("There's more to life than this class, I'm still a good person who is good at other things . . ."). Obviously, before the exam, the stress-reduction-by-studying strategy should dominate, while you should hold off on the stress-reduction-by-reframing approach until after the exam. As a more meaningful example, consider a major illness in the family, complete with a bunch of brutally difficult decisions looming, versus a death in the family. Typically, problem-solving approaches work better in the illness scenario; emotion- and relationship-based coping works better in the case of a death.

Another version of this need for switching strategies crops up in the work of Martin Seligman. Amid all the good press that an inner locus of control gets, we just saw from the John Henryism example how counterproductive it can be. Seligman's work has demonstrated how useful and healthy it is to be able to switch loci of control. When something good happens, you want to believe that this outcome arose from your efforts, and has broad, long-lasting implications for you. When the outcome is bad, you want to believe that it was due to something out of your control, and is just a transient event with very local, limited implications.

Implicit in switching to the optimal strategy for the particular circumstance is having the cognitive flexibility to switch strategies, period. This was something emphasized by Antonovsky, one of the pioneers of SES and health research. For him, what was the predictor of health in a person? Coping responses built around fixed rules and flexible strategies. This requires that we fight a reflex common to most of us. If something bad is happening and our attempts to cope are not working, one of our most common responses is to, well, go back in there and just try twice as hard to cope in the usual way. Although that sometimes does the trick, that's rare. During times of stress, finding the resources to try something new is really hard and is often just what's needed.

 ## WHAT WAS HE GOING ON ABOUT WITH *THAT*?

Here's an additional idea that doesn't even feel half-baked yet. One of the themes of this book is the goal of contrasts. Physical stressor, you want to activate a stress-response; psychological stressor, you don't. Basal conditions, as little glucocorticoid secretion as possible; real stressor, as much as possible. Onset of stress, rapid activation; end of stress, rapid recovery.

Consider a schematic version of this, based on those Norwegian soldiers learning to parachute: the first time they jumped, their blood pressure was through the roof at the time of the jump (Part B). But in addition it was up for hours before with anticipatory terror (Part A), and for hours after—still weak-kneed (Part C).

By the zillionth time they jumped, what was the profile like? The same massive stress-response during the jump (Part B), but two seconds before and after, nothing—the parachuters are just thinking about what they're going to have for lunch.

This is what "conditioning" is about. Sharpening the contrasts between on and off, between foreground and background. Increasing the signal-to-noise ratio. Framed in the context of this book, when someone has gotten a zillion jumps' worth of experience, they turn on the stress-response only during the actual stressor. As discussed earlier, what have been winnowed away by that experience are parts A and C—the psychological stress-response.

This is great. But what I'm grasping at is an idea about a subtler goal. This thinking owes a lot to conversations with Manjula Waldron of Ohio State University, an engineering professor who also happens to be a hospital chaplain. This feels embarrassingly Zen-ish for me to spout, being a short, hypomanic guy with a Brooklyn accent, but here goes:

Maybe the goal isn't to maximize the contrast between a low baseline and a high level of activation. Maybe the idea is to have both *simultaneously*. Huh? Maybe the goal would be for your baseline to be something more than the mere absence of activation, a mere default, but to instead be an energized calm, a proactive choice. And for the ceiling to consist of some sort of equilibrium and equanimity threading through the crazed arousal. I have felt this a few times playing soccer, inept as I am at it, where there's a moment when, successful outcome or not, every physiological system is going like mad, and my body does something that my mind didn't even dream of, and the two seconds when that happened seemed to take a lot longer than it should have. But this business about the calm amid the arousal isn't just another way of talking about "good stress" (a stimulating challenge, as opposed to a threat). Even when the stressor is bad and your heart is racing in crisis, the goal should be to somehow make the fraction of a second between each heartbeat into an instant that expands in time and allows you to regroup.

There, I have no idea what I'm talking about, but I think there might be something important lurking there. Enough said.

JUST DO IT: THE 80/20 QUALITY
OF STRESS MANAGEMENT

There's this idea in a number of disciplines called the 80/20 rule. In retail business, it takes the form of, "20 percent of the customers account for 80 percent of the complaints." In criminology, it's, "20 percent of the criminals account for 80 percent of the crime." Or, "20 percent of the research and design team accounts for 80 percent of the new ideas." The numbers are not meant to be literal; it's just a way of stating that causality is not equally distributed in a population of causal agents.

I would apply the 80/20 rule to stress management: 80 percent of the stress reduction is accomplished with the first 20 percent of effort. What do I mean by this? Suppose you're a Type-A nightmare, this hostile, curt, tightly wound misery to those around you. No number of times that friends and loved ones sit you down, warmly look you in the eyes, and then yell at you about your being a pain in the ass will cause anything to change. No number of doctor visits with elevated blood pressure readings are going to make a difference. It's not going to happen until you've decided to change, and *really* decided, not just decided to try to make everyone else stop hassling you over some nonexistent problem.

This is an essential truth for mental health professionals—the whole family that's in therapy is desperately trying to get the one individual to make some changes, and nothing is going to happen if all he's doing is staring sullenly at the Siggie Freud action figure on the shrink's bookshelf. But once you sincerely want to change, the mere act of making an effort can do wonders. For example, clinically depressed people feel significantly better simply by scheduling a first appointment to see a therapist—it means they've recognized there's a problem, it means they've fought their way up through the psychomotor quagmire to actually do something, it means they've turned a corner.

This has obvious relevance for stress management. This section has examined characteristics of the most effective forms of stress management. But don't get crazed, holding off on doing something until you figure out *the* perfect approach for you. On a certain level, it doesn't matter what management technique you use (beyond it not being abusive to those around you). If your special stress reduction trick is to stand on a busy street corner in a toga reciting Teletubbies monologues, you're going to benefit from that, simply because you've decided that making a change is enough of a priority that you're willing to say no to all the things that can't be said no to, in

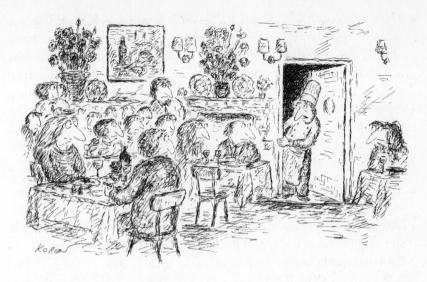

"Is there anyone here who specializes in stress management?"

order to do that Tinkie-Winkie soliloquy. Don't save your stress management for the weekend, or for when you're on hold on the phone for thirty seconds. Take the time out to do it almost daily. And if you manage that, change has become important enough to you that you're already a lot of the way there—maybe not really 80 percent, but at least a great start.

 ## A SUMMING UP

So what have we learned?

- In the face of terrible news beyond control, beyond prevention, beyond healing, those who are able to find the means to deny tend to cope best. Such denial is not only permitted, it may be the only means of sanity; truth and mental health often go hand in hand, but not necessarily in situations like these. In the face of lesser problems, one should hope, but protectively and rationally. Find ways to view even the most stressful of situations as holding the promise of improvement but do not deny the possibility that things will not improve. Balance these two opposing trends carefully. Hope for the best and let that dominate most of your emotions, but at the same time let one small piece of you prepare for the worst.

- Those who cope with stress successfully tend to seek control in the face of present stressors but do not try to control things that have already come to pass. They do not try to control future events that are uncontrollable and do not try to fix things that are not broken or that are broken beyond repair. When faced with the large wall of a stressor, it is great if there emerges one singular solution that makes the wall crumble. But often, a solution instead will be a series of footholds of control, each one small but still capable of giving support, that will allow you to scale the wall.

- It is generally helpful to seek predictable, accurate information. However, such information is not useful if it comes too soon or too late, if it is unnecessary, if there is so much information that it is stressful in and of itself, or if the information is about news far worse than one wants to know.

- Find that outlet for your frustrations and do it regularly. Make the outlet benign to those around you—one should not give ulcers in order to avoid getting them. Read the fine print and the ingredient list on each new form of supposed anti-stress salvation, be skeptical of hype, figure out what works for you.

- It is important to find sources of social affiliation and support. Even in our obsessively individualistic society, most of us yearn to feel part of something larger than ourselves. But one should not mistake true affiliation and support for mere socializing. A person can feel vastly lonely in a vast crowd or when faced with a supposed intimate who has proved to be a stranger. Be patient; most of us spend a lifetime learning how to be truly good friends and spouses.

Some of these ideas are encompassed in Reinhold Niebuhr's famous prayer, adopted by Alcoholics Anonymous:

God grant me the serenity to accept the things I cannot change, courage to change the things I can, and wisdom to know the difference.

Have the wisdom to pick your battles. And once you have, the flexibility and resiliency of strategies to use in those battles is summarized in something I once heard in a Quaker meeting:

In the face of strong winds, let me be a blade of grass.
In the face of strong walls, let me be a gale of wind.

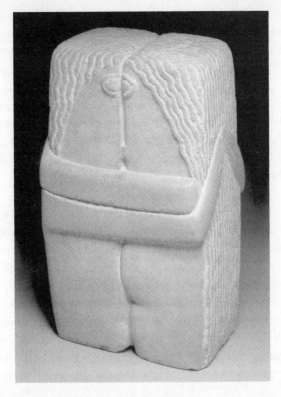

Constantin Brancusi, The Kiss, *limestone, 1912.*

Sometimes, coping with stress consists of blowing down walls. But sometimes it consists of being a blade of grass, buffeted and bent by the wind but still standing when the wind is long gone.

Stress is not everywhere. Every twinge of dysfunction in our bodies is not a manifestation of stress-related disease. It is true that the real world is full of bad things that we can finesse away by altering our outlook and psychological makeup, but it is also full of awful things that cannot be eliminated by a change in attitude, no matter how heroically, fervently, complexly, or ritualistically we may wish. Once we are actually sick with the illness, the fantasy of which keeps us anxiously awake at two in the morning, the things that will save us have little to do with the content of this book. Once we have that cardiac arrest, once a tumor has metastasized, once our brain has been badly deprived of oxygen, little about our psychological outlook is likely to help. We have entered the realm where someone else—a highly trained physician—must use the most high-tech of appropriate medical interventions.

These caveats must be emphasized repeatedly in teaching what cures to seek and what attributions to make when confronted with many diseases. But amid this caution, there remains a whole realm of health and disease that is sensitive to the quality of our minds—our thoughts and emotions and behaviors. And sometimes whether or not we become sick with the diseases that frighten us at two in the morning will reflect this realm of the mind. It is here that we must turn from the physicians and their ability to clean up the mess afterward and recognize our own capacity to *prevent* some of these problems beforehand in the small steps with which we live our everyday lives.

Perhaps I'm beginning to sound like your grandmother, advising you to be happy and not to worry so much. This advice may sound platitudinous, trivial, or both. But change the way even a rat perceives its world, and you dramatically alter the likelihood of its getting a disease. These ideas are no mere truisms. They are powerful, potentially liberating forces to be harnessed. As a physiologist who has studied stress for many years, I clearly see that the physiology of the system is often no more decisive than the psychology. We return to the catalogue at the beginning of the first chapter, the things we all find stressful— traffic jams, money worries, overwork, the anxieties of relationships. Few of them are "real" in the sense that that zebra or that lion would understand. In our privileged lives, we are uniquely smart enough to have invented these stressors and uniquely foolish enough to have let them, too often, dominate our lives. Surely we have the potential to be uniquely wise enough to banish their stressful hold.

NOTES

CHAPTER 1: WHY DON'T ZEBRAS GET ULCERS?

PAGE 1 For years, in lectures, I've rhetorically compared disease patterns in humans with those of zebras, and when sitting down to write this book, it suddenly scared the willies out of me that I wasn't sure about the business with zebras and ulcers. And then where would we be? What good is a book entitled something like *Why Do Zebras Get Ulcers Less Frequently Than We Do and for Some Fairly Different Reasons, Although It's Complicated*? However, according to M. Fowler, *Zoo and Wild Animal Medicine*, 2d ed. (Philadelphia: Saunders, 1986) and phone calls to the zebra vets at the Brookfield, Bronx, National, Philadelphia, and San Diego zoos, ulcers are extremely uncommon in zebras. They occur in animals undergoing severe and unnatural stress (e.g., when they are first transported into a zoo), but that is about the only circumstance. Stated in the framework of this book, when left to their own devices (either in the wild or in reasonably large enclosures in a zoo), zebras don't develop ulcers.

PAGE 1 Many of the ideas in this chapter have a long history in stress physiology. The main point was stated well by Walter Cannon over half a century ago: "A highly important change has occurred in the incidence of disease in our country . . . serious infections, formerly extensive and disastrous, have markedly decreased or almost disappeared, . . . meanwhile, conditions involving strain in the nervous system have been greatly augmented" ("The role of emotion in disease," *Annals of Internal Medicine* 9, no. 2 [May 1936]).

PAGE 2 Viewed through the eclipse of World War II, we seem to remember World War I with odd fondness—Irving Berlin tunes, colorful uniforms, rickety motorcars, and heads of states with silly titles and big mustaches. Eight and a half million people were killed in the pointless bloodbath we know as World War I (D. Fromkin, *A Peace to End All Peace* [New York: Avon Books, 1989], 379). The flu that swept the planet at the same time, by contrast, killed 20 million (W. McNeill, *Plagues and Peoples* [New York: Doubleday Books, 1976], 255). "The sum of American sailors and soldiers who died of flu and pneumonia in 1918 is over 43,000, about 80 percent of American battle deaths in the war" (A. Crosby, *Epidemic and Peace* [London: Greenwood Press, 1918, 1976], 36). Also: Kolata, G., *Flu* (New York: Farrar, Straus and Giroux, 1999).

PAGE 5 Footnote: The von Karajan story can be found in A. Damasio, *Descartes's Error: Emotion, Reason, and the Human Brain* (New York: Quill, 1994).

PAGE 5 The definitive study on chess players was carried out by the physiologist Leroy DuBeck and his graduate student Charlotte Leedy. They wired up chess players in order to measure their breathing rates, blood pressure, muscle contractions, and so on, and monitored the players before, during, and after major tournaments. They found tripling of breathing rates, muscle contractions, systolic blood pressures that soared to over 200—exactly the sort of thing seen in athletes during physical competition. See the original report, Leedy's thesis, "The effects of tournament chess playing on selected physiological responses in players of varying aspirations and abilities" (Temple University, 1975) or their brief report (Leedy, C., and DuBeck, L., "Physiological changes during tournament chess," *Chess Life and Review* [1971]: 708). In a telephone conversation, DuBeck also tells the story of the international match in the early 1970s between grand masters Bent Larson and Bobby Fischer, in which the former had to be given antihypertensive medication in the middle of his losing match; his blood pressure remained elevated for days afterward. The Kasparov-Karpov report is from the *New York Times*, 20 December 1990. And for that special chess fan out there who just can't get enough of this subject, may I suggest as the perfect gift a copy of Glezerov, V., and Sobol, E., "Hygienic evaluation of the changes in work capacity of young chess players during training," *Gigiena i Sanitariia* 24 (1987), in the original Russian.

PAGE 6 The brain having evolved to seek homeostasis: McMillan, F. D., "Stress, distress, and emotion: distinctions and implications for animal well-being," in McMillan, F. D., ed., *Mental Health and Well-being in Animals* (Ames, Iowa: Iowa State Press, in press).

PAGE 7 Selye published numerous autobiographical articles and books, many of which contain the story of the ovarian extract and his discovery of the nonspecific stress-response; a good example is *The Stress of My Life* (New York: Van Nostrand, 1979). The book also contains Selye's claim that he was the first to use the word *stress* in a biomedical, rather than an engineering, sense. Actually, Walter Cannon beat him to it by decades ("The interrelations of emotions as suggested by recent physiological researches," *American Journal of Psychology* 25 [1914]: 256). This point was brought up in a colorful debate between Selye and John Mason, a psychiatrist whose pioneering work on the psychological stress-response is discussed later (Mason, J., "A historical view of the stress field," *Journal of Human Stress* 1, no. 6 [1975]: part II, 1, 22. Selye, H., "Confusion and controversy in the stress field," *Journal of Human Stress* 1 [1975]: 37).

PAGE 9 For an entrée to the world of allostasis, see Sterling, P., and Eyer, J., "Allostasis: a new paradigm to explain arousal pathology," in Fisher, S., and Reason, J., eds., *Handbook of Life Stress, Cognition, and Health* (New York: Wiley, 1988). Also see Sterling, P., "Principles of allostasis: optimal design, predictive regulation, pathophysiology and rational therapeutics," in Schulkin, J., ed., *Allostasis, Homeostasis, and the Costs of Adaptation* (Cambridge: MIT Press, 2003). Also see: McEwen, B., *The End of Stress* (New York: Joseph Henry Press, 2002); Schulkin, J., "Allostasis: a neural behavioral perspective," *Hormones and Behavior* 43 (2003): 21. For a contrarian view of the allostasis concept, see Dallman, M., "Stress by any other name . . . ?" *Hormones and Behavior* 43 (2003): 18.

PAGE 15 Descriptions of Addison's disease can be found in all endocrinology textbooks, as it is one of the best-studied endocrine disorders. Shy-Drager is rarer and more recent, first described in 1960. For a description right from the horses' mouths, see Shy, G., and Drager, G., "A neurological syndrome associated with orthostatic hypotension," *A.M.A. Archives of Neurology* 2 (1960): 41–511. Also see Low, P., *Seminars in Neurology* 7, no. 1 (March 1987): 53; and Bannister, R., and Mathios, C., *Autonomic Failure* (New York: Oxford University Press, 1992).

PAGE 16 For a review of syndromes in which there is an insufficient stress-response, see: Raison, C., and Miller, A., "When not enough is too much: the role of insufficient glucocorticoid signaling in the pathophysiology of stress-related disorders," *American Journal of Psychiatry* 160 (2003): 1554.

CHAPTER 2: GLANDS, GOOSEFLESH, AND HORMONES

PAGE 19 The D. H. Lawrence quotation is from *Lady Chatterley's Lover* (Cutchogue, N.Y.: Buccaneer Books, 1983). The idea for this example comes from a colleague, the British immunologist Nick Hall. He regularly lectures to halls of distracted scientists clicking away with their three-color pens; he starts off with some really steamy passage of Lawrence recited in his impressive English accent, and rivets their attention.

PAGE 24 The testicular injection mania began in 1889, with a paper published by the formidable Charles-Edouard Brown-Sequard, entitled "On the physiological and therapeutic role of a juice extracted from the testicles of animals according to a number of facts observed in man," *Archives de physiologie normale et pathologique*, 5e series (1889): 1, 739.

A lot of the facts Brown-Sequard collected had been observed in one man, himself. Brown-Sequard was arguably the most august physiologist in the world at the time, age seventy-two and with somewhat declining energies. He had theorized that some features of senescence of humans were due to declining gonadal function (the more global statements about such decline as the cause of aging came from later followers). He felt that the testes contained some sort of active secreted substance, and he started injecting himself subcutaneously with extracts of testes from dogs and guinea pigs. He was absolutely right that the testes secreted a substance—testosterone (which had not yet been discovered; the term *hormone* did not even exist then)—but his experiment couldn't possibly work, since he made his extracts in water; testosterone, because of its chemical nature, does not dissolve in water.

Despite that, he reported wondrous results (increased physical vitality, increased length of his jet of urine—the latter no doubt being the sort of thing we all hope to retain into our golden years). All placebo. The reproductive physiologist Roger Gosden of Leeds University in the United Kingdom suspects that Brown-Sequard was probably depressed at the time of his experiments and thus was particularly vulnerable to such a placebo effect (see page 148 in Gosden, R., *Cheating Time: Science, Sex and Ageing* [London: Macmillan, 1996]). Nevertheless, doctors were thrilled at the report, and within two years, organotherapy, as it was called, was being used worldwide. Brown-Sequard took particular umbrage at the charlatans making quick money using his (altogether incorrect and ineffectual) discovery, particularly the American hucksters soon selling "Dr. Brown-Sequard's Elixir of Life." He also expanded his theory a bit, noting that loss of semen resulted in loss of strength (twenty years earlier he had speculated on the rejuvenative effects of intravenous injections of sperm into men, an idea fortunately not tried), citing the well-known physical and mental weaknesses of men who masturbated frequently or who had frequent intercourse. (For the original citations and a thorough review of the subject, see Borell, M., "Brown-Sequard's organotherapy and its appearance in America at the end of the nineteenth century," *Bulletin of the History of Medicine* 50 [1976]: 309, as well as the very entertaining section on the subject in Gosden's book.)

PAGE 27 The history of hypothalamic hormones (Harris's theory that the brain was an endocrine organ, and the work of Guillemin and Schally) has been well documented, especially in the aftermath of the award of the Nobel Prize to the latter pair. This is because of the ferocity and colorfulness of the Guillemin-Schally race, and because the huge, "corporate" lab that each evolved in the process seemed the wave of the scientific future at the time. For a particularly readable account, see Wade, N., *The Nobel Duel: Two Scientists' 21-Year Race to Win the World's Most Coveted Research Prize* (Garden City, N.Y.: Anchor Press, 1981). The quotation from Schally about the competition with Guillemin is in Wade's book, page 7. For a dauntingly academic account of the sociology of Guillemin's lab (although it is not identified as Guillemin's by name), see Latour, B., and Woolgar, S., *Laboratory Life: The Social Construction of Scientific Facts* (Beverly Hills, Calif.: Sage Publications, 1979).

New releasing and inhibiting factors continue to be isolated, still often in sprints to the finish line by research groups in frenzied competition with one another. An exception to this pattern came in 1981 with the isolation of what was perhaps the most sought-after of the brain hormones. This hormone, which will be discussed throughout the book, is the main way in which the brain controls a principal branch of the stress-response. Corticotropin releasing hormone (CRH), as it is called, was the first brain hormone whose existence was inferred (in 1955) but one of the last ones isolated, because it turned out to be among the most chemically complex. In a wrinkle on the old Guillemin-Schally dichotomy, its isolation was carried out by a team headed by Wylie Vale, once Guillemin's right-hand man. Vale and his band of renegades, in a lab of their own, had the audacity to look for CRH in places none of the other researchers had tried in the twenty-five years of investigation, by considering very unlikely chemical structures for CRF. One turned out to be the right one, and they beat the competition by miles. See Vale, W., Speiss, J., Rivier, C., and Rivier, J., "Characterization of a 41-residue ovine hypothalamic peptide that stimulates the secretions of corticotropin and beta-endorphin," *Science* 213 (1983): 1394.

PAGE 33 For the tend and befriend concept, see: Taylor, S., Klein, L., Lewis, B., Gruenewald, T., Gurung, R., Updegraff, J., "Biobehavioral responses to stress in females: tend-and-befriend, not fight-or-flight," *Psychological Review* 107 (2000): 411. For a critique of it, see: Geary, D., Flinn, M., "Sex differences in behavioral and hormonal response to social threat: commentary on Taylor et al.," *Psychological Reviews* 109 (2002): 745.

PAGE 34 For a consideration of how glucocorticoids prepare you for a subsequent stress-response, see: Sapolsky, R., Romero, M., Munck, A., "How do glucocorticoids influence the stress-response?: integrating permissive, suppressive, stimulatory, and preparative actions," *Endocrine Reviews* 21 (2000): 55.

PAGE 35 Hormonal "signatures" of different stressors: Henry, J. P., *Stress, Health, and the Social Environment* (New York: Springer-Verlag, 1977); Frankenhaeuser, M., "The sympathetic-adrenal and pituitary-adrenal response to challenge," in Dembroski, T., Schmidt, T., and Blumchen, G., eds., *Biobehavioral Basis of Coronary Heart Disease* (Basel: Karger, 1983), 91. For some more recent studies concerning stress signatures, see: Schommer, N., Hellhammer, D., Kirschbaum, C., "Dissociation between reactivity of the hypothalamus-pituitary-adrenal axis and the sympathetic-adrenal-medullary system to repeated psychosocial stress," *Psychosomatic Medicine* 65 (2003): 450; Dayas, C., Buller, K., Crane, J., Day, T., "Stressor categorization: acute physical and psychological stressors elicit distinctive recruitment patterns in the amygdala and in medullary noradrenergic cell groups," *European Journal of Neuroscience* 14 (2001): 1143; Pacak, K., Palkovits, M., "Stressor specificity of central neuroendocrine responses: implications for stress-related disorders," *Endocrine Reviews* 22 (2001): 502. For a particularly odd example of stress signatures (laboratory rats having different patterns of stress-responses depending on which human handled them), see Dobrakovova, M., Kvetnansky, R., Oprsalova, Z., and Jezova, D., "Specificity of the effect of repeated handling on sympathetic-adrenomedullary and pituitary-adrenocortical activity in rats," *Psychoneuroendocrinology* 18 (1993): 163. For a review of the hypothalamic stress signature for different types of psychological stress, see Romero, L., and Sapolsky, R., "Patterns of ACTH secretagog secretion in response to psychological stimuli," *Journal of Neuroendocrinology* 8 (1996): 243.

PAGE 35 Stress signatures arising from changes in tissue sensitivity to stress hormones: Avitsur, R., Stark, J., Sheridan, J., "Social stress induces glucocorticoid resistance in subordinate animals," *Hormones and Behavior* 39 (2001): 247.

CHAPTER 3: STROKE, HEART ATTACKS, AND VOODOO DEATH

PAGE 37 Good general overviews of what the cardiovascular system does during stress can be found in most physiology textbooks, although the information is rarely explicitly organized under the topic of "stress." Instead, it can usually be found in a chapter on the heart itself, or on the physiological response to exercise. Those reviews typically focus on the role of the sympathetic nervous system in regulating the cardiovascular system. The role of glucocorticoids (which make cardiovascular tissue more sensitive to the sympathetic nervous system) is reviewed in Whitworth, J., Brown, M., Kelly, J., Williamson, P., "Mechanisms of cortisol-induced hypertension in humans," *Steroids* 60 (1995): 76. Also see Sapolsky, R., and Share, L., "Rank-related differences in cardiovascular function among wild baboons: role of sensitivity to glucocorticoids," *American Journal of Primatology* 32 (1994): 261.

PAGE 37 Glucocorticoids activate neurons in the brain stem: Rong, W., Wang, W., Yuan, W., and Chen, Y., "Rapid effects of corticosterone on cardiovascular neurons in the rostral ventrolateral medulla of rats," *Brain Research* 815 (1999): 51. Glucocorticoids enhancing epinephrine effects: Sapolsky, R., Share, L., "Rank-related differences in cardiovascular function among wild baboons: role of sensitivity to glucocorticoids," *American Journal of Primatology* 32 (1994): 261. For a mechanism for how glucocorticoids can cause hypertension: Wallerath, T., Witte, K., Schafeer, S., Schwarz, P., Prellwitz, W., Wohlfart, P., Kleinert, H., Lehr, H., Lemmer, B., Forstermann, U., "Down-regulation of the expression of eNOS is likely to contribute to glucocorticoid-mediated hypertension," *Proceedings of the National Academy of Sciences, USA* 96 (1999), 13357.

PAGE 38 The 1833 study showing that emotional stress would shut down blood flow to the guts of the Native American with the gunshot wound: Beaumont, W., *Experiments and Observations on the Gastric Juice and the Physiology of Digestion* (Plattsburgh, N.Y.: F. P. Allen, 1833).

PAGE 38 For a discussion of the role of kidneys in increasing blood pressure during stress, see Guyton, A., "Blood pressure control—special role of the kidneys and body fluids," *Science* 252 (1991): 1813.

PAGE 39 The Patton story: Ambrose, S., *Citizen Soldiers* (New York: Simon and Schuster, 1997). The Korean War story: Weintraub, S., *MacArthur's War* (New York: Prentice Hall, 2000).

PAGE 39 Enuresis footnote: Anand, S., Berkowitz, C., "Enuresis," in Fink, G., ed., *Encyclopedia of Stress* (San Diego: Academic Press, 2000), vol. 3, 49.

PAGE 40 The difference in cardiovascular responses to overt physical stressors and to quiet vigilance: Fisher, L., "Stress and cardiovascular physiology in animals," in Brown, M., Koob, G., and Rivier, C., eds., *Stress: Neurobiology and Neuroendocrinology* (New York: Marcel Dekker, 1991). 2 hours, 10 minutes; black and white. With Claude Rains, Lily Pons, and the young Robert Mitchum as the descending aorta.

PAGE 41 Detailed discussions about how damage to the vascular lining, various hormones, and high levels of fat in the bloodstream interact to cause atherosclerosis: Lusis, A., "Atherosclerosis," *Nature* 407 (2000): 233. The clumping of platelets during stress is discussed in Allen, M., and Patterson, S., "Hemoconcentration and stress: a review of physiological mechanisms and relevance for cardiovascular disease risk," *Biological Psychology* 41 (1995): 1. Also Rozanski, A., Krantz, D., Klein, J., and Gottdiener, J., "Mental stress and the induction of myocardial ischemia," in Brown et al., *Stress: Neurobiology and Neuroendocrinology* (New York: Marcel Dekker, 1991). Also see Fuster, V., Badimon, L., Badimon, J., and Chesebro, J., "The pathogenesis of coronary artery disease and the acute coronary syndromes," *New England Journal of Medicine* 326 (1992): 242.

PAGE 42 Stress-induced thickening of muscles around blood vessels: Folkow, B., "Physiological aspects of primary hypertension," *Physiological Reviews* 62 (1982): 374.

PAGE 42 Left ventricular hypertrophy: Baker, G., Suchday, S., Krantz, D., "Heart disease/attack," in Fink, G., ed., *Encyclopedia of Stress* (San Diego: Academic Press, 2000), vol. 2, 326.

PAGE 43 Stress-induced increase in blood viscosity: Von Kanel, R., Mills, P., Fainman, C., Dimsdale, J., "Effects of psychological stress and psychiatric disorders on blood coagulation and fibrinolysis: a biobehavioral pathway to coronary artery disease?" *Psychosomatic Medicine* 63 (2001): 531. Platelet aggregation: Wentworth, P., Nieva, J., Takeuchi, C., Galve, R., "Evidence for ozone formation in human atherosclerotic arteries," *Science* 302 (2003): 1053.

PAGE 43 Heart attacks with normal cholesterol levels: Gorman, C., Park, A., "The fires within," *Time* (23 February 2004). The importance of inflammation and of C reactive protein: Taubes, G., "Does inflammation cut to the heart of the matter?" *Science* 296 (2002): 242.

PAGE 44 The work regarding social stress and heart disease in rodents can be found in Henry, J. P., *Stress, Health, and the Social Environment* (New York: Springer-Verlag, 1977). Also, social subordination in rodents increasing the risk of cardiac arrhythmia: Sgoifo, A., Koolhaas, J., De Boer, S., Musso, E., Stilli, D.,

Buwalda, B., Meerlo, P., "Social stress, autonomic neural activation, and cardiac activity in rats," *Neuroscience and Biobehavioral Reviews* 23 (1999): 915. The work regarding social stress and plaque formation in primates is reviewed in Manuck, S., Marsland, A., Kaplan, J., and Williams, J., "The pathogenicity of behavior and its neuroendocrine mediation: an example from coronary artery disease," *Psychosomatic Medicine* 57 (1995): 275. The work regarding interactions of the hormones of the metabolic stress-response in causing atherosclerosis can be found in Brindley, D., "Role of glucocorticoids and fatty acids in the impairment of lipid metabolism observed in the metabolic syndrome," *International Journal of Obesity and Related Metabolic Disorders* 19 (1995): supp. 1, S69.

PAGE 45 Stress and stroke: May, M., McCarron, P., Stansfeld, S., Ben-Shlomo, Y., Gallacher, J., Yarnell, J., Smith, G., Elwood, P., Ebrahim, S., "Does psychological distress predict the risk of ischemic stroke and transient ischemic attack?" *Stroke* 33 (2002): 7; Williams, J., Nieto, F., Sanford, C., Couper, D., Tyroler, H., "The association between trait anger and incident stroke risk," *Stroke* 33 (2002): 13; Everson, S., Lynch, J., Kaplan, G., Lakka, T., Silvenius, J., Salonen, J., "Stress-induced blood pressure reactivity and incident stroke in middle-aged men," *Stroke* 32 (2001): 1263.

PAGE 46 Myocardial ischemia, damaged heart muscle, and its subsequent vulnerability to stress: M. Brown et al., *Stress: Neurobiology and Neuroendocrinology* (New York: Marcel Dekker, 1991) contains a number of chapters with useful information. These include chapters 20 (Verrier, R., "Stress, sleep and vulnerability to ventricular fibrillation"), 21 (Fisher, L., "Stress and cardiovascular physiology in animals"), 22 (Brodsky, M., and Allen, B., "Effects of psychological stress on cardiac rate and rhythm"), and 23 (Rozanski, A., Krantz, D., Klein, J., and Gottdiener, J., "Mental stress and the induction of myocardial ischemia"). Chapters 20 and 23 contain good reviews of ambulatory electrocardiography; the former chapter details Verrier's own studies showing that psychological stress in humans and dogs can cause acute ischemia in damaged heart tissue. (Also see Rozanski, A., and Berman, D., "Silent myocardial ischaemia. I. Pathophysiology, frequency of occurrence and approaches toward detection," *American Heart Journal* 114 [1987]: 615.) For a review of the paradoxical vasoconstriction, rather than vasodilation, during stress in damaged coronary arteries, see Fuster, V., Badimon, L., Badimon, J., and Chesebro, J., "The pathogenesis of coronary artery disease and the acute coronary syndromes, part II," *New England Journal of Medicine* 326 (1992): 310. Also see Schwartz, C., Valente, A., and Hildebrandt, E., "Prevention of atherosclerosis and end-organ damage: a basis for antihypertensive interventional strategies," *Journal of Hypertension* 12 (1994): S3. Cardiologists are beginning to get some sense of what causes this paradoxical vasoconstriction. In healthy tissue, when the heart starts working hard, hormones called EDRF (endothelium-derived relaxant factors) and prostacyclin are secreted, causing the vasodilation. When cardiac tissue is made ischemic on a regular basis, it loses the capacity to release EDRF and prostacyclin for some reason. In addition, hormones called endothelin and serotonin, which cause vasoconstriction, seem to be released. As a result, epinephrine and norepinephrine now cause constriction instead of dilation. Interestingly, this paradoxical vasoconstriction is also observed in the socially stressed monkeys, discussed above, who developed atherosclerosis. One way to dilate coronary arteries during angina pectoris is to take a synthetic version of EDRF—nitroglycerin. For epidemiological evidence that stress is more likely to worsen preexisting heart disease than to cause it outright, see Greenwood, D., Muir, K., Packham, C., and Madeley, R., "Coronary heart disease: a review of the role of psychosocial stress and social support," *Journal of Public Health Medicine* 18 (1996): 221. For more examples of ischemia in heart patients being brought on by subtle psychological stressors (in this case, public speaking), see Taggert, P., Carruthers, M., and Somerville, W., "Electrocardiogram, plasma catecholamines, and their modification by oxyprenolol when speaking before an audience," *The Lancet* 2 (1973): 341. In another demonstration, patients were shown to have as much myocardial ischemia when describing a personal problem to a stranger as they did during exercise: Rozanski, A., "Mental stress and the induction of silent myocardial ischemia in patients with coronary artery disease," *New England Journal of Medicine* 318 (1988): 1005. For reviews of some of the special features linking stress and heart disease in women, see Brezinka, V., Kittel, F., "Psychosocial factors of coronary heart disease in women; a review," *Social Science and Medicine* 42 (1996): 1351, and Elliott, S., "Psychosocial stress, women and heart health; a critical review," *Social Science and Medicine* 40 (1995): 105.

PAGE 48 Variability in the interbeat interval: Porges, S., "Cardiac vagal tone: a physiological index of stress," *Neuroscience and Biobehavioral Reviews* 19 (1995): 225.

PAGE 49 Instances of sudden cardiac death during stress in humans: Engel, G., "Sudden and rapid death during psychological stress: folklore or folk wisdom?" *Annals of Internal Medicine* 74 (1971): 771. A report shows a tripling in the incidence of myocardial infarctions of the Tel Aviv population during the first three days of the SCUD attacks, as compared with the same three days of January the year before: Meisel, S., Kutz, I., Dayan, K., Pauzner, H., Chetboun, I., Arbel, Y., and David, D., "Effect of Iraqi missile war on incidence of acute myocardial infarction and sudden death in Israeli civilians," *The Lancet* 338 (1991): 660. For data regarding the L.A. earthquake, see Leor, J., Poole, W., Kloner, R., "Sudden cardiac death triggered by an earthquake," *New England Journal of Medicine* 334 (1996): 413. The elderly couple is discussed in a letter from Dr. Paul Morrow, chief medical examiner, state of Vermont. The mechanisms underlying sudden cardiac death: Davis, A., Natelson, B., "Brain-heart interactions: the neurocardiology of arrhythmia and sudden cardiac death," *Texas Heart Institute Journal* 20 (1993): 158; also Meerson, F., "Stress-induced arrhythmic disease of the heart—part I," *Clinical Cardiology* 17 (1994): 362; this paper also describes stress making rat hearts more vulnerable to fibrillation. Anger as increasing the risks of cardiac infarct: Mittleman, M., Maclure, M., Sherwood, J., Mulry, R., Tofler, R., Jacobs, S., Friedman, R., Benson, H., Muller, J., "Triggering of acute myocardial infarction onset by episodes of anger," *Circulation* 92 (1995): 1720.

PAGE 49 Heart attacks in NYC: Christenfeld, N., Glynn, L., Phillips, D., Shrira, I., "Exposure to New York City as a risk factor for heart attack mortality," *Psychosomatic Medicine* 61 (1999): 740.

PAGE 51 Heart disease as leading cause of death in women: *Time,* cover story, 28 April 2003. Smoking rates declining slowly in women: "Morbidity and Mortality Weekly Report," Report of the CDC, 51 (RR12) 1 (30 August 2002); Women and smoking: *A Report of the Surgeon General*. Women working outside the home and the risk of heart disease: Haynes, S., Feinleib, M., "Women, work and coronary disease: prospective findings from the Framingham Heart Study," *American Journal of Public Health* 700 (1980): 133.

PAGE 52 Papers leading to the revisionism about the cardiovascular benefits of estrogen: Rossouw, J., Anderson, G., Prentice, R., et al., "Risks and benefits of estrogen and progesterone in healthy post-menopausal women: principal results from the Women's Health Initiative randomized controlled trial," *Journal of the American Medical Association* 288 (2002): 321. Manson, J. E., Hsia, J., Johnson, K. C., Rossouw, J. E., Assaf, A. R., Lasser, N. L., Trevisan, M., Black, H. R., Heckbert, S. R., Detrano, R., Strickland, O. L., Wong, N. D., Crouse, J. R., Stein, E., Cushman, M., Women's Health Initiative Investigators, "Estrogen plus progestin and the risk of coronary heart disease," *New England Journal of Medicine* 349 (2003): 523; Hodis, H. N., Mack, W. J., Azen, S. P., Lobo, R. A., Shoupe, D., Mahrer, P. R., Faxon, D. P., Cashin-Hemphill, L., Sanmarco, M. E., French, W. J., Shook, T. L., Gaarder, T. D., Mehra, A. O., Rabbani, R., Sevanian, A., Shil, A. B., Torres, M., Vogelbach, K. H., Selzer, R. H., Women's Estrogen-Progestin Lipid-Lowering Hormone Atherosclerosis Regression Trial Research Group, "Hormone therapy and the progression of coronary-artery atherosclerosis in postmenopausal women," *New England Journal of Medicine* 349 (2003): 535.

A recent review of the Kaplan work with primates, suggesting that estrogen is protective: Kaplan, J., Manuck, S., Anthony, M., Clarkson, T., "Premenopausal social status and hormone exposure predict postmenopausal atherosclerosis in female monkeys," *Obstetrics and Gynecology* 99 (2002): 381–88.

For a review of the controversy, see: J. Couzin, "The great estrogen conundrum," *Science* 302 (2003): 1136.

PAGE 54 Psychophysiological death: Davis, W., and DeSilva, R., "Psychophysiological death: a cross-cultural and medical appraisal of voodoo death," *Anthropologia,* in press. Walter Cannon contacted a variety of missionaries, anthropologists, and medical people working in the third world, collecting their descriptions of voodoo death in order to decide that it sounded like too much sympathetic nervous system activity to him ("'Voodoo' death," *American Anthropologist* 44 [1942]: 169). Curt Richter, by contrast, didn't gather any firsthand accounts of his own. Instead, he noted the similarity between the accounts in Cannon's paper and cases of parasympathetic-induced death in rats undergoing severe stressors in his own laboratory (he noted that the phenomenon occurred much more readily in wild rats captured and brought to his lab than in the lab-bred strains, and made comparisons between "uncivilized primitive humans" and undomesticated wild rats). ("On the phenomenon of sudden death in animals and man," *Psychosomatic Medicine* 19 [1957]: 191.) Also see Morse, D., Martin, J., and Moshonov, J., "Psychosomatically induced death: relative to stress, hypnosis, mind control, and voodoo: review and possible mechanisms," *Stress Medicine* 7 (1991): 213. (Note: at no extra cost, this review also includes an excerpt of a scene describing a voodoo death, complete with descriptions of dancers "making obscene gestures with their buttocks" in what appears to be a fairly schlocky novel by the first author, something unique to any scientific paper I've seen.)

As he described in *The Serpent and the Rainbow* (New York: Warner Books, 1985), Wade Davis believed he had isolated the critical substance—a poison called tetrodotoxin, isolated from puffer fish—that the Haitian witch doctors use to put someone in a zombified state. This is the same poison found in the fugu fish, used in Japanese cooking. (When the fugu chef leaves a smidgen of the tetrodotoxin gland in the fish, the well-paying customer gets a mild buzz. When the chef leaves too much in, the well-paying customer goes into a coma. Fugu chefs, by the way, are carefully licensed.) Davis made a fascinating argument that zombification in Haiti reflected the intersection of the biology of tetrodotoxin action and the anthropology of traditional Haitian religion: when a Japanese businessman gets major tetrodotoxin poisoning and recovers, he sues the chef and switches restaurants. When a Haitian villager gets the same tetrodotoxin poisoning and recovers, he realizes that his village hired a shaman to poison him because he has done something terrible—he awakes as an ostracized zombie with no will, and then is often used for slave labor (although in some cases, the zombified person's passive state is promoted by continually drugging him). It's a charming story, although the isolation of tetrodotoxin remains controversial. Davis and tetrodotoxin zombification became so trendy in the 1980s that in Garry Trudeau's *Doonesbury,* Uncle Duke was zombified at one point, and *Miami Vice* used the zombie motif in an episode about drug runners from Haiti.

CHAPTER 4: STRESS, METABOLISM, AND LIQUIDATING YOUR ASSETS

PAGE 57 Energy storage and mobilization: the basics of this vastly complicated subject—involving storage tissues throughout the body, a variety of different hormonal messengers, and the liver as Grand Central Station for various nutrients coming and going—are covered in any physiology textbook. A fairly lucid presentation of the subject on an introductory college level can be found in Vander, A., Sherman, J., and Luciano, D., *Human Physiology: The Mechanisms of Body Function,* 6th ed. (New York: McGraw-Hill, 1994). For a discussion of how stress causes energy mobilization, see Mizock, B., "Alterations in carbohydrate metabolism during stress; a review of the literature," *American Journal of Medicine* 98 (1995): 75. Note that this discusses big-time stressors in humans (sepsis, burns, and trauma); the same principles hold for the more subtle ones that dominate this book.

PAGE 59 Secreting insulin in anticipation of eating: Schwartz, M. W., Woods, S. C., Porte, D., Seeley, R. J., Baskin, D. G., "Central nervous system control of food intake," *Nature* 404 (2000): 661–72.

PAGE 61 Recent findings about the workings of gluconeogenesis: Herzig, S., Hedrick, S., Morantte, I., Koe, S., Galimi, F., and Montminy, M., "CREB controls hepatic lipid metabolism through nuclear hormone receptor PPAR-gamma," *Nature* 426 (2003): 190; Yoon, J., Puigserver, P., Chen, G., Donovan, J., Wu, Z., et al., "Control of hepatic gluconeogenesis through the transcriptional coactivator PGC-1," *Nature* 413 (2001): 131.

PAGE 61 Low glucocorticoid levels in chronic fatigue syndrome: Raison, C., Miller, A., "When not enough is too much: the role of insufficient glucocorticoid signaling in the pathophysiology of stress-related disorders," *American Journal of Psychiatry* 160 (2003): 1554.

PAGE 62 The inefficiency of the repeated activation of the metabolic stress-response: this is horrendously complicated. The introductory reference given above will teach the general principle that it is inefficient to repeatedly store away energy and then reverse the process by mobilizing it. However, in order to gain a detailed, quantitative understanding of it, one must become something of an accountant—learning what the currency of energy is in the body and how much it costs to make all those deposits and withdrawals in the body's metabolic banks. For this, one must consult biochemistry texts (typically, of the early graduate school level of difficulty); among the best is Stryer, L., *Biochemistry*, 4th ed. (New York: W. H. Freeman, 1995).

PAGE 62 Chronic glucocorticoid exposure causes muscle wastage: for a classic demonstration of this, see Kaplan, S., and Nagareda Shimizu, C., "Effects of cortisol on amino acid in skeletal muscle and plasma," *Endocrinology* 72 (1963): 267. (Cortisol is the glucocorticoid found in humans and primates.) For some recent findings, see Hong, D., and Forsberg, N., "Effects of dexamethasone on protein degradation and protease gene expression in rat L8 myotube cultures," *Molecular and Cellular Endocrinology* 108 (1995): 199.

PAGE 63 Footnote: Stoney, C., West, S., "Lipids, personality, and stress: mechanisms and modulators," in Hillbrand, M., Spitz, R., eds., *Lipids and Human Behavior* (Washington, D.C.: APA Books, 1997).

PAGE 63 The workings of the two types of diabetes mellitus dominate chapters of every endocrinology textbook. For a review of the autoimmune features of insulin-dependent diabetes, see Andre, I., Gonzalez, A., Wang, B., Katz, J., Benoist, C., Mathis, D., "Checkpoints in the progression of autoimmune disease: lessons from diabetes models," *Proceedings of the National Academy of Sciences USA* 93 (1996): 2260. For a classic demonstration that type 2 (adult-onset) diabetes involves impaired sensitivity to insulin, rather than impaired secretion of insulin, see: Reaven, G., Bernstein, R., Davis, B., and Olefsky, J., "Nonketotic diabetes mellitus: insulin deficiency or insulin resistance?" *American Journal of Medicine* 60 (1976): 80. For demonstrations that the insulin resistance arises from a loss of insulin receptors see: Gavin, J., Roth, J., Neville, D., DeMeyts, P., and Buell, D., "Insulin-dependent regulation of insulin receptor concentrations: a direct demonstration in cell culture," *Proceedings of the National Academy of Sciences USA* 71 (1974): 84. For a discussion of how the insulin resistance also arises from the remaining insulin receptors' not working properly (what is called a "post-receptor" defect), see Flier, J., "Insulin receptors and insulin resistance," *Annual Review of Medicine* 34 (1983): 145. Finally, despite the primary defect of target tissue resistance to insulin's actions, a subset of patients also has a defect in the secretion of insulin. The mechanisms underlying this are reviewed by Unger, R., "Role of impaired glucose transport by cells in the pathogenesis of diabetes," *Journal of NIH Research* 3 (1991): 77.

PAGE 64 One of the puzzles of how diabetes affects your health has been solved. It is relatively easy to understand how extra glucose in the bloodstream can clog blood vessels and cause damage. One of the mysteries, however, is why high levels of circulating glucose damage the eye (diabetes is the leading cause of blindness in this country). It turns out that glucose can stick to all sorts of proteins, causing them to form aggregates; indeed, because of its structure, glucose can stick onto proteins without the aid of enzymes to mediate the process, something called nonenzymatic modification. Once glucose fuses these proteins, they have to be broken apart and replaced. However, in some tissues—such as the lens of the eye—proteins are not recycled very frequently, and those cells are stuck with the fused mess. For a discussion of the nonenzymatic chemistry of sugars, focusing on its implications for aging and adult-onset diabetes, see Lee, A., and Cerami, A., "Modifications of proteins and nucleic acids by reducing sugars: possible role in aging," in Schneider, E., and Rowe, J., eds., *Handbook of the Biology of Aging,* 3d ed. (New York: Academic Press, 1990).

Hyperglycemia can cause vascular damage even in nondiabetics: this is because of the nonenzymatic modification of glucose just discussed. See: Schmidt, A., Hori, O., Brett, J., Yan, S., Wautier, J., and Stern, D., "Cellular receptors for advanced glycation end products: implications for induction of oxidant stress and cellular dysfunction in the pathogenesis of vascular lesions," *Arteriosclerosis and Thrombosis* 14 (1994): 1521. For more mechanisms by which hyperglycemia can be damaging, see: Brownlee, M., "Biochemistry and molecular cell biology of diabetic complications," *Nature* 414 (2001): 813.

PAGE 64 Glucocorticoids promote insulin resistance: Rizza, R., Mandarino, L., and Gerich, J., "Cortisol-induced insulin resistance in man: impaired suppression of glucose production and stimulation of glucose utilization due to a postreceptor defect of insulin action," *Journal of Clinical Endocrinology and Metabolism* 54 (1982): 131. Stress promotes insulin resistance: Brandi, L., Santoro, D., Natali, A., Altomonte, F., Baldi, S., Frascerra, S., Ferrannini, E., "Insulin resistance of stress: sites and mechanisms," *Clinical Science* 85 (1993): 525.

PAGE 64 Fat cells releasing hormones that influence muscle and the liver: Saltiel, A., Kahn, C., "Insulin signaling and the regulation of glucose and lipid metabolism," *Nature* 414 (2001): 799; Steppan, C., Bailey, S., Bhat, S., Brown, E., Banerjee, R., Wright, C., Patel, H., Ahima, R., Lazar, M., "The hormone resistin links obesity to diabetes," *Nature* 409 (2001): 307; Abel, E., Peroni, O., Kim, J., Kim, Y., Boss, O., Hadro, E., Minnemann, T., Shulman, G., Kahn, B., "Adipose-selective targeting of the Glut4 gene impairs insulin action in muscle and liver," *Nature* 409 (2001): 729.

PAGE 65 Stress disrupts metabolic control in insulin-dependent diabetics: Moberg, E., Kollind, M., Lins, P., Adamson, U., "Acute mental stress impairs insulin sensitivity in IDDM patients" [IDDM means "insulin-dependent diabetes mellitus"], *Diabetologia* 37 (1994): 247. This presents a special challenge, in terms of stress management, for adolescents with insulin-dependent diabetes: Davidson, M., Boland, E., and Grey, M., "Teaching teens to cope: coping skills training for adolescents with insulin-dependent diabetes mellitus," *Journal of the Society of Pediatric Nurses* 2 (1997): 65. Controlled versus uncontrolled diabetics and stress: Dutour, A., Boiteau, V., Dadoun, F., Feissel, A., Atlan, C., and Oliver, C., "Hormonal response to stress in brittle diabetes," *Psychoneuroendocrinology* 21 (1996): 525.

PAGE 65 High blood glucose levels in people with the strongest emotional reactions to stressors: Stabler, B., Morris, M., Litton, J., Feinglos, M., Surwit, R., "Differential glycemic response to stress in Type A and Type B individuals with IDDM," *Diabetes Care* 9 (1986): 550.

PAGE 65 Stressors preceding diabetes onset: Robinson, N., Fuller, J., "Role of life events and difficulties in the onset of diabetes mellitus," *Journal of Psychosomatic Research* 29 (1985): 583.

PAGE 66 In westernized societies, rates of glucose intolerance and insulin resistance rise with age: Andres, R., "Aging and diabetes," *Medical Clinics of North*

America 55 (1971): 835; Davidson, M., "The effect of aging on carbohydrate metabolism: a review of the English literature and a practical approach to the diagnosis of diabetes mellitus in the elderly," *Metabolism* 28 (1979): 687.

Insulin-resistant diabetes seems not to be an obligatory part of aging: aging rats and aging humans in our own society do not become more glucose-intolerant with age, so long as they are active and lean: Reaven, G., and Reaven, E., "Age, glucose intolerance and non-insulin-dependent diabetes mellitus," *Journal of the American Geriatrics Society* 33 (1985): 286. Also see Goldberg, A., and Coon, P., "Non-insulin-dependent diabetes mellitus in the elderly: influence of obesity and physical inactivity," *Endocrinology and Metabolism Clinics* 16 (1987): 843.

PAGE 66 Fat cells become less responsive to insulin: Hirosumi, J., Tuncman, G., Chang, L., Gorgun, C., Uysal, K., Maeda, K., Karin, M., Hotamisligil, G., "A central role for JNK in obesity and insulin resistance," *Nature* 420 (2002): 333; Santaniemi, M., "Adiponectin: a link between excess adiposity and associated co-morbidities?" *Journal of Molecular Medicine* 80 (2002): 696; Alper, J., "New insights into type 2 diabetes," *Science* 289 (2000): 37.

PAGE 66 Juvenile diabetes triggered by adult-onset diabetes. The mechanisms by which this might happen can be found in: Bell, G., Polonsky, K., "Diabetes mellitus and genetically programmed defects in B-cell function," *Nature* 414 (2001): 788; Mathis, D., Vence, L., Benoist, C., "B-cell death during progression to diabetes," *Nature* 414 (2001): 792.

PAGE 67 Glucocorticoids and stress can exacerbate the symptoms of insulin-resistant diabetes: Surwit, R., Ross, S., and Feingloss, M., "Stress, behavior, and glucose control in diabetes mellitus," in McCabe, P., Schneidermann, N., Field, T., and Skyler, J., eds., *Stress, Coping and Disease* (Hillsdale, N.J.: L. Erlbaum Assoc., 1991), 97; Surwit, R., and Williams, P., "Animal models provide insight into psychosomatic factors in diabetes," *Psychosomatic Medicine* 58 (1996): 582. For a study that does not show an association between stress and worsening of symptoms, see Pipernik-Okanovic, M., Roglic, G., Prasek, M., and Metelko, Z., "War-induced prolonged stress and metabolic control in type 2 diabetic patients," *Psychological Medicine* 23 (1993): 645.

PAGE 67 Stress causes insulin resistance and metabolic imbalances even in non-diabetics: Raikkonen, K., Keltikangas-Jarvinen, L., Adlercreutz, H., and Hautanen, A., "Psychosocial stress and the insulin resistance syndrome," *Metabolism: Clinical and Experimental* 45 (1996): 1533; Nilsson, P., Moller, L., Solstad, K., "Adverse effects of psychosocial stress on gonadal function and insulin levels in middle-aged males," *Journal of Internal Medicine* 237 (1995): 479.

Stress worsens metabolic control in nondiabetics who are at genetic risk for diabetes: Esposito-Del Puente, A., Lillioja, S., Bogardus, C., McCubbin, J., Feinglos, M., Kuhn, C., and Surwit, R., "Glycemic response to stress is altered in euglycemic Pima Indians," *International Journal of Obesity and Related Metabolic Disorders* 18 (1994): 766.

PAGE 67 The epidemic of adult-onset diabetes: Wickelgren, I., "Obesity: how big a problem?" *Science* 280 (1998): 1364; Friedman, J., "A war on obesity, not the obese," *Science* 299 (2003): 856; *Time,* cover story (4 September 2000).

PAGE 68 Cultural reasons for the onset of diabetes with a westernized diet: Sterling, P., "Principles of allostasis: optimal design, predictive regulation, pathophysiology and rational therapeutics," in Schulkin, J., ed., *Allostasis, Homeostasis, and the Costs of Adaptation* (Cambridge, Mass.: MIT Press, 2003).

PAGE 68 Genetic reasons for the onset of diabetes with a westernized diet: for a demonstration of extremely low rates of insulin-resistant diabetes in nonwesternized populations, for example, the Inuit and other Native Americans, New Guinea islanders, inhabitants of rural India, and North African nomads, see table 5 in Eaton, S., Konner, M., and Shostak, M., "Stone agers in the fast lane: chronic degenerative diseases in evolutionary perspective," *American Journal of Medicine* 84 (1988): 739.

The low rates of insulin-resistant diabetes in nonwesternized populations pose a fascinating mystery. If these people begin eating westernized diets, they get astonishingly high rates of insulin-resistant diabetes. Part of this has an obvious explanation; once these various groups gain entrée into our world of packaged food and processed sugars, they tend to eat themselves into obesity (and, thus, high rates of this diabetes). However, the mystery is that given the same diet and degree of obesity, most people in the developing world are at greater risk for such diabetes than people in Western societies. Diabetes rates soar among Mexicans and Japanese after they emigrate to the United States, among Asian Indians moving to Britain, and among Yemenite Jews moving to Israel. In the most striking cases, about half the adult residents of the Pacific island of Nauru have diabetes (fifteen times the rate in the United States), while more than 70 percent of the Pima people of Arizona over age fifty-five have diabetes. In the absence of a Western diet, there is virtually no diabetes—as a striking correlate of this, Pima in Arizona weigh an average of 60 pounds more than Pima living in Mexico, with a more traditional diet. Kopelman, P., "Obesity as a medical problem," *Nature* 404 (2000): 635.

Why should those in the developing world be at such risk for diabetes once they start consuming a Western diet? One fascinating theory is that the gene for a propensity to diabetes is adaptive in nonwesternized settings. Normally, westerners are inefficient at handling dietary sugar; not all of it is absorbed from the circulation, getting lost in the urine. The notion is that people of the developing world are more efficient at utilizing sugar; the second they get any in their circulation, they have a burst of insulin secretion and every bit of the sugar gets stored, instead of urinated away. This makes sense, given tough environments with intermittent food sources, where every little bit must be exploited. And it is easy to imagine this as a genetic trait—for example, genes might alter the sensitivity with which the pancreas senses circulating glucose concentrations and releases insulin, or the sensitivity with which target tissues respond to insulin. These have been termed "thrifty genes," and at least one such candidate in fat cells has been found to have a mutation among Pima Indians. Reviewed in Ezzell, C., "Fat times for obesity research," *Journal of NIH Research* 7, no. 10 (1995): 39. Another has been related to cholesterol transport in populations in northern India (Holden, C., "Race and medicine," *Science* 302 [2003]: 594.)

With traditional diets in the developing world, this trigger-happy insulin secretion keeps the body from wasting any sugar. Once people begin eating a westernized, high-sugar diet, this tendency leads to constant bursts of insulin secretion, which is more likely to cause storage tissues to become insulin resistant, leading to insulin-resistant diabetes. People in Western countries, in contrast, are theorized to have more sluggish insulin responses to sugar; the net result is less efficient storing of sugar from the circulation, but lower risk of diabetes. And why are people in westernized societies theorized to be genetically less efficient in handling blood sugar? Because a few centuries back, as we first began eating typical westernized diets, those people with the greatest tendency toward insulin secretion failed to survive and pass on their genes. This predicts that populations like the Nauru islanders and Pima are undergoing the same process now; in a few centuries, most of their descendants will be the offspring of the rare individuals now with the lower diabetes risk. In support of this prediction, the rate of diabetes is already beginning to decline among the Nauru islanders. Diamond, J., "The double puzzle of diabetes," *Nature* 423 (2003): 599.

But at present the existence of thrifty genes, and their differential presence in different human populations, is mostly speculative. For a nontechnical discussion of these ideas, see Diamond, J., "Sweet death," *Natural History* (February 1992): 2. For technical discussions from the originator of the idea, see Neel, J., "Diabetes mellitus: a 'thrifty' genotype rendered detrimental by 'progress'?" *American Journal of Human Genetics* 14 (1962): 353; Neel, J., "The thrifty genotype revisited," in Kobberling, J., and Tattersall, R., eds., *The Genetics of Diabetes Mellitus* (London: Academic Press, Proceedings of the Serono Symposia, 1982), vol. 47, 283. For some technical discussions of the change in the incidence of diabetes with westernization, see Bennett, P., LeCompte, P., Miller, M., and Rushforth, N., "Epidemiological studies of diabetes in the Pima Indians," *Recent Progress in Hormone Research* 32 (1976): 333; O'Dea, K., Spargo, R., and Nestle, P., "Impact of westernization on carbohydrate and lipid metabolism in Australian Aborigines," *Diabetologia* 22 (1976): 148; Cohen, A., Chen, B., Eisenberg, S., Fidel, J., and Furst, A., "Diabetes, blood lipids, lipoproteins and change of environment: restudy of the 'new immigrant Yemenites' in Israel," *Metabolism* 28 (1979): 716. For information on the rate of diabetes having peaked among the Nauru islanders, see Diamond, J., "Diabetes running wild," *Nature* 357 (1992): 362. For a discussion of other cases of thrifty genes, see the chapter, "The Dangers of Fallen Soufflés in the Developing World," in Sapolsky, R., *"The Trouble with Testosterone" and Other Essays on the Biology of the Human Predicament* (New York: Scribner, 1997). And for evidence of the "thriftiness" of metabolism among people such as Nauru islanders, see Robinson, S., Johnston, D., "Advantage of diabetes?" *Nature* 375 (1995): 640.

PAGE 68 For a general review of Metabolic syndrome, see: Zimmel, P., Alberti, K., Shaw, J., "Global and societal implications of the diabetes epidemic," *Nature* 414 (2001): 782. Metabolic syndrome in baboons: Banks, W., Altmann, J., Sapolsky, R., Phillips-Conroy, J., Morley J., "Serum leptin levels as a marker for a Syndrome X-like condition in wild baboons," *Journal of Clinical Endocrinology and Metabolism* 88 (2003): 1234.

PAGE 68 Sterling, "Principles of allostasis," in *Allostasis,* op. cit.

PAGE 69 The interrelationship of risk factors in Metabolic syndrome: Vitaliano, P., Scanlan, J., Zhang, J., Savage, M., Hirsch, I., Siegler, I., "A path model of chronic stress, the metabolic syndrome, and CHD," *Psychosomatic Medicine* 64 (2002): 418–35.

PAGE 69 The Seeman study: Seeman, T., McEwen, B., Rowe, J., Singer, B., "Allostatic load as a marker of cumulative biological risk: MacArthur studies of successful aging," *Proceedings of the National Academy of Sciences, USA* 98 (2001): 4770.

CHAPTER 5: ULCERS, THE RUNS, AND HOT FUDGE SUNDAES

PAGE 71 Elevated stress-response in anorexia: Jimerson, D., "Eating disorders and stress," in Fink, G., ed., *Encyclopedia of Stress* (San Diego: Academic Press, 2000), vol. 2, 4.

PAGE 72 The effects of CRH in the brain including the effect on appetite and feeding: Turnbull, A., and Rivier, C., "CRF and endocrine responses to stress; CRF receptors, binding protein, and related peptides," *Proceedings of the Society for Experimental Biology and Medicine* 215 (1997): 1. The effects of glucocorticoids on appetite are discussed in McEwen, B., de Kloet, E., and Rostene, W., "Adrenal steroid receptors and actions in the nervous system," *Physiological Reviews* 66 (1986): 1121. I am not aware of any publication in which the opposing effects of CRF and glucocorticoids on appetite are analyzed in the manner done in this chapter. However, a similar flavor (viewing some glucocorticoid actions as mediating the "recovery" from the stress-response, rather than the "mediation" of the stress-response) can be found in a very influential paper: Munck, A., Guyre, P., and Holbrook, N., "Physiological functions of glucocorticoids during stress and their relation to pharmacological actions," *Endocrine Reviews* 5 (1984): 25. Some examples of glucocorticoids increasing transcription of the ob gene and increasing circulating leptin levels: Reul, B., Ongemba, L., Pottier, A., Henquin, J., and Brichard, S., "Insulin and insulin-like growth factor I antagonize the stimulation of ob gene expression by dexamethasone in cultured rat adipose tissue," *Biochemical Journal* 324 (1997): 605; Considine, R., Nyce, M., Kolaczynski, J., Zhang, P., Ohannesian, J., Moore, J., Fox, J., and Caro, J., "Dexamethasone stimulates leptin release from human adipocytes: unexpected inhibition by insulin," *Journal of Cellular Biochemistry* 65 (1997): 254; Miell, J., Englaro, P., and Blum, W., "Dexamethasone induces an acute and sustained rise in circulating leptin levels in normal human subjects," *Hormone and Metabolic Research* 28 (1996): 704. Glucocorticoids blunt the efficacy of leptin: Zakrzewska, K., Cusin, I., Sainsbury, A., Rohner-Jeanrenaud, F., and Jeanrenaud, B., "Glucocorticoids as counterregulatory hormones of leptin: toward an understanding of leptin resistance," *Diabetes* 46 (1997): 717. Chronic glucocorticoid exposure might cause leptin resistance: Ur, E., Grossman, A., and Despres, J., "Obesity results as a consequence of glucocorticoid induced leptin resistance," *Hormones and Metabolic Research* 28 (1997): 744.

PAGE 72 Glucocorticoids and appetite: Dallman, M., Pecoraro, N., Akana, S., le Fleur, S., Gomez, F., Houshyar, H., Bell, M., Bhatnagar, S., Laugero, K., Manalo, S., "Chronic stress and obesity: a new view of 'comfort food,'" *Proceedings of the National Academy of Sciences, USA* 100 (2003): 11696.

PAGE 73 Beta-endorphins increase appetite: Smith, K., Goodwin, G., "Food intake and stress, human," in Fink, G., ed., *Encyclopedia of Stress* (New York: Academic Press, 2000), vol. 2, 158.

PAGE 75 Epel's work: Epel, E., Lapidus, R., McEwen, B., Brownell, K., "Stress may add bite to appetite in women: a laboratory study of stress-induced cortisol and eating behavior," *Psychoneuroendocrinology* 26 (2000): 37.

PAGE 75 Emotional eaters: Greeno, C., Wing, R., "Stress-induced eating," *Psychological Bulletin* 115 (1994): 444. Restrained eaters and stress: Bjorntorp, P., "Behavior and metabolic disease," *International Journal of Behavioral Medicine* 3 (1997): 285.

PAGE 76 Glucocorticoids promote apple-shaped obesity: Rebuffe-Scrive, M., "Steroid hormones and distribution of adipose tissue," *Acta Medical Scandinavia* 723 (1998): supp. 143; including in monkeys: Jayo, J., Shively, C., Kaplan, J., Manuck, S., "Effects of exercise and stress on body fat distribution in male cynomologus monkeys," *International Journal of Obstetrics Related to Metabolic Disorders* 17 (1993): 597. Glucocorticoid receptor patterns in fat cells: Rebuffe-Scrive, M., Bronnegard, M., Nilsson, A., Eldh, J., Gustafsson, J., Bjorntorp, P., "Steroid hormone receptors in human adipose tissues," *Journal of Clinical Endocrinology and Metabolism* 71 (1990): 1215.

PAGE 77 Applish people preferentially at disease risk: Welin, L., Svardsudd, K., Wilhelmsen, L., Larsson, B., Tibblin, G., "Family history and other risk factors for stroke: the study of men born 1913," *New England Journal of Medicine* 317 (1987): 521.

PAGE 78 Prolonged glucocorticoid secretion in applish people: Epel, E., McEwen, B., Seeman, T., Matthews, K., Castellazzo, G., Brownell, K., Bell, J., Ickovics, J., "Stress and body shape: stress-induced cortisol secretion is consistently greater among women with central fat," *Psychosomatic Medicine* 62 (2000): 623. There may also be a subset of applish people with normal glucocorticoid profiles, but abdominal fat cells that, for a peculiar reason, generate excessive glucocorticoids locally: Masuzaki, M., Paterson, J., Shinyama, H., Morton, N., Mullins, J., Seckl, J., Flier, J., "A transgenic model of visceral obesity and the metabolic syndrome," *Science* 294 (2001): 2166. So a different mechanism but the same involvement of excessive glucocorticoids. And there may also be applish people with normal glucocorticoid levels but with a genetic variant of glucocorticoid receptor that increases its sensitivity to the hormone: Tremblay, A., Bouchard, L., Bouchard, C., Despres, J. P., Drapeau, V., Perusse, L., "Long-term adiposity changes are related to a glucocorticoid receptor polymorphism in young females," *Journal of Clinical Endocrinology and Metabolism* 88 (2003): 3141.

PAGE 78 Dallman, M., et al. "Chronic stress and obesity," *Proceedings of the National Academy of Sciences,* op. cit.

PAGE 78 Footnote: some of these new, exotic hormones: Gura, T., "Uncoupling proteins provide new clue to obesity's causes," *Science* 280 (1998): 1369; Comuzzie, A., Allison, D., "The search for human obesity genes," *Science* 280 (1998): 1374; Schwartz, M., Woods, S., Porte, D., Seeley, R., Baskin, D., "Central nervous system control of food intake," *Nature* 404 (2000): 661; Broglio, F., Gottero, C. Arvat, E., Ghigo, E., "Endocrine and non-endocrine actions of ghrelin.1," *Hormone Research* 59 (2003): 109; Fu, J., Gaetani, S., Oveisi, F., et al., "Oleylethanolamide regulates feeding and body weight through activation of the nuclear receptor PPAR-alpha," *Nature* 425 (2003): 90.

PAGE 79 The cost of digestion: Secor, S., and Diamond, J., *Journal of Experimental Biology* 198 (1995): 1313. Those authors also report that animals that really do some energetic digesting—such as pythons and boa constrictors, who may swallow up some antelope far larger than themselves and spend the next week digesting it—use a third of their calories on the process.

PAGE 79 Stressors tend to inhibit gastrointestinal function: Desiderato, O., MacKinnon, J., and Hissom, R., "Development of gastric ulcers following stress termination," *Journal of Comparative and Physiological Psychology* 87 (1974): 208;

Hess, W., *Diencephalon; Autonomic and Extrapyramidal Functions* (New York: Grune and Stratton, 1957); Kiely, W., "From the symbolic stimulus to the pathophysiological response," in Lipowski, Z., Lipsitt, D., and Whybrow, P., eds., *Current Trends and Clinical Applications* (New York: Oxford University Press, 1977); Murison, R., and Bakke, H., "The role of corticotropin-releasing factor in rat gastric ulcerogenesis," in Hernandez, D., and Glavin, G., eds., *Neurobiology of Stress Ulcers* (New York: Annals of the New York Academy of Sciences, 1990), vol. 597, 71; Tache, Y., "Effect of stress on gastric ulcer formation," in Brown, M., Koob, G., and Rivier, C., eds., *Stress: Neurobiology and Neuroendocrinology* (New York: Marcel Dekker, 1991), 549.

PAGE 79 Stress decreases contractions in the small intestines: Thompson, D., Richelson, E., and Malagelada, J., "Perturbation of gastric emptying and duodenal motility through the central nervous system," *Gastroenterology* 83 (1982): 1200; Thompson, D., Richelson, E., and Malagelada, J., "Perturbation of upper gastrointestinal function by cold stress," *Gut* 24 (1983): 277; O'Brien, J., Thompson, D., Holly, J., Burnham, W., and Walker, E., "Stress disturbs human gastrointestinal transit via a beta-1 adrenoreceptor mediated pathway," *Gastroenterology* 88 (1985): 1520. Stress increases contractions in the large intestines: Almy, T., "Experimental studies on irritable colon," *American Journal of Medicine* 10 (1951): 60; Almy, T., and Tulin, M., "Alterations in colonic function in man under stress: experimental production of changes simulating the 'irritable colon,'" *Gastroenterology* 8 (1947): 616; Narducci, F., Snape, W., Battle, W., London, R., and Cohen, S., "Increased colonic motility during exposure to a stressful situation," *Digestive Disease Science* 30 (1985): 40.

PAGE 80 Chemical mediators of the sympathetic stress-response bring about the changes in contractions: Williams, C., Peterson, J., Villar, R., and Burks, T., "Corticotropin-releasing factor directly mediates colonic responses to stress," *American Journal of Physiology* 253 (1987): G582. Also Burks, T., "Central nervous system regulation of gastrointestinal motility," in Hernandez, D., and Glavin, G., eds., *Neurobiology of Stress Ulcers* (New York: Annals of the New York Academy of Sciences, 1990), vol. 597, 36. Glucocorticoids are not mediators of the contractions: Williams, C., Villar, R., Peterson, J., and Burks, T., "Stress-induced changes in intestinal transit in the rat: a model for irritable bowel syndrome," *Gastroenterology* 94 (1988): 611.

PAGE 80 Mayer, E., "The neurobiology of stress and gastrointestinal disease," *Gut* 47 (2000): 861.

PAGE 81 Stress and IBS: Whitehead, W., Crowell, M., Robinson, J., "Effects of stressful life events on bowel symptoms: subjects with irritable bowel syndrome compared with subjects without bowel dysfunction," *Gut* 33 (1992): 825; Bennett, E., Tennant, C., Piesse, C., "Level of chronic life stress predicts clinical outcome in irritable bowel syndrome," *Gut* 43 (1998): 256; Gwee, K., "The role of psychological and biological factors in postinfective gut dysfunction," *Gut* 44 (1999): 400; Stamm, R., Akkermans, L., Wiegant, V., "Interactions between stressful experience and intestinal function," *Gut* 40 (1997): 704.

PAGE 82 No gut contractions in IBS during sleep: Murison, R., "Gastrointestinal effects," in Fink, G., ed., *Encyclopedia of Stress* (San Diego: Academic Press, 2000), vol. 2, 191.

PAGE 83 IBS and sympathetic nervous system activity: Heitkemper, M., Jarrett, M., Cain, K., "Increased urine catecholamines and cortisol in women with irritable bowel syndrome," *American Journal of Gastroenterology* 91 (1996): 906. Confusion about glucocorticoids levels: Heitkemper, ibid.; Munakata, J., Mayer, E., Chang, L., "Autonomic and neuroendocrine responses to recto-sigmoid stimulation," *Gastroenterology* 114 (1998): 808.

PAGE 83 Traumatic stress early in life increases the risk of IBS in adulthood: Drossman, D., Talley, N., Leserman, J., "Sexual and physical abuse and gastrointestinal illness: review and recommendations," *Annals of Internal Medicine* 123 (1995): 782; Walker, E., Katon, W., Roy-Byrne, P., "Histories of sexual victimization in patients with irritable bowel syndrome or inflammatory bowel disease," *American Journal of Psychiatry* 150 (1993): 1502.

PAGE 83 For the classic psychoanalytic view of these diseases, see Alexander, F., *Psychosomatic Medicine* (New York: W. W. Norton, 1950). See also Aronowitz, R., and Spiro, H., "The rise and fall of the psychosomatic hypothesis in ulcerative colitis," *Journal of Clinical Gastroenterology* 10 (1988): 298; Ramchandani, D., Schindler, B., and Katz, J., "Evolving concepts of psychopathology in inflammatory bowel disease," *Medical Clinics of North America* 78 (1994): 1321.

PAGE 83 Some studies that have not found a stress link in colitis (note that the first two studies are from the same group): Helzer, J., Stillings, W., and Chammas, S., "A controlled study of the association between ulcerative colitis and psychiatric diagnoses," *Digestive Disease Science* 27 (1982): 513. North, C., Alpers, D., and Helzer, J., "Do life events or depression exacerbate inflammatory bowel disease? A prospective study," *Annals of Internal Medicine* 114 (1991): 381. Tartar, R., Switala, J., and Carra, J., "Inflammatory bowel disease: psychiatric status of patients before and after disease onset," *International Journal of Psych Medicine* 17 (1987): 173; Drossman, D., McKee, D., and Sandler, R., "Psychosocial factors in the irritable bowel syndrome: a multivariate study of patients and nonpatients with irritable bowel syndrome," *Gastroenterology* 95 (1988): 701; Camilleri, M., and Neri, M., "Motility disorders and stress," *Digestive Disease Science* 34 (1989): 1777.

PAGE 83 A study using time-series analysis to show a stress-symptom link: Greene, B., Blanchard, E., and Wan, C., "Long-term monitoring of psychosocial stress and symptomatology in inflammatory bowel disease," *Behaviour Research and Therapy* 32 (1994): 217. A discussion of some of the methodological problems in stress research in this area: Whitehead, W., "Assessing the effects of stress on physical symptoms," *Health Psychology* 13 (1994): 99. People are bad at accurately reporting events more than three months old: Jenkins, C., Hurst, W., and Rose, R., "Life changes: do people really remember?" *Archives of General Psychiatry* 36 (1979): 379.

PAGE 84 Selye was the first to note that stress could cause peptic ulcers ("A syndrome produced by diverse nocuous agents," *Nature* 138 [1936]: 32). The first researchers to systematically explore the role of psychological stress in causing ulcers were Brady, J., Porter, D., Conrad, D., and Mason, J., "Avoidance behavior and the development of gastroduodenal ulcers," *Journal of Experimental Analysis of Behavior* 1 (1958): 69; and Weiss, J., "Effects of coping responses on stress," *Journal of Comparative and Physiological Psychology* 65 (1968): 251.

The evidence that major and short-term traumas in humans can cause rapidly emerging stress ulcers can be found in Skillman, J., Bushnell, L., Goldman, H., and Silen, W., "Respiratory failure, hypotension, sepsis, and jaundice: a clinical syndrome associated with lethal hemorrhage from acute stress ulceration of the stomach," *American Journal of Surgery* 117 (1969): 523; Lucas, C., Sugawa, C., Riddle, J., Rector, F., Rosenberg, B., and Walt, A., "Natural history and surgical dilemma of 'stress' gastric bleeding," *Archives of Surgery* 102 (1971): 266; Butterfield, W., "Experimental stress ulcers: a review," *Surgical Annual* 7 (1975): 261. For evidence that more subtle psychological stress can cause gradually emerging peptic ulcers in humans, see Feldman, M., Walker, P., Green, J., and Weingarden, K., "Life events, stress and psychosocial factors in men with peptic ulcer disease: a multidimensional case-controlled study," *Gastroenterology* 91 (1986): 1370. Also see Weiner, H., *Perturbing the Organism: The Biology of Stressful Experience* (Chicago: University of Chicago Press, 1992).

PAGE 85 The bacteria-ulcer revolution: Warren, J., Marshall, B., "Unidentified curved bacilli on gastric epithelium in active chronic gastritis," *The Lancet* 1 (1983): 1273. Also, Wyatt, J., Rathbone, B., Dixon, M., and Heatley, R., "Campylobacter pylorides and acid induced gastric metaplasia in the pathogenesis of duodenitis," *Journal of Clinical Pathology* 40 (1987): 841. (Campylobacter pylorides was an earlier name for Helicobacter). Dooley, C., and Cohen, H., "The clinical significance of Campylobacter pylori," *Annals of Internal Medicine* 108 (1988): 70. For a breathless account of the discovery with Marshall (and occasionally Warren) as the heroic underdogs, see Monmaney, T., "Marshall's hunch," *The New Yorker* (20 September 1993): 64. The bacteria's resistance to acidity: Doolittle, R., "A bug with excess gastric avidity," *Nature* 388 (1997): 515; Tom, J., White, O., Kerlavage, A., et al. [there's a total of 42 authors—no kidding], "The complete genome sequence of the gastric pathogen Helicobacter pylori," *Nature* 388 (1997): 539.

PAGE 86 The efficacy of antibiotics with duodenal ulcers is reviewed in Konturek, P., "Physiological, immunohistochemical and molecular aspects of gastric adaptation to stress, aspiring and to H. pylori-derived gastrotoxins," *Journal of Physiology and Pharmacology* 48 (1997): 3.

PAGE 87 The decline of ulcer-stress research: Melmed, R., and Gelpin, Y., "Duodenal ulcer: the helicobacterization of a psychosomatic disease?" *Israeli Journal of Medical Science* 32 (1996): 211. The CDC's mailing: Levenstein, S., "Stress and peptic ulcer: life beyond Helicobacter," *British Medical Journal* 316 (1998): 538. Ulcers, but no bacteria: McColl, K., El-Nujami, A., and Chittajallu, R., "A study of the pathogenesis of Helicobacter pylori negative chronic duodenal ulceration," *Gut* 34 (1993): 762. Bacteria but no ulcers: Tompkins, L., and Falkow, S., "The new path to preventing ulcers," *Science* 267 (1995): 1621.

PAGE 87 Stress as an additional factor: Levenstein, S., "Stress and peptic ulcer," *British Medical Journal* 316 (1998): 538; Aoymama, N., Kinoshita, Y., Fujimoto, S., Himeno, S., Todo, A., Kasuga, M., Chiba, T., "Peptide ulcers after the Hanshin-Awaji earthquake: increased incidence of bleeding gastric ulcers," *American Journal of Gastroenterology* 93 (1998): 311.

PAGE 88 The rodent studies showing no bacteria, no stress ulcers: Pare, W., Burken, M., Allen, E., and Kluczynski, J., "Reduced incidence of stress ulcer in germ-free Sprague Dawley rats," *Life Sciences* 53 (1993): 1099. The interactions of stress, bacterial load, and other risk factors in human ulcer cases: Levenstein, S., Prantera, C., Varvo, V., Scribano, M., Berto, E., Spinella, S., and Lanari, G., "Patterns of biologic and psychologic risk factors in duodenal ulcer patients," *Journal of Clinical Gastroenterology* 21 (1995): 110.

PAGE 88 Stress-related ulcers are predominantly formed during the poststress recovery period, rather than during the stressor itself: Overmier, J., Murison, R., and Ursin, H., "The ulcerogenic effect of a rest period after exposure to water-restraint stress," *Behavioral and Neural Biology* 46 (1986): 372; Vincent, G., and Pare, W., "Post stress development and healing of supine-restraint induced stomach lesions in the rat," *Physiology and Behavior* 29 (1982): 721; Desiderato, O., MacKin-non, J., and Hissom, H., "Development of gastric ulcers in rats following stress termination," *Journal of Comparative and Physiological Psychology* 87 (1974): 208; Glavin, G., "Restraint ulcer: history, current research and future implications," *Brain Research Bulletin* 5 (1980): supp. 1, 51. For the evidence for how this is due to rebound of the parasympathetic nervous system, see the Glavin paper just cited; also see Klein, H., Gheorghiu, T., and Hubner, G., "Morphological and functional gastric changes in stress ulcer," in Gheorghiu, T., ed., *Experimental Ulcer: Models, Methods and Clinical Validity* (Baden-Baden: Witzstrock, 1975).

Back to hydrochloric acid digesting the stomach in which it is secreted: if the mucous layer prevents the acid from penetrating it, how can acid, first secreted by the stomach wall, ever get through the mucous layer to digest food? This conundrum is answered by Bhaskar, K., Garik, P., Turner, B., Bradley, J., Bansil, R., Stanley, H., and Lamont, J., "Viscous fingering of hydrochloric acid through gastric mucin," *Nature* 360 (1992): 458.

Bicarbonate secretion decreases in ulcer patients: Isenberg, J., Selling, J., Hogan, D., and Koss, M., "Impaired proximal duodenal mucosal bicarbonate secretion in duodenal ulcer patients," *New England Journal of Medicine* 316 (1987): 374. Bicarbonate secretion decreases with sustained stress in an animal ulcer model: Takeuchi, K., Furukawa, O., and Okabe, S., "Induction of duodenal ulcers in rats under water-immersion stress conditions: influence on gastric acid and duodenal alkaline secretion," *Gastroenterology* 91 (1986): 554. Mucus secretion decreases with stress and with glucocorticoid administration: Schuster, M., "Irritable bowel syndrome," in Sleisenger, M., and Fordtron, J., eds., *Gastrointestinal Disease: Pathophysiology, Diagnosis, Management*, 4th ed. (Philadelphia: Saunders, 1989), 1402. In approximately half the cases, during this rebound period the amount of gastric acid secreted is normal, implying that the problem is that the stomach wall is relatively more vulnerable, since the acidic attack is not stronger than usual: Dayal, Y., and DeLellis, R., "The gastrointestinal tract," in Robbins, S., Cotran, R., and Kumar, V., eds., *Pathologic Basis of Disease*, 4th ed. (Philadelphia: Saunders, 1989), 827; also Weiner, H., "From simplicity to complexity (1950–1990): the case of peptic ulceration—I. Human studies," *Psychosomatic Medicine* 53 (1991): 467; and Weiner, H., "From simplicity to complexity (1950–1990): the case of peptic ulceration—II. Animal studies," *Psychosomatic Medicine* 53 (1991): 491; Grossman, M., "Abnormalities of acid secretion in patients with duodenal ulcer," *Gastroenterology* 75 (1978): 524; also Brodie, D., Marshall, R., and Moreno, O., "The effect of restraint on gastric acidity in the rat," *American Journal of Physiology* 202 (1962): 812.

As noted, an interesting implication of the rebound phenomenon is that in a person at risk for a stress ulcer, continuous stress may protect against the formation of an ulcer (although, as noted, this is not a good prescriptive idea for many other reasons). As a building block of that idea, sustained administration of CRH will protect against ulcer formation: Murison, R., and Bakke, H., "The role of corticotropin-releasing factor in rat gastric ulcerogenesis," in Hernandez, D., and Glavin, G., eds., *Neurobiology of Stress Ulcers* (New York: Annals of the New York Academy of Sciences, 1990), vol. 597, 71.

PAGE 89 Ulcers form as a result of decreased blood flow to the stomach, causing ischemic lesions, due to both acid accumulation and to formation of oxygen radicals. These ideas are reviewed in Tsuda, A., and Tanaka, M., "Neurochemical characteristics of rats exposed to activity stress," in Hernandez, D., and Glavin, G., eds., *Neurobiology of Stress Ulcers*, op. cit., vol. 597, 146; also Yabana, T., and Yachi, A., "Stress-induced vascular damage and ulcer," *Digestive Disease Science* 33 (1988): 751; also Menguy, R., "The prophylaxis of stress ulceration," *New England Journal of Medicine* 302 (1980): 461; also Robert, A., and Kauffman, G., "Stress ulcers, erosions and gastric motility injury," in Sleisenger, M., and Fordtron, J., eds., *Gastrointestinal Disease: Pathophysiology, Diagnosis, Management*, 4th ed. (Philadelphia: Saunders, 1989), 1402. Original data regarding how hemorrhage stress can cause oxidative damage: Itoh, M., and Guth, P., "Role of oxygen-derived free radicals in hemorrhagic shock-induced gastric lesions in the rat," *Gastroenterology* 88 (1985): 1162.

PAGE 90 Although glucocorticoids may cause ulcer formation by suppressing the immune system during stress via this route, it is not clear how important this is for mild stressors. During mild or infrequent stressors, the levels of glucocorticoids secreted do not predict whether ulcers form: Murison, R., and Overmeir, J., "Adrenocortical activity and disease, with reference to gastric pathology in animals," in Hellhammer, D., Florin, I., and Weiner, H., eds., *Neurobiological Approaches to Human Disease* (Toronto: Hans Huber, 1988), 335. Moreover, removal of glucocorticoids by adrenalectomizing a rat actually protects against ulcers: Brodie, D., "Experimental peptic ulcer," *Gastroenterology* 55 (1968): 125.

All this suggests that glucocorticoids are unlikely to be the cause of ulcers during stress. However, with more sustained or repeated stressors, the amount of glucocorticoids secreted does predict the severity of ulceration: Weiss, J., "Somatic effects of predictable and unpredictable shock," *Psychosomatic Medicine* 32 (1980): 397; Weiss, J., "Effects of coping behavior in different warning signal conditions on stress pathology in rats," *Journal of Comparative and Physiological Psychology* 77 (1981): 1; Murphy, H., Wideman, C., and Brown, T., "Plasma corticosterone levels and ulcer formation in rats with hippocampal lesions," *Neuroendocrinology* 28 (1979): 123. In addition, supraphysiological levels of glucocorticoids (levels that are higher in the bloodstream than the body can normally generate, even during stress, but are induced by taking glucocorticoid medication) can cause ulcers: Robert, A., and Nezmis, J., "Histopathology of steroid-induced ulcers: an experimental study in the rat," *Archives of Pathology* 77 (1964): 407.

Footnote regarding speculations about the benefits of *Helicobacter*: Whitfield, J., "Gut reaction," *Nature* 423 (2003): 583.

PAGE 90 The role of prostaglandins in ulcerogenesis: the protective effects of prostaglandins are discussed in Kauffman, G., Zhang, L., Xing, L., Seaton, J., Colony, P., and Demers, L., "Central neurotensin protects the mucosa by a prostaglandin-mediated mechanism and inhibits gastric acid secretion in the rat," in Hernandez, D., and Glavin, G., eds., *Neurobiology of Stress Ulcers* (New York: Annals of the New York Academy of Sciences, 1990), vol. 597, 175. See also Schepp, W., Steffen, B., Ruoff, H., Schusdziarra, V., and Classen, M., "Modulation of rat gastric mucosal prostaglandin E2 release by dietary linoleic acid: effects on gastric acid secretion and stress-induced mucosal damage," *Gastroenterology* 95 (1988): 18.

Aspirin is ulcerogenic by blocking prostaglandin synthesis: Adcock, J., Hernandez, D., Nemeroff, C., and Prang, A., "Effect of prostaglandin synthesis inhibitors on neurotensin and sodium salicylate-induced gastric cytoprotection in rats," *Life Science* 32 (1983): 2905. Glucocorticoids block prostaglandin synthesis: Flowers, R., and Blackwell, G., "Anti-inflammatory steroids induce biosythesis of a phospholipase A2 inhibitor which prevents prostaglandin generation," *Nature* 278 (1979): 456.

PAGE 90 The role of stomach contractions in causing ulcers is discussed at length in Weiner, H., "From simplicity to complexity (1950–1990): the case of peptic ulceration—II. Animal studies," *Psychosomatic Medicine* 53 (1991): 491.

PAGE 90 Levenstein, S., "The very model of a modern etiology: a biopsychosocial view of peptic ulcer," *Psychosomatic Medicine* 62 (2000): 176. Her footnoted quote is from: Levenstein, S., "Wellness, health, Antonovsky," *Advances* 10 (1994): 26.

CHAPTER 6: DWARFISM AND THE IMPORTANCE OF MOTHERS

PAGE 92 The mechanisms of growth and its regulation by various hormones can be found in any basic endocrine or physiology textbook. A relatively accessible version for nonspecialists can be found in Vander, A., Sherman, J., and Luciano, D., *Human Physiology: The Mechanisms of Body Function*, 6th ed. (New York: McGraw-Hill, 1994).

PAGE 94 For introductions to this massive topic of metabolic imprinting, see: Hales, C., Barker, D., "Type 2 (non-insulin-dependent) diabetes mellitus: the thrifty phenotype hypothesis," *Diabetologia* 35 (1992): 595; Barker, D., Hales, C., "The thrifty phenotype hypothesis," *British Medical Bulletin* 60 (2001): 5.

PAGE 95 Fetal undernourishment followed by postnatal nutritional plenty: Ozanne, S., Hales, C., "Catch-up growth and obesity in male mice," *Nature* 427 (2004): 411.

PAGE 95 Fetal imprinting applying to less dramatic nutritional states: Gluckman, P., "Nutrition, glucocorticoids, birth size, and adult disease," *Endocrinology* 142 (2001): 1689; Reynolds, R. M., Walker, B. R., Syddall, H. E., Andrew, R., Wood, P. J., Whorwood, C. B., Phillips, D. I., "Altered control of cortisol secretion in adult men with low birth weight and cardiovascular risk factors," *Journal of Clinical Endocrinology and Metabolism* 86 (2001): 245. Low birth weight predicting adult diabetes and hypertension risk: Levitt, N. S., Lambert, E. V., Woods, D., Hales, C. N., Andrew, R., Seckl, J. R., "Impaired glucose tolerance and elevated blood pressure in low birth weight, nonobese, young South African adults: early programming of cortisol axis," *Journal of Clinical Endocrinology and Metabolism* 85 (2000): 4611.

PAGE 96 Magnitude of these imprinting effects: Hales and Barker, "Type 2 (noninsulin dependent) diabetes," *Diabetologia,* op. cit.; Leon, D., Lithell, H., Vagero, D., Loupilova, L., Mohsen, R., Berglund, L., Lithell, U., McKeigue, P., "Reduced fetal growth rate and increased risk of death from ischaemic heart disease: cohort study of 15,000 Swedish men and women born 1915–29," *British Medical Journal* 317 (1998): 241.

Footnote: Ravelli, A. J., van der Meulen, J., "Absence of an imprinting effect of fetuses from the Siege of Leningrad," *The Lancet* 351 (1998): 173.

PAGE 96 Fetal programming of adult glucocorticoid levels: Lesage, J., Dufourmy, L., Laborie, C., Bernet, F., Blondeau, B., Avril, I., Breant, B., Dupouy, J., "Perinatal malnutrition programs sympathoadrenal and HPA axis responsiveness to restraint stress in adult male rats," *Journal of Neuroendocrinology* 14 (2002): 135; Huizink, A., Mulder, E., Buitelaar, J., "Prenatal stress and risk for psychopathology: specific effects or induction of general susceptibility?" *Psychological Bulletin* 130 (2002): 115; Welberg, L., Seckl, J., "Prenatal stress, glucocorticoids, and the programming of the brain," *Journal of Neuroendocrinology* 13 (2001): 113. This effect is mediated by maternal glucocorticoid secretion: Matthews, S., "Antenatal glucocorticoids and programming of the developing CNS," *Pediatric Research* 47 (2000): 291; Uno, H., Lohmiller, L., Thieme, C., Kemnitz, J., Engle, M., Roecker, E., Farrell, P., "Brain damage induced by prenatal exposure to dexamethasone in fetal rhesus macaques; I. Hippocampus," *Developmental Brain Research* 53 (1990): 157.

PAGE 97 Prenatal programming of adult glucocorticoid levels in humans: Clark, P., "Programming of the HPA axis and the fetal origins of adult disease hypothesis," *European Journal of Pediatrics* 157 (1998): S7. This is worsened by premature birth: Kajantie, E., Phillips, D., Andersson, S., Barker, D., Dunkel, L., Forsen, T., Osmond, C., Tuominen, J., Wood, P., Eriksson, J., "Size at birth, gestational age and cortisol secretion in adult life: foetal programming of both hyper- and hypocortisolism?" *Clinical Endocrinology* 57 (2002): 635.

PAGE 97 Fetal programming of Metabolic syndrome risk: Dodic, M., Peers, A., Coghlan, J., Wintour, M., "Can excess glucocorticoid, in utero, predispose to cardiovascular and metabolic disease in middle age?" *Trends in Endocrinology and Metabolism* 10 (1999): 86; Dodic, M., Moritz, K., Koukoulas, I., Wintour, E., "Programmed hypertension: kidney, brain or both?" *Trends in Endocrinology and Metabolism* 13 (2002): 405; Welberg and Seckl, "Prenatal stress, glucocorticoids, and the programming of the brain," *Journal of Neuroendocrinology,* op. cit.

PAGE 97 Fetal programming of adult reproduction: Charmandari, E., Kino, T., Souvatzoglou, E., Chrousos, G., "Pediatric stress: hormonal mediators and human development," *Hormone Research* 59 (2003): 161; Huizink et al., "Prenatal stress and risk," *Psychological Bulletin,* op. cit.

PAGE 98 Fetal programming of adult anxiety: Matthews, op. cit.; Welberg and Seckl, op. cit., Huizink et al., op. cit. More of a pro-anxiety neurotransmitter, fewer receptors for anti-anxiety: Avishai-Eliner, S., Brunson, K., Sandman, C., Baram, T., "Stress-out, or in (utero)," *Trends in Neuroscience* 25 (2002): 518; Teicher, M., Andersen, S., Plcari, A., Anderson, C., Navalta, C., Kim, D., "The neurobiological consequences of early stress and childhood maltreatment," *Neuroscience and Biobehavioral Reviews* 27 (2003): 33.

PAGE 98 Programming of brain function: Vallee, M., Maccari, S., Dellu, F., Simon, H., Le Moal, M., Mayo, W., "Long-term effects of prenatal stress and postnatal handling on age-related glucocorticoid secretion and cognitive performance: a longitudinal study in the rat," *European Journal of Neuroscience* 11 (1999):

2906; Lou, H., Hansen, D., Nordentoft, M., Pryds, O., Jensen, F., Nim, J., Hem-mingsen, R., "Prenatal stressors of human life affect fetal brain development," *Developmental Medicine and Child Neurology* 36 (1994): 826; Coe, C. L., Kramer, M., Czeh, B., Gould, E., Reeves, A. J., Kirschbaum, C., Fuchs, E., "Prenatal stress diminishes neurogenesis in the dentate gyrus of juvenile rhesus monkeys," *Biological Psychiatry* 54 (2003): 1025; Mathew, S. J., Shungu, D. C., Mao, X., Smith E. L., Perera, G. M., Kegeles, L. S., Perera, T., Lisanby, S. H., Rosenblum, L. A., Gorman, J. M., Coplan, J. D., "A magnetic resonance spectroscopic imaging study of adult nonhuman primates exposed to early-life stressors," *Biological Psychiatry* 4 (2003): 727.

PAGE 99 Multigenerational effects of programming: Lumey, L., "Decreased birth weights in infants after maternal in utero exposure to the Dutch famine of 1944–1945," *"Paeditra perinatal," Epidemology* 6 (1992): 240; Van Assche, F., and Aerts, L., "Long-term effect of diabetes and pregnancy in the rat," *Diabetes* 34 (1985): 116; Laychock, S., Vadlamudi, S., Patel, M., "Neonatal rat dietary carbohydrate affects pancreatic islet insulin secretion in adults and progeny," *American Journal of Physiology* 269 (1995): E739–744; Marx, J., "Unraveling the causes of diabetes," *Science* 296 (2002): 686.

PAGE 100 Consequences of maternal separation: Hunt, R., Ladd, C., Plotsky, P., "Maternal deprivation," in Fink, G., ed., *Encyclopedia of Stress* (San Diego: Academic Press, 2000), vol. 2, 699. Bennett, A., Lesch, K., Heils, A., Loing, J., Lorenz, J., Shoaf, S., Champoux, M., Suomi, S., Linnoila, M., Higley, J., "Early experience and serotonin transporter gene variation interact to influence primate CNS function," *Molecular Psychiatry* 7 (2002): 118; Liu, D., Diorio, J., Tannenbaum, B., Caldji, C., Francis, D., Feedman, A., Sharma, S., Pearson, D., Plotsky, P., Meaney, J., "Maternal care, hippocampal glucocorticoid receptors, and HPA responses to stress," *Science* 277 (1997): 1659. For a study showing that social isolation in an infant rat decreases the birth of new neurons, see: Lu, L., Bao, G., Chen, H., Xia, P., Fan, X., Zhang, J., Pei, G., Ma, L., "Modification of hippocampal neurogenesis and neuroplasticity by social environments," *European Journal of Neuroscience* 183 (2003): 600.

PAGE 101 Early trauma increasing risk of irritable bowel syndrome in humans: Murison, R., "Gastrointestinal effects," in Fink, G., ed., *Encyclopedia of Stress* (San Diego: Academic Press, 2000), vol. 2, 191. Romanian orphanage children: Gunnar, M., Mirison, S., Chisholm, K., Schuder, M., "Salivary cortisol levels in children adopted from Romanian orphanages," *Development and Psychopathology* 13 (2001): 611. Childhood abuse: de Bellis, M., Thomas, L., "Biologic findings of PTSD and child maltreatment," *Current Psychiatry Reports* 5 (2003): 108; Carrion, V., Weems, C., Ray, R., Glaser, B., Hessl, D., Reiss, A., "Diurnal salivary cortisol in pediatric PTSD," *Biological Psychiatry* 51 (2002): 575.

PAGE 102 Short summaries of stress dwarfism and of failure to thrive can be found in most endocrine or pediatric textbooks. A relatively recent technical summary of the subject can be found in Green, W., Campbell, M., and David, R., "Psychosocial dwarfism: a critical review of the evidence," *Journal of the American Academy of Child Psychiatry* 23 (1984): 1. A somewhat dated but very readable nontechnical account can be found in Gardner, L., "Deprivation dwarfism," *Scientific American* 227 (1972): 76. A specific discussion of the intellectual impairments found in such children can be found in Dowdney, L., Skuse, D., Heptinstall, E.,

Puckering, C., and Zur-Szpiro, S., "Growth retardation and developmental delay amongst inner-city children," *Journal of Child Psychology and Psychiatry* 28 (1987): 529. A demonstration that removing stress dwarfism children from their stressful environments normalizes growth and growth hormone: Albanese, A., Hamill, G., Jones, J., Skuse, D., Matthews, D., and Stanhope, R., "Reversibility of physiological growth hormone secretion in children with psychosocial dwarfism," *Clinical Endocrinology* 40 (1994): 687.

PAGE 103 Catch-up growth after stress dwarfism: Boersma, B., and Wit, J., "Catch-up growth," *Endocrine Reviews* 18 (1997): 646.

PAGE 103 Fairly consistent versions of the King Frederick story are reported by a number of his biographers, including Kingston, T., *History of Frederick the Second, Emperor of the Romans* (Cambridge, England: Macmillan, 1862), Allshorn, L., *Stupor Mundi: The Life and Times of Frederick II, Emperor of the Romans, King of Sicily and Jerusalem 1194–1250* (London: Martin Secker, 1912), and Kantorowicz, E., *Frederick the Second, 1194–1250* (London: Constable, 1931). The quotation by Salimbene comes from Montagu, A., *Touching: The Human Significance of the Skin* (New York: Harper and Row, 1978).

PAGE 104 The tale of the two orphanages: Widdowson, E., "Mental contentment and physical growth," *The Lancet* (16 June 1951): 1316. The information on the appalling survivorship in orphanages comes from Chapin, H., "A plea for accurate statistics in children's institutions," *Transactions of the American Pediatric Society* 27 (1915): 180. The quotation comes from Gardner, L., "Deprivation dwarfism," *Scientific American* 227 (1972): 76.

PAGE 105 J. M. Barrie and stress dwarfism: the discussion of Barrie that so caught my attention during my student days can be found in Martin, J., and Reichlin, S., *Clinical Neuroendocrinology*, 1st ed. (Philadelphia: Davis Company, 1977). I am particularly grateful to Seymour Reichlin, one of the giants of endocrinology and my teacher at the time, for remembering this source.

In preparing this book, I decided to read up a bit more on Barrie. I was surprised to discover a vast number of Barrie biographies; this now fairly obscure man was once the most popular author and playwright in Britain. The details of his life are both fascinating and grotesque. He retained a lifelong obsession with his mother, forever attempting to win her love. In one remarkable passage that encapsulated both his Oedipal wooing of her and his pathological identification with her, he predicted that in his later years, "when age must dim my mind and the past comes sweeping back like the shades of night over the bare road of the present, it will not, I believe, be my youth I shall see but hers, not a boy clinging to his mother's skirt and crying, 'Wait till I'm a man, and you'll lie on feathers,' but a little girl in a magenta frock and a white pinafore." He also had a lifelong obsession with young boys, and his private writing includes passages of sadomasochism and pedophilia.

What is perhaps most fascinating is the transition of Barrie from a rather pathetic and sympathetic loner as a young man to a far-from-sympathetic manipulator in his later years, all because his writing success brought him the power and wealth to disrupt lives around him. As he grew older, alone and childless, he inveigled his way into the lives of a succession of young couples, appearing as a generous benefactor and gradually coming to dominate them more and more, especially the fates of the sons in these families (one boy, Peter Davies, became the model for Peter Pan; he loathed the association all his adult life and, probably unrelated to that, threw himself in front of a London subway at age sixty-three). For the most interesting of the Barrie biographies (from which the above quotation was taken), I recommend Birkin, A., *J. M. Barrie and the Lost Boys* (London: Constable, 1979). Also see the elegiac piece by Lurie, Alison, "The boy who couldn't grow up," *New York Review of Books* (6 February 1975): 11.

PAGE 106 In addition to the references given above on the clinical profiles of kids with various deprivation syndromes, the following could be checked for details of the endocrinology of the disruption of growth: chapter 20 (Rose, R. "Psychoendocrinology") in Wilson, J., and Foster, D., eds., *Williams Textbook of Endocrinology*, 7th ed. (Philadelphia: Saunders, 1985); Reichlin, S. "Prolactin and growth hormone secretion in stress," in Chrousos, G., Loriaux, D., and Gold, P., eds., *Mechanisms of Physical and Emotional Stress* (New York: Plenum Press, 1988). These references also discuss the differences between growth hormone regulation in the adult versus the developing child, and in primates and humans versus rodents.

PAGE 107 The data from the study of the child with stress dwarfism whose nurse went on vacation comes from Saenger, P., Levine, L., Wiedemann, E., Schwartz, E., Korth-Schutz, S., Pareira, J., Heinig, B., and New, M., "Somatomedin and growth hormone in psychosocial dwarfism," *Padiatrie und Padologie* (1977): supp. 5, 1.

PAGE 107 For a review of the regulation of growth factors by psychological factors, see Schanberg, S., Evoniuk, G., and Kuhn, C., "Tactile and nutritional aspects of maternal care: specific regulators of neuroendocrine function and cellular development," *Proceedings of the Society for Experimental Biology and Medicine* 175 (1984): 135. Information on the requirement of active contact with the mother to normalize growth hormone levels in infant rats can be found in Kuhn, C., Paul, J., and Schanberg, S., "Endocrine responses to mother-infant separation in developing rats," *Developmental Psychobiology* 23 (1990): 395. For a discussion of the effects of maternal separation on glucocorticoid levels, see the Kuhn et al. paper just cited, plus the earlier work by Stanton, M., Guitierrez, Y., and Levine, S., "Maternal deprivation potentiates pituitary-adrenal stress responses in infant rats," *Behavioral Neuroscience* 102 (1988): 692. For the classic demonstration of the effects of neonatal handling in rats on growth rates see any of the following three reports by Denenberg, V., and Karas, G., "Effects of differential handling upon weight gain and mortality in the rat and mouse," *Science* 130 (1959): 629; "Interactive effects of age and duration of infantile experience on adult learning," *Psychological Reports* 7 (1960): 313; "Interactive effects of infant and adult experience upon weight gain and mortality in the rat," *Journal of Comparative and Physiological Psychology* 54 (1961): 658.

PAGE 108 The importance of touch in rat development: Hofer, M., "Relationships as regulators," *Psychosomatic Medicine* 46 (1984): 183.

PAGE 108 The work on touching of premature human infants is described in Field, T., Schanberg, S., Scarfidi, F., Bauer, C., Vega-Lahr, N., Garcia, R., Nystrom, J., and Kuhn, C., "Tactile/kinesthetic stimulation effects on preterm neonates," *Pediatrics* 77 (1986): 654. Also Scarfidi, F., Field, T., Schanberg, S., Bauer, C., Vega-Lahr, N., Garcia, R., Poirier, J., Nystrom, J., and Kuhn, C., "Effects of tactile-kinesthetic stimulation on the clinical course and sleep-wake behavior of pre-term infants," *Infant Behavior and Development* 9 (1986): 71. A similar experiment was carried out some years earlier in a much sketchier form with only five infants, as reported in Sokoloff, N., Yaffe, S., Weintraub, D., and Blase, G., "Effects of handling on the subsequent development of premature infants," *Developmental Psychology* 1 (1969): 765. That work, in turn, was inspired by the research of some pioneers in the field: the developmental biologist Rene Spitz and the famed pediatrician T. Berry Brazelton.

The estimate of $1 billion in savings is based on the following (admittedly very crude) analysis. A federal report in 1987 ("Neonatal Intensive Care for Low Birthweight Infants: Costs and Effectiveness," Health Technology Case Study 38, Office of Technology Assessment, Washington, D.C.) reported 150,000–200,000 infants admitted annually to neonatal intensive care units, of whom approximately 20 percent were of very low weight (less than 3 pounds). The average length of stay for that most vulnerable group was approximately 48 days at a cost of $41,000; for the other 80 percent, average stay was approximately 28 days at a cost of $24,000. Total hospitalization bills thus come to something in excess of $5 billion, based on an average individual stay of approximately 32 days (weighting the two different groups). Thus an average reduction of one week's stay in the intensive care unit constitutes an approximate 20 percent reduction and (assuming, probably incorrectly, that the rate of expense incurred is constant over time) produces savings something in excess of a billion dollars. This does not even count savings on the considerable costs of outpatient care lasting months to years for preemies after discharge (discussed in Blackman, J., "Neonatal intensive care: is it worth it?" *Pediatric Clinics of North America,* 38, no. 6 [1991]).

PAGE 109 The ability of glucocorticoids (and stress) to stimulate growth hormone release in humans in the short run, yet inhibit it in the long run, is reviewed in: Thakore, J., and Dinan, T., "Growth hormone secretion: the role of glucocorticoids," *Life Sciences* 55 (1994): 1083.

PAGE 111 The cross-cultural studies of the stressfulness of developmental rituals: Landauer, T., and Whiting, J., "Infantile stimulation and adult stature of human males," *American Anthropologist* 66 (1964): 1007. A similar theme emerges from their later studies showing that the physical stressor of immunization (and the subsequent brief illness) of children under two years of age resulted in taller adults. The population was Americans who had been children in the 1930s, a time when immunization was far from universal: Whiting, J., Landauer, T., and Jones, T., "Infantile immunization and adult stature," *Child Development* 39 (1968): 59.

PAGE 112 A single round of glucocorticoids is benign: "Antenatal Corticosteroids Revisited: Repeat Courses," *NIH Consensus Statement Online* 17 (17–18 August 2000): 1–10.

PAGE 113 Critics of the importance of the FOAD concept: Zimmel, P., Alberti, K., Shaw, J., "Global and societal implications of the diabetes epidemic," *Nature* 414 (2001): 782.

PAGE 113 Reversibility of FOADish effects: Maccari, S., Piazza, P., Kabbaj, M., Barbazanges, A., Simon, H., Le Moal, M., "Adoption reverses the long-term impairment in glucocorticoid feedback induced by prenatal stress," *Journal of Neuroscience* 15 (1995): 110.

PAGE 114 Small, M., *Our Babies, Ourselves* (New York: Anchor Books, 1999).

PAGE 114 Most basic physiology textbooks include descriptions of bone growth and resorption in the adult and its hormonal regulation. A particularly clear discussion can be found in Rhoades, R., and Pflanzer, R., *Human Physiology* (Philadelphia: Saunders College Publishing, 1989). A good recent review of how glucocorticoids cause osteoporosis: Canalis, E., "Mechanisms of glucocorticoid action in bone: implications to glucocorticoid-induced osteoporosis," *Journal of Clinical Endocrinology and Metabolism* 81 (1996): 3441. The first report of bone fractures in patients with Cushing's syndrome came, of course, from Dr. Harvey Cushing himself: "The basophil adenomas of the pituitary body and their clinical manifestations as basophilism," *Bulletin of the Johns Hopkins Hospital* 1 (1932): 137. A report on how patients being treated with glucocorticoids to control a disease (in this case, asthma) will get osteoporosis: Adinoff, A., and Hollister, J., "Steroid-induced fractures and bone loss in patients with asthma," *New England Journal of Medicine* 309 (1983): 265. Sustained social stress is associated with loss of bone mass in female primates: Kaplan, J., and Manuck, S., "Behavioral and evolutionary considerations in predicting disease susceptibility in nonhuman primates," *American Journal of Physical Anthropology* 78 (1989): 250; and Shively, C., Jayo, M., Weaver, D., and Kaplan, J., "Reduced vertebral bone mineral density in socially subordinate female cynomolgus macaques," *American Journal of Primatology* 24 (1991): 135.

PAGE 115 Footnote: JFK and glucocorticoids: Robert Dallek, *Atlantic Monthly* (December 2002).

PAGE 116 The discussion of child-rearing practices at the time can be found in Montagu, A., *Touching: The Human Significance of the Skin*, op. cit. The authoritative "expert" who advised against such unscientific practices as handling infants too much was Dr. Luther Holt, professor of pediatrics at Columbia University and the author of *The Care and Feeding of Children* (East Norwalk, Conn.: Appleton-Century), which went through fifteen editions between 1894 and 1915. For a discussion of the impact of this child-rearing policy on pediatric medicine, see: Sapolsky, R., "How the other half heals," *Discover* (April 1998): 46.

PAGE 117 Some Harlow papers: "The nature of love," *American Psychologist* 13 (1958): 673. More technical reports of his work can be found in Harlow, H., and Zimmerman, R., "Affectional responses in the infant monkey," *Science* 130 (1959): 421; Harlow, H., Harlow, M., Dodsworth, R., and Arling, G., "Maternal behavior of rhesus monkeys deprived of mothering and peer associations in infancy," *Proceedings of the American Philosophical Society* 110 (1966): 58.

Footnote: Deborah Blum, *Love at Goon Park: Harry Harlow and the Science of Affection* (New York: Perseus, 2002).

CHAPTER 7: SEX AND REPRODUCTION

PAGE 120 Basic male reproductive endocrinology and the effects of the various hormonal changes described during stress on reproduction are covered in most basic textbooks. General reviews of male reproductive physiology during stress: Rivier, C., "Luteinizing-hormone-releasing hormone, gonadotropins, and gonadal steroids in stress," *Annals of the New York Academy of Sciences* 771 (1995): 187; Negro-Vilar, A., "Stress and other environmental factors affecting fertility in men and women: overview," *Environmental Health Perspectives* 101 (1993): S2, 59.

PAGE 120 Some of the original papers showing how physical stressors (such as surgery, immobilization, drought for a wild primate population, foot shock, or forced swimming) will suppress hormones of the male reproductive system: Bardin, C., and Peterson, R., "Studies of androgen production by the rat: Testosterone and androstenedione content of blood," *Endocrinology* 80 (1967): 38; Free, M., and Tillson, S., "Secretion rate of testicular steroids in conscious and halothane-anesthetized rat," *Endocrinology* 93 (1973): 874; Matsumoto, K., Takeyasu, K., Mizutani, S., Hamanaka, Y., and Uozumi, T., "Plasma testosterone levels following surgical stress in male patients," *Acta Endocrinology* 65 (1970): 11; Sapolsky, R., "Endocrine and behavioral correlates of drought in the wild baboon," *American Journal of Primatology* 2 (1986): 217. Some more recent papers: Jain, S., Bruot, B., and Stevenson, J., "Cold swim stress leads to enhanced splenocyte responsiveness to concanavalin A, decreased serum testosterone, and increased serum corticosterone, glucose and protein," *Life Sciences* 59 (1996): 209; Ellison, P., and Panter-Brick, G., "Salivary testosterone levels among Tamang and Kami males of central Nepal," *Human Biology* 68 (1996): 955.

PAGE 122 Psychological stressors will also suppress these hormones; examples follow. A drop in social rank for a male primate: Rose, R., Bernstein, I., and Gordon, T., "Consequences of social conflict on plasma testosterone levels in rhesus monkeys," *Psychosomatic Medicine* 37 (1975): 50; Mendoza, S., Coe, C., Lowe, E., and Levine, S., "The physiological response to group formation in adult male squirrel monkeys," *Psychoneuroendocrinology* 3 (1979): 221. A difficult learning task for a primate: Mason, J., Kenion, C., and Collins, D., "Urinary testosterone response to 72-hour avoidance sessions in the monkey," *Psychosomatic Medicine* 30 (1968): 721. A first parachute jump: Davidson, J., Smith, E., and Levine, S., "Testosterone," in Ursin, H., Baade, E., and Levine, S., eds., *Psychobiology of Stress* (New York: Academic Press, 1978), 57. Social instability for primates: Sapolsky, R., "Endocrine aspects of social instability in the olive baboon," *American Journal of Primatology* 5 (1983): 365; Curtin, F., and Steimer, T., "Lower sex hormones in men during anticipatory stress," *NeuroReport* 7 (1996): 3, 101. The suppressive effects of Officer Candidate School on testosterone levels: Kreuz, L., Rose, R., and Jennings, J., "Suppression of plasma testosterone levels and psychological stress," *Archives of General Psychiatry* 26 (1972): 479.

A recent paper reports a fascinating example of the reproductive suppression caused by a combination of physical and psychological stressors in a population of wild animals. A population of male elephants in a national park in Africa were orphaned by poachers, and as a result, grew up without role models. When, as adolescents, they came into heat (called "musth" in male elephants), they turned into elephant hoodlums—hyperaggressive, hypersexual (if I recall correctly, trying to forcibly mate with anything of an appropriate size, including the rhinos). Adult males were introduced into the study to stress and harass these rogue males out of musth: Slotow, R., Van Dyk, G., Poole, J., Page, B., Klocke, A., "Older bull elephants control young males," *Nature* 408 (2000): 425.

PAGE 122 Opiate drugs and opioid-like hormones (for instance, beta-endorphin) block the release of LHRH: Delitala, G., Devilla, L., and Arata, L., "Opiate receptors and anterior pituitary hormone secretion in man. Effect of naloxone infusion," *Acta Endocrinology* (Copenhagen) 97 (1981): 150; Jacobs, M., and Lightman, S., "Studies in the opioid control of anterior pituitary hormones," *Journal of Physiology* (London) 300 (1980): 53; Rasmussen, D., Liu, J., Wolf, P., and Yen, S.,

"Endogenous opioid regulation of gonadotropin-releasing hormone release from the human fetal hypothalamus in vitro," *Journal of Clinical Endocrinology and Metabolism* 57 (1983): 881; Hulse, G., and Coleman, G., "The role of endogenous opioids in the blockade of reproductive function in the rat following exposure to acute stress," *Pharmacology, Biochemistry, and Behavior* 19 (1983): 795.

Exercise stimulates beta-endorphin release: Colt, E., Wardlaw, S., and Frantz, A., "The effect of running on plasma beta-endorphin," *Life Science* 28 (1981): 1637. For an interesting demonstration of the potential for this release to disrupt reproduction, see McArthur, J., Bellen, B., Beitins, T., Pagaon, M., Badger, T., and Klibanski, A., "Hypothalamic amenorrhea in runners of normal body composition," *Endocrine Research Communications* 7 (1980): 13. This study examined an amenorrheic runner with low LH levels; when she was given a drug (naloxone) that blocked beta-endorphin's actions, LH levels rose. Also see Samuels, M., Sanborn, C., Hofeldt, F., and Robbins, R., "The role of endogenous opiates in athletic amenorrhea," *Fertility and Sterility* 55 (1991): 507.

A moderate amount of exercise will stimulate testosterone levels: Elias, M., "Cortisol, testosterone and testosterone-binding globulin responses to competitive fighting in human males," *Aggressive Behavior* 7 (1981): 215. By contrast, sustained major exercise suppresses the system: Dessypris, A., Kuoppasalmi, K., and Adlercreutz, H., "Plasma cortisol, testosterone, androstenedione and luteinizing hormone (LH) in a non-competitive marathon run," *Journal of Steroid Biochemistry* 7 (1976): 33; MacConnie, S., Barkan, A., Lampman, R., Schorok, M., and Beitins, I., "Decreased hypothalamic gonadotropin releasing hormone secretion in male marathon runners," *New England Journal of Medicine* 315 (1986): 411; Grandi, M., and Celani, M., "Effects of football on the pituitary-testicular axis: differences between professional and non-professional soccer players," *Experimental and Clinical Endocrinology* 96 (1990): 253; De Souza, M., Arce, J., Pescatello, L., Scherzer, H., and Luciano, A., "Gonadal hormones and semen quality in male runners: a volume threshold effect of endurance training," *International Journal of Sports Medicine* 15 (1994): 383. Abnormalities in glucocorticoid function in men who exercise heavily: Duclos, M., Corcuff, J., Pehourcq, F., Tabarin, A., "Decreased pituitary sensitivity to glucocorticoids in endurance-trained men," *European Journal of Endocrinology* 144 (2001): 363.

Similarly, major amounts of exercise suppress reproductive physiology in women. As one example, highly active ballet dancers have their onset of puberty delayed: Warren, M., "The effects of exercise on pubertal progression and reproductive function in girls," *Journal of Clinical Endocrinology and Metabolism* 51 (1980): 1150; Frisch, R., Wyshak, G., and Vincent, L., "Delayed menarche and amenorrhea in ballet dancers," *New England Journal of Medicine* 303 (1980): 17; Bale, P., Doust, J., and Dawson, D., "Gymnasts, distance runners, anorexics: body composition and menstrual status," *Journal of Sports Medicine and Physical Fitness*, 36 (1996): 49. Amenorrhea occurs among women who exercise heavily: Kiningham, R., Apgar, B., and Schwenk, T., "Evaluation of amenorrhea," *American Family Physician* 53 (1996): 1185; Dale, E., Gerlach, D., and Wilhite, A., "Menstrual dysfunction in distance runners," *Obstetrics and Gynecology* 54 (1996): 47. In these cases, the degree of dysfunction is tightly coupled with body weight or body fat content: Sanborn, C., Martin, B., and Wagner, W., "Is athletic amenorrhea specific to runners?" *American Journal of Obstetrics and Gynecology* 143 (1982): 859; Shangold, M., and Levine, H., "The effect of marathon training upon menstrual function," *American Journal of Obstetrics and Gynecology* 143 (1982): 862. As more examples of the roughly 50 percent amenorrhea rate: Buskirk, E., Mendez, J., Durfee, S., "Effects of exercise on the body composition of women," *Seminars in Reproductive Endocrinology* 3 (1985): 9; Shangold, M., "Exercise and amenorrhea," *Seminars in Reproductive Endocrinology* 3 (1985): 35.

Some of the additional effects of overexercising. A moderate amount of exercise will increase bone density, particularly in the bones most heavily utilized in the exercise: Nilsson, B., and Westlin, N., "Bone density in athletes," *Clinical Orthopedics* 77 (1971): 179; Lanyon, L., "Bone loading, exercise, and the control of bone mass; the physiological basis for the prevention of osteoporosis," *Bone* 6 (1989): 19. Nevertheless, extremes of exercise can reverse this trend, leading to bone thinning, increased risk of osteoporosis, scoliosis, and stress fractures: Myburgh, K., Hutchins, J., Fataar, A., Hough, S., and Koakes, T., "Low bone density is an etiologic factor for stress fractures in athletes," *Annals of Internal Medicine* 113 (1990): 754; Drinkwater, B., Nilson, K., and Chesnut, C., "Bone mineral content of amoenorrheic and eumenorrheic athletes," *New England Journal of Medicine* 311 (1984): 277; Marcus, R., Cann, C., Madvig, P., Minkoff, J., Goddard, M., Bayer, M., Martin, M., Gaudiani, L., Haskell, W., and Genant, H., "Menstrual function and bone mass in elite women distance runners: endocrine and metabolic factors," *Annals of Internal Medicine* 102 (1985): 158; Barrow, G., and Saha, S., "Menstrual irregularity and stress fractures in collegiate female distance runners," *American Journal of Sports Medicine* 16 (1988): 209. The same occurs in male athletes: Bennell, K., Brukner, P., and Malcolm, S., "Effect of altered reproductive function and lowered testosterone levels on bone density in male endurance athletes," *British Journal of Sports Medicine* 30 (1996): 205. In prepubescent female athletes, the risks also include scoliosis: Warren, M., Brooks-Gunn, J., Hamilton, J., Warren, L., and Hamilton, G., "Scoliosis and fractures in young ballet dancers: relation to delayed menarche and secondary amenorrhea," *New England Journal of Medicine* 314 (1986): 1348.

These deleterious effects may be due, in part, to the elevated levels of glucocorticoids seen in serious athletes: Luger, A., Deuster, P., Kyle, S., Gallucci, W., Montgomery, L., Gold, P., Loriaux, L., and Chrousos, G., "Acute hypothalamic-pituitary-adrenal responses to the stress of treadmill exercise," *New England Journal of Medicine* 316 (1987): 1309; Willaneuva, A., Schlosser, C., Hopper, B., Liu, J., Hoffman, D., and Rebar, R., "Increased cortisol production in women runners," *Journal of Clinical Endocrinology and Metabolism* 63 (1986): 133; Loucks, A., Mortola, J., Girton, L., and Yen, S., "Alterations in the hypothalamic-pituitary-ovarian and the hypothalamic-pituitary-adrenal axes in athletic women," *Journal of Clinical Endocrinology and Metabolism* 68 (1989): 402. These cases documented pretty substantial increases in the levels of these hormones.

PAGE 123 Glucocorticoids work at the pituitary and the testes to block LH and testosterone release, respectively: Cummings, D., Quigley, M., and Yen, S., "Acute suppression of circulating testosterone levels by cortisol in men," *Journal of Clinical Endocrinology and Metabolism* 57 (1983): 671; Bambino, T., and Hseuh, A., "Direct inhibitory effect of glucocorticoids upon testicular luteinizing hormone receptors and steroidogenesis in vivo and in vitro," *Endocrinology* 108 (1981): 2142; Johnson, B., Welsh, T., and Juniewicz, P., "Suppression of luteinizing hormone and testosterone secretion in bulls following adrenocorticotropin hormone treatment," *Biology of Reproduction* 26 (1982): 305; Vierhapper, H., Waldhausl, W., and Nowotny, P., "Gonadotropin-secretion in adrenocortical insufficiency:

impact of glucocorticoid substitution," *Acta Endocrinology* (Copenhagen) (1982): 580; Sapolsky, R., "Stress-induced suppression of testicular function in the wild baboon: role of glucocorticoids," *Endocrinology* 116 (1985): 2273.

Stress-induced reproductive suppression need not involve CRH, however: Jeong, K., Jacobson, L., Widmaier, E., Majzoub, J., "Normal suppression of the reproductive axis following stress in CRH-deficient mice," *Endocrinology* 140 (1999): 1702.

Prolactin inhibits multiple steps in the male reproductive system: Bartke, A., Smith, M., Michael, S., Peron, F., and Dalterio, S., "Effects of experimentally-induced chronic hyperprolactinemia on testosterone and gonadotropin levels in male rats and mice," *Endocrinology* 100 (1977): 182; Bartke, A., Goldman, B., Bex, F., and Dalterio, S., "Effects of prolactin on pituitary and testicular function in mice with hereditary prolactin deficiency," *Endocrinology* (1977): 1760; McNeilly, A., Sharpe, R., and Fraser, H., "Increased sensitivity to the negative feedback effect of testosterone induced by hyperprolactinemia in the adult male rat," *Endocrinology* 112 (1983): 22.

PAGE 123 A good introductory summary of the basic workings of erections and ejaculation can be found in Previte, J., *Human Physiology* (New York: McGraw-Hill, 1983). A more detailed version is found in Guyton, A., *Textbook of Medical Physiology,* 7th ed. (Philadelphia: Saunders, 1986), 959. The parasympathetic neurotransmitter acetylcholine promotes erections: Saenz de Tejada, I., Blanco, R., Goldstein, I., Azadzoi, K., De Las Morenas, A., and Krane, R., "Cholinergic neurotransmission in human corpus cavernosum. I. Responses of isolated tissue," *American Journal of Physiology* 254 (1988): H459. The sympathetic neurotransmitter noradrenaline (norepinephrine) inhibits erections: Saenz de Tejada, I., Kim, N., Lagan, I., Krane, R., and Goldstein, I., "Regulation of adrenergic activity in penile corpus cavernosum," *Journal of Urology* 142 (1989): 1117. Just to make life and sex more complicated, researchers are coming to recognize that there are mechanisms for inducing erections that do not involve the parasympathetic nervous system. These are poorly understood, but it appears that these nerve endings make the arteries into the penis dilate (and thus engorge the penis with blood) by way of nitric oxide, a newly identified gaseous neurotransmitter that is closely related to nitrous oxide (laughing gas): Ignarro, L., "Nitric oxide as the physiological mediator of penile erection," *Journal of NIH Research* 4 (1992): 59.

Footnote: The Da Vinci quote is from: Goldstein, I., "Male sexual circuitry," *Scientific American* (August 2000): 70.

PAGE 125 Incidences of psychogenic impotency: it remains controversial just how common this disorder is. Older studies reported that 90 to 95 percent of all cases of impotency were psychogenic in origin. For example, see Strauss, E., "Impotence from a psychiatric standpoint," *British Medical Journal* 1 (1950): 697; or Kaplan, H., *The New Sex Therapy: Active Treatment of Dysfunctions* (New York: Brunner-Mazel, 1974). These numbers are almost certainly high, as they come from a time when many subtle organic causes of impotency were not yet understood. Some more recent studies report extremely low rates (perhaps 10 to 15 percent) of psychogenic impotency. For example, see Spark, R., White, R., and Connolly, P., "Impotence is not always psychogenic," *Journal of the American Medical Association* 243 (1980): 750. In general, recent studies indicate rates ranging from 14 percent of cases of impotency being psychogenic in nature to one study showing that 55 percent were, with another 15 percent being of unknown origin.

These are summarized in Leiblum, S., and Rosen, R., *Principles and Practices of Sex Therapy* (New York: Guilford Press, 1989).

PAGE 126 The occasional resistance of the reproductive system to stress is reviewed in: Wingfield, J., Sapolsky, R., "Reproduction and resistance to stress: when and how," *Journal of Neuroendocrinology* 15 (2003): 711.

PAGE 127 For an introduction to revisionist ecology about hyenas (their role as hunters, rather than just scavengers) see Kruuk, H., *The Spotted Hyena: A Study of Predation and Social Behavior* (Chicago: University of Chicago Press, 1972). For studies of their anatomy, physiology, and behavior, see Frank, L., "Social organization of the spotted hyena: II. Dominance and reproduction," *Animal Behavior* 35 (1986): 1510; Frank, L., Glickman, S., and Licht, P., "Fatal sibling aggression, presocial development and androgens in neonatal spotted hyenas," *Science* 252 (1991): 702; Frank, L., "The evolution of female masculinization in hyenas: why does a female hyena have such a large penis?" *Trends in Ecology and Evolution* 12 (1997): 58.

The final reference discusses the possible evolution of the unique hyena anatomy and social system. The most plausible scenario revolves around the fact that most large carnivores in Africa, such as lions, have large litters; relatively few of the offspring survive. Most starve to death, and this is because a lioness and her cubs are usually excluded from feeding on a kill until the males are sated (despite that the females do the bulk of the hunting—there, one less feature to admire lions for).

By contrast, hyenas tend to have fewer progeny than these other carnivores. Suddenly the pressure is on to get those few to survive. Somewhere back when, a female hyena had a wondrous mutation—her ovaries started secreting huge amounts of the male sex hormone androstenedione, in addition to the normal estrogen. As a result, when she was pregnant, her female fetuses were exposed to the hormone, and as a result, they grew up more muscular and aggressive than typical female mammals; and the tables got turned. Within a few generations, the starving, intimidated male hyenas go and kill something, and just as they are about to gorge, the females boot them off. The kids of high-ranking moms eat before any adult males do; they survive. Thus the tendency in females toward secreting large amounts of androstenedione is highly adaptive, likely to be passed on over the generations.

There is one problem with this, however. Your average female mammal, exposed to those sorts of male sex hormone levels at birth, won't be having kids. The androstenedione would have "masculinized" her hypothalamus, which is to say that, as an adult, her hypothalamus would secrete LHRH at a roughly constant rate (as males do) instead of in the cyclic pattern that females need to ovulate. In any other species, this "perinatal androgenization" (masculinization around the time of birth) would make it impossible to reproduce.

Therefore, female hyenas are speculated to have a second mutation, one that protects the reproductive part of the hypothalamus from the masculinizing effects of the hormones. (By contrast, the "aggressive" part of the brain—a phrase that is obviously simplistic—is plenty sensitive to the androstenedione: the female hyenas are terrifyingly aggressive.) At present, no one has a clue what that second mutation may be.

PAGE 129 General reviews of stress and female reproduction: Rivier, C., "Luteinizing-hormone-releasing hormone, gonadotropins, and gonadal steroids in stress," *Annals of the New York Academy of Sciences* 771 (1995): 187; Negro-Vilar, A., "Stress and other environmental factors affecting fertility in men and women: overview," *Environmental Health Perspectives* 101 (1993): S2, 59.

The subject of the effects of starvation, fat depletion, and muscle-to-fat ratios on female reproduction is reviewed in Frisch, R., *Female fertility and the Body Fat Connection* (Chicago: University of Chicago Press, 2000); Williams, N., Helmreich, D., Parfitt, D., Caston-Balderrama, A., "Evidence for a causal role of low energy availability in the induction of menstrual cycle disturbances during strenuous exercise training," *Journal of Clinical Endocrinology and Metabolism* 86 (2001): 5184–93.

These reviews also give a good introduction to the reproductive abnormalities seen in anorexia nervosa. Anorexia and the related eating disorder bulimia are peculiar in that more is going on than just loss of weight. Specifically, reproductive suppression occurs even before there is substantial weight loss; in other words, the reproductive systems of anorexics and bulimics are more vulnerable to such suppression than those of healthy women and girls. For a recent finding linking metabolism and female fertility, see: Burks, D., de Mora, J., Schubert, M., Withers, D., Myers, M., Towery, H., Altamuro, S., Flint, C., White, M., "IRS-2 pathways integrate female reproduction and energy homeostasis," *Nature* 407 (2000): 377.

Weight regain doesn't always reinstate cyclicity: Suri, R., Altshuler, L., "Menstrual cycles and stress," in Fink, G., ed., *Encyclopedia of Stress* (San Diego: Academic Press, 2000), vol. 2, 736.

PAGE 131 Opiates and opioids inhibit LHRH release in the female: Pfeiffer, A., and Herz, A., "Endocrine actions of opioids," *Hormone and Metabolic Research* 16 (1984): 386; Ching, M., "Morphine suppresses the proestrus surge of GnRH in pituitary portal plasmas of rats," *Endocrinology* 112 (1983): 2209. (GnRH, LHRH, and LHRF all refer to the same hypothalamic hormone, which causes release of LH and FSH from the pituitary.) For an interesting example of how this is relevant to female athletes, see McArthur, J., Bullen, B., Beitins, T., Pagaon, M., Badger, T., and Klibanski, A., "Hypothalamic amenorrhea in runners of normal body composition," *Endocrine Research Communications* 7 (1980): 13. This study examined an amenorrheic runner with low LH levels; when she was given a drug (naloxone) that blocked the action of beta-endorphin, LH levels rose. See the above male section for additional references regarding disrupted reproductive physiology in female athletes. An additional neurotransmitter seems to be implicated in stress-induced suppression of LHRH release: Akema, T., Chiba, A., Shinozaki, R., Oshida, M., Kimura, F., and Toyoda, J., "Acute stress suppresses the N-methyl-D-aspartate-induced LH release in the ovariectomized estrogen-primed rat," *Neuroendocrinology* 62 (1995): 270. (The authors did not measure LHRH directly, but were able to infer it indirectly through a complicated trick in their LH measurements.)

Glucocorticoids suppress the responsiveness of the pituitary to LHRH: Suter, D., and Schwartz, N., "Effects of glucocorticoids on secretion of luteinizing hormone and follicle-stimulating hormone by female rat pituitary cells in vitro," *Endocrinology* 117 (1985): 849. References above show how glucocorticoid levels are elevated in female athletes who exercise heavily.

The follicular stage of the menstrual cycle is more vulnerable to disruption than the luteal phase: this is reported in many places. For an accessible version, see Hatcher, R., *Contraceptive Technology, 1984–85* (New York: Irvington Publishers, 1984). For a more detailed account, see Speroff, L., Glass, R., and Kase, N., *Clinical Gynecologic Endocrinology and Infertility* (Baltimore: Williams and Wilkins, 1989).

PAGE 132 The assertion that breast-feeding prevents more pregnancies than any other type of contraception comes from Carl Djerassi, the chemist who invented the pill and has spent much of the rest of his extraordinary career studying the social, economic, and political consequences of the revolution he caused, in *The Politics of Contraception* (San Francisco: W. H. Freeman, 1979).

PAGE 132 Nursing, prolactin, and the Kalahari Bushmen: Konner, M., and Worthman, C., "Nursing frequency, gonadal function, and birth spacing among !Kung hunter-gatherers," *Science* 207 (1980): 788. The paper reviews what is known about how quickly prolactin rises in response to breast feeding and how long it stays up following the end of an episode of nursing. The Kalahari !Kung have been the darlings of anthropologists for decades, and they are often considered to be the prototypical hunter-gatherer society. Their "affluent" preagricultural life has been described in Lee, R., *!Kung San: Men, Women and Work in a Foraging Society* (New York: Cambridge University Press, 1979); Lee, R., and DeVore, I., *Kalahari Hunter-Gatherers* (Cambridge, Mass.: Harvard University Press, 1976); Jenkins, T., and Nurse, G., *Health and the Hunter-Gatherers* (Basel: Karger, 1978); Marshall, L., *The !Kung of Nyae Nyae* (Cambridge, Mass.: Harvard University Press, 1976); Shostak, M., *Nisa: The Life and Words of a !Kung Woman* (Cambridge, Mass.: Harvard University Press, 1981). There has been some questioning of just how typical they are of hunter-gatherers: Lewin, R., "New views emerge on hunters and gatherers," *Science* 240 (1988): 1146. The link among westernized women between a large number of menstrual cycles and a proclivity toward gynecological diseases is discussed by MacDonald, P., Dombroski, R., and Casey, M., "Recurrent secretion of progesterone in large amounts: an endocrine/metabolic disorder unique to young women?" *Endocrine Reviews* 12 (1991): 372.

The increased incidence of certain reproductive diseases in westernized women because of fewer and later pregnancies is documented in most gynecology textbooks.

Footnote: The increased rate in some zoo animals is found in: Vogel, G., "A fertile mind on wildlife conservation's front lines," *Science* 294 (2001): 1271.

PAGE 134 The effects of stress on female libido are discussed in two chapters by Sue Carter, "Neuroendocrinology of sexual behavior in the female" and "Hormonal influences on human sexual behavior," both in Becker, J., Breedlove, S., and Crews, D., eds., *Behavioral Endocrinology* (Cambridge, Mass.: MIT Press, 1992). Also see Rose, R., "Psychoendocrinology," in Wilson, J., and Foster, D., eds., *Williams Textbook of Endocrinology*, 7th ed. (Philadelphia: Saunders, 1985).

PAGE 136 Stressfulness of infertility: Domar, A., Zuttermeister, P., and Friedman, R., "The psychological impact of infertility: a comparison with patients with other medical conditions," *Journal of Psychosomatic Obstetrics and Gynaecology* 14 (1993): S45. These authors found depression rates equal to those seen in women with cancer, although less than in those with AIDS. Also see: Van Balen, F., and Trimbos-Kemper, T., "Long-term infertile couples: a study of their well-being," *Journal of Psychosomatic Obstetrics and Gynaecology* 14 (1993): S53.

Stressfulness of IVF procedures: Boivin, J., and Takefman, J., "Impact of the in vitro fertilization process on emotional, physical and relational variables," *Human Reproduction* 11 (1996): 903; Harlow, C., Fahy, U., Talbot, W., Wardle, P., and Hull, M., "Stress and stress-related hormones during in vitro fertilization treatment," *Human Reproduction* 11 (1996): 274.

More stressed or depressed women are less likely to have successful IVFs: Facchinetti, F., Matteo, M., Artini, G., Volpe, A., and Genazzani, A., "An increased vulnerability to stress is associated with a poor outcome of in vitro fertilization-embryo transfer treatment," *Fertility and Sterility* 67 (1997): 309; Boivin, J., and Takefman, J., "Stress level across stages of in vitro fertilization in subsequently pregnant and nonpregnant women," *Fertility and Sterility* 64 (1995): 802; Thiering, P., Beaurepaire, J., Jones, M., Saunders, D., and Tennant, C., "Mood state as a predictor of treatment outcome after in vitro fertilization/embryo transfer technology," *Journal of Psychosomatic Research* 37 (1993): 481; Demyttenaere, K., Nijs, P., Evers-Kiebooms, G., Koninckx, P., "Personality characteristics, psychoendocrinological stress and outcome of IVF depend upon the etiology of infertility," *Gynecological Endocrinology* 8 (1994): 233. This last study was the one that showed that the stress-success link depended on the type of infertility. No relationship between stress and IVF outcome: Harlow, C., Fahy, U., Talbot, W., Wardle, P., and Hull, M., "Stress and stress-related hormones during in vitro fertilization treatment," *Human Reproduction* 11 (1996): 274.

PAGE 138 Hippocrates' advice to pregnant women is noted in Huisjes, H., *Spontaneous Abortion* (Edinburgh: Churchill Livingstone, 1984), 108. Anne Boleyn's attribution is found in Ives, E., *Anne Boleyn* (Oxford: Basil Blackwell, 1986). George Eliot's *Middlemarch* (London: Zodiac Press, 1982), 557. Miscarriage and the job environment: Lobel, M., "Conceptualizations, measurements and effects of prenatal maternal stress on birth outcomes," *Journal of Behavioral Medicine* (1994): 225. Cited in Mendelsohn, M., and Albertini, R., eds., *Mutation and the Environment*, Part B (New York: Wiley-Liss, 1990), 467. Much of this paper reviews the links between various occupational hazards and increased risk of miscarriage; however, it also presents epidemiologic data linking stressful lifestyles to increased rates of miscarriage. For further links between stress and either pregnancy complications or miscarriage, see Vartiainen, H., Suonio, S., Halonen, P., and Rimon, R., "Psychosocial factors, female fertility and pregnancy: a prospective study—Part II: Pregnancy," *Journal of Psychosomatic Obstetrics and Gynaecology* 15 (1994): 77; O'Hare, T., and Creed, F., "Life events and miscarriage," *British Journal of Psychiatry* 167 (1995): 799; Lederman, R., "Relationship of anxiety, stress and psychosocial development to reproductive health," *Behavioral Medicine* 21 (1995): 101.

PAGE 139 Competitive infanticide in animals is reviewed in Hausfater, G., and Hrdy, S., *Infanticide: Comparative and Evolutionary Perspectives* (Hawthorne, N.Y.: Aldine, 1984). Harassment and abortion: Berger, J., "Induced abortion and social factors in wild horses," *Nature* 303 (1983): 59; Pereira, M., "Abortion following the immigration of an adult male baboon (Papio cynephalus)," *American Journal of Primatology* 4 (1983): 93; Alberts, S., Sapolsky, R., and Altmann, J., "Behavioral, endocrine, and immunological correlates of immigration by an aggressive male into a natural primate group," *Hormones and Behavior* 26 (1992): 167–78. Olfactory-induced abortions in rodents: Bruce, H., "An exteroceptive block to pregnancy in the mouse," *Nature* 184 (1959): 105; De Cantanzaro, D., Muir, C., O'Brien, J., and

Williams, S., "Strange-male-induced pregnancy disruption in mice: reduction of vulnerability by 17 beta-estradiol antibodies," *Physiology and Behavior* 58 (1995): 401.

Footnote: The gigolo appellation comes from Sarah Hrdy of the University of California at Davis, who first described competitive infanticide.

PAGE 140 Miscarriages typically occur many days to weeks after the death of the fetus: chapter 24, "Abortions," in Pritchard, J., MacDonald, P., and Gant, N., *Williams Obstetrics,* 17th ed. (East Norwalk, Conn.: Appleton-Century-Crofts, 1985). For a good review of the possible mechanisms of stress-induced miscarriage, see Myers, R., "Maternal anxiety and fetal death," in Ziochella, L., and Pancheri, P., eds., *Psychoneuroendocrinology in Reproduction* (New York: Elsevier, 1979). The notion that decreased blood flow to the fetus can be the mechanism underlying miscarriage is found in Lapple, M., "Stress as an explanatory model for spontaneous abortions and recurrent spontaneous abortions," *Zentralblatt für Gynakologie* 110 (1988): 325 (in German).

PAGE 141 Stress and preterm births: De Haas, I., Harlow, B., Cramer, D., Frigoletto, F., "Spontaneous preterm birth: a case-control study," *American Journal of Obstetrics and Gynecology* 165 (1991): 1290.

PAGE 141 The Kenyan birth rate: Hatcher, J., Kowal, N., Guest, S., Trussell, J., Stewart, M., Stewart, N., Bowen, T., and Cates, J., *Contraceptive Technology: International Edition* (Atlanta, Ga.: Printed Matter, 1989), 21. Hutterite studies: Eaton, J., and Mayer, A., "The social biology of very high fertility among the Hutterites: the demography of a unique population," *Human Biology* 25 (1953): 206 (for an estimate of nine children per family). See Frisch, R., "Population, food intake and fertility," *Science* 199 (1978): 22 (for an estimate of ten to twelve kids per family).

The Nazi studies of the women in the Theresienstadt death camp are discussed, without attribution, in Reichlin, S., "Neuroendocrinology," in Williams, R., ed., *Textbook of Endocrinology,* 6th ed. (Philadelphia: Saunders, 1974).

CHAPTER 8: IMMUNITY, STRESS, AND DISEASE

PAGE 144 For an introduction to psychoimmunology, or psychoneuroimmunology (the study of the links among the nervous, endocrine, and immune systems), there is the bible in the field: Ader, R., Felten, D., and Cohen, N., *Psychoneuroimmunology,* 3d ed. (San Diego: Academic Press, 2001).

Projections from the autonomic nervous system to immune organs, and presence of receptors for autonomic hormones in immune cells: Downing, J., Miyan, J., "Neural immunoregulation: emerging roles for nerves in immune homeostasis and disease," *Immunology Today* 21 (2000): 277; Bellinger, D., Lorton, D., Lubahn, C., Felten, D., "Innervation of lymphoid organs—association of nerves with cells of the immune system and their implications in disease," in Ader et al., op. cit., 55.

Psychoimmunology of trained actors: Futterman, A., Kemeny, M., Shapiro, D., and Fahey, J., "Immunological and physiological changes associated with induced positive and negative mood," *Psychosomatic Medicine* 56 (1994): 499.

PAGE 145 Most college physiology textbooks will have introductions to the workings of the immune system. For those who want even more, a good introductory text for immunology is Benjamini, E., and Leskowitz, S., *Immunology: A Short Course,* 2d ed. (New York: Wiley-Liss, 1991).

PAGE 150 A review about innate immunity: Gura, T., "Innate immunity: ancient system gets new respect," *Science* 291 (2001): 2068.

PAGE 151 Reviews on the ability of stress to inhibit the immune system: Cohen, S., and Herbert, T., "Health psychology: psychological factors and physical disease from the perspective of human psychoneuroimmunology," *Annual Review of Psychology* 47 (1996): 113; Coe, C., "Psychosocial factors and immunity in nonhuman primates: a review," *Psychosomatic Medicine* 55 (1993): 298; Herbert, T., and Cohen, S., "Stress and immunity in humans: a meta-analytic review," *Psychosomatic Medicine* 55 (1993): 364; Chiappelli, F., Hodgson, D., "Immune suppression," in Fink, G., ed., *Encyclopedia of Stress* (San Diego: Academic Press, 2000), vol. 2, 531.

Effects of glucocorticoids on the immune system: the most up-to-date and masterly of reviews can be found in McEwen, B., Biron, C., Brunson, K., Bulloch, K., Chambers, W., Dhabhar, F., Goldfarb, R., Kitson, R., Miller, A., Spencer, R., and Weiss, J., "The role of adrenocorticoids as modulators of immune function in health and disease: neural, endocrine and immune interactions," *Brain Research Reviews* 23 (1997): 79. For some of the most recent molecular findings regarding how glucocorticoids suppress the release of immune messengers, see Scheinman, R., Cogswell, P., Lofquist, A., and Baldwin, A., "Role of transcriptional activation of IkNFkappaB in mediation of immunosuppression by glucocorticoids," *Science* 270 (1995): 283; and Auphan, N., DiDonato, J., Rosette, C., Helmberg, A., and Karin, M., "Immunosuppression by glucocorticoids: inhibition of NF-KB activity through induction of IkB synthesis," *Science* 270 (1995): 286. (Note that this is another case of a pair of papers—from two groups on opposite sides of the globe—reporting the same novel finding in the same week.)

Glucocorticoids kill cells of the immune system in many species and do so by causing the DNA to be chopped into small pieces. This has been shown in many studies; some of the classic ones are Wyllie, A., "Glucocorticoid-induced thymocyte apoptosis is associated with endogenous endonuclease activation," *Nature* 284 (1980): 555; Cohen, J., and Duke, R., "Glucocorticoid activation of a calcium-dependent endonuclease in thymocyte nuclei leads to cell death," *Journal of Immunology* 132 (1984): 38; Compton, M., and Cidlowski, J., "Rapid in vivo effects of glucocorticoids on the integrity of rat lymphocyte genomic DNA," *Endocrinology* 118 (1986): 38. As noted throughout the chapter, a frequent question runs along the line of "Okay, so if you inject an animal with a ton of glucocorticoids and you mess up its immune system in some way (in this case, by killing lymphocytes), is that a 'physiological' effect—will the smaller amounts of glucocorticoids secreted during stress (or stress itself) do the same thing?" The previous paper also presents a small amount of data suggesting that stress will damage lymphocytes in the same way: Compton, M., Haskill, J., and Cidlowski, J., "Analysis of glucocorticoid actions on rat thymocyte DNA by fluorescence-activated flow cytometry," *Endocrinology* 122 (1988): 2158. For some recent advances in the mechanisms underlying glucocorticoid-induced apoptosis, see: Nocentini, G., Giunchi, L., Ronchetti, S., Krausz, L., Bartoli, A., Moraca, R., Migliorati, G., Riccardi, C., "A new member of the tumor NF/NGF receptor family inhibits T cell receptor-induced apoptosis," *Proceedings of the National Academy of Sciences, USA* 94 (1997): 6216.

PAGE 152 Sympathetic role in suppressing immunity: Hori, T., Katafuchi, T., Take, S., Shimizu, N., and Nijima, A., "The autonomic nervous system as a communication channel between the brain and the immune system," *Neuroimmunomodulation* 2 (1995): 203; role of beta-endorphin: Shavit, Y., Lewis, J., and Terman, G., "Opioid peptides mediate the suppressive effect of stress on natural killer cell cytotoxicity," *Science* 188 (1984): 233; role of CRH: Irwin, M., Vale, W., and Rivier, C., "Central CRF mediates the suppressive effect of footshock stress on natural cytotoxicity," *Endocrinology* 126 (1990): 2837. Glucocorticoids don't play a role in some instances of immunosuppression: Gust, D., Gordon, T., and Wilson, M., "Removal from natal social group to peer housing affects cortisol levels and absolute numbers of T cell subsets in juvenile rhesus monkeys," *Brain Behavior and Evolution* 6 (1992): 189; Manuck, S., Cohen, S., Rabin, B., Muldoon, M., and Bachen, E., "Individual differences in cellular immune response to stress," *Psychological Sciences* 2 (1991): 111; Keller, S., Weiss, J., Schleifer, S., Miller, N., and Stein, M., "Stress-induced suppression of immunity in adrenalectomized rats," *Science* 221 (1983): 1301.

PAGE 153 The idea that not all the traits of an organism are necessarily sculpted by evolution to be adaptive runs through much of Stephen Jay Gould's writing. It is most succinctly presented in "The spandrels of San Marco and the Panglossian paradigm: a critique of the adaptationist programme," written with the geneticist Richard Lewontin, *Proceedings of the Royal Society of London B* (1979): 205.

PAGE 153 Interleukin-1 causes the release of CRH from the hypothalamus: Sapolsky, R., Rivier, C., Yamamoto, G., Plotsky, P., and Vale, W., "Interleukin-1 stimulates the secretion of hypothalamic corticotropin-releasing factor," *Science* 238 (1987): 522; Berkenbosch, F., van Oers, J., del Rey, A., Tilders, F., and Besedovsky, H., "Corticotropin-releasing factor-producing neurons in the rat activated by interleukin-1," *Science* 238 (1987): 524. Footnote: Just to make things worse, the same issue contained a report that IL-1 works at the level of the pituitary, rather than the hypothalamus in the brain, to stimulate the stress-response: Bernton, E., Beach, J., Holaday, J., Smallridge, R., and Fein, H., "Release of multiple hormones by a direct action of interleukin-1 on pituitary cells," *Science* 238 (1987): 519. I think a vague consensus is emerging in the field that the effect on the hypothalamus occurs reproducibly in an animal, whereas the pituitary effect depends on the use of pituitary cells in a petri dish (rather than in the living animal) and on the conditions under which the cells are grown in the dish. For recent advances in this area, see: Bethin, K. E., Vogt, S. K., Muglia, L. J., "Interleukin-6 is an essential, corticotropin-releasing hormone-independent stimulator of the adrenal axis during immune system activation," *Proceedings of the National Academy of Sciences, USA* 97 (2000): 9317.

PAGE 154 Short-term stress stimulates immunity: Berkenbosch, F., Heijnen, C., and Croiset, G., "Endocrine and immunological responses to acute stress," in Plotnikoff, N., Faith, R., Murgo, A., and Good, R., eds., *Enkephalins and Endorphins: Stress and the Immune System* (New York: Plenum Press, 1986); Croiset, G., Heijnen, C., and Veldhuis, H., "Modulation of the immune response by emotional stress," *Life Sciences* 40 (1987): 775; Dhabhar, F., and McEwen, B., "Stress-induced enhancement of antigen-specific cell-mediated immunity," *Journal of Immunology* 156 (1996): 2608; Weiss, J., Sundar, S., Becker, K., and Cierpial, M., "Behavioral and neural influences on cellular immune responses: effects of stress and interleukin-1," *Journal of Clinical Psychiatry* 50 (1989): 43; Herbert, T., Cohen, S., Marsland, A., Bachen, E., and Rabin, B., "Cardiovascular reactivity and the course of immune response to an acute psychological stressor," *Psychosomatic Medicine* 56 (1994): 337; Herbert, T., and Cohen, S., "Stress and immunity in humans: a meta-analytic review," *Psychosomatic Medicine* 55 (1993): 364 (see tables 2 and 3); Carlson, S., "Neural influences on cell adhesion molecules and lymphocyte trafficking," in Ader et al., op. cit., 231; Dhabhar, F., McEwen, B., "Bidirectional effects of stress and glucocorticoid hormones on immune function: Possible explanation for paradoxical observations," in Ader et al., op. cit., 301.

Why this transient increase actually makes sense: Moynihan, J., Sevens, S., "Mechanisms of stress-induced modulation of immunity in animals," in Ader et al., op. cit., vol. 2, 227. Antibody release into the saliva: Wood, P., Karol, M., Kusnecov, A., Rabin, B., "Enhancement of antigen-specific humoral and cell-mediated immunity by electric footshock stress in rats," *Brain Behavior and Immunity* 7 (1993): 121; Carroll, D., Ring, C., Winzer, A., "Stress and mucosal immunity," in Fink, G., ed., *Encyclopedia of Stress* (San Diego: Academic Press, 2000), vol. 2, 781; Booth, R., "Antibody response," in Fink, op. cit., vol. 1, 206.

This short-term increase is mediated by sympathetic hormones: Bachen, E., Manuck, S., Cohen, S., Muldoon, M., and Raible, R., "Adrenergic blockage ameliorates cellular immune responses to mental stress in humans," *Psychosomatic Medicine* 64 (1995): 15; Landmann, R., Muller, F., and Perini, C., "Changes of immunoregulatory cells induced by psychological and physical stress: relationship to plasma catecholamines," *Clinical and Experimental Immunology* 58 (1984): 127; Ernstrom, U., and Sandberg, G., "Effects of alpha- and beta-receptor stimulation on the release of lymphocytes and granulocytes from the spleen," *Scandinavian Journal of Hematology* 11 (1973): 275. Involvement of glucocorticoids: Bateman, A., Singh, A., Kral, T., and Solomon, S., "The immune hypothalamic-pituitary-adrenal axis," *Endocrine Reviews* 10 (1989): 92; McEwen, B., Biron, C., Brunson, K., Bulloch, K., Chambers, W., Dhabhar, F., Goldfarb, R., Kitson, R., Miller, A., Spencer, R., and Weiss, J., "The role of adrenocorticoids as modulators of immune function in health and disease: neural, endocrine and immune interactions," *Brain Research Reviews* 23 (1997): 79.

Approximate 40–70 percent declines: Dhabhar, F., "Immune cell distribution, effects of stress on," in Fink, op. cit., vol. 2, 507.

PAGE 156 Munck's ideas: Munck, A., Guyre, P., and Holbrook, N., "Physiological actions of glucocorticoids in stress and their relation to pharmacological actions," *Endocrine Reviews* 5 (1984): 25. This is probably the most influential paper written about glucocorticoids in the last quarter-century. This reorientation has been updated recently in: Sapolsky, R., Romero, M., Munck, A., "How do glucocorticoids influence the stress-response?: integrating permissive, suppressive, stimulatory, and preparative actions," *Endocrine Reviews* 21 (2000): 55.

Blockade of the glucocorticoid-mediated recovery from stress-induced activation of the immune system is associated with autoimmunity: Wick, G., Hu, Y., Schwarz, S., and Kroemer, G., "Immunoendocrine communication via the hypothalamo-pituitary-adrenal axis in autoimmune diseases," *Endocrine Reviews* 14 (1993): 539; Sternberg, E., Chrousos, G., Wilder, R., and Gold, P., "The stress response and regulation of inflammatory disease," *Annals of Internal Medicine* 117 (1992): 854; Rose, N., Bacon, L., and Sundick, R., "Genetic determinants of thyroiditis in the OS chicken," *Transplantation Reviews* 31 (1976): 264–70; Heim, C., Ehlert, U., Hellhammer, D., "The potential role of hypocortisolism in the pathophysiology of stress-related bodily disorders," *Psychoneuroendocrinology* 25 (2000): 1; Wilder, R., "Arthritis," in Fink, op. cit., vol. 1, 251; Takasu, N., Komiya,

I., Nagasawa, Y., Aaswa, T., and Yamada, T., "Exacerbation of autoimmune thyroid dysfunction after unilateral adrenalectomy in patients with Cushing's syndrome due to adrenocortical adenoma," *New England Journal of Medicine* 322 (1990): 1708–12; Harbuz, S., and Lightman, S., "Stress and the hypothalamo-pituitary-adrenal axis: acute, chronic and immunological activation," *Journal of Endocrinology* 134 (1992): 327–39; Green, M., and Lim, K., "Bronchial asthma with Addison's disease," *The Lancet* 1 (1971): 1159–65. Decreased sensitivity of immune cells to glucocorticoids, and the mechanisms mediating it: Farrell, R. J., Kelleher, D., "Glucocorticoid resistance in inflammatory bowel disease," *Journal of Endocrinology* 178 (2003): 339; Franchimont, D., Martens, H., Hagelstein, M., Louis, E., Dewe, W., Chrousos, G., Belaiche, J., Geenen, V., "TNF alpha decreases, and IL-10 increases, the sensitivity of human monocytes to dexamethasone: potential regulation of the GR," *Journal of Clinical Endocrinology and Metabolism* 84 (1999): 2834; Pariante, C., Pearce, B., Pisell, T., Sanchez, C., Po, C., Su, C., Miller, A., "The proinflammatory cytokine, IL-1a, reduces glucocorticoid receptor translocation and function," *Endocrinology* 140 (1999): 4359.

There is also evidence of underactivity of the sympathetic nervous system in some autoimmune flare-ups: Madden, K., "Catecholamines, sympathetic nerves, and immunity," in Ader et al., *Psychoneuroimmunology,* 3rd ed., op. cit., 197.

PAGE 157 The notion of glucocorticoids sculpting the immune response can be found in Besedovsky, H., Del Ray, S., Sorkin, E., and Dinarello, C., "Immuno-regulatory feedback between interleukin-1 and glucocorticoid hormones," *Science* 233 (1986): 652; Besedovsky, H., and Del Ray, A., "Immuno-neuro-endocrine interactions: facts and hypotheses," *Endocrine Reviews* 17 (1996): 64.

PAGE 158 Glucocorticoids as causing a salutary redistribution of lymphocytes: Dhabhar, F., and McEwen, B., "Stress-induced enhancement of antigen-specific cell-mediated immunity," *Journal of Immunology* 156 (1996): 2608; McEwen, B., Biron, C., Brunson, K., Bulloch, K., Chambers, W., Dhabhar, F., Goldfarb, R., Kitson, R., Miller, A., Spencer, R., and Weiss, J., "The role of adrenocorticoids as modulators of immune function in health and disease: neural, endocrine and immune interactions," *Brain Research Reviews* 23 (1997): 79; Dhabhar, F., McEwen, B., "Bidirectional effects of stress and glucocorticoid hormones on immune function: possible explanation for paradoxical observations," in Ader et al., *Psychoneuroimmunology,* 3rd ed., op. cit., 301.

PAGE 158 Prolonged stressors can protect against autoimmunity: Kuroda, Y., Mori, T., Hori, T., "Restraint stress suppresses experimental allergic encephalomyelitis," *Brain Research Bulletin* 34 (1994): 15.

PAGE 158 Patient reports about stress worsening autoimmunity: Affleck, G., et al., "Attributional processes in rheumatoid arthritis patients," *Arthritis and Rheumatology* 30 (1987): 927. Documentation that stress can exacerbate some autoimmune diseases: Leclere, J., and Weryha, G., "Stress and auto-immune endocrine diseases," *Hormone Research* 31 (1989): 90; Weiner, H., "Social and psychobiological factors in autoimmune diseases," in Ader, R., Felten, D., and Cohen, N., eds., *Psychoneuroimmunology,* 2d ed. (San Diego: Academic Press, 1991); Chiovato, L., and Pinchera, A., "Stressful life events and Graves' disease," *European Journal of Endocrinology* 134 (1996): 68; Rosch, P., "Stressful life events and Graves' disease," *The Lancet* 342 (1993): 566; Rimon, R., Belmaker, R., and Ebstein, R., "Psychosomatic aspects of juvenile rheumatoid arthritis," *Scandina-*

vian Journal of Rheumatology 6 (1977): 1; Dancey, C., Taghavi, M., and Fox, R., "The relationship between daily stress and symptoms of irritable bowel," *Journal of Psychosomatic Research* 44 (1998): 537; Homo-Delarche, F., Fitzpatrick, F., Christeff, N., Nunez, E., Bach, J., and Dardenne, M., "Sex steroids, glucocorticoids, stress and autoimmunity," *Journal of Steroid Biochemistry and Molecular Biology* 40 (1991): 619; Potter, P., and Zautra, A., "Stressful life events' effects on rheumatoid arthritis disease activity," *Journal of Consulting and Clinical Psychology* 65 (1997): 319; Zautra, A., Burleson, M., Matt, K. I., Roth, S., Burrows, L., "Interpersonal stress, depression, and disease activity in rheumatoid arthritis and osteoarthritis patients," *Health Psychology* 13 (1994): 139; Sekas, G., and Wile, M., "Stress-related illnesses and sources of stress: comparing M.D.-Ph.D., M.D., and Ph.D. students," *Journal of Medical Education* 55 (1980): 440; Buske-Kirschbaum, A., von Auer, K., Krieger, S., Weis, S., Rauh, W., Hellhammer, D., "Blunted cortisol responses to psychosocial stress in asthmatic children: a general feature of atopic disease?" *Psychosomatic Medicine* 65 (2003): 806; Harbuz, M. S., Korendowych, E., Jessop, D. S., Crown, A. L., Li, S. L., Kirwan, J. R., "Hypothalamo-pituitary-adrenal axis dysregulation in patients with rheumatoid arthritis after the dexamethasone/corticotrophin releasing factor test," *Journal of Endocrinology* 178 (2003): 55. A report of no effect of stress: Nispeanu, P., and Korczyn, A., "Psychological stress as risk factor for exacerbations in multiple sclerosis," *Neurology* 43 (1993): 1311. In contrast: Warren, S., Greenhill, S., and Warren, K., "Emotional stress and the development of multiple sclerosis: case-control evidence of a relationship," *Journal of Chronic Disease* 35 (1982): 821; Ackerman, K., Heyman, R., Rabin, B., Anderon, B., Houck, P., Frank, E., Baum, A., "Stress life events precede exacerbations of multiple sclerosis," *Psychosomatic Medicine* 64 (2002): 916. For criticisms of the link between stress and these diseases, see: Reder, A., "Multiple sclerosis," in Fink, op. cit., vol. 2, 791.

Stress can worsen autoimmunity in animal models: Chandler, N., Jacobson, S., Esposito, P., Connolly, R., Theoharides, T., "Acute stress shortens the time to onset of experimental allergic encephalomyelitis in SJL/J mice," *Brain Behavior and Immunity* 16 (2002): 757; Lehman, C., Rodin, J., McEwen, B., Brinton, R., "Impact of environmental stress on the expression of insulin-dependent diabetes mellitus," *Behavioral Neuroscience* 2 (1991): 241; Joachim, R., Ouarcoo, D., Arck, P., Herz, U., Renz, H., Klapp, B., "Stress enhances airway reactivity and airway inflammation in an animal model of allergic bronchial asthma," *Psychosomatic Medicine* 65 (2003): 811.

PAGE 164 Social relationships are associated with decreased mortality rates: House, J., Landis, K., and Umberson, D., "Social relationships and health," *Science* 241 (1988): 540. Social stressors are particularly immunosuppressive: Herbert, T., and Cohen, S., "Stress and immunity in humans: a meta-analytic review," *Psychosomatic Medicine* 55 (1993): 364; Berkman, L., *Health and Ways of Living: Findings from the Alameda County Study* (New York: Oxford University Press, 1983). Lonelier individuals had less natural killer cell activity: Kiecolt-Glaser, J., Garner, W., Speicher, C., Penn, G., and Glaser, R., "Psychosocial modifiers of immunocompetence in medical students," *Psychosomatic Medicine* 46 (1984): 7. The socially isolated rate themselves as lonely: Kiecolt-Glaser, J., McGuire, L., Robles, T., Glaser, R., "Psychoneuroimmunology and psychosomatic medicine: back to the future," *Psychosomatic Medicine* 64 (2002): 15–28; Cohen, S., Frank, E., Doyle, W., Skoner, D., Rabin, B., Gwaltney, J., "Types of stressors that increase susceptibility to the common cold in healthy adults," *Health Psychology* 17 (1998): 214.

Factors like divorce or marital discord are associated with suppressed aspects of immune function. Reviewed in Robles, T., Kiecolt-Glaser, J., "The physiology of marriage: pathways to health," *Physiology and Behavior* 79 (2003): 409.

Isolation damping immune function: reviewed in Kiecolt-Glaser et al., op. cit.; Leserman, J., Petitto, J., Golden, R., Gaynes, B., Gu, H., Perkins, D., Silva, S., Folds, J., Evans, D., "Impact of stressful life events, depression, social support, coping, and cortisol on progression to AIDS," *American Journal of Psychiatry* 157 (2000): 1221.

Some subtle confounds in lifestyle-disease relationships: some particularly thoughtful discussions can be found in House, J., Landis, K., and Umberson, D., "Social relationships and health," *Science* 241 (1988): 540. Less medical compliance among the socially isolated: Williams, C., "The Edgecomb County high blood pressure control program: III. Social support, social stressors, and treatment dropout," *American Journal of Public Health* 75 (1985): 483.

Social support helps the immune system of primates: Cohen, S., Kaplan, J., Cunnick, J., Manuck, S., and Rabin, B., "Chronic social stress, affiliation, and cellular immune response in nonhuman primates," *Psychological Science* 3 (1992): 301. Social isolation suppresses primate immunity: Laudenslager, M., Capitano, J., and Reite, M., "Possible effects of early separation experiences on subsequent immune function in adult macaque monkeys," *American Journal of Psychiatry* 142 (1985): 862; Coe, C., "Psychosocial factors and immunity in nonhuman primates: a review," *Psychosomatic Medicine* 55 (1993): 298. The SIV study: Capitano, J., Mendoza, S., Lerche, N., Mason, W., "Social stress results in altered glucocorticoid regulation and shorter survival in SIV syndrome," *Proceedings of the National Academy of Sciences, USA* 95 (1998): 4714; also: Capitano, J., Mendoza, S., Baroncelli, S., "The relationship of personality dimensions in adult male rhesus macaques to progression of SIV disease," *Brain, Behavior and Immunity* 13 (1999): 138; Capitano, J., Lerche, N., "Social separation, housing relocation, and survival in simian AIDS: a retrospective analysis," *Psychosomatic Medicine* 60 (1998): 235–44.

PAGE 166 Bereavement: Bereavement decreases immune function and increases the risk for mortality: Kiecolt-Glaser, J., and Glaser, R., "Stress and immune function in humans," in Ader, R., Felten, D., and Cohen, N., eds., *Psychoneuroimmunology*, 2d ed. (San Diego: Academic Press, 1991); Levav, I., Friedlander, Y., Kark, J., and Peritz, E., "An epidemiological study of mortality among bereaved parents," *New England Journal of Medicine* 319 (1988): 457; Clayton, P., "Bereavement," in Fink, G., ed., *Encyclopedia of Stress*, vol. 1, 304.

PAGE 166 Stress and the common cold: Cohen, S., Tyrrell, D., and Smith, A., "Psychological stress and susceptibility to the common cold," *New England Journal of Medicine* 325 (1991): 606; Cohen, S. W., and Doyle, W., "Social ties and susceptibility to the common cold," *Journal of the American Medical Association* 277 (1997): 1940; Cohen, S., Frank, E., Doyle, W., Skoner, D., Rabin, B., and Gwaltney, J., "Types of stressors that increase susceptibility to the common cold in healthy adults," *Health Psychology* 17 (1998): 214. Fewer antibodies in saliva and nasal passageways: Carroll, D., Ring, C., and Winzer, A., "Mucosal immunity, stress and," in Fink, G., ed., *Encyclopedia of Stress*, vol. 2, 781. Footnote: Roach, M., "How I blew my summer vacation," *Health* (January–February 1990): 73.

Stress and the common cold in nonhuman primates: Cohen, S., Line, S.,

Manuck, S., Rabin, B., Heise, E., and Kaplan, J., "Chronic social stress, social status and susceptibility to upper respiratory infections in nonhuman primates," *Psychosomatic Medicine* 59 (1997): 213.

PAGE 168 Stress and HIV progression—petri dish studies: Antoni, M., Cruess, D., "AIDS," in Fink, *Encyclopedia of Stress*, vol. 2, 118. The SIV study: Capitano et al., "Social separation," op. cit. Human studies: Cole, S., Kemeny, M. "Psychosocial influences on the progression of HIV infection," in Ader et al., *Psychoneuroimmunology*, 3d ed., vol. 2, 583. Elevated activity of the sympathetic nervous system: Cole, S., Naliboff, B., Kemeny, M., Griswold, M., Fahey, J., Zack, J., "Impaired response to HAART in patients with high autonomic nervous system activity," *Proceedings of the National Academy of Sciences, USA* 98 (2001): 12695; Leserman et al., "Impact of stressful life events," op. cit. Bereavement among HIV patients: Goodkin, K., Feaster, D., Tuttle, R., Blaney, N., Kumar, M., Baum, M., Shapshak, P., and Fletcher, M., "Bereavement is associated with time-dependent decrements in cellular immune function in asymptomatic HIV type 1-seropositive homosexual men," *Clinical and Diagnostic Laboratory Immunology* 3 (1996): 109; Kemeny, M., Weiner, H., Duran, R., Taylor, S., Visscher, B., and Fahey, J., "Immune system changes after the death of a partner in HIV-positive gay men," *Psychosomatic Medicine* 57 (1995): 547; Kemeny, M., and Dean, L., "Effects of AIDS-related bereavement on HIV progression among New York City gay men," *AIDS Education and Prevention* 7 (1995): 36.

PAGE 169 Reactivation of latent viruses by stress or glucocorticoids: Padgett, D., Sheridan, J., Dorne, J., Berntson, G., Candelora, J., Glaser, R., "Social stress and the reactivation of latent herpes simplex virus type," *Proceedings of the National Academy of Sciences, USA* 95 (1998): 7231; Padgett, D., Sheridan, J., "Herpesviruses," in Fink, G., ed., *Encyclopedia of Stress*, vol. 2, 357; Glaser, R., Friedman, S., Smyth, J., Ader, R., Bijur, P., Brunell, P., Cohen, N., Krilov, L., Lifrak, S., Stone, A., "The differential impact of training stress and final examination stress on herpesvirus latency at the U.S. Military Academy at West Point," *Brain, Behavior and Immunity* 13 (1999): 240; Hudnall, S., Rady, P., Tyring, S., Fish, J., "Hydrocortisone activation of human herpesvirus 8 viral DNA replication and gene expression in vitro," *Transplantation* 67 (1999): 648. Latent viruses reactivate by measuring glucocorticoid levels: Hardwicke, M., Schaffer, P., "Differential effects of NGF and dexamethasone on herpes simplex virus type 1 oriL- and oriS-dependent DNA replication in PC12 cells," *Journal of Virology* 71 (1997): 3580. Herpes stimulates glucocorticoid secretion: Bonneau, R., Sheridan, J., Feng, N., Glaser, R., "Stress-induced modulation of the primary cellular immune response to HSV infection is mediated by both adrenal-dependent and independent mechanisms," *Journal of Neuroimmunology* 42 (1993): 167.

PAGE 171 Studies showing stress-cancer links with laboratory animals—stress increases the rate of spontaneous tumors in mice: Henry, J., Stephens, V., and Watson, F., "Forced breeding, social disorder, and mammary tumor formation in CBA/USC mouse colonies: a pilot study," *Psychosomatic Medicine* 37 (1975): 277. Stress accelerates tumor growth in rats: Sklar, L., and Anisman, H., "Stress and coping factors influence tumor growth," *Science* 205 (1979): 513; Riley, V., "Psychoneuroendocrine influences on immunocompetence and neoplasia," *Science* 212 (1981): 1100. Visintainer, M., Volpicelli, J., and Seligman, M., "Tumor rejection in rats after inescapable or escapable shock," *Science* 216 (1982): 437.

Sapolsky, R., and Donnelly, T., "Vulnerability to stress-induced tumor growth increases with age in rats: role of glucocorticoids," *Endocrinology* 117 (1985): 662. Tumor growth rates in rodents can be accelerated by housing them in stressful conditions, giving them rotational stress, and giving them glucocorticoids: Riley, V., "Psychoneuroendocrine influences on immunocompetence and neoplasia," *Science* 212 (1981): 1100. Tumor growth can also be accelerated by inescapable shock: Visintainer, M., Volpicelli, J., and Seligman, M., "Tumor rejection in rats after inescapable or escapable shock," *Science* 216 (1982): 437. Discussions of some of the limits of this literature: the links between stress and cancer mostly involve induced tumors, acceleration of tumor growth rather than initial establishment of tumors, and virally derived tumors: Fitzmaurice, M., "Physiological relationships among stress, viruses, and cancer in experimental animals," *International Journal of Neuroscience* 39 (1988): 307; Justice, A., "Review of the effects of stress on cancer in laboratory animals: importance of time of stress application and type of tumor," *Psychological Bulletin* 98 (1985): 108.

The effects of stress make sense in the context of the biology of tumorigenesis. Stress and glucocorticoid effects on natural killer cell activity: Munck, A., and Guyre, P., "Glucocorticoids and immune function," in Ader et al., *Psychoneuroimmunology,* 2d ed.; Wu, W. J., Yamaura, T., Murakami, K., Murata, J., Matsumoto, K., Watanabe, H., Saiki, I., "Social isolation stress enhanced liver metastasis of murine colon 26-L5 carcinoma cells by suppressing immune responses in mice," *Life Sciences* 66 (2000): 1827. Effects on angiogenesis: Folkman, J., Langer, R., Linhardt, R., Haudenschild, C., and Taylor, S., "Angiogenesis inhibition and tumor regression caused by heparin or a heparin fragment in the presence of cortisone," *Science* 221 (1983): 719. Effects of glucocorticoids on tumor metabolism: Romero, L., Raley-Susman, K., Redish, K., Brooke, S., Horner, H., and Sapolsky, R., "A possible mechanism by which stress accelerates growth of virally-derived tumors," *Proceedings of the National Academy of Sciences, USA* 89 (1992): 11084.

PAGE 172 Minimal link between a history of stress and cancer in humans reviewed in: Turner-Cobb, J., Sephton, S., Spiegel, D., "Psychosocial effects on immune function and disease progression in cancer A: human studies," in Ader et al., *Psychoneuroimmunology,* vol. 2, 565. The stress-colon cancer link: Courtney, J., Longnecker, M., Theorell, T., Gerhardsson-de-Verdier, M., "Stressful life events and the risk of colorectal cancer," *Epidemiology* 4 (1993): 407; Kune, S., Kune, G., Watson, L., Rahe, R., "Recent life changes and large bowel cancer: data from the Melbroune Colorectal Cancer Study," *Journal of Clinical Epidemiology* 44 (1991): 57. The Western Electric study: Shekelle, R., Raynor, W., Ostfeld, A., Garron, D., Bieliauskas, L., Liu, S., Maliza, C., and Paul, O., "Psychological depression and 17-year risk of death from cancer," *Psychosomatic Medicine* 43 (1981): 117; Persky, V., Kempthorne-Rawson, J., and Shekelle, R., "Personality and risk of cancer: 20-year follow-up of the Western Electric Study," *Psychosomatic Medicine* 49 (1987): 435. Its revisionist debunking: Fox, B., "Depressive symptoms and risk of cancer," *Journal of the American Medical Association* 262 (1989): 1231. Other studies showing no depression-cancer link: Kaplan, G., and Reynolds, P., "Depression and cancer mortality and morbidity: prospective evidence from the Alameda County Study," *Journal of Behavioral Medicine* 11 (1988): 1; Hahn, R., and Petitti, D., "Minnesota Multiphasic Personality Inventory-rated depression and the incidence of breast cancer," *Cancer* 61 (1988): 845. One review (McGee, R., Williams, S., and

Elwood, M., "Depression and the development of cancer; a meta-analysis," *Social Science and Medicine* 38 [1993]: 187) surveyed all the studies in the field at the time and concluded that there was a tiny but significant link between depression and cancer, with depression increasing the cancer risk about 14 percent. However, one of the strongest effects in that meta-analysis was found in the since-discredited Western Electric study; once it is removed, any effect disappears.

The lack of links between other types of stressors and subsequent cancer is reviewed in Hilakivi-Clarke, L., Rowland, J., Clarke, R., and Lippman, M., "Psychosocial factors in the development and progression of breast cancer," *Breast Cancer Research and Treatment* 29 (1993): 141. This business of trying to find links between lifestyle or personality and some disease outcome years later is extremely tricky. For example, it was widely reported that cancer rates went up in the surrounding areas following the Three Mile Island nuclear accident in 1979. However, it involved all types of cancers, including those not thought to be sensitive to the radiation released. In that case, the subtle confound was probably that people were more anxious and thus more vigilant, taking more trips to the doctors, who, aware of the accident history, checked things more carefully—and thus spotted more cancer. Pool, R., "A stress-cancer link following accident?" *Nature* 351 (1991): 429.

Cancer, working night shifts, and the likely role of melatonin: Schernhammer, E., Laden, F., Speizer, F., Willett, W., Hunter, D., Kawachi, I., Colditz, G., "Rotating night shifts and risk of breast cancer in women participating in the nurses' health study," *Journal of the National Cancer Institute* 93 (2001): 1563; Hansen, J., "Light at night, shiftwork, and breast cancer risk," *Journal of the National Cancer Institute* 93 (2001): 1513.

Glucocorticoid treatment and skin cancer incidence: Karagas, M., Cushing, G., Greenberg, E., Mott, L., Spencer, S., Nierenberg, D., "Non-melanoma skin cancers and glucocorticoid therapy," *British Journal of Cancer* 85 (2001): 683.

PAGE 174 Breast cancer assumed most often to be stress-related: Petticrew, M., Fraser, J., Regan, M., "Adverse life-events and risk of breast cancer: a meta-analysis," *British Journal of Health Psychology* 4 (1999): 1. Cancer and personality—one of the most influential papers showing a link is: Temoshok, L., Heller, B., Sagebiel, R., Blois, M., Sweet, D., and DiClemente, R., "The relationship of psychosocial factors to prognostic indicators in cutaneous malignant melanoma," *Journal of Psychosomatic Research* 29 (1985): 139. Other papers on the subject are reviewed carefully in Spiegel, D., and Kato, P., "Psychosocial influences on cancer incidence and progression," *Harvard Review of Psychiatry* 4 (1996): 10; also Bryla, C., "The relationship between stress and the development of breast cancer: literature review," *Oncology Nursing Forum* 23 (1996): 441; Hilakivi-Clarke, L., Rowland, J., Clarke, R., and Lippman, M., "Psychosocial factors in the development and progression of breast cancer," *Breast Cancer Research and Treatment* 29 (1993): 141.

PAGE 175 Stress and cancer relapse: Ramirez, A., Craig, T., Watson, J., Fentiman, I., North, W., Rubens, R., "Stress and relapse of breast cancer," *British Medical Journal* 298 (1989): 291; Barraclough, J. K., Pinder, P., Cruddas, M., Osmond, C., Perry, M., "Life events and breast cancer prognosis," *British Medical Journal* 304 (1992): 1078.

PAGE 175 Once cancer has occurred, the helpful effects of a fighting spirit: Temoshok, L., and Fox, B., "Coping styles and other psychosocial factors related to medical status and to prognosis in patients with cutaneous malignant melanoma," in Fox, B., and Newberry, B., eds., *Impact of Psychoneurocrine System in Cancer and Immunity* (Toronto: Hogrefe, 1984), 86. These authors talk about the depression-prone individuals who collapse in the face of cancer as having a "Type C" personality, a term that has caught on in this field to some extent. In many ways, these closely resemble the repressive individuals who appear to be somewhat cancer-prone in the first place. Just to add to the confusion, in addition to a fighting spirit, denial has been shown in some studies to be helpful as well (reviewed in Bauer, S., "Psychoneuroimmunology and cancer: an integrated review," *Journal of Advanced Nursing* 19 [1994]: 1114).

The Spiegel study concerning cancer survival and being in a support group: Spiegel, D., Bloom, J., and Kraemer, H., "Effect of psychosocial treatment on survival of patients with metastatic breast cancer," *The Lancet* 2 (1989): 888. The latest and most visible study that failed to replicate this finding: Goodwin, P., Leszcz, M., Ennis, M., Koopmans, J., Vincent, L., Guther, H., Drysdale, E., Hundleby, M., Chochinov, H., Navarro, M., Speca, M., Hunter, J., "The effect of group psychosocial support on survival in metastatic breast cancer," *New England Journal of Medicine* 345 (2001): 1767. Spiegel's commentary on the Goodwin findings: Spiegel, D., "Mind matters: group therapy and survival in breast cancer," *New England Journal of Medicine* 345 (2001): 1767. The percentages of doctors telling patients they had cancer: Holland, J., "History of psycho-oncology: overcoming attitudinal and conceptual barriers," *Psychosomatic Medicine* 64 (2002): 206–21.

PAGE 175 Psychosocial interventions blunt the stress-response: Van der Polmpe, G., Duivenvoorden, H., Antoni, M., Visser, A., Heijnen, C., "Effectiveness of a short-term group psychotherapy program on endocrine and immune function in breast cancer patients: an exploratory study," *Journal of Psychosomatic Research* 42 (1997): 453; Schedlowski, M., Jung, C., Schimanski, G., Tewes, U., Schmoll, H., "Effects of behavioral intervention on plasma cortisol and lymphocytes in breast cancer patients: an exploratory study," *Psychooncology* 3 (1994): 181.

Footnote regarding our study of glucocorticoid rhythmicity: Sephton, S., Sapolsky, R., Kraemer, H., Spiegel, D., "Diurnal cortisol rhythm as a predictor of breast cancer survival," *Journal of the National Cancer Institute* 92 (2000): 994.

Cancer patients with more stress had lower natural killer cell activity: Anderson, *Journal of the National Cancer Institute* 90 (1998): 30. Despite higher NK cell activity with social support, no prediction of survival time with NK activity: Spiegel, D., "Cancer," in Fink, *Encyclopedia of Stress*, vol. 1, 368; Fawzy, F. I., Fawzy, N. W., Hyun, C. S., "Malignant melanoma: effects of an early structured psychiatric intervention, coping, and affective state on recurrence and survival 6 years later," *Archives of General Psychiatry* 50 (1993): 681; Fawzy, F., Kemeny, M., Fawzy, N., Elashoff, R., Morton, D., Cousins, N., Fahey, J., "A structured psychiatric intervention for cancer patients: II. Changes over time in immunological measures," *Archives of General Psychiatry* 47 (1990): 729.

PAGE 177 The issue of compliance is discussed in: Spiegel, D., and Kato, P., "Psychosocial influences on cancer incidence and progression," *Harvard Review of Psychiatry* 4 (1996): 10.

PAGE 178 Some similar sentiments to those in Bernie Siegel's 1986 magnum opus, *Love, Medicine and Miracles*, can be found in other books, including one by

Simonton, one of Siegel's mentors: Simonton, O., Matthews-Simonton, S., and Creighton, J., *Getting Well Again* (Los Angeles: Tarcher, 1978). The lack of an effect of Siegel's program on survivorship can be found in Morgenstern, H., Gellert, G., Walter, S., Ostfeld, A., and Siegel, B., "The impact of a psychosocial support program on survival with breast cancer: the importance of selection bias in program evaluation," *Journal of Chronic Disease* 37 (1984): 273; and Gellert, G., Maxwell, R., and Siegel, B., "Survival of breast cancer patients receiving adjunctive psychosocial support therapy: a 10-year follow-up study," *Journal of Clinical Oncology* 11 (1993): 66. The program's lack of efficacy is pointed out in a 1992 debate between Siegel and David Spiegel (the physician whose work is discussed earlier in this chapter and who owns up to having sustained a fair amount of discomfort by having a name readily confused with Siegel's): "Psychosocial interventions and cancer," *Advances* 8 (1992): 2.

PAGE 180 The Herbert Weiner quotation comes from his book, *Perturbing the Organism: The Biology of Stressful Experience* (Chicago: University of Chicago Press, 1992).

PAGE 181 The lapsarian in the Reagan administration: in an extraordinary episode, a top appointee in the Department of Education turned out to hold lapsarian views. "There is no injustice in the universe," she wrote. "As unfair as it may seem, a person's external circumstances do fit his level of inner spiritual development. . . . [The handicapped] falsely assume that the lottery of life has penalized them at random. This is not so. 'Nothing comes to an individual that he has not [at some point in his development] summoned.'" (Second set of brackets her own.) She extended this philosophy to explaining why James Brady, Reagan's press secretary, had been seriously wounded in John Hinckley's assassination attempt. Her policy advice included terminating any special educational programs for the handicapped. Fortunately, she lasted three days in her new position before being returned to the conservative fundamentalist think tank from which she had emerged.

Testimony by and about the woman, Eileen Gardner of the conservative Heritage Foundation, can be found in the Senate Hearings Before the Committee on Appropriations, 99th Congress, First Session, 1986, HR 3424, part 3, Appropriations Hearings for the Departments of Labor, HHS, and Education, pp. 74 and 177. The fiery hearings were reported in newspapers throughout the country (for example, *New York Times*, 17–19 April 1985; *Washington Post*, 17 May 1985). In the Senate, Gardner expressed her view that sometimes congenital illnesses are visited upon newborn infants not so much on account of their own sinfulness as because of the sinfulness of the parents—all the while apparently unaware that the senator presiding over her hearings, Lowell Weicker of Connecticut, is the father of a congenitally retarded, institutionalized child and a passionate supporter of research into retardation and congenital abnormalities. Weicker, a veteran politician who probably is as knowledgeable as anyone can be about the corridors of power, described her testimony as "the most incredible thing I have read in my career in the United States Senate. I have never seen such callousness" (*New York Times*, 17 April 1985).

The 2001 study about breast cancer attribution: Stewart, D. E., Cheung, A. M., Duff, S., Wong, F., McQuestion, M., Cheng, T., Purdy, L., Bunston, T., "Attributions of cause and recurrence in long-term breast cancer survivors," *Psychooncology* 10 (2001): 179.

PAGE 182 The history of status thymicolymphaticus was originally published by me under the title "Poverty's remains," *The Sciences* (September–October 1991): 8. The original observation of "enlarged" thymuses in SIDS infants was reported in 1830 by Kopp, J., "Denkwurdigkeiten in der artzlichen Praxis," and was greatly expanded in 1889 by Paltauf, A., *Plotzlicher Thymus Tod,* Wiener klin. Woechesucher, Berlin 46 and 9. The supposed disease was named a few years later in Escherich, T., *Status thymico-lymphaticus,* Berlin klin. Woechesucher 29 (1896). By the late 1920s it was in all the textbooks, complete with radiation advice (how much to administer, where to aim it, and so on). See, for example, Lucas, W., *Modern Practise of Pediatrics* (New York: Macmillan, 1927). Amid this generally grim story, I was amused to note that by the time of this textbook, the "disease" was so well established that the author now broke ground by describing the distinctive and striking behavioral features of infants who would later be found to have died of thymicolymphaticus. They were characterized as having "phlegmatic" dispositions—presumably because these were normal kids and thus were phlegmatic about their imaginary illnesses. It is a chilling experience to wander the dusty lower floor of a medical library, reading these forgotten texts and their confident discussions of this supposed disease. Page after page of errors. What similar mistakes are we making now?

Lost amid this consensus of the savants was a 1927 study by E. Boyd ("Growth of the thymus, its relation to status thymicolymphaticus and thymic symptoms," *American Journal of Diseases of Children* 33 [1927]: 867), which should have put the whole thing to rest. Boyd showed for the first time that a stressor (malnutrition, in this case) caused thymic shrinking. She demonstrated, moreover, that some children who died of accidents turned out, upon autopsy, to be "suffering" from thymicolymphaticus, and suggested for the first time that the whole thing might be an artifact. It was not until the 1930s that the first of the pediatric textbooks began to voice the opinion that this conclusion might be correct; not until 1945 did the leading textbook in the field emphatically state that treating this "disease" was a disastrous thing to do (Nelson, W., *Nelson's Textbook of Pediatrics,* 4th ed. [Philadelphia: Saunders, 1945]). In researching this subject, I had the pleasure of talking with the same Dr. Nelson, now in his nineties, still seeing inner-city children at the University of Pennsylvania Hospital every day and basking in the positive reviews of the recent edition of his classic textbook. He recalled how, by the early 1930s, the Young Turk pediatricians (one of whom he most surely was) were already contemptuous of the old guard for advocating something as crazy and outdated as radiating kids to prevent an imaginary disease. Despite that, the practice continued widely well into the 1950s.

For a discussion of how status thymicolymphaticus was a "progressive" advance in medicine in the 1800s (by substituting for simply blaming the parents), see Guntheroth, W., "The thymus, suffocation, and sudden infant death syndrome—social agenda or hubris?" *Perspectives in Biology and Medicine* 37 (1993): 2.

CHAPTER 9: STRESS AND PAIN

PAGE 186 The extended quotation comes from page 178 of Joseph Heller's *Catch-22* (New York: Simon and Schuster, 1955).

PAGE 187 Pain asymbolia (the inability to feel pain): Appenzeller, O., and Kornfeld, M., "Indifference to pain: a chronic peripheral neuropathy with mosaic

Schwann cells," *Archives of Neurology* 27 (1972): 322; Murray, T., "Congenital sensory neuropathy," *Brain 96* (1973): 387; Fox, J., Belvoir, F., and Huott, A., "Congenital hemihypertrophy with indifference to pain," *Archives of Neurology* 30 (1974): 490.

PAGE 187 A general review of pain pathways can be found in Hopkin, K., "Show me where it hurts: tracing the pathways of pain," *Journal of the National Institutes of Health Research* 9 (10) (1997): 37. The pain of a distended bladder: Cockayne, D., Hamilton, S., Zhu, Q., Dunn, P., Novakovic, S., Malmberg, A., Cain, G., Berson, A., Kassotakis, L., Hedley, L., Lachnit, W., Burnstock, G., McMahon, S., Ford, A., "Urinary bladder hyporeflexia and reduced pain-related behaviour in P2X3-deficient mice," *Nature* 407 (2000): 1011. How injury causes inflammation: Samad, T., Moore, K., Sapirstein, A., Billet, S., Allchorne, A., Poole, S., Bonventre, J., Woolf, C., "Interleukin-1beta-mediated induction of cox-2 in the CNS contributes to inflammatory pain hypersensitivity," *Nature* 410 (2001): 471; Blackburn-Munro, G., Blackburn-Munro, R., "Chronic pain, chronic stress, and depression; coincidence or consequence?" *Journal of Neuroendocrinology* 13 (2001): 1009; Woolf, C., Salter, M., "Neuronal plasticity: Increasing the gain in pain," *Science* 288 (2000): 1765.

PAGE 188 Footnote regarding capsaicin: Caterina, M., Leffler, A., Malmberg, A., Martin, W., Trafton, J., Petersen-Zeitz, K., Koltzenburg, M., Basbaum, A., Julius, D., "Impaired nociception and pain sensation in mice lacking the capsaicin receptor," *Science* 288 (2000): 306. I am pleased to note that one of the authors of this key paper, Jodie Trafton, was once a stellar member of my own lab. The horseradish component of pain: Jordt, S., Bautista, D., Chuang, H., McKemy, D., Zygmunt, P., Hogestatt, E., Meng, I., Julius, D., "Mustard oils and cannabinoids excite sensory nerve fibres through the TRP channel ANKTM1," *Nature* 427 (2004): 260.

PAGE 189 The interactions of fast and slow pain fibers were first described in the classic paper by Melzack, R., and Wall, P., "Pain mechanisms: a new theory," *Science* 150 (1965): 971. They are elaborated in Wall, P., and Melzack, R., *Textbook of Pain*, 2d ed. (Edinburgh, UK: Churchill Livingstone, 2003). Yeomans's framing of the functions of fast and slow fibers: personal communication.

PAGE 191 Mechanisms of pain hypersensitivity are reviewed in: Julius, D., Basbaum, A., "Molecular mechanisms of nociception," *Nature* 413 (2001): 203. Neuroma formation is reviewed in Blackburn-Munro et al., "Chronic pain, chronic stress," op. cit. A hyperexcitable spinal cord: Woolf et al., "Neuronal plasticity," op. cit.; Samad et al., "Interleukin-1beta mediated induction," op. cit.; Tsuda, M., Shigemoto-Mogami, Y., Koizumi, S., Mizokoshi, A., Kohsaka, S., Salter, M., Inoue, K., "P2X4 receptors induced in spinal microglia gate tactile allodynia after nerve injury," *Nature* 424 (2003): 778; Ikeda, H., Heinke, B., Ruscheweyh, R., Sandkuhler, J., "Synaptic plasticity in spinal lamina 1 projection neurons that mediate hyperalgesia," *Science* 299 (2003): 1237.

PAGE 193 Pain medication requests by gallbladder surgery patients: Ulrich, R., "View through a window may influence recovery from surgery," *Science* 224 (1984): 420.

PAGE 193 Contextual setting of pain as critical: Price, D., "Psychological and neural mechanisms of the affective dimension of pain," *Science* 288 (2000): 1769.

Hypnosis and the anatomy of pain responses: Rainville, P., Duncan, D., Price, D., Carrier, B., Bushnell, M., "Pain affect encoded in human anterior cingulated but not somatosensory cortex," *Science* 177 (1997): 968.

PAGE 194 Most clinicians concerned with chronic pain syndromes are anecdotally familiar with stress-induced analgesia, and many basic neurology, neuroscience, or physiological psychology texts cover the subject—for example, see the chapter on pain by Dennis Kelly in Kandel, E., and Schwartz, J., eds., *Principles of Neural Science* (New York: Elsevier, 1985). This also contains the famous description of the phenomenon by Dr. David Livingstone upon the occasion of his being mauled by a lion. Also see Fields, H., *Pain* (New York: McGraw-Hill, 1987).

Requests for morphine by soldiers versus civilians: Beecher, H., "Relationship of significance of wound to pain experienced," *Journal of the American Medical Association* 161 (1956): 17.

Stress-induced analgesia in animals: Terman, G., Shavit, Y., Lewis, J., Cannon, J., and Liebeskind, J., "Intrinsic mechanisms of pain inhibition: activation by stress," *Science* 226 (1984): 1270; Helmstetter, F., "The amygdala is essential for the expression of conditioned hypoalgesia," *Behavioral Neuroscience* 106 (1992): 518.

PAGE 195 Footnote: Analgesia in female versus male jocks: Sternberg, W., Bokat, C., Kass, L.O., Alboyadjian, A., Gracely, R., "Sex-dependent components of the analgesia produced by athletic competition," *Journal of Pain* 2 (2001): 65.

PAGE 195 Opiates, opiate receptors, and opioids: for technical reviews on this subject, see Akil, H., Watson, S., Young, E., Lewis, M., Khachaturian, H., and Walker, J., "Endogenous opioids: biology and function," *Annual Review of Neuroscience* 7 (1984): 223; Basbaum, A., and Fields, H., "Endogenous pain control systems: brain stem spinal pathways and endorphin circuitry," *Annual Review of Neuroscience* 7 (1984): 309. For a surprisingly readable account of the history of this field, see Snyder, S., *Brainstorming: The Science and Politics of Opiate Research* (Cambridge, Mass.: Harvard University Press, 1989). Snyder, one of the discoverers of the opiate receptor and a leading figure in the field, is an excellent nontechnical writer.

PAGE 196 The effects of acupuncture are mediated by opiate receptors: Mayer, D., Price, D., Barber, J., and Rafii, A., "Acupuncture analgesia: evidence for activation of a pain inhibitory system as a mechanism of action," in Bonica, J., and Albe-Fessard, D., eds., *Advances in Pain Research and Therapy*, vol. 1 (New York: Raven Press, 1976), 751; Mayer, D., and Hayes, R., "Stimulation-produced analgesia: development of tolerance and cross-tolerance to morphine," *Science* 188 (1975): 941.

PAGE 197 The meta-analysis of when placebos are useful: Hrobjartsson, A., and Gotzsche, P., "Is the placebo powerless?" *New England Journal of Medicine* 344 (2001): 1594. Painkillers are less effective when administered with the patient unawares: Holden, C., "Drugs and placebos look alike in the brain," *Science* 295 (2002): 947. Placebo effects are opioid-dependent: Petrovic, P., Kalso, E., Petersson, K., Ingvar, M., "Placebo and opioid analgesia—imaging a shared neuronal network," *Science* 295 (2002): 1737.

PAGE 198 First demonstration of endorphin release during stress: Guillemin, R., Vargo, T., and Rossier, J., "Beta-endorphin and adrenocorticotropin are secreted concomitantly by pituitary gland," *Science* 197 (1977): 1367. Its stimulation by a variety of stressors: Colt, E., Wardlaw, S., and Frantz, A., "The effect of running on plasma beta-endorphin," *Life Sciences* 28 (1981): 1637; Cohen, M., Pickar, D., and Dubois, M., "Stress-induced plasma beta-endorphin immunoreactivity may predict postoperative morphine usage," *Psychiatry Research* 6 (1982): 7; Katz, E., Sharp, B., and Kellermann, J., "Beta-endorphin immunoreactivity and acute behavioral distress in children with leukemia," *Journal of Nervous and Mental Disease* 170 (1982): 72; Jungkunz, G., Engel, R., and King, U., "Endogenous opiates increase pain tolerance after stress in humans," *Psychiatry Research* 8 (1983): 13. Efficacy of opioids at skin and organs: Stein, C., Schafer, M., Machwelska, H., "Attacking pain at its source: new perspectives on opioids," *Nature Medicine* 9 (2003): 1003.

Nonopioid mediated analgesia during stress: Mogil, J., Sternberg, W., Marek, P., Sadowski, B., Belknap, J., and Liebeskind, J., "The genetics of pain and pain inhibition," *Proceedings of the National Academy of Sciences, USA* 93 (1996): 3048; Mogil, J., Marek, P., Yirmiya, R., Balian, H., Sadowski, B., Taylor, A., and Liebeskind, J., "Antagonism of the non-opioid component of ethanol-induced analgesia by the NMDA receptor antagonist MK-801," *Brain Research* 602 (1993): 126; Nakao, K., Takahashi, M., Kaneto, H., "Implications of ATP-sensitive K+ channels in various stress-induced analgesia in mice," *Japanese Journal of Pharmacology* 71 (1996): 269.

PAGE 199 Anti-anxiety drugs blocking stress hyperalgesia: Price, "Psychological and neural mechanisms," op. cit.

PAGE 200 Fibromyalgia: Kalb, C., "Taking a new look at pain," *Newsweek*, 19 May 2003.

CHAPTER 10: STRESS AND MEMORY

PAGE 204 For some primers into the biology and neuropsychology of how memory works: Squire, L., *Memory and Brain* (New York: Oxford University Press, 1987); Gazzaniga, M., *The Cognitive Neurosciences* (Cambridge, Mass.: MIT Press, 1995; warning: this book is almost 1,500 pages long); Hebb, D. O., *The Organization of Behavior* (New York: Wiley, 1947). This last book is something of a cult classic. Hebb was one of the great neuroscientists of all time and, in this one book, predicted how long-term potentiation and neural networks were going to work—long before any of the underlying biology had been sorted out. Basically, anything new that has come along in this field for decades was outlined somewhere in this 1947 book.

PAGE 206 The Squire book gives a good overview of H.M. and his extraordinary history. For insights into the very different workings of short-term memory, see: Egorov, A., Hamam, B., Fransen, E., Hasselmo, M., Alonso, A., "Graded persistent activity in entorhinal cortex neurons," *Nature* 420 (2002): 173.

PAGE 207 One of the Nobel Prize–winning classics of Hubel and Wiesel: Hubel, D., and Wiesel, T., "Receptive fields, binocular interaction and functional architecture in the cat's visual cortex," *Journal of Physiology* (London) 160 (1962): 106.

PAGE 208 For an introduction to neural networks (and a lesson in how distorted and simplified this chapter's version of a network is) see Arbib, M., *The Handbook* of *Brain Theory and Neural Networks* (Cambridge, Mass.: MIT Press, 1995); also Taylor, J., *Neural Networks and Their Applications* (Chichester, England: Wiley, 1996). Also see: Fitzsimonds, R., Song, H., and Poo, M., "Propagation of activity-dependent synaptic depression in simple neural networks," *Nature* 388 (1997): 439.

PAGE 210 For introductions to long-term potentiation, see Gluck, M., and Meyers, C., "Psychobiological models of hippocampal function in learning and memory," *Annual Review of Psychology* 48 (1997): 481.

PAGE 210 Memory and the formation of new synapses: Trachtenberg, J., Vhen, B., Knott, G., Feng, G., Sanes, J., Welker, E., Svoboda, K., "Long-term in vivo imaging of experience-dependent synaptic plasticity in adult cortex," *Nature* 420 (2003): 788; Grutzendler, J., Kasthuri, N., Gan, W., "Long-term dendritic spine stability in the adult cortex," *Nature* 420 (2003): 812. Memory and the formation of new neurons: Shors, T., Miesegaes, G., Beylin, A., Zhao, M., Rydel, T., and Gould, E., "Neurogenesis in the adult is involved in the formation of trace memories," *Nature* 410 (2001): 372–76.

PAGE 210 For broad overviews of stress and memory, see: McGaugh, J., *Memory and Emotion* (New York: Weidenfeld and Nicolson, 2003); Sauro, M., Jorgensen, R., Pedlow, C., "Stress, glucocorticoids and memory: a meta-analytic review," *Stress* 6 (2004): 235; Lupien, S., McEwen, B., "The acute effects of corticosteroids on cognition: integration of animal and human model studies," *Brain Research Reviews* 24 (1997): 1; Garcia, R., "Stress, hippocampal plasticity, and spatial learning," *Synapse* 40 (2001): 180; Kim, J. J., Diamond, D., "The stressed hippocampus, synaptic plasticity and lost memories," *Nature Reviews Neuroscience* 3 (2002): 4534–62; Roozendaal, B., "Glucocorticoids and the regulation of memory consolidation," *Psychoneuroendocrinology* 25 (2000): 213–38; Sapolsky, R., "Stress and cognition," in Gazzaniga, M., ed., *The Cognitive Neurosciences*, 3rd ed. (Cambridge, Mass.: MIT Press, in press, due 2005). The book by McGaugh and the reviews by Roozendaal, and by Kim and Diamond, are particularly strong in discussing the realm in which memory is improved by stress.

Cahill and McGaugh: Cahill, L., Prins, B., Weber, M., McGaugh, J., "Beta-adrenergic activation and memory for emotional events," *Nature* 371 (1994): 702. The larger context of this study, especially the involvement of the amygdala, is discussed in McGaugh, *Emotion and Memory*, op. cit., and in Roozendaal, "Glucocorticoids and the regulation of memory consolidation," op. cit.

PAGE 213 A general review of the disruptive effects of stress can be found in Sapolsky, "Stress and cognition," op. cit.

PAGE 214 Memory problems in Cushing's disease: Starkman, M., Gebarski, S., Berent, S., and Schteingart, D., "Hippocampal formation volume, memory dysfunction, and cortisol levels in patients with Cushing's syndrome," *Biological Psychiatry* 32 (1992): 756–65. Memory problems in people treated with synthetic glucocorticoids: Keenan, P., Jacobson, M., Soleymani, R., Mayes, M., Stress, M., Yaldoo, D., "The effect on memory of chronic prednisone treatment in patients with systemic disease," *Neurology* 47 (1996): 1396–1403.

PAGE 214 Glucocorticoids disrupt memory in healthy humans: Wolkowitz, O., Reuss, V., Weingartner, H., "Cognitive effects of corticosteroids," *American Journal of Psychiatry* 147 (1990): 1297–1310; Wolkowitz, O., Weingartner, H., Rubinow, D., Jimerson, D., Kling, M., Berretini, W., Thompson, K., Breier, A., Doran, A., Reus,

V., Pickar, D., "Steroid modulation of human memory: biochemical correlates," *Biological Psychiatry* 33 (1993): 744–51; Wolkowitz, O., Reus, V., Canick, J., Levin, B., Lupien, S., "Glucocorticoid medication, memory and steroid psychosis in medical illness," *Annals of the New York Academy of Sciences* 823 (1997): 81–96; Newcomer, J., Craft, S., Hershey, T., Askins, K., Bardgett, M., "Glucocorticoid-induced impairment in declarative memory performance in adult human," *Journal of Neuroscience* 14 (1994): 2047–53. Disruptions with naturally high levels of glucocorticoids: Newcomer, J., Selke, G., Melson, A., Hershey, T., Craft, S., Richards, K., and Alderson, A., "Decreased memory performance in healthy humans induced by stress-level cortisol treatment," *Archives of General Psychiatry* 56 (1999): 527–33.

Stress impairs executive function: Arnsten, A., "Stress impairs prefrontal cortical function in rats and monkeys: role of dopamine D1 and norepinephrine alpha-1 receptor mechanisms," *Progress in Brain Research* 126 (2000): 183–92.

PAGE 214 Stress disrupts long-term potentiation and enhances long-term depression: stress levels of glucocorticoids inhibit long-term potentiation: Diamond, D., Bennet, M., Fleshner, M., and Rose, G., "Inverted-U relationship between the level of peripheral corticosterone and the magnitude of hippocampal primed burst potentiation," *Hippocampus* 2 (1992): 421; Joels, M., "Steroid hormones and excitability in the mammalian brain," *Frontiers in Neuroendocrinology* 18 (1997): 2. Stress enhances long-term depression: Xu, L., Anwyl, R., and Rowan, M., "Behavioural stress facilitates the induction of long-term depression in the hippocampus," *Nature* 387 (1997): 497. For a recent demonstration of how forgetting, and suppressing the formation of new memories, is an active process: Anderson, M., Ochsner, K., Kuhl, B., Cooper, J., Robertson, E., Gabrieli, S., Glover, G., Gabrieli, J., "Neural systems underlying the suppression of unwanted memories," *Science* 303 (2004): 232. Stress disrupts these forms of memory amid preserving implicit memory: Woodson, J., Macintosh, D., Fleshner, M., Diamond, D. Emotion-induced amnesia in rats: working memory-specific impairment, corticosterone-memory correlation and fear versus arousal effects on memory," *Learning and Memory* 10 (2003): 326.

The two receptor systems for glucocorticoids: Reul, J., de Kloet, E., "Two receptor systems for corticosterone in rat brain: microdistribution and differential occupation," *Endocrinology* 117 (1985): 2505. The relevance of the two receptor systems to memory is discussed in Kim and Diamond, "The stressed hippocampus," op. cit.

The need for amygdaloid activation for stress to disrupt hippocampal function: discussed in Roozendaal, op. cit., and McGaugh, "Glucocorticoids and the regulation of memory consolidation," *Memory and Emotion*, op. cit. Sex raises glucocorticoid levels without disrupting hippocampal function: Woodson, J., et al., "Emotion-induced amnesia in rats," op. cit.

PAGE 215 For a review of long-term depression, see Stevens, C., "Strengths and weaknesses in memory," *Nature* 381 (1996): 471; Nicoll, R., and Malenka, R., "Long-distance long-term depression," *Nature* 388 (1997): 427.

PAGE 217 Atrophy of hippocampal neuronal connections with stress: Woolley, C., Gould, E., and McEwen, B., "Exposure to excess glucocorticoids alters dendritic morphology of adult hippocampal pyramidal neurons," *Brain Research* 531 (1990): 225; Magarinos, A., and McEwen, B., "Stress-induced atrophy of apical dendrites of hippocampal CA3c neurons: comparison of stressors," *Neuroscience* 69 (1995): 83; Magarinos, A., and McEwen, B., "Stress-induced atrophy of apical dendrites of hippocampal CA3c neurons: involvement of glucocorticoid secretion and excitatory amino acid receptors," *Neuroscience* 69 (1995): 88; Magarinos, A., McEwen, B., Flugge, G., and Fuchs, E., "Chronic psychosocial stress causes apical dendritic atrophy of hippocampal CA3 pyramidal neurons in subordinate tree shrews," *Journal of Neuroscience* 16 (1996): 3534.

PAGE 217 Stress inhibits neurogenesis: Gould, E., Gross, C., "Neurogenesis in adult mammals: some progress and problems," *Journal of Neuroscience* 22 (2002): 619. This paper is a strong supporter of the idea that there is considerable neurogenesis in the adult hippocampus. The new neurons are needed for certain types of learning: Shors et al., "Neurogenesis in the adult," op. cit. For a review of the field by one of its strongest skeptics, see: Rakic, P., "Neurogenesis in adult primate neocortex: an evaluation of the evidence," *Nature Reviews Neuroscience* 3 (2002): 65–71.

Footnote concerning pregnancy-induced neurogenesis: Shingo, T., et al., "Pregnancy-stimulated neurogenesis in the adult female forebrain mediated by prolactin," *Science* 299 (2003): 117.

PAGE 218 Glucocorticoids inhibit glucose utilization and transport in the hippocampus and in hippocampal neurons and glia: Kadekaro, M., Masonori, I., and Gross, P., "Local cerebral glucose utilization is increased in acutely adrenalectomized rats," *Neuroendocrinology* 47 (1988): 329; Horner, H., Packan, D., and Sapolsky, R., "Glucocorticoids inhibit glucose transport in cultured hippocampal neurons and glia," *Neuroendocrinology* 52 (1990): 57; Virgin, C., Ha, T., Packan, D., Tombaugh, G., Yang, S., Horner, H., and Sapolsky, R., "Glucocorticoids inhibit glucose transport and glutamate uptake in hippocampal astrocytes: implications for glucocorticoid neurotoxicity," *Journal of Neurochemistry* 57 (1991): 1422.

The concept of neuroendangerment by glucocorticoids is discussed in Sapolsky, R., "Stress, glucocorticoids, and damage to the nervous system: the current state of confusion," *Stress* 1 (1996): 1. Also see Sapolsky, R., *Stress, the Aging Brain, and the Mechanisms of Neuron Death* (Cambridge, Mass.: MIT Press, 1992).

Glucocorticoids worsen the hippocampal damage caused by seizure in the rat: Sapolsky, R., "A mechanism for glucocorticoid toxicity in the hippocampus: increased neuronal vulnerability to metabolic insults," *Journal of Neuroscience* 5 (1995): 1227; and by lack of oxygen caused by cardiac arrest: Sapolsky, R., and Pulsinelli, W., "Glucocorticoids potentiate ischemic injury to neurons: therapeutic implications," *Science* 229 (1985): 1397; vulnerability to damage caused by the amyloid fragment of Alzheimer's disease: Behl, C., Lezoualc'h, F., Trapp, T., Widmann, M., Skutella, T., and Holsboer, F., "Glucocorticoids enhance oxidative stress-induced cell death in hippocampal neurons in vitro," *Endocrinology* 138 (1997): 101; Goodman, Y., Bruce, A., Cheng, B., and Mattson, M., "Estrogens attenuate and corticosterone exacerbates excitotoxicity, oxidative injury, and amyloid beta-peptide toxicity in hippocampal neurons," *Journal of Neurochemistry* 66 (1996): 1836; gp120-induced damage in neurons: Brooke, S., Chan, R., Howard, S., and Sapolsky, R., "Endocrine modulation of the neurotoxicity of gp120 implications for AIDS-related dementia complex," *Proceedings of the National Academy of Sciences, USA* 94 (1997): 9457–62.

PAGE 219 Glucocorticoids as neurotoxic: the first report of glucocorticoid neurotoxicity: Aus der Muhlen, K., and Ockenfels, H., "Morphologische veranderungen im diencephalon und telenceaphlin nach storngen des regelkreises adenohypophyse-nebennierenrinde III. Ergebnisse beim meerschweinchen nach verabreichung von cortison und hydrocortison," *Z Zellforsch* 93 (1969): 126. The first report of the hippocampus as a glucocorticoid target site: McEwen, B., Weiss, J., and Schwartz, I., "Selective retention of corticosterone by limbic structures in rat brain," *Nature* 220 (1968): 911. Glucocorticoids and stress and accelerating hippocampal neuron loss: Sapolsky, R., Krey, L., and McEwen, B., "Prolonged glucocorticoid exposure reduces hippocampal neuron number: implications for aging," *Journal of Neuroscience* 5 (1985): 1221; Kerr, D., Campbell, L., Applegate, M., Brodish, A., and Landfield, P., "Chronic stress-induced acceleration of electrophysiologic and morphometric biomarkers of hippocampal aging," *Journal of Neuroscience* 11 (1991): 1316. Removing glucocorticoids or decreasing their secretion delays hippocampal neuron loss: Landfield, P., Baskin, R., and Pitler, T., "Brain-aging correlates: retardation by hormonal–pharmacological treatments," *Science* 214 (1981): 581; Meaney, M., Aitken, D., Bhatnager, S., van Berkel, C., and Sapolsky, R., "Effect of neonatal handling on age-related impairments associated with the hippocampus," *Science* 239 (1988): 766.

Stress and glucocorticoids damage the nonhuman primate hippocampus: Uno, H., Tarara, R., Else, J., Suleman, M., and Sapolsky, R., "Hippocampal damage associated with prolonged and fatal stress in primates," *Journal of Neuroscience* 9 (1989): 1705; Sapolsky, R., Uno, H., Rebert, C., and Finch, C., "Hippocampal damage associated with prolonged glucocorticoid exposure in primates," *Journal of Neuroscience* 10 (1990): 2897; Uno, H., Eisele, S., Sakai, A., Shelton, S., Baker, E., DeJesus, O., and Holden, J., "Neurotoxicity of glucocorticoids in the primate brain," *Hormones and Behavior* 28 (1994): 336.

PAGE 220 Hippocampal atrophy in Cushing's disease: Starkman, M., Gebarski, S., Berent, S., and Schteingart, D., "Hippocampal formation volume, memory dysfunction, and cortisol levels in patients with Cushing's syndrome," *Biological Psychiatry* 32 (1992): 756.

PAGE 221 Hippocampal atrophy in PTSD: Bremner, J., Randall, P., Scott, T., Bronen, R., et al., "MRI-based measurement of hippocampal volume in patients with combat-related PTSD," *American Journal of Psychiatry* 152 (1995): 973; Gurvits, T., Shenton, M., Hokama, H., Ohta, H., Lasko, N., Gilbertson, M., et al., "Magnetic resonance imaging study of hippocampal volume in chronic, combat-related posttraumatic stress disorder," *Biological Psychiatry* 40 (1996): 1091; Bremner, J., Randall, P., Vermetten, E., Staib, L., Bronen, A., et al., "Magnetic resonance imaging-based measurement of hippocampal volume in PTSD related to childhood physical and sexual abuse—a preliminary report," *Biological Psychiatry* 41 (1997): 23. Most in the field think of the hippocampal volume loss in PTSD as being irreversible. However, a recent report suggests that may not be the case: Vermetten, E., Vythilingam, M., Southwick, S. M., Charney, D. S., and Bremner, J. D., "Long-term treatment with paroxetine increases verbal declarative memory and hippocampal volume in posttraumatic stress disorder," *Biological Psychiatry* 54 (2003): 693.

PAGE 221 Hippocampal atrophy in depression: Sheline, Y., Wang, P., Gado, M., Csernansky, J., Vannier, M., "Hippocampal atrophy in recurrent major depression,"

Proceedings of the National Academy of Sciences, USA 93 (1996): 3908–4003; Sheline, Y., Sanghavi, M., Mintun, M., Gado, M., "Depression duration but not age predicts hippocampal volume loss in medical healthy women with recurrent major depression," *Journal of Neuroscience* 19 (1999): 5034–41; Bremner, J., Narayan, M., Anderson, E., Staib, L., Miller, H., Charney, D., "Hippocampal volume reduction in major depression," *American Journal of Psychiatry* 157 (2000): 115–27; Sheline, Y., Gado, M., Kraemer, H., "Untreated depression and hippocampal volume loss," *American Journal of Psychiatry* 160 (2003): 1516; MacQueen, G., Campbell, S., McEwen, B., Macdonald, K., Amano, S., Joffe, R., Nahmias, C., Young, L., "Course of illness, hippocampal function, and hippocampal volume in major depression," *Proceedings of the National Academy of Sciences, USA* 100 (2002): 1387.

PAGE 221 Jet lag and hippocampal atrophy: Cho, K., "Chronic 'jet lag' produces temporal lobe atrophy and spatial cognitive deficits," *Nature Neuroscience* 4 (2001): 567.

PAGE 221 Normative aging: Lupien, S., de Leon, M., de Santi, S., Convit, A., Tarshish, C., Nair, N., Thakur, M., McEwen, B., Hauger, R., Meaney, M., "Cortisol levels during human aging predict hippocampal atrophy and memory deficits," *Nature Neuroscience* 1 (1998): 69–73.

PAGE 222 Glucocorticoid interactions with neurological insults: higher glucocorticoid levels associated with worse outcome to a stroke in humans: Astrom, M., Olsson, T., and Asplund, K., "Different linkage of depression to hypercortisolism early versus later after stroke," *Stroke* 24 (1993): 52.

Problems and complications reviewed in: Sapolsky, R., "Glucocorticoids and hippocampal atrophy in neuropsychiatric disorders," *Archives of General Psychiatry* 57 (2000): 925.

Atrophy in Cushing's syndrome as reversible: Bourdeau, I., Gbard, C., Noel, B., Leclerc, I., Cordeau, M., Belair, M., Lesage, J., Lafontaine, L., Lacroix, A., "Loss of brain volume in endogenous Cushing's syndrome and its reversibility after correction of hypercortisolism," *Journal of Clinical Endocrinology and Metabolism* 87 (2002): 1949.

PAGE 223 Glucocorticoids as pro-inflammatory in the injured nervous system: Dinkel, K., Ogle, W., Sapolsky, R., "Glucocorticoids and CNS inflammation," *Journal of NeuroVirology* 8 (2002): 513; Dinkel, K., MacPherson, A., Sapolsky, R., "Novel glucocorticoid effects on acute inflammation in the central nervous system," *Journal of Neurochemistry* 84 (2003): 705; Dinkel, K., Dhabhar, F., Sapolsky, R., "Neurotoxic effects of polymorphonuclear granulocytes on hippocampal primary cultures," *Proceedings of the National Academy of Sciences, USA* 101 (2004): 331.

PAGE 224 Glucocorticoids and their clinical use with AIDS patients: Bozzette, S., Sattler, F., Chiu, J., Wu, A., Gluckstein, D., et al., "A controlled trial of early adjunctive treatment with corticosteroids for Pneumocystis carinii pneumonia in the acquired immunodeficiency syndrome," *New England Journal of Medicine* 323 (1990): 1451; Gagnon, S., Boota, A., Fischl, M., Baier, H., Kirksey, O., La Voie, L., "Corticosteroids as adjunctive therapy for severe pneumocystis carinii pneumonia in the acquired immunodeficiency syndrome: a double-blind, placebo-controlled trial," *New England Journal of Medicine* 323 (1990): 1444.

PAGE 224 Huge stress response after neurological insults in humans: Feibel, J., Hardi, P., Campbell, M., Goldstein, N., and Joynt, R., "Prognostic value of the stress response following stroke," *Journal of the American Medical Association* 238 (1977): 1374. Blocking glucocorticoid secretion after a stroke or seizure in a rat is neuroprotective: Stein, B., and Sapolsky, R., "Chemical adrenalectomy reduces hippocampal damage induced by kainic acid," *Brain Research* 473 (1988): 175; Morse, J., and Davis, J., "Chemical adrenalectomy protects hippocampal cells following ischemia," *Society for Neuroscience Abstracts* 15 (1989): 149.4.

PAGE 225 The Woody Allen quote is from *Sleeper*.

CHAPTER 11: STRESS AND A GOOD NIGHT'S SLEEP

PAGE 227 Basics of sleep: Pace-Schott, E., Hobson, J., "The neurobiology of sleep; genetics, cellular physiology and subcortical networks," *Nature Reviews Neuroscience* 3 (2002): 591; Siegel, J., "Why we sleep," *Scientific American* (November 2003): 92.

Footnote: mallards: Rattonborg, N., Lima, S., Amlaner, C., "Half-awake to the risk of predation," *Nature* (1999): 397. Dolpins and birds: Siegel, "Why we sleep," op. cit.

PAGE 228 Brain function during different sleep stages: Braun, A., Balkin, T., Wesensten, N., Gwadry, F., Carson, R., Varga, M., Baldwin, P., Belenky, G., Herscovitch, P., "Dissociated patterns of activity in visual cortices and their projections during human rapid eye movement sleep," *Science* 279 (1998): 91. Energy depletion as a signal for sleep: Benington, J., Heller, H., "Restoration of brain energy metabolism as the function of sleep," *Progress in Neurobiology* 45 (1995): 347. Why dreams are dreamlike: Sapolsky, R., "Wild dreams," *Discover* 22 (2001): 36.

PAGE 230 What is sleep for? Fruit flies' sleep: Shaw, P., Tononni, G., Greenspan, R., Robinson, D., "Stress response genes protect against lethal effects of sleep deprivation in Drosophila," *Nature* 417 (2002): 287. Theories about the purpose of sleep: Maquet, P., "The role of sleep in learning and memory," *Science* 294 (2001): 1048.

PAGE 231 Sleep and cognition: Stickgold, R., lecture at University of Wisconsin, April 2002. Consolidating information from the previous day: Fenn, K., Nusbaum, H., Margoliash, D., "Consolidation during sleep of perceptual learning of spoken language," *Nature* 425 (2003): 614. Sleep deprivation disrupts consolidation: reviewed in McGaugh, J., *Memory and Emotion* (New York: Weidenfeld and Nicolson, 2003). Sleep deprivation is not merely stress: Maquet, "Role of sleep," op. cit. Patterns of sleep stages predict patterns of memory consolidation: Wagner, U., Gais, S., Borm, J., "Emotional memory formation is enhanced across sleep intervals with high amounts of rapid eye movement sleep," *Learning and Memory* 8 (2001): 112; Stickgold, op. cit.; Pace-Schott and Hobson, "Neurobiology of sleep," op. cit.

PAGE 232 McNaughton's work: Wilson, M., McNaughton, B., "Reactivation of hippocampal ensemble memories during sleep," *Science* 265 (1994): 676. Skaggs, W., McNaughton, B., "Replay of neuronal firing sequences in rat hippocampus during sleep following spatial experience," *Science* 271 (1996): 1870. Similar studies in humans: Maquet, op. cit. Gene activation during sleep: Pace-Schott and Hobson, op. cit. Elevated metabolism in the hippocampus: Siegel, op. cit.

Facilitation of one type of learning by sleep deprivation: Hairston, I., Little, M., Scanlon, M., Lutan, C., Barakat, M., Palmer, T., Sapolsky, R., Heller, H., "Sleep deprivation enhances memory?" *Society for Neuroscience Annual Meeting* (2003): abstract 616.19.

Remarkably, a nap can benefit cognition as much as does a good night's sleep: Mednick, S., Nakayama, K., Stickgold, R., "Sleep-dependent learning: a nap is as good as a night," *Nature Neuroscience* 6 (2003): 697.

PAGE 233 Delta sleep-inducing factor as a CIF: Okajima, T., Hertting, G., "Delta-sleep-inducing peptide inhibited CRF-induced ACTH secretion from rat anterior pituitary gland in vitro," *Hormones and Metabolic Research* 18 (1986): 497.

PAGE 233 Good overview of the subject: VanReeth, O., Weibel, L., Spiegel, K., Leproult, R., Dugovic, C., Maccari, S., "Interactions between stress and sleep: from basic research to clinical situations," *Sleep Medicine Reviews* 4 (2000): 201. Activation of the stress-response during sleep deprivation: Meerlo, P., Koehl, M., van der Borght, K., Turek, F., "Sleep restriction alters the HPA response to stress," *Journal of Neuroendocrinology* 14 (2002): 397–402; Cauter, E., Spiegel, K., "Sleep as a mediator of the relationship between socioeconomic status and health: a hypothesis," *Annals of the New York Academy of Sciences* 896 (1999): 254. The dry quote about sleep deprivation and death: Vgontzas, A., Bixler, E., Kales, A., "Sleep, sleep disorders, and stress," in Fink, ed., *Encyclopedia of Stress* (San Diego: Academic Press, 2000), vol. 3, 449.

Glucocorticoids break down glycogen during sleep deprivation: Gip, P., Hagiwara, G., Sapolsky, R., Cao, V., Heller, H., Ruby, N., "Glucocorticoids influence brain glycogen levels during sleep deprivation," *American Journal of Physiology*, in press. The frontal cortex recruiting other cortical regions for problem solving during sleep deprivation: Drummond, S., Brown, G., Gillin, J., Stricker, J., Wong, E., Buxton, R., "Altered brain response to verbal learning following sleep deprivation, *Nature* 403 (2000): 655.

PAGE 235 Health consequences of night work and shift work: van Cauter, E., "Sleep loss, jet lag, and shift work," in Fink, ed., *Encyclopedia of Stress*, vol. 3, 447. Jet-lag study: Cho, K., "Chronic 'jet lag' produces temporal lobe atrophy and spatial cognitive deficits," *Nature Neuroscience* 4 (2001): 567. Amounts of sleep now and in 1910: Vgontzas, "Sleep, sleep disorders, and stress," op. cit.

PAGE 236 Stress as a disruptor of sleep. Effects of CRH infusion: Vgontzas, A., Chrousos, G., "Sleep, the HPA axis, and cytokines: multiple interactions and disturbances in sleep disorders," *Endocrinology and Metabolism Clinics of North America* 31 (2002): 15. Activated stress-response in many poor sleepers: Vgontzas and Chrousos, op. cit. Stress-producing fragmented sleep: Dugovic, C., Maccari, S., Weibel, L., Turek, F., Van Reeth, O., "High corticosterone levels in prenatally stressed rats predict persistent paradoxical sleep alterations," *Journal of Neuroscience* 19 (1999): 8656. Less delta sleep with stress: Prinz, P. N., Bailey, S. L., Woods, D. L., "Sleep impairments in healthy seniors: roles of stress, cortisol and interleukin-1 beta," *Chronbiology International* 17 (2000): 391. Glucocorticoids impair memory consolidation during sleep: Plihal, W., Pietrowsky, R., Born, J., "Dexamethasone blocks sleep-induced improvement of declarative memory," *Psychoneuroendocrinology* 24 (1999): 313–31.

PAGE 237 The study showing the interaction of the two halves: Borm, J., Hansen, K., Marshall, L., Malle, M., Fehm, H., "Timing the end of nocturnal sleep," *Nature* 397 (1999): 29.

CHAPTER 12: AGING AND DEATH

PAGE 242 Aging as not so bad. Vaillant, G., Mukamal, K., "Successful aging," *American Journal of Psychiatry* 158 (2001): 839. The quality of social networks retained: Carstensen, L., Lockenhoff, C., "Aging, emotion, and evolution: the bigger picture," *Annals of the New York Academy of Sciences* 1000 (2003): 152. Improved cognitive skills: Helmuth, L., "The wisdom of the wizened," *Science* 299 (2003): 1300. Average aged person feels healthier than average: Vaillant, op. cit. Happiness increases with age: Carstensen, op. cit. Impact of negative images: Mather, M., and Carstensen, L., "Aging and attentional biases for emotional faces," *Psychological Sciences* 14 (2003): 409; Iadaka, T., Opkada, T., Murata, T., Omori, M., "Age-related differences in the medial temporal lobe responses to emotional faces as revealed by MRI," *Hippocampus* 12 (2002): 352–62.

PAGE 243 The aged stress-response on a cellular level: Horan, M., Barton, R., Lithgow, G., "Aging and stress, biology of," in Fink, ed., *Encyclopedia of Stress* (San Diego: Academic Press, 2000), vol. 1, 111.

PAGE 243 A detailed discussion of all the ways in which the cardiovascular system functions similarly in young and old healthy subjects in the absence of stress can be found in Lakatta, E., "Heart and circulation," in Schneider, E., and Rowe, J., eds., *Handbook of the Biology of Aging,* 3d ed. (San Diego: Academic Press, 1990). Decrease in maximal heart rate and work capacity with age: Gerstenblith, G., Lakatta, E., and Weisfeldt, M., "Age changes in myocardial function and exercise response," *Progress in Cardiovascular Disease* 19 (1976): 1. Decreased ejection volume during exercise with age: Rodeheffer, R., Gerstenblith, G., Becker, L., Fleg, J., Weisfeldt, M., and Lakatta, E., "Exercise cardiac output is maintained with advancing age in healthy human subjects: cardiac dilatation and increased stroke volume compensate for diminished heart rate," *Circulation* 69 (1984): 203. Increased cardiac muscle stiffness with force as a function of age: Spurgeon, H., Thorne, P., Yin, F., Shock, N., and Weisfeldt, M., "Increased dynamic stiffness of tabeculae carneae from senescent rats," *American Journal of Physiology* 232 (1977): H373. Easier immunosuppression in aged primates: Ershler, W., Coe, C., and Gravenstein, S., "Aging and immunity in nonhuman primates. I. Effects of age and gender on cellular immune function in rhesus monkeys," *American Journal of Primatology* 15 (1988): 181.

PAGE 244 Energetics of old and young brains, the effect of age on the vulnerability of cerebral metabolism to a metabolic stressor: Benzi, G., Pastoris, O., Vercesi, L., Gorini, A., Viganotti, C., and Villa, R., "Energetic state of aged brain during hypoxia," *Gerontology* 33 (1987): 207; Hoffman, W., Pelligrino, D., Miletich, D., and Albrecht, R., "Brain metabolic changes in young versus aged rats during hypoxia," *Stroke* 16 (1985): 860.

Aging and body temperature—functioning in old organisms is disrupted by stress more than in young ones. The classic studies on temperature dysregulation during aging can be found in Shock, N., "Systems integration," in Finch, C., and Hayflick, L., eds., *Handbook of the Biology of Aging,* 1st ed. (New York: Van Nostrand, 1977), 200.

PAGE 244 The effect of age on performance on intelligence tests: in Birren, J., and Schaie, K., *Handbook of the Psychology of Aging*, 3d ed. (New York: Van Nostrand, 1990). This vast subject is reviewed in a number of chapters: Cerella, J. "Aging and information-processing rate"; Kausler, D., "Motivation, human aging and cognitive performance"; Hultsch, D., and Dixson, R., "Learning and memory in aging." See also Katzman, R., and Terry, R., *The Neurology of Aging* (Philadelphia: Davis, 1983).

PAGE 244 Elevated epinephrine and norepinephrine concentrations during exercise as a function of age: Fleg, J., Tzankoff, S., and Lakatta, E., "Age-related augmentation of plasma catecholamines during dynamic exercise in healthy males," *Journal of Applied Physiology* 59 (1985): 1033. Decreased cardiovascular sensitivity to adrenaline and noradrenaline with age: Lakatta, E., "Cate-cholamines and cardiovascular function in aging," *Endocrinology and Metabolism Clinics of North America* 16 (1987): 877.

Slower epinephrine-norepinephrine recovery after the end of stress: McCarty, R., "Age-related alterations in sympathetic-adrenal medullary responses to stress," *Gerontology* 32 (1986): 172. Slower glucocorticoid recovery after the end of stress: Sapolsky, R., Krey, L., and McEwen, B., "The adrenocortical stress-response in the aged male rat: impairment of recovery from stress," *Experimental Gerontology* 18 (1983): 55; Ida, Y., Tanaka, M., and Tsuda, A., "Recovery of stress-induced increases in noradrenaline turnover is delayed in specific brain regions of old rats," *Life Sciences* 34 (1984): 2357. The delayed glucocorticoid recovery may accelerate tumor growth: Sapolsky, R., and Donnelly, T., "Vulnerability to stress-induced tumor growth increases with age in the rat: role of glucocorticoid hypersecretion," *Endocrinology* 117 (1985): 662.

Resting epinephrine and norepinephrine levels increase with age: Fleg, J., Tzankoff, S., and Lakatta, E., "Age-related augmentation of plasma catechola-mines during dynamic exercise in healthy males," *Journal of Applied Physiology* 59 (1985): 1033; also Rowe, J., and Troen, B., "Sympathetic nervous system and aging in man," *Endocrine Reviews* 1 (1980): 167. Resting glucocorticoid levels rise with age in the rat: reviewed in Sapolsky, R., "Do glucocorticoid concentrations rise with age in the rat?" *Neurobiology of Aging* 13 (1991): 171. In the aged human: reviewed in Sapolsky, R., "The adrenocortical axis," in Schneider, E., and Rowe, J., eds., *Handbook of the Biology of Aging*, 3d ed. (New York: Academic Press, 1990). In the wild baboon: Sapolsky, R., and Altmann, J., "Incidences of hypercorti-solism and dexamethasone resistance increase with age among wild baboons," *Biological Psychiatry* 30 (1991): 1008.

PAGE 244 Impaired neurogenesis: Cameron, H., McKay, R., "Restoring produc-tion of hippocampal neurons in old age," *Nature Neuroscience* 2 (1999): 894. The elevated glucocorticoid levels disrupt the ability of the brain for sprouting after injury: Scheff, S., and Cotman, C., "Chronic glucocorticoid therapy alters axon sprouting in the hippocampal dentate gyrus," *Experimental Neurology* 76 (1982): 644; DeKosky, S., Scheff, S., and Cotman, C., "Elevated corticosterone levels: a possible cause of reduced axon sprouting in aged animals," *Neuroendocrinology* 38 (1984): 33.

PAGE 245 For a discussion of why programmed aging (and aging in general) may have evolved, see Sapolsky, R., and Finch, C., "On growing old: not every creature ages, but most do. The question is why," *The Sciences* (March–April

1991): 30. For the original demonstration of what goes wrong in the salmon, see Robertson, O., and Wexler, B., "Pituitary degeneration and adrenal tissue hyperplasia in spawning Pacific salmon," *Science* 125 (1957): 1295. For a comparison of the effects of salmon aging with the effects of glucocorticoid excess, see Wexler, B., "Comparative aspects of hyperadrenocorticism and aging," in Everitt, A., and Burgess, J., eds., *Hypothalamus, Pituitary and Aging* (Springfield, Ill.: Charles C. Thomas, 1976). For an introduction to the marsupial mouse aging literature, see McDonald, I., Lee, A., and Bradley, A., "Endocrine changes in dasyurid marsupials with differing mortality patterns," *General and Comparative Endocrinology* 44 (1981): 292, and McDonald, I., Lee, A., and Than, K., "Failure of glucocorticoid feedback in males of a population of small marsupials (Antechinus swainsonii) during the period of mating," *Journal of Endocrinology* 108 (1986): 63. Beta-amyloid in salmon brains: Maldonado, T., Jones, R., Norris, D., "Distribution of beta-amyloid and amyhloid precursor protein in the brain of spawning (senescent) salmon: a natural, brain-aging model," *Brain Research* 858 (2000): 237.

A brief digression: what about those children who senesce incredibly rapidly and die of old age when they are twelve? Progeria, as the disease is called, is extremely rare. Those afflicted go bald, have bony chins, beaked noses, and dry, scratchy voices; they lose their hearing, get hardening of the arteries and heart disease (which is what usually kills them). When you try to grow some of their cells in a petri dish, you have as much trouble as you would with the cells of a seventy-year-old. Despite that, not everything about progeric kids is prematurely aged: they don't become demented, nor do they get cancer—two diseases typically linked with aging (although not necessary features of it, obviously). General consensus in the field is that progeria is a disease of some facets of aging being accelerated, rather than the entire aging process (which indirectly demonstrates that aging involves the ticking of multiple and independent clocks in the body). For a discussion of progeria and its relationship to aging, see Finch, C., *Longevity, Senescence and the Genome* (Chicago: University of Chicago Press, 1991); Mills, R., and Weiss, A., "Does progeria provide the best model of accelerated aging in humans?" *Gerontology* 36 (1990): 84.

PAGE 247 Can stress accelerate the aging process? For those who want to go straight to the horse's mouth (in German), there is Rubner, M., *Das problem der lebensdauer und seine beziehungen zum wachstum und ernahrung* (Munich: Oldenbourg, 1908). Also see Pearl, R., *The Rate of Living* (New York: Knopf, 1928) for the most detailed exploration of rate-of-living hypotheses. For some of Selye's ideas about stress and aging, see Selye, H., and Tuchweber, B., "Stress in relation to aging and disease," in Everitt, A., and Burgess, J., eds., *Hypothalamus, Pituitary and Aging* (Springfield, Ill.: Charles C. Thomas, 1976). For a scholarly discussion of the whole topic by one of the wisest thinkers in gerontology, see chapter 5 ("Rates of living and dying: correlations of life span with size, metabolic rates, and cellular and biochemical characteristics") in Finch, C., *Longevity, Senescence, and the Genome* (Chicago: University of Chicago Press, 1990).

PAGE 248 Old humans, primates, and rats tend to become dexamethasone-resistant with age: reviewed in Sapolsky, R., "The adrenocortical axis," in Schneider, E., and Rowe, J., eds., *Handbook of the Biology of Aging*, 3d ed., op. cit. In the wild baboon: Sapolsky, R., and Altmann, J., "Incidences of hypercortisolism and dexamethasone resistance increase with age among wild baboons," *Biological Psychiatry* 30 (1991): 1008.

PAGE 249 The hippocampus plays a role in inhibiting glucocorticoid secretion: reviewed in Jacobson, L., and Sapolsky, R., "The role of the hipocampus in feedback regulation of the hypothalamic-pituitary-adrenocortical axis," *Endocrine Reviews* 12 (1991): 118.

PAGE 249 The interaction between the effects of glucocorticoids on the hippocampus and the effects of the hippocampus on glucocorticoid secretion: Sapolsky, R., Krey, L., and McEwen, B., "The neuroendocrinology of stress and aging: the glucocorticoid cascade hypothesis," *Endocrine Reviews* 7 (1986): 284. For an update on these ideas, see: Sapolsky, R., "Stress, glucocorticoids, and their adverse neurological effects: relevance to aging," *Experimental Gerontology* 34 (1999): 721; Reagan, L., McEwen, B., "Controversies surrounding glucocorticoid-mediated cell death in the hippocampus," *Journal of Chemical Neuroanatomy* 13 (1997): 149.

PAGE 251 For a somewhat dated review of this entire topic in unreadably technical detail, the truly masochistic may want to buy a dozen copies of Sapolsky, R., *Stress, the Aging Brain and the Mechanisms of Neuron Death* (Cambridge, Mass.: MIT Press, 1992).

CHAPTER 13: WHY IS PSYCHOLOGICAL STRESS STRESSFUL?

PAGE 252 Footnote: Teddy Roosevelt's childhood lament can be found in Morris, E., *The Rise of Theodore Roosevelt* (New York: Ballantine Books, 1979).

PAGE 253 For a history of the field of stress research, as well as the celebrated debate between Selye and Mason, see Selye, H., "Confusion and controversy in the stress field," *Journal of Human Stress* 1 (1975): 37; Mason, J., "A historical view of the stress field," *Journal of Human Stress* 1 (1975): 6.

PAGE 255 Outlets for frustration: for a nontechnical review of Weiss's work, see Weiss, J., "Psychological factors in stress and disease," *Scientific American* 226 (June 1972): 104. The demonstration that social support networks are associated with lower glucocorticoid concentrations can be found in Ray, J., and Sapolsky, R., "Styles of male social behavior and their endocrine correlates among high-ranking wild baboons," *American Journal of Primatology* 28 (1992): 231; Virgin, C., and Sapolsky, R., "Styles of male social behavior and their endocrine correlates among low-ranking baboons," *American Journal of Primatology* 42 (1997): 25.

PAGE 256 Support and rodents: Ruis, M., te Brake, J., Buwalda, B., De Boer, S., Meerlo, P., Korte, S., Blokhuis, H., Koolhaas, J., "Housing familiar male wild-type rats together reduces the long-term adverse behavioural and physiological effects of social defeat," *Psychoneuroendocrinology* 24 (1999): 285. Support and nonhuman primates in a novel setting: Gust, D., Gordon, T., Brodie, A., and McClure, H., "Effect of companions in modulating stress associated with new group formation in juvenile rhesus macaques," *Physiology and Behavior* 59 (1996): 941; Smith, T., McGreer-Whitworth, B., French, J., "Close proximity of the heterosexual partner reduces the physiological and behavioral consequences of novel-cage housing in black tufted-ear marmosets (*Callithrix kuhli*)," *Hormones and Behavior* 34 (1998): 211; Sapolsky, R., Alberts, S., Altmann, J., "Hypercortisolism associated with social subordinance or social isolation among wild baboons," *Archives of General Psychiatry* 54 (1997): 1137; Aureli, F., Preston, S., de Waal, F.,

"Heart rate responses to social interactions in free-moving rhesus macaques: a pilot study," *Journal of Comparative Psychology* 113 (1999): 59.

PAGE 257 Supportive friend during human stressors: Lepore, S., Allen, K., and Evans, G., "Social support lowers cardiovascular reactivity to an acute stressor," *Psychosomatic Medicine* 55 (1993): 518; Edens, J., Larkin, K., and Abel, J., "The effect of social support and physical touch on cardiovascular reactions to mental stress," *Journal of Psychosomatic Research* 36 (1992): 371; Gerin, W., Pieper, C., Levy, R., and Pickering, T., "Social support in social interaction: a moderator of cardiovascular reactivity," *Psychosomatic Medicine* 54 (1992): 324; Kamarck, T., Manuck, S., and Jennings, J., "Social support reduces cardiovascular reactivity to psychological challenge: a laboratory model," *Psychosomatic Medicine* 52 (1990): 42. Glucocorticoids in stepchildren: Flinn, M., and England, B., "Social economics of childhood glucocorticoid stress response and health," *American Journal of Physical Anthropology* 102 (1997): 33. Breast cancer study: Turner-Cobb, J., Sephton, S., Koopman, C., Blake-Mortimer, J., and Spiegel, D., "Social support and salivary cortisol in women with metastatic breast cancer," *Psychosomatic Medicine* 62 (2000): 337.

Social support and sympathetic nervous system: Fleming, R., "Mediating influence of social support on stress at Three Mile Island," *Journal of Human Stress* 8 (1982): 14. Social support and cardiovascular disease: Williams, R., and Littman, A., "Psychosocial factors: role in cardiac risk and treatment strategies," *Cardiology Clinics* 14 (1996): 97.

The health benefits of grooming (in nonhuman primates) and touch (in humans) can be found in: Boccia, M., Reite, N. M., Laudenslager, M., "On the physiology of grooming in a pigtail macaque," *Physiology and Behavior* 45 (1989): 667; Drescher, V., Gantt, W., Whitehead, W., "Heart rate response to touch," *Psychosomatic Medicine* 42 (1980): 559.

Social support at the community level: Boydell, J., van Os, J., McKenzie, K., "Incidence of schizophrenia in ethnic minorities in London: ecological study into interactions with environment," *British Journal of Medicine* 323 (2001): 1336; Neeleman, J., Wilson-Jones, C., Wessely, S., "Ethnic density and deliberate self-harm; a small area study in south east London," *Journal of Epidemiology and Community Health* 55 (2001): 85.

Finally, a recent paper shows that the health benefits of sociality extend into some unexpected realms; among wild baboons, the more social a female is (independent of ecological factors or social rank), the better the survival chances of her offspring: Silk, J., Alberts, S., Altmann, J., "Social bonds of female baboons enhance infant survival," *Science* 302 (2003): 1231.

PAGE 258 Importance of predictability: Abbott, B., Schoen, L., and Badia, P., "Predictable and unpredictable shock: behavioral measures of aversion and physiological measures of stress," *Psychological Bulletin* 96 (1984): 45; Davis, H., and Levine, S., "Predictability, control, and the pituitary-adrenal response in rats," *Journal of Comparative and Physiological Psychology* 96 (1982): 393; Seligman, M., and Meyer, B., "Chronic fear and ulcers with rats as a function of the unpredictability of safety," *Journal of Comparative and Physiological Psychology* 73 (1970): 202. Predictability: an analysis similar to mine (a warning signal tells you when to worry and, even more important, when you can relax) has been termed the safety-signal hypothesis by psychologist Martin Seligman, *Helplessness: On Depression, Development and Death* (San Francisco: W. H. Freeman and Co., 1975).

Parachute jumpers habituating: Ursin, H., Baade, E., and Levine, S., *Psychobiology of Stress: A Study of Coping Men* (New York: Academic Press, 1978).

The stress-response in migrating birds, reviewed in: Wingfield, J., Sapolsky, R., "Reproduction and resistance to stress: when and how," *Journal of Neuroendocrinology* 15 (2003): 711.

PAGE 260 Ulcers and bombings in World War II: Stewart, D., and Winser, D., "Incidence of perforated peptic ulcer: effect of heavy air-raids," *The Lancet* (28 February 1942): 259.

PAGE 260 Control: you don't actually need to exercise control in order to get its benefits: Glass, D., and Singer, J., *Urban Stress: Experiments on Noise and Social Stressors* (New York: Academic Press, 1972). Effects of uncontrollability on tumor growth: Visintainer, M., Volpicelli, J., and Seligman, M., "Tumor rejection in rats after inescapable or escapable shock," *Science* 216 (1982): 437. General references for control being helpful: Houston, B., "Control over stress, locus of control, and response to stress," *Journal of Personality and Social Psychology* 21 (1972): 249; Lundberg, U., and Frankenhaeuser, M., "Psychophysiological reactions to noise as modified by personal control over stimulus intensity," *Biological Psychology* 6 (1978): 51; Brier, A., Albus, M., Pickar, D., Zahn, T. P., Wolkowitz, O., and Paul, S., "Controllable and uncontrollable stress in humans: alterations in mood and neuroendocrine and psychophysiological function," *American Journal of Psychiatry* 144 (1987): 1419; Manuck, S., Harvey, A., Lechleiter, S., and Neal, K., "Effects of coping on blood pressure responses to threat of aversive stimulation," *Psychophysiology* 15 (1978): 544. Rats forced to exercise: Moraska, A., Deak, T., Spencer, R., Roth, D., Fleshner, M., "Treadmill running produces both positive and negative physiological adaptations in Sprague-Dawley rats," *American Journal of Physiology: Regulatory, Integrative and Comparative Physiology* 279 (2000): R1321. A masterful review can be found in: Haidt, J., Rodin, J., "Control and efficacy as interdisciplinary bridges," *Review of General Psychology* 3 (2000): 317.

PAGE 261 Stress and control in the workplace: Karasek, R., Theorell, T., *Health, Work, Stress, Productivity, and the Reconstruction of Working Life* (New York: Basic Books, 1990); Schnall, P., Pieper, C., Schwartz, J., Karasek, R., Schlussel, Y., Devereux, R., Ganau, A., Alderman, M., Warren, K., Pickering, T., "Relationship between job strain, workplace diastolic blood pressure, and left ventricular mass index," *Journal of the American Medical Association* 263 (1990): 1929; Steptoe, A., Kunz-Ebrecht, S., Owen, N., Feldman, P., Rumley, A., Lowe, G., Marmot, M., "Influence of socioeconomic status and job control on plasma fibrinogen responses to acute mental stress," *Psychosomatic Medicine* 65 (2003): 137. Job stress only occurs in certain domains: Kohn, M., Schooler, C., *Work and Personality; An Inquiry into the Impact of Social Stratification* (Norwood, N.J.: Ablex, 1983). Stressed orchestra musicians: Levine, R., Levine, S., "Why they are not smiling: stress and discontent in the orchestral workplace," *Harmony* 2 (1996): 15–25.

PAGE 263 The perception of things worsening or improving: baboons rising or declining in the hierarchy: Sapolsky, R., "Cortisol concentrations and the social significance of rank instability among wild baboons," *Psychoneuroendocrinology* 17 (1992): 701 (cortisol is glucocorticoid found in the bloodstream of primates and humans). Parents of children with cancer: Wolff, C., Friedman, S., Hofer, M., and Mason, J., "Relationship between psychological defenses and mean urinary

17-hydroxycorticosteroid excretion rates," *Psychosomatic Medicine* 26 (1964): 576 (17-hydroxycorticosteroids are the versions of glucocorticoids that humans excrete).

PAGE 264 The use of random terror among competitive baboons: Silk, J., "Practice random acts of aggression and senseless acts of intimidation: the logic of status contest in social groups," *Evolutionary Anthropology* 11 (2002): 221.

PAGE 264 Change as stressful, even if good: Shively, C., Laber-Laird, K., Anton, R., "Behavior and physiology of social stress and depression in female cynomolgus monkeys," *Biological Psychiatry* 41 (1997): 871.

PAGE 266 Predictive information doesn't work with long lag time: Pitman, D., Natelson, B., Ottenweller, J., McCarty, R., Pritzel, T., and Tapp, W., "Effects of exposure to stressors of varying predictability on adrenal function in rats," *Behavioral Neuroscience* 109 (1995): 767; Arthur, A., "Stress of predictable and unpredictable shock," *Psychological Bulletin* 100 (1986): 379.

PAGE 267 Subtleties of control: DeGood, D., "Cognitive control factors in vascular stress responses," *Psychophysiology* 12 (1975): 399; Houston, B., "Control over stress, locus of control, and response to stress," *Journal of Personality and Social Psychology* 21 (1972): 249; Lundberg, U., and Frankenhaeuser, M., "Psychophysiological reactions to noise as modified by personal control over stimulus intensity," *Biological Psychology* 6 (1978): 51.

PAGE 269 Executive stress syndrome and ulcerating monkeys: technical and nontechnical versions of the famous experiment with executive monkeys can be found, respectively, in Brady, J., Porter, R., Conrad, D., and Mason, J., "Avoidance behavior and the development of gastroduodenal ulcers," *Journal of the Experimental Analysis of Behavior* I (1958): 69; and Brady, J., "Ulcers in 'executive' monkeys," *Scientific American* 199 (1958): 95. Technical and nontechnical critiques by Weiss of this experiment can be found, respectively, in Weiss, J., "Effects of coping response on stress," *Journal of Comparative and Physiological Psychology* 65 (1968): 251, and Weiss, J., "Psychological factors in stress and disease," *Scientific American* 226 (1972): 104. A technical critique is also offered by Natelson, B., Dubois, A., and Sodetz, F., "Effect of multiple stress procedures on monkey gastro-duodenal mucosa, serum gastrin and hydrogen ion kinetics," *American Journal of Digestive Diseases* 22 (1977): 888.

Many of the ideas in this chapter will be returned to in the final chapter on stress management, along with additional references.

CHAPTER 14: STRESS AND DEPRESSION

PAGE 271 Five to 20 percent of the population will suffer from a major depression: Robins, L., Helzer, J., Weissman, M., Orvaschel, H., Gruenberg, E., Burke, J., and Regier, D., "Lifetime prevalence of specific psychiatric disorders in three sites," *Archives of General Psychiatry* 41 (1984): 949; Weissman, M., and Myers, J., "Rates and risks of depressive symptoms in a United States urban community," *Acta Psychiatrica Scandinavica* 57 (1978): 219; Helgason, T., "Epidemiological investigation concerning affective disorders," in Schor, M., and Stromgren, M., eds., *Origin, Presentation and Treatment of Affective Disorders* (London: Academic

Press, 1979), 241. The rate is increasing: Klerman, G., Weissman, M., "Increasing rates of depression," *Journal of the American Medical Association* 261 (1989): 2229. Second leading cause of disability: *Science* 288, 39.

PAGE 272 Good descriptions of the symptoms found in different depressive subtypes can be found in the bible on the subject, the *Diagnostic and Statistical Manual of Mental Disorders* (DSM-III-R), 3d ed., rev. (Washington, D.C.: American Psychiatric Association, 1987). Also see Gold, P., Goodwin, F., and Chrousos, G., "Clinical and biochemical manifestations of depression: relation to the neurobiology of stress," *New England Journal of Medicine* 319 (1988): 348. Positive and negative emotions are not mere opposites: Zautra, A., *Emotions, Stress and Health* (New York: Oxford University Press, 2003).

PAGE 274 Re 800,000 suicides a year: "Spirit of the age," *The Economist* (18 December 1998): 113.

PAGE 274 Footnote: who is at risk for depression: Whooley, M., and Simon, G., "Managing depression in medical outpatients," *New England Journal of Medicine* 343 (2000): 1942.

PAGE 275 For the classic discussion of depression as a cognitive disorder, see Beck, A., *Cognitive Therapy and the Emotional Disorders* (New York: International Universities Press, 1976).

PAGE 275 Vegetative symptoms: for the first report of sleep changes in many depressives: Diaz-Guerrero, R., Gottlieb, J., and Knott, J., "The sleep of patients with manic-depressive psychosis, depressive type: an electroencephalographic study," *Psychosomatic Medicine* 8 (1946): 399. Also see Coble, P., Foster, F., and Kupfer, D., "Electroencephalographic sleep diagnosis of primary depression," *Archives of General Psychiatry* 33 (1976): 1124; Gillin, J., Duncan, W., Pettigrew, K., Frankel, B., and Snyder, F., "Successful separation of depressed, normal and insomniac subjects by EEG sleep data," *Archives of General Psychiatry* 36 (1979): 85. Cortisol (glucocorticoid) levels are elevated in many depressives; for an early demonstration of this, see Sachar, E., "Neuroendocrine abnormalities in depressive illness," in Sachar, E., ed., *Topics of Psychoendocrinology* (New York: Grune and Stratton, 1975), 135. For a more recent review, see Sapolsky, R., and Plotsky, P., "Hypercortisolism and its possible neural bases," *Biological Psychiatry* 27 (1990): 937.

PAGE 276 Memory problems in depression: Austin, M., Mitchell, P., Goodwin, G., "Cognitive deficits in depression," *British Journal of Psychiatry* 178 (2001): 200.

PAGE 277 Depressive symptomatology can follow cyclic patterns over time; a classic demonstration of this can be found in Richter, C., "Two-day cycles of alternating good and bad behavior in psychotic patients," *Archives of Neurology and Psychiatry* 39 (1938): 587. For a good review of seasonal affective disorders, see Rosenthal, N., Sack, D., Gillin, C., Lewy, A., Goodwin, F., Davenport, Y., Mueller, P., Newsome, D., and Wehr, T., "Seasonal affective disorder," *Archives of General Psychiatry* 41 (1984): 72. For demonstrations of the use of light therapy for SADs, see Rosenthal, N., Sack, D., Carpenter, C., Parry, B., Mendelson, W., and Wehr, T., "Antidepressant effects of light in seasonal affective disorder," *American Journal of Psychiatry* 142 (1985): 163; Wehr, T., Jacobsen, F., Sack, D., Arendt, J., Tamarkin, L., and Rosenthal, N., "Phototherapy of seasonal affective disorder," *Archives of Gen-*

eral Psychiatry 43 (1986): 870. Retinal cells sending information to the limbic system: Barinaga, M., "How the brain's clock gets daily enlightenment," *Science* 295 (2002): 955.

PAGE 278 The neurochemistry of depression is a vast subject with a dizzying number of papers, many of them contradicting one another. For an authoritative and relatively accessible discussion of the current confusion about whether it is a neuroepinephrine, dopamine, or serotonin problem, involving too much or too little of the neurotransmitters, or too much or too little of the receptors, see Kandel, E., "Disorders of mood," in Kandel, E., Schwartz, J., and Jessell, T., eds., *Principles of Neural Sciences*, 3d ed. (New York: Elsevier, 1991). An excellent and accessible introduction to the topic of neurotransmitters can be found in Barondes, S., *Molecules and Mental Illness* (New York: Scientific American Library, W. H. Freeman, 1993).

PAGE 280 Footnote: St. John's wort as effective: DiCarlo, G., Borrelli, F., Ernst, E., Izzo, A., "St. John's wort: Prozac from the plant kingdom," *Trends in Pharmacological Sciences* 22 (2001): 292. St. John's wort disrupting efficacy of other medications: Vogel, G., "How the body's 'garbage disposal' may inactivate drugs," *Science* 291 (2001): 35.

PAGE 282 A brief tirade about ECT: few medical procedures of our time have a worse popular image. In the past, ECT involved sufficient amounts of electricity to cause brain damage and memory loss, and to induce convulsions, causing body injury. Far worse, ECT's use for all sorts of things besides intractable depression— behavior disorders, juvenile delinquency, and so on—smacked of medicopolitical control and punishment. However, ECT is now conducted very differently—far less electricity is used, and there is no evidence that the modern form of ECT causes brain damage or permanent memory loss. Moreover, people are now typically sedated during ECT sessions, which virtually eliminates the danger of physical injury from convulsing. Most important, when it is administered correctly, ECT can save lives. For people who have been through every type of psychotherapy, every known antidepressant, and every combination of the two, yet are still suicidally depressed, ECT may be the only known technique that will ever get them functioning again. It can be an extraordinarily helpful procedure, and many former depressives swear by it. For a discussion of the history of ECT and its rather safe record as currently used, see Fink, M., "Convulsive therapy: fifty years of progress," *Convulsive Therapy* I (1985): 204. Mechanisms of ECT action: some papers showing effects of ECT on numbers of receptors for norepinephrine and related neurotransmitters: Kellar, K., and Stockmeier, C., "Effects of electroconvulsive shock and serotonin axon lesions on beta-adrenergic and serotonin-2 receptors in rat brain," *Annals of the New York Academy of Sciences* 462 (1986): 76; Chiodo, L., and Antelman, S., "Electroconvulsive shock: progressive dopamine autoreceptor subsensitivity independent of repeated treatment," *Science* 210 (1980): 799; Reches, A., Wagner, H., Barkai, A., Jackson, V., Yablonskaya-Alter, E., and Fahn, S., "Electroconvulsive treatment and haloperidol: effects on pre- and postsynaptic dopamine receptors in rat brain," *Psychopharmacology* 83 (1984): 155. Devan, D., Dwork, A., Hutchinson, E., Bolwig, T., Sackeim, H., "Does ECT alter brain structure?" *American Journal of Psychiatry* 151 (1994): 957. Also see: Fink, M., *Electroshock: Restoring the Mind* (New York: Oxford University Press, 1999).

PAGE 283 Pleasure pathways in the brain; for a history of the start of this field by one of its two discoverers, see Milner, P., "The discovery of self-stimulation and other stories," *Neuroscience and Biobehavioral Reviews* 13 (1989): 61. For another general overview of the field, see Routtenberg, A., "The reward system of the brain," *Scientific American* (November 1978). For a demonstration that stimulation of these pathways can be more reinforcing than food, see Routtenberg, A., and Lindy, J., "Effects of the availability of rewarding septal and hypothalamic stimulation on bar pressing for food under conditions of deprivation," *Journal of Comparative and Physiological Psychology* 60 (1965): 158. For an early study implicating norepinephrine in the pleasure pathway, see Stein, L., "Effects and interactions of imipramine, chlorpromzaine, reserpine, and amphetamine on self-stimulation: possible neurophysiological basis of depression," in Wortis, J., ed., *Recent Advances in Biological Psychiatry,* vol. 4 (New York: Plenum, 1962), 288. This study showed that norepinephrine depletion in the rat decreases self-stimulation of the pleasure pathways. In recent years, there has been a shift in this field away from considering norepinephrine to be the principal neurotransmitter of the pleasure pathways, much as there has been a shift away from considering it the sole culprit in depression. A neurotransmitter called dopamine is moving toward the forefront as the first neurotransmitter among equals involved in pleasure signaling. This makes some sense, as cocaine works mostly on dopamine synapses. However, although norepinephrine is probably not the most important neurotransmitter of pleasure perception, a defect in norepinephrine regulation in that part of the brain still has a great deal of potential for wreaking havoc. In considering how multiple neurotransmitters are used in many synaptic steps in these pleasure pathways, an analogy might help: a long cable may be made of stronger and weaker materials at different points; nevertheless, severing the cable in any place causes problems, and the norepinephrine link might be where the severing occurs. This is reviewed in Milner, P., "Brain-stimulation reward: a review," *Canadian Journal of Psychology* 45 (1991): 1.

A review of the human literature regarding pleasure pathways and self-stimulation can be found in Heath, R., "Electrical self-stimulation of the brain in man," *American Journal of Psychiatry* 120 (1963): 571.

PAGE 284 Substance P blockers as antidepressants: Bondya, B., Baghaia, T., Minova, C., Schulea, C., Schwarza, M., Zwanzgera, P., Rupprechta, R., Mullera, H., "Substance P serum levels are increased in major depression: preliminary results," *Biological Psychiatry* 53 (2003): 538. Also, discussed in: Fava, M., Kendler, K., "Major depressive disorder," *Neuron* 28 (2000): 335.

PAGE 286 For a discussion of the cons and surprising number of pros concerning cingulotomy (and for a thoughtful discussion of psychosurgical controversies in general), see Konner, M., "Too desperate a cure?" originally published in *The Sciences* (May 1988): 6; reprinted in Konner, M., *Why the Reckless Survive* (New York: Viking Penguin, 1990). For a technical discussion of the outcome of cingulotomies, see Ballantine, H., Bouckoms, A., Thomas, E., and Giriunas, I., "Treatment of psychiatric illness by stereotactic cingulotomy," *Biological Psychiatry* 22 (1987): 807. For a history of psychosurgery and its accompanying controversies, see Valenstein, E., *Great and Desperate Cures: The Rise and Decline of Psychosurgery and Other Radical Treatments for Mental Illness* (New York: Basic Books, 1986). Interestingly, a 1992 study supports the rough picture of "the cortex whispering too many depressing thoughts to the limbic system" and demonstrates that depressed patients have enhanced metabolism (relative to nondepressed patients) in the prefrontal cortex and the amygdala: Drevets, W., Videen, T., Price, J., Preskorn, S., Carmichael, S., and Raichle, M., "A functional anatomical study of unipolar depression," *Journal of Neuroscience* 12 (1992): 3628.

PAGE 286 The anterior cingulate cortex; positive emotions inhibit ACC: Aalto, S., Naatanen, P., Wallius, E., Metsahonkaala, L., Stenman, H., Niemi, P., Karlsson, H., "Neuroanatomical substrate of amusement and sadness: a PET activation study using film stimuli," *NeuroReport* 13 (2002): 67–73. ACC stimulation and a sense of foreboding: Drevets, W., "Neuroimaging and neuropathological studies of depression: implications for the cognitive-emotional features of mood disorders," *Current Opinion in Neurobiology* 11 (2001): 240. Hypnotism and ACC activation: Rainville, P., Duncan, D., Price, D., Carrier, B., Bushnell, M., "Pain affect encoded in human anterior cingulated but not somatosensory cortex," *Science* 277 (1997): 968. ACC activated by pain: Hutchison, W., Davis, K., Lozano, A., Tasker, R., Dostrovsky, J., "Pain-related neurons in the human cingulated cortex," *Nature Neuroscience* 2 (1999): 403. Widows and ACC activation: O'Connor, M., Littrell, L., Fort, C., Lane, R., "Functional neuroanatomy of grief: an MRI study," *American Journal of Psychiatry* 160 (2003): 1946. ACC activated when excluded in a game: Eisenberger, N., Lieberman, M., Williams, K., "Does rejection hurt? An fMRI study of social exclusion," *Science* 302 (2003): 290. Sad faces cause exaggerated ACC responses: Drevets, op. cit. Davidson's work on laterality of ACC activation: Davidson, R., Jackson, D., Kalin, N., "Emotion, plasticity, context, and regulation: perspectives from affective neuroscience," *Psychological Bulletin* 126 (2000): 890. ACC activation patterns in infant monkey: Rilling, J., Winslow, J., O'Brien, D., Gutman, D., Hoffman, J., Kilts, C., "Neural correlates of maternal separation in rhesus monkeys," *Biological Psychiatry* 49 (2001): 146.

PAGE 288 The genetics of depression is reviewed in Kendler, K., Prescott, C., Myers, J., Neale, M., "The structure of genetic and environmental risk factors for common psychiatric and substance use disorders in men and women," *Archives of General Psychiatry* 60 (2003): 929.

PAGE 289 Immune activation and depression: Dantzer, R., "Cytokines and depression: an update," *Brain Behavior and Immunity* 16 (2002): 501; Anisman, H., Merali, Z., "Cytokines, stress, and depressive illness," *Brain, Behavior and Immunity* 16 (2002): 513.

PAGE 289 Thyroid hormone insufficiency can lead to depression: Denko, J., and Kaelbling, R., "Psychiatric aspects of hypoparathyroidism," *Acta Psychiatrica Scandinavica* 38 (1962): supp. 164, 7; Whybrow, P., Prange, A., and Treadway, C., "Mental changes accompanying thyroid gland dysfunction," *Archives of General Psychiatry* 20 (1969): 47. One way in which this may occur comes with the finding that thyroid hormones influence norepinephrine processing in the brain: Prange, A., Meek, J., and Lipton, M., "Catecholamines: diminished rate of synthesis in rat brain and heart after thyroxine pretreatment," *Life Sciences* 9 (1970): 901. Many patients with depression turn out to have an underlying thyroid hormone deficiency: Lipton, M., Breese, G., Prange, A., Wilson, I., and Cooper, B., "Behavioral effects of hypothalamic polypeptide hormones in animals and man," in Sacher, E., ed., *Hormones, Behavior and Psychopathology* (New York: Raven Press, 1976), 15.

Hypothyroidism can cause resistance to antidepressants: Bauer, M., Heinz, A., Whybrow, P., "Thyroid hormones, serotonin and mood: of synergy and significance in the adult brain," *Molecular Psychiatry* 7 (2002): 140–56; Cole, D., Thase, M., Mallinger, A., Soares, J., Luther, J., Kupfer, D., Frank, E., "Slower treatment response in bipolar depression predicted by lower pretreatment thyroid function," *American Journal of Psychiatry* 159 (2002): 116.

PAGE 290 Higher rates of depression in women than in men: Murphy, M., Sobol, A., Neff, R., Olivier, D., and Leighton, A., "Stability of prevalence," *Archives of General Psychiatry* 41 (1984): 990. More depressive episodes in bipolar women than men: Gater, R., Tansella, M., Korten, A., Tiemens, B., Mavreas, V., Olatawura, M., "Sex differences in the prevalence and detection of depressive and anxiety disorders in general health care settings: report from the World Health Organization Collaborative Study on psychological problems in general health care," *Archives of General Psychiatry* 55 (1998): 405. Sex differences in the rates of depression: the best overview of some of the nonhormonal theories can be found in Nolen-Hoeksma, S., "Sex differences in depression: theory and evidence," *Psychological Bulletin* 101 (1987): 259. Hormonal aspects of sex differences in depression: women have particularly high incidences of depression around the time of menstruation: Abramowitz, E., Baker, A., and Fleischer, S., "Onset of depressive psychiatric crises and the menstrual cycle," *American Journal of Psychiatry* 139 (1982): 475. The immediate postparturition period is one of great risk for depression: Campbell, S., and Cohn, J., "Prevalence and correlates of postpartum depression in first-time mothers," *Journal of Abnormal Psychology* 100 (1991): 594; O'Hara, M., Schlechte, J., Lewis, D., and Wright, E., "Prospective study of postpartum blues: biologic and psychosocial factors," *Archives of General Psychiatry* 48 (1991): 801. What is generally viewed to be a heretical idea was voiced in a recent study, namely, that fathers have the same rate of postpartum depression as mothers do: Richman, J., Raskin, V., and Gaines, C., "Gender roles, social support, and postpartum depressive symptomatology," *Journal of Nervous and Mental Disease* 179 (1991): 139.

PAGE 290 Issues of gender differences in control and in substance abuse in traditional societies. Loewenthal, K., Goldblatt, V., "Gender and depression in Anglo-Jewry," *Psychological Medicine* 25 (1995): 1051. I found this study to be quite confusing, or at least challenging of my expectations. This paper initially seemed to test the idea that the gender difference was an artifact of men being more likely than women to mask their depression in alcoholism and other forms of substance abuse (i.e., the depressed alcoholic is more likely to get categorized as an alcoholic than as a depressive). Thus, the authors examined a population of Orthodox Jews, among whom rates of alcohol and drug abuse are exceedingly low. If in the general population, men have a depression rate of X and women 2X, one would expect the rates of depression in these Orthodox women and men to both be 2X (in other words, in the general population, men actually had 2X rates of depression, but half of those cases were categorized as substance abuse). The paper did indeed report equivalent rates of depression in women and in men among Orthodox Jews, in sharp contrast to the general population. However, rather than everyone having the 2X rate of the general population, everyone was more like X. Thus, it wasn't the lack of alcoholism unmasking the higher rate of depression in men. Rather, it was something about Orthodoxy lowering the depression rate in women to the lower levels seen in men. The authors suggested that this was due to the honored and socially meaningful role of women in Orthodox Jewish society. As someone who was raised in such a community, I find myself to be a bit skeptical of this interpretation, but cannot offer a better one.

PAGE 291 Estrogen and progesterone have effects on the brain; as just some examples of these, estrogen will change the electrical excitability of the brain (Teyler, T., Vardaris, R., Lewis, D., and Rawitch, A., "Gonadal steroids: effects on excitability of hippocampal pyramidal cells," *Science* 209 [1980]: 1017) and the number of receptors for some of the major neurotransmitters (Schumacher, M., "Rapid membrane effects of steroid hormones: an emerging concept in neuroendocrinology," *Trends in Neurosciences* 13 [1990]: 359; see also Weiland, N., "Sex steroids alter N-methyl-D-aspartate receptor binding in the hippocampus," *Society for Neuroscience Abstracts* 16 [1990]: 959), as well as the number of receiving sites on dendrites ("dendritic spines") that form synapses with axon terminals. This last observation is particularly interesting, as it has been shown that the number of dendritic spines fluctuates in parts of the brain of the rat as a function of the reproductive cycle of the female (Woolley, C., Gould, E., Frankfurt, M., and McEwen, B., "Naturally occurring fluctuation in dendritic spine density on adult hippocampal pyramidal neurons," *Journal of Neuroscience* 10 [1990]: 4035; Young, E., Korszun, A., "Psychoneuroendocrinology of depression: Hypothalamic-pituitary-gonadal axis," *Psychiatric Clinics of North America* 21 [1999]: 309).

Progesterone also has effects, in that one of its breakdown products (metabolites) can bind to one of the main neurotransmitter receptor types in the brain and alter its functioning: Majewska, M., Harrison, N., Schwartz, R., Barker, J., and Paul, S., "Steroid hormone metabolites are barbiturate-like modulators of the GABA receptor," *Science* 232 (1986): 1004. This is particularly interesting for two reasons. First, the fact that the critical agent there is not progesterone but its metabolite (called 3-alpha-hydroxy-5-alpha-dihydroprogesterone by its close friends) means that one must keep track of not only how much progesterone there is on the scene but how much of it gets converted to the metabolite. Of particular interest in terms of the menstrual cycle, progesterone, mood, and depression is the fact that these progesterone metabolites bind to the same receptor complex that binds the benzodiazepine tranquilizers (like those marketed as Valium and Librium) as well as barbiturate anesthetics ("downers"). Moreover, at proper doses, this progesterone metabolite can work as an anesthetic itself (such "steroid anesthetics" have even been used on humans during surgery). No one has quite sorted out the functional significance of this yet, but everyone assumes that something extremely interesting is going on.

Finally, for a way in which estrogen and progesterone can alter the action of antidepressant drugs in the brain, see Wilson, M., Dwuyer, K., and Roy, E., "Direct effects of ovarian hormones on antidepressant binding sites," *Brain Research Bulletin* 22 (1989): 181. For a demonstration that females break down antidepressant drugs in the bloodstream more slowly than males, so that more gets into the brain, see Biegon, A., and Samuel, D., "The in vivo distribution of an antidepressant drug (DMI) in male and female rats," *Psychopharmacology* 65 (1979): 259. For a fascinating discussion of the ways in which people of different ethnic backgrounds vary in their sensitivity to various psychoactive drugs, see Holden, C., "New center to study therapies and ethnicity," *Science* 251 (1991): 748.

PAGE 291 For broad discussions of the connections between stress and depression, see Gold, P., Goodwin, F., and Chrousos, G., "Clinical and biochemical manifestations of depression: relation to the neurobiology of stress," *New England Journal of Medicine* 319 (1988): 348 (outlines a model, similar to that proposed in this chapter, of the genetic defect in depression as a failure for stress to induce tyrosine hydroxylase); Zis, A., and Goodwin, F., "Major affective disorders as a recurrent illness: a critical review," *Archives of General Psychiatry* 36 (1979): 385; Anisman, H., and Zacharko, R., "Depression: the predisposing influence of stress," *Behavioral and Brain Science* 5 (1982): 89; Turner, R., and Beiser, M., "Major depression and depressive symptomatology among the physically disabled: assessing the role of chronic stress," *Journal of Nervous and Mental Disease* 178 (1990): 343. Stress generation among depressives: Roberts, J., Ciesla, J., "Stress generation in the context of depressive disorders," in Fink, G., ed., *Encyclopedia of Stress*, vol. 3, 512.

Major stressors preceding first major depression: Brown, G., Harris, T., *Social Origins of Depression* (New York: Free Press, 1978); Brown, G., Harris, T., Hepworth, C., "Loss, humiliation and entrapment among women developing depression: a patient and non-patient comparison," *Psychological Medicine* 25 (1995): 7. For some studies examining factors that predict who becomes depressed in response to major stressors, see: Maciejewiski, P., Prigerson, H., Mazure, C., "Self-efficacy as a mediator between stressful life events and depressive symptoms: differences based on history of prior depression," *British Journal of Psychiatry* 176 (2000): 373; Mitchell, P., Parker, G., Gladstone, G., Wilhelm, K., Austin, V., "Severity of stressful life events in first and subsequent episodes of depression: the relevance of depression subtype," *Journal of Affective Disorders* 73 (2003): 245.

PAGE 293 A predisposing gene: Caspi, A., Sugden, K., Moffitt, T., Taylor, A., Craig, I., Harrington, H., McClay, J., Mill, J., Martin, J., Braithwait, A., Poulton, R., "Influence of life stress on depression: moderation by a polymorphism in the 5-HTT gene," *Science* 301 (2003): 386. A similar finding in nonhuman primates: Bennett, A., Lesch, K., Heils, A., Long, J., Lorenz, J., Shoaf, S., Champoux, M., Suomi, S., Linnoila, M., Higley, J., "Early experience and serotonin transporter gene variation interact to influence primate CNS function," *Biological Psychiatry* 7 (2002): 118.

PAGE 294 Low glucocorticoid levels in atypical depression: Gold, P., Chrousos, G., "Organization of the stress system and its dysregulation in melancholic and atypical depression: high versus low CRH/NE states," *Molecular Psychiatry* 7 (2002): 254–75.

PAGE 294 Feedback problems in depression, for review, see: Pariante, C., Miller, A., "Glucocorticoid receptors in major depression: relevance to pathophysiology and treatment," *Biological Psychiatry* 49 (2001): 391.

PAGE 295 Stress alters neurochemistry relevant to depression: reviewed in; Tafet, G., Bernardini, R., "Psychoneuroendocrinological links between chronic stress and depression," *Progress in Neuro-Psychopharmacology and Biological Psychiatry* 27 (2003): 893; Sabban, E., Kvetnansky, R., "Stress-triggered activation of gene expression in catecholaminergic systems: dynamics of transcriptional events," *Trends in Neurosciences* 24 (2001): 91. For an immensely interesting link between glucocorticoids and the neurochemistry of serotonin, see: Glatz, K., Mossner, R., Heils, A., Lesch, K., "Glucocorticoid-regulated human serotonin transporter (5-HTT) expression is modulated by the 5-HTT gene-promoter-linked polymorphic

Ahlers, S., Salander, M., Shurtleff, D., and Thomas, J., "Tyrosine pretreatment alleviates suppression of schedule-controlled responding produced by CRF in rats," *Brain Research Bulletin* 29 (1992): 567; Sabban and Kvetnansky, "Stress-triggered activation," op. cit.

PAGE 307 Glatz et al., "Glucocorticoid-regulated human serotonin transporter," op. cit.; Koch, C., Stratakis, C. "Genetic factors and stress," in Fink, G., ed., *Encyclopedia of Stress*, vol. 2, 205.

CHAPTER 15: PERSONALITY, TEMPERAMENT, AND THEIR STRESS-RELATED CONSEQUENCES

PAGE 311 Animal personality: Koolhaas, J., Korte, S., De Boer, S., Van der Vegt, B., Van Reenen, Hopster, H., De Jong, I., Ruis, M., Blokhuis, H., "Coping styles in animals: current status in behavior and stress-physiology," *Neuroscience and Biobehavioral Review* 23 (1999): 925. For a review of primate personality, see Clarke, A., and Boinski, S., "Temperament in nonhuman primates," *American Journal of Primatology* 37 (1995): 103. Personality in sunfish: Wilson, D., Coleman, K., Clark, A., and Biderman, L., "Shy-bold continuum in pumpkinseed sunfish (Lepomis gibbosus): an ecological study of a psychological trait," *Journal of Comparative Psychology* 107 (1993): 250. Personality in geese: Pfeffer, K., Fritz, J., Kotrschal, K., "Hormonal correlates of being an innovative greylag goose, *Anser anser*," *Animal Behavior* 63 (2002): 687.

PAGE 312 Baboons, personality, and physiology: Sapolsky, R., and Ray, J., "Styles of dominance and their physiological correlates among wild baboons," *American Journal of Primatology* 18 (1989): 1. Ray, J., and Sapolsky, R., "Styles of male social behavior and their endocrine correlates among high-ranking baboons," *American Journal of Primatology* 28 (1992): 231. Sapolsky, R., "Why should an aged male baboon transfer troops?" *American Journal of Primatology* 39 (1996): 149. Virgin, C., and Sapolsky, R., "Styles of male social behavior and their endocrine correlates among low-ranking baboons," *American Journal of Primatology* 42 (1997): 25. Also see: Suomi, S., "Early determinants of behaviour: evidence from primate studies," *British Medical Bulletin* 53 (1997): 270.

PAGE 317 Before approaching the question of what personality types are associated with particular types of stress-responses, one must first ask whether there are even stable individual differences in qualities of the stress-response among people. This is documented in: Cohen, S., and Hamrick, N., "Stable individual differences in physiological response to stressors: implications for stress-elicited changes in immune related health," *Brain, Behavior, and Immunity* 17 (2003): 407. For the most detailed review of the literature on psychogenic abortions, see Huisjes, H., *Spontaneous Abortion* (New York: Churchill Livingstone, 1984).

PAGE 318 The reader is referred back to chapter 13 for references on the cognitive and endocrine profile of depression.

PAGE 319 Overview of stress and anxiety: Ohman, A., "Anxiety," in Fink, G., ed., *Encyclopedia of Stress* (San Diego: Academic Press, 2000), vol. 1, 226. Anxiety and catecholamines: Friedman, B., Thayer, J., Borkovec, T., Tyrrell, R., Johnson, B., and Columbo, R., "Autonomic characteristics of nonclinical panic and blood phobia,"

region," *Journal of Neurochemistry* 86 (2003): 1072. Also: van Riel, E., Meijer, O., Steenbergen, P., Joels, M., "Chronic unpredictable stress causes attenuation of serotonin responses in cornu ammonis 1 pyramidal neurons," *Neuroscience* 120 (2003): 649. For a demonstration that uncontrollable, but not controllable, stress alters serotonin neurochemistry, see: Bland, S., Twining, C., Watkins, L., Maier, S., "Stressor controllability modulates stress-induced serotonin but not dopamine efflux in the nucleus accumbens shell," *Synapse* 49 (2003): 206.

PAGE 295 The consequences of the elevated glucocorticoid levels in depression: Immunity: Irwin, M., "Depression and immunity," in Ader, R., Felten, D., Cohen, N., eds., *Psychoneuroimmunology*, 3d ed. (San Diego: Academic Press, 2001), vol. 2, 383. Osteoporosis: Cizza, G., Ravn, P., Chrousos, G., Gold, P., "Depression: a major, unrecognized risk factor for osteoporosis?" *Trends in Endocrinology and Metabolism* 12 (2001): 198. Heart disease: Penninx, B., Beekman, A., Honig, A., Deeg, D., Schoevers, R., van Eijk, J., van Tilburg, W., "Depression and cardiac mortality: results from a community-based longitudinal study," *Archives of General Psychiatry* 58 (2001): 229; Ferketich, A., Schwartzbaum, J., Frid, J., Moeschberger, M., "Depression as an antecedent to heart disease among women and men in the NHANES I study," *National Health and Nutrition Examination Survey, Archives of Internal Medicine* 9 (2000): 1261; Grippoa, A., Johnson, A., "Biological mechanisms in the relationship between depression and heart disease," *Neuroscience and Biobehavioral Reviews* 26 (2002): 941.

PAGE 295 Hippocampal atrophy in depression: Sheline, Y., Wang, P., Gado, M., Csernansky, J., Vannier, M., "Hippocampal atrophy in recurrent major depression," *Proceedings of the National Academy of Sciences, USA* 93 (1996): 3908–4003; Sheline, Y., Sanghavi, M., Mintun, M., Gado, M., "Depression duration but not age predicts hippocampal volume loss in medical healthy women with recurrent major depression," *Journal of Neuroscience* 19 (1999): 5034–41; Bremner, J., Narayan, M., Anderson, E., Staib, L., Miller, H., Charney, D., "Hippocampal volume reduction in major depression," *American Journal of Psychiatry* 157 (2000): 115–27; Sheline, Y., Gado, M., Kraemer, H., "Untreated depression and hippocampal volume loss," *American Journal of Psychiatry* 160 (2003): 1516; MacQueen, G., Campbell, S., McEwen, B., Macdonald, K., Amano, S., Joffe, R., Nahmias, C., Young, L., "Course of illness, hippocampal function, and hippocampal volume in major depression," *Proceedings of the National Academy of Sciences, USA* 100 (2002): 1387.

Frontal cortical atrophy: Lai, T., Payne, M. E., Byrum, C. E., Steffens, D. C., Krishnan, K. R., "Reduction of orbital frontal cortex volume in geriatric depression," *Biological Psychiatry* 48 (2000): 971; Rajkowska, G., Miguel-Hidalgo, J., Wei, J., Pittman, S., Dilley, G., Overholser, J., Meltzer, H., Stockmeier, C., "Morphometric evidence for neuronal and glial prefrontal cell pathology in major depression," *Biological Psychiatry* 45 (1999): 1085. Frontal cortical sensitivity to glucocorticoids: Sanchez, M., Young, L., Plotsky, P., Insel, T., "Distribution of corticosteroid receptors in the rhesus brain: relative absence of GR in the hippocampal formation," *Journal of Neuroscience* 20 (2000): 4657.

PAGE 296 Footnote regarding neurogenesis and depression: Kempermann, G., Kronenberg, G., "Depressed new neurons—adult hippocampal neurogenesis and a cellular plasticity hypothesis of major depression," *Biological Psychiatry* 54 (2003): 499. A late 2004 issue of *Biological Psychiatry* will feature a debate between two of the principal groups in this controversy (Duman, Vollmayr, Henn), mediated by myself.

PAGE 296 Antidepressant effects of steroidogenesis inhibitors: Wolkowitz, O., Reus, V., Chan, T., Manfredi, F., Raum, W., Johnson, R., Canick, J., "Antiglucocorticoid treatment of depression: double-blind ketoconazole," *Biological Psychiatry* 45 (1999): 1070; McQuade, R., Young, A., "Future therapeutic targets in mood disorders: the glucocorticoid receptor," *British Journal of Psychiatry* 177 (2000): 390; Sapolsky, R., "Taming stress," *Scientific American* (September 2003): 86. Efficacy of glucocorticoid receptor blockers: Belanoff, J., Rothschild, A., Cassidy, F., DeBattista, C., Baulieu, E., Schold, C., Schatzberg, A., "An open label trial of C-1073 (Mifepristone) for psychotic major depression," *Biological Psychiatry* 52 (2002): 386–92.

DHEA as an antidepressant: McQuade, "Future therapeutic agents," op. cit.

PAGE 297 Normalizing glucocorticoid levels as a prerequisite for antidepressant efficacy: Holsboer, F., "The corticosteroid receptor hypothesis of depression," *Neuropsychopharmacology* 23 (2000): 477. Normalization of glucocorticoid levels precede lifting of depression: Yau, J., Seckl, J., "Antidepressant actions on glucocorticoid receptors," in Fink, G., ed., *Encyclopedia of Stress*, vol. 1, 212. As an offshoot of this thinking, some researchers are suggesting that antidepressants are working, primarily, not so much by changing the levels of glucocorticoid receptors as by changing the activity of a protein that regulates how much glucocorticoids penetrate into a neuron. This is an interesting but definitely minority view and is reviewed in: Pariante, C., Thomas, S., Lovesteon, S., Makoff, A., Kerwin, R., "Do antidepressants regulate how cortisol affects the brain?," *Psychoneuroendocrinology* 29 (2004): 423.

PAGE 299 Freud's classic essay, "Mourning and melancholia," can be found in *The Collected Papers*, vol. 4 (New York: Basic Books, 1959).

PAGE 300 Psychological features of learned helplessness: the definitive book on the subject is by Martin Seligman (from which the various quotations are taken): *Helplessness: On Depression, Development and Death* (San Francisco: W. H. Freeman, 1975). This monumental (and quite readable) work is one of the most influential books ever published in psychology. The specific human experiments cited in this section are Hiroto, D., "Locus of control and learned helplessness," *Journal of Experimental Psychology* 102 (1974): 187 (uncontrollable noise induces helplessness with a noise-avoidance task); Hiroto, D., and Seligman, M., "Generality of learned helplessness in man," *Journal of Personality and Social Psychology* 31 (1974): 311 (uncontrollable noise disrupts learning of simple word puzzles, and unsolvable tasks induce helplessness); Seligman, *Helplessness*, p. 35 (unsolvable tasks induce social helplessness).

For a discussion of learned helplessness as a cognitive or affective phenomenon, see Seligman, M., *Helplessness*. For a discussion of learned helplessness as a phenomenon of psychomotor retardation, see Weiss, J., Bailey, W., Goodman, P., Hoffman, L., Ambrose, M., Salman, S., and Charry, J., "A model for neurochemical study of depression," in Spiegelstein, M., and Levy, A., eds., *Behavioral Models and the Analysis of Drug Action* (Amsterdam: Elsevier, 1982). "Learned laziness" in animals given noncontingent reward: the use of the term "spoiled brat" is cited by Seligman, *Helplessness*, p. 35. The published version of those findings can be found in Engberg, L., Hansen, G., Welker, R., and Thomas, D., "Acquisition of

key-pecking via autoshaping as a function of prior experience: 'learned laziness?'" *Science* 178 (1973): 1002.

PAGE 302 Biological features of learned helplessness, where rats show altered grooming, social behavior, sexual behavior, feeding, plus many of the vegetative symptoms: Stone, E., "Possible grooming deficit in stressed rats," *Research Communication in Psychology, Psychiatry and Behavior* 3 (1978): 109; Weiss, J., Simson, P., Ambrose, M., Webster, A., and Hoffman, L., "Neurochemical basis of behavioral depression," in Katkin, E., and Manuck, S., eds., *Advances in Behavioral Medicine*, vol. 1 (Greenwich, Conn.: JAI Press, 1985); Weiss, J., Goodman, P., Losito, P., Corrigan, S., Charry, J., and Bailey, W., "Behavioral depression produced by an uncontrolled stressor: relation to norepinephrine, dopamine and serotonin levels in various regions of the rat brain," *Brain Research Reviews* 3 (1981): 167. For an explicit comparison between the symptoms of depression (DSM-III criteria) and learned helplessness, see Weiss, J., Bailey, W., Goodman, P., Hoffman, L., Ambrose, M., Salman, S., and Charry, J., "A model for neurochemical study of depression," in Spiegelstein, M., and Levy, A., eds., *Behavioral Models and the Analysis of Drug Action*.

Learned helplessness can be lessened by antidepressants or ECT: Dorworth, T., and Overmier, J., "On learned helplessness: the therapeutic effects of electroconvulsive shocks," *Physiological Psychology* 5 (1977): 355; Leshner, A., Remler, H., Biegon, A., and Samuel, D., "Desmethylimipramine counteracts learned helplessness in rats," *Psychopharmacology* 66 (1979): 207; Petty, F., and Sherman, A., "Reversal of learned helplessness by imipramine," *Communications in Psychopharmacology* 3 (1980): 371; Sherman, A., Allers, G., Petty, F., and Henn, F., "A neuropharmacologically-relevant animal model of depression," *Neuropharmacology* 18 (1979): 891.

PAGE 303 Internal locus of control as protective: Maciejewiski et al., "Self-efficacy as a mediator," op. cit.

PAGE 304 Rozin, P., Poritsky, S., and Sotsky, R., "American children with reading problems can easily learn to read English represented by Chinese characters," *Science* 171 (1971): 1264.

PAGE 304 Early parental loss increases the risk of adulthood depression: this subject is reviewed in Breier, A., Kelso, J., Kirwin, P., Beller, S., Wolkowitz, O., and Pickar, D., "Early parental loss and development of adult psychopathology," *Archives of General Psychiatry* 45 (1988): 987; Amato, P., Keith, B., "Consequences of parental divorce for the well-being of children: a meta-analysis," *Psychological Bulletin* 110 (1991): 26; Gutman, D., Nemeroff, C., "Persistent CNS effects of an adverse early environment: clinical and preclinical studies," *Physiology and Behavior* 79 (2003): 471.

PAGE 306 Stress depletes parts of the brain of norepinephrine, while also increasing the activity of tyrosine hydroxylase: Stone, E., and McCarty, R., "Adaptation to stress: tyrosine hydroxylase activity and catecholamine release," *Neuroscience and Biobehavioral Reviews* 7 (1983): 29. Glucocorticoids have something to do with this: Dunn, A., Gildersleeve, N., and Gray, H., "Mouse brain tyrosine hydroxylase and glutamic acid decarboxylase following treatment with adrenocorticotropic hormone, vasopressin or corticosterone," *Journal of Neurochemistry* 31 (1978): 977. In addition, CRH may have something to do with this:

Biological Psychiatry 34 (1993): 298. For a discussion of the dichotomy between still striving to cope (accompanied by catecholamine secretion) and having given up (characterized by glucocorticoid hypersecretion), see: Frankenhaeuser, M., "The sympathetic-adrenal and pituitary-adrenal response to challenge," in Dembroski, T., Schmidt, T., and Blumchen, G., eds., *Biobehavioral Basis of Coronary Heart Disease* (Basel: Karger, 1983), 91. Shorter lifespan in anxious rats: Cavigelli, S., and McClintock, M., *Proceedings of the National Academy of Sciences*, 100 (December 2003). The footnoted quote is from Aragno, A., *Forms of Knowledge: A Psychoanalytic of Human Communication* (Madison, Conn.: International Universities Press, 2004).

PAGE 319 Animal models of anxiety: Davis, M., "Functional neuroanatomy of anxiety and fear: a focus on the amygdala," in Charney, D., Nestler, E., and Bunney, B., *Neurobiology of Mental Illness* (New York: Oxford University Press, 1999), 463.

PAGE 320 McGaugh, J., *Memory and Emotion* (New York: Weidenfeld and Nicolson, 2003); Roozendaal, B., "Glucocorticoids and the regulation of memory consolidation," *Psychoneuroendocrinology* 25 (2000): 213–38.

PAGE 322 Heart racing before conscious awareness: Dolan, R., "Emotion, cognition and behavior," *Science* 298 (2002): 1191. The sympathetic nervous system biases the amygdala: Critchley, H., Mathias, C., and Dolan, R., "Fear conditioning in humans: the influence of awareness and autonomic arousal on functional neuroanatomy," *Neuron* 33 (2002): 653–63.

PAGE 323 Footnote: The disturbing, footnoted finding about race and amygdala activation: Hart, A., Whalen, P., Shin, L., McInerney, C., Fischer, H., and Rauch, S., "Differential response in the human amygdala to racial outgroup vs ingroup face stimuli," *NeuroReport* 11 (2000): 2351; Golby, A., Gabrieli, J., Chiao, J., and Eberhardt, J., "Differential responses in the fusiform region to same-race and other-race faces," *Nature Neuroscience* 4 (2001): 845. Close readers of this latter paper will note that it is not really the amygdala that activates, but a related area that is very responsive to faces.

PAGE 323 People with anxiety disorders slow down even more: Ohman, op. cit.

PAGE 323 The amygdala becomes hyperexcitable: Karst, H., Nair, S., Velzing, E., Rumpff-van Essen, L., Slagter, E., Shinnick-Gallagher, P., and Joels, M., "Glucocorticoids alter calcium conductances and calcium channel subunit expression in basolateral amygdala neurons," *European Journal of Neuroscience* 16 (2002): 1083–89; Diamond, D., Park, C., Puls, M., and Rose, G., "Differential effects of stress on hippocampal and amygdaloid LTP," in Holscher, C., *Neuronal Mechanisms of Memory Formation* (New York: Cambridge University Press, 2001), 379. New connections: Vyas, A., Mitra, R., Rao, B., and Chattarji, S., "Chronic stress induces contrasting patterns of dendritic remodeling in hippocampal and amygdaloid neurons," *Journal of Neuroscience* 22 (2002): 6810. Make a rat's amygdala more excitable: Rosen, J., Hammerman, E., Sitcoske, M., Glowa, J., and Schulkin, J., "Hyperexcitability and exaggerated fear-potentiated startle produced by partial amygdala kindling," *Behavioral Neuroscience* 110 (1996): 43. LeDoux's model: LeDoux, J., *The Emotional Brain* (New York: Simon and Schuster, 1996).

PAGE 324 Type A: the definitive prospective study showing a link between Type-A personality and coronary heart disease is Rosenman, R., Brand, R.,

Jenkins, C., Friedman, M., Straus, R., and Wurm, M., "Coronary heart disease in the Western Collaborative Group Study: final follow-up experience of 8 1/2 years," *Journal of the American Medical Association* 233 (1975): 872. See also Friedman, M., and Rosenman, R., *Type A Behavior and Your Heart* (New York: Knopf, 1974). The blue-ribbon panel that endorsed the Type-A concept published its report as: Cooper, T., Detre, T., and Weiss, S., "Coronary prone behavior and coronary heart disease; a critical review," *Circulation* 63 (1981): 1199.

Problems with replicating the original Type-A finding: the most influential study was Shekelle, R., Billings, J., and Borhani, N., "The MRFIT behavior pattern study. II. Type-A behavior and incidence of coronary heart disease," *American Journal of Epidemiology* 122 (1985): 599. Others are discussed in Barefoot, J., Peterson, B., Harrell, F., et al., "Type A behavior and survival: a follow-up study of 1,467 patients with coronary artery disease," *American Journal of Cardiology* 64 (1989): 427.

The demonstration that Type-A behavior is associated with better survivorship: the Barefoot study just cited, plus Ragland, D., and Brand, R., "Type A behavior and mortality from coronary heart disease," *New England Journal of Medicine* 313 (1988): 65. That finding is a good lesson in how incredibly subtle some confounds can be in epidemiology research. Why should being Type A be associated with better survivorship, once you are diagnosed with coronary heart disease? Some possibilities: Type-A people, because of their driven and disciplined nature, are more likely to comply with the medicine, dieting, and exercise schedules given them by their doctors. Or certain people may immediately be recognized as being Type A by their doctors, who then think "Aha, here's this Type-A patient with coronary heart disease. I know all about Friedman and Rosenman's studies; I'd better take extra good care of this person." Or Type-A people may be more disciplined about annual checkups with doctors, and thus be diagnosed with coronary heart disease earlier than average, when it is still pretty mild—leading to seemingly better survivorship. This last factor has probably been ruled out, but no one is sure about the other possible confounds yet, as the studies showing better Type-A survivorship are quite recent. Some of the possible sources of confounds in these findings are discussed in Matthews, K., and Haynes, S., "Type A behavior pattern and coronary disease risk," *American Journal of Epidemiology* 123 (1986): 923.

PAGE 324 The importance of hostility as a predictor of heart disease: the demonstration of this by reanalysis of the original Friedman and Rosenman data: Hecker, M., Chesney, M. N., Black, G., and Frautsch, N., "Coronary-prone behaviors in the Western Collaborative Group Study," *Psychosomatic Medicine* 50 (1988): 153. Hostility in medical students: Barefoot, J., Dahlstrom, W., and Williams, R., "Hostility, CHD incidence, and total mortality: a 25-year follow-up study of 255 physicians," *Psychosomatic Medicine* 45 (1983): 59. In lawyers: Barefoot, J., Dodge, K., Peterson, B., Dahlstrom, W., and Williams, R., "The Cook-Medley Hostility scale: item content and ability to predict survival," *Psychosomatic Medicine* 51 (1989): 46. In Finnish twins: Koskenvuo, M., Kaprio, J., Rose, R., Kesaniemi, A., Sarna, S., Heikkila, K., and Langinvainio, H., "Hostility as a risk factor for mortality and ischemic heart disease in men," *Psychosomatic Medicine* 50 (1988): 330. In Western Electric employees: Shekelle, R., Gale, M., Ostfeld, A., and Paul, O., "Hostility, risk of coronary disease, and mortality," *Psychosomatic Medicine* 45 (1983): 219. For general reviews, see Miller, T., Smith, T., Turner, C., Guijarro, M., and Hallet, A., "A meta-analytic review of research on hostility and physical health," *Psychological Bulletin* 119 (1996): 322; Williams, R., and Littman, A., "Psychosocial factors: role in cardiac risk and treatment strategies," *Cardiology Clinics* 14 (1996): 97. Hostility as a predictor of overall mortality: Houston, B., Babyak, M., Chesney, M., Black, G., and Ragland, D., "Social dominance and 22-year all-cause mortality in men," *Psychosomatic Medicine* 50 (1997): 5. Yan, L. L., Liu, K., Matthews, K. A., Daviglus, M. L., Ferguson, T. F., and Kiefe, C. I., "Psychosocial factors and risk of hypertension: the Coronary Artery Risk Development in Young Adults (CARDIA) study," *Journal of the American Medical Association* 290 (2003): 2190. Hostility in different cities: Marmot, M., "Epidemiology of SES and health: are determinants within countries the same as between countries?" *Annals of the New York Academy of Sciences* 896 (1999): 16. Hostility and stroke: Williams, J., Nieto, F., Sanford, C., Couper, D., and Tyroler, H., "The association between trait anger and incident stroke risk," *Stroke* 33 (2002): 13.

Insecurity as the key to Type A-ness: Price, V., Friedman, M., Ghandour, G., and Fleischmann, N., "Relation between insecurity and Type A behavior," *American Heart Journal* 129 (1995): 488.

PAGE 326 The studies of James Gross concerning the intentional inhibition of emotional expression can be found in Gross, J., and Levenson, R., "Emotional suppression: physiology, self-report, and expressive behavior," *Journal of Personality and Social Psychology* 64 (1993): 870. See also Gross, J., and Levenson, R., "Hiding feelings: the acute effects of inhibiting negative and positive emotion," *Journal of Abnormal Psychology* 106 (1997): 95. For a vote in favor of expression of hostility as being most injurious: Siegman, A., "Cardiovascular consequences of expressing, experiencing, and repressing anger," *Journal of Behavioral Medicine* 16 (1993): 539.

PAGE 326 Hormonal and cardiovascular function in hostile versus non-hostile people. Demonstration that hostile and non-hostile people do not differ in hormone and blood pressure measures during rest or during nonsocial stressors: Sallis, J., Johnson, C., Treverow, T., Kaplan, R., and Hovell, M., "The relationship between cynical hostility and blood pressure reactivity," *Journal of Psychosomatic Research* 31 (1987): 111. See also Smith, M., and Houston, B., "Hostility, anger expression, cardiovascular responsivity, and social support," *Biological Psychology* 24 (1987): 39. Also Krantz, D., and Manuck, S., "Acute psychophysiologic reactivity and risk of cardiovascular disease: a review and methodological critique," *Psychological Bulletin* 96 (1984): 435; Suarez, E., Kuhn, C., Schanberg, S., Williams, R., and Zimmermann, E., "Neuroendocrine, cardiovascular, and emotional responses of hostile men: the role of interpersonal challenge," *Psychosomatic Medicine* 60 (1998): 78.

Demonstration of larger responses in hostile people to social provocations: being interrupted during a task: Suarez, E., and Williams, R., "Situational determinants of cardiovascular and emotional reactivity in high and low hostile men," *Psychosomatic Medicine* 51 (1989): 404. During a rigged game against a disparaging opponent: Glass, D., Krakoff, L., and Contrada, R., "Effect of harassment and competition upon cardiovascular and catecholamine responses in Type A and Type B individuals," *Psychophysiology* 17 (1980): 453. During a role-play of social conflict: Hardy, J., and Smith, T., "Cynical hostility and vulnerability to disease: social support, life stress, and physiological response to conflict," *Health Psychology* 7 (1988): 477. Unsolvable tasks with bad instructions: Weidner, G., Friend, R.,

Ficarrotto, T., and Mendell, N., "Hostility and cardiovascular reactivity to stress in women and men," *Psychosomatic Medicine* 51 (1989): 36; also see Suls, J., and Wan, C., "The relationship between trait hostility and cardiovascular reactivity: a quantitative review and analysis," *Psychophysiology* 30 (1993): 615. Note that many of these studies were done when everyone was still dichotomizing between Type-A and Type-B people, rather than hostile and non-hostile.

PAGE 327 If you can change Type-A tendencies, you decrease the risk of coronary heart disease: Friedman, M., Thoresen, C., and Gill, J., "Alteration of Type A behavior and its effect on cardiac recurrences in post-myocardial infarction patients: summary results of the Recurrent Coronary Prevention Project," *American Heart Journal* 112 (1986): 653; Friedman, M., Breall, W., Goodwin, M., Sparagon, B., Ghandour, G., and Fleischmann, N., "Effect of Type A behavioral counseling on frequency of episodes of silent myocardial ischemia in coronary patients," *American Heart Journal* 132 (1996): 933.

Finally, for an analysis of the medical histories and the significantly shortened life spans of the American presidents, in which the author concludes that they have died disproportionately from stress-related cardiovascular disease: Gilbert, R., "Travails of the chief," *The Sciences* (January–February 1993): 8.

PAGE 328 The story the (non)-discovery of Type A-ness can be found in: Sapolsky, R., "The role of upholstery in cardiovascular physiology," *Discover* (November 1997): 58.

PAGE 330 A more extensive discussion of Friedman's life can be found in: Sapolsky, R., "All the rage," *Men's Health* (April 2002): 104.

PAGE 331 Optimists versus pessimists: Cohen, F., Kearney, K., Zegans, L., Kemeny, M., Neuhaus, J., and Stites, D., "Differential immune system changes with acute and persistent stress for optimists vs pessimists," *Brain, Behavior and Immunity* 13 (1999): 155. Shyer individuals: Dettling, A., Gunnar, M., Donzella, B., "Cortisol levels of young children in full-day childcare centers: relations with age and temperament," *Psychoneuroendocrinology* 24 (1999): 519.

PAGE 331 Repressive personality: they really are happy: Brandtstadter, J., Balte, S., Gotz, B., Kirschbaum, C., and Hellhammer, D., "Developmental and personality correlates of adrenocortical activity as indexed by salivary cortisol: observations in the age range of 35 to 65 years," *Journal of Psychosomatic Research* 35 (1991): 173. Weinberger, D., Schwartz, G., and Davidson, R., "Low-anxious, high-anxious, and repressive coping styles: psychometric patterns and behavioral and physiological responses to stress," *Journal of Abnormal Psychology* 88 (1979): 369; Shaw, R., Cohen, F., Fishman-Rosen, R., Murphy, M., Stertzer, S., Clark, D., and Myler, K., "Psychologic predictors of psychosocial and medical outcomes in patients undergoing coronary angioplasty," *Psychosomatic Medicine* 48 (1986): 582; Shaw, R., Cohen, F., Doyle, B., and Palesky, J., "The impact of denial and repressive style on information gain and rehabilitation outcomes in myocardial infarction patients," *Psychosomatic Medicine* 47 (1985): 262.

Patterns of repressives: Brown, L., Tomarken, A., Orth, D., Loosen, P., Kalin, N., and Davidson, R., "Individual differences in repressive-defensiveness predict basal salivary cortisol levels," *Journal of Personality and Social Psychology* 70 (1996): 362. Such individuals have impaired immune profiles: Jamner, L., Schwartz, G., and Leigh, H., "The relationship between repressive and defensive coping styles and monocyte, eosinophile, and serum glucose levels: support for the opioid peptide hypothesis of repression," *Psychosomatic Medicine* 50 (1988): 567. Tomarken, A., and Davidson, R., "Frontal brain activation in repressors and non-repressors," *Journal of Abnormal Psychology* 103 (1994): 339. Sociopathy and the frontal cortex: Damasio, A., Tranel, D., and Damasio, H., "Individuals with socio-pathic behavior caused by frontal damage fail to respond autonomically to social stimuli," *Behavioural Brain Research* 41 (1990): 81.

CHAPTER 16: JUNKIES, ADRENALINE JUNKIES, AND PLEASURE

PAGE 335 Blakemore, S., Wolpert, D., and Frith, C., "Why can't you tickle your-self?" *NeuroReport* 11 (2000): R11. Sex and its effects on glucocorticoid levels: Woodson, J., Macintosh, D., Fleshner, M., and Diamond, D., "Emotion-induced amnesia in rats: working memory-specific impairment, corticosterone-memory correlation, and fear versus arousal effects on memory," *Learning and Memory* 10 (2003): 326.

PAGE 337 Dopamine and the tegmentum/accumbens pathway: good, if techni-cal reviews can be found in: Kelley, A., and Berridge, K., "The neuroscience of natural rewards: relevance to addictive drugs," *Journal of Neuroscience* 22 (2002): 3306–11; Koob, G. F., "Allostatic view of motivation: implications for psy-chopathology," in: Bevins, R., and Bardo, M. T., eds., *Motivational Factors in the Etiology of Drug Abuse*, Nebraska Symposium on Motivation, vol. 50 (Lincoln, Neb.: University of Nebraska Press), in press.

PAGE 337 Schultz's work: Schultz, W., Tremblay, L., and Holerman, J., "Reward processing in primate orbitofrontal cortex and basal ganglia," *Cerebral Cortex* 10 (2000): 272; Waelti, P., Dickinson, A., and Schultz, W., "Dopamine responses com-ply with basic assumptions of formal learning theory," *Nature* 412 (2001): 43.

PAGE 339 Phillips's work: Phillips, P., Stuber, G., Heien, M., Wightman, R., and Carelli, R., "Subsecond dopamine release promotes cocaine seeking," *Nature* 422 (2003): 614.

PAGE 339 Recent work by Schultz: Fiorillo, C., Tobler, P., and Schultz, W., "Dis-crete coding of reward probability and uncertainty by dopamine neurons," *Sci-ence* 299 (2003): 1998; this and the previous study are discussed in Sapolsky, R., "The pleasures (and pain) of 'maybe,'" *Natural History* (September 2003): 22.

PAGE 340 The study about one's true love is described in Helmuth, L., "Caudate-over-heels in love," *Science* 302 (2003): 1320.

PAGE 341 Animal play: Spinka, M., Newberry, R., and Bekoff, M., "Mammalian play: training for the unexpected," *Quarterly Review of Biology* 76 (2001): 141. For a good review of the differences between challenge (i.e., stimulation) and threat, see: Epel, E., McEwen, B., and Ockovics, J., "Embodying psychological thriving: physical thriving in response to stress," *Journal of Social Issues* 54 (1998): 301.

PAGE 341 Glucocorticoids and dopamine: Piazza, P., and Le Moal, M., "Glu-cocorticoids as a biological substrate of reward: physiological and patho-physiological implications," *Brain Research Reviews* 25 (1997): 359; Rouge-Pont, F., Abrous, D., Le Moal, M., and Piazza, P., "Release of endogenous dopamine in cultured mesencephalic neurons: influence of dopaminergic agonists and glucocorticoid antagonists," *European Journal of Neuroscience* 1 (1999): 2343; Piazza, P., and Le Moal, M., "The role of stress in drug self-administration," *Trends in Pharmacological Sciences* 19 (1998): 6. Deroche-Gamonet, V., Sillaber, I., Aouizerate, B., Izawa, R., Jaber, M., Ghozland, S., Kellendonk, C., Le Moal, M., Spanagel, R., Schutz, G., Tronche, F., and Piazza, P. V., "The glucocorticoid receptor as a potential target to reduce cocaine abuse," *Journal of Neuroscience* 23 (2003): 4785.

Stress and dopamine depletion: Gambarana, C., Masi, F., Tagliamonte, A., Scherggi, S., Ghiglieri, O., and De Monti, M., "A chronic stress that impairs reactivity in rats also decreases dopaminergic transmission in the nucleus accumbens: a microdialysis study," *Journal of Neurochemistry* 72 (1999): 2039. Stress and amygdala release of dopamine: Wolak, M., Gold, P., and Chrousos, G., "Stress system: emphasis on CRF in physiologic stress responses and the endocrinopathies of melancholic and atypical depression," *Endocrine Reviews* 11 (2002), in press.

PAGE 342 Neurons that are unresponsive to dopamine signals: Ding, Y., Chi, H., Grady, D., Morishima, A., Kidd, J., Kidd, K., Flodman, P., Spence, M., Schuck, S., Swanson, J., Zhang, Y., and Moyzis, M., "Evidence of positive selection acting at the human dopamine receptor D4 gene locus," *Proceedings of the National Academy of Sciences* 99 (2002): 309.

PAGE 343 Commonalities across addictions: Holden, C., "'Behavioral' addictions; Do they exist?" *Science* 294 (2001): 980. For a discussion of whether the neurobiology of addiction applies to a very different realm, see Insel, T., "Is social attachment an addictive disorder?" *Physiology and Behavior* 79 (2003): 351.

PAGE 343 Correlation between pathway activation and subjective pleasure: Stein, Elliott, lecture, University of Wisconsin, April 2002. Thousand-fold increase in dopamine: Abbott, A., "Addicted," *Nature* 419 (2002): 872.

PAGE 344 Opponent process: Ahmed, S., Lin, D., Koob, G., and Parsons, L., "Escalation of cocaine self-administration does not depend on altered cocaine-induced nucleus accumbens dopamine levels," *Journal of Neurochemistry* 86 (2003): 102.

PAGE 345 Endogenous opiates and "wanting": Kelley and Berridge, op. cit. Porn films: Stein, op. cit.

PAGE 346 Context-dependent relapse: Grimm, J., Hope, B., Wise, R., and Shaham, Y., "Incubation of cocaine craving after withdrawal," *Nature* 412 (2001): 141; Schulteis, G., Ahmed, S., Morse, A., Koob, G., and Everitt, B., "Conditioning and opiate withdrawal," *Nature* 405 (2000): 1013.

PAGE 346 Potentation of projections onto dopamine neurons: Ungless, M., Whistler, J., Malenka, R., and Bonci, A., "Single cocaine exposure in vivo induces LTP in dopamine neurons," *Nature* 411 (2001): 583; Bao, S., Chan, V., and Merzenich, M., "Cortical remodeling induced by activity of ventral tegmental dopamine neurons," *Nature* 412 (2001): 79; Nestler, E., "Total recall—the memory of addiction," *Science* 292 (2001): 2266; Hyman, S., and Malenka, R., "Addiction and the brain: the neurobiology of compulsion and its persistence," *Nature Neuroscience* 2 (2001): 695. Electrically stimulate the pathway: Vorel, S., Liu, X., Hayes, R., Spector, J., and Gardner, E., "Relapse to cocaine-seeking after hippocampal theta burst stimulation," *Science* 292 (2001): 1175.

PAGE 347 Alcohol raising glucocorticoid levels: Taylor, A., and Pilati, M., "Alcohol, alcoholism and stress: a psychobiological perspective," in Fink, G., ed., *Encyclopedia of Stress* (San Diego: Academic Press, 2000), vol. 1, 131; alcohol damping CRH effects: Valdez, G. R., Roberts, A. J., Chan, K., Davis, H., Brennan, M., Zorrilla, E. P., and Koob, G. F., "Increased ethanol self-administration and anxiety-like behavior during acute withdrawal and protracted abstinence: regulation by corticotropin-releasing factor," *Alcoholism: Clinical and Experimental Research* 26 (2002):1494–1501.

PAGE 347 Predictable versus unpredictable stress: Piazza and Le Moal, "The role of stress," op. cit. Social subordinance: Morgan, D., Grant, K., Gage, H., Mach, R., Kaplan, J., Prioleau, O., Nader, S., Buchheimer, N., Ehrenkaufer, R., and Nader, M., "Social dominance in monkeys: dopamine D2 receptors and cocaine self-administration," *Nature Neuroscience* 5 (2002): 169–74; Ellison, G., "Stress and alcohol intake: the socio-pharmacological approach," *Physiology and Behavior* 40 (1987): 387. Stress increases alcohol consumption: Taylor, op. cit. Stressor must come just before the drug exposure: Piazza and Le Moal, "The role of stress," op. cit.

PAGE 348 Prenatal stress, adult drug propensity: DeTurck, K., and Pohorecky, L., "Ethanol sensitivity in rats: effect of prenatal stress," *Physiology and Behavior* 40 (1987): 407. Birth complication: Brake, W., Sullivan, R., and Gratton, A., "Perinatal distress leads to lateralized medial prefrontal cortical dopamine hypofunction in adult rats," *Journal of Neuroscience* 20 (2000): 5538. Ditto in infancy: Taylor and Pilati, op. cit. Separation in monkeys: Bennet et al., op. cit. "Separation in humans," cited in Taylor and Pilati, op. cit.; Bohman, M., Sigvardsson, S., Cloninger, R., and Von Knorring, A., "Alcoholism: lessons from population, family and adoption studies," *Alcohol and Alcoholism* (1987): supp. 1, 55.

PAGE 348 Stress increases the extent of abuse: Piazza, P., and Le Moal, M., "Interactions between stress and drugs of abuse," in Fink, G., ed., *Encyclopedia of Stress* (San Diego: Academic Press, 2000), vol. 2, 586. CRH elevated during withdrawal: Service, R., "Probing alcoholism's dark side," *Science* 285 (1999): 1473. Glucocorticoid levels elevated in withdrawal: Leshner, A., "Drug use and abuse," in Fink, G., ed., *Encyclopedia of Stress* (San Diego: Academic Press, 2000), vol. 1, 755. Stress just before the return to the cage: Leshner, ibid.

PAGE 350 High reactor rats: Piazza, P., Deminiere, J., Le Moal, M., and Simon, H., "Factors that predict individual vulnerability to amphetamine self-administration," *Science* 245 (1989): 1511; Kabbaj, M., Devine, D. P., Savage, V. R., and Akil, H., "Neurobiological correlates of individual differences in novelty-seeking behavior in the rat: differential expression of stress-related molecules," *Journal of Neuroscience* 20 (2000): 6983.

PAGE 351 Sterling, P., "Principles of allostasis: optimal design, predictive regulation, pathophysiology and rational therapeutics," in Schulkin, J., ed., *Allostasis, Homeostasis, and the Costs of Adaptation* (Cambridge, Mass.: MIT Press, 2003).

CHAPTER 17: THE VIEW FROM THE BOTTOM

PAGE 354 Rudolph Virchow: Rosen, G., "The evolution of social medicine," in Freeman, H., Levine, S., and Reeder, L., eds., *Handbook of Medical Sociology*, 2d ed. (Englewood Cliffs, N.J.: Prentice-Hall, 1972). This is also the source of the Virchow quotes.

PAGE 355 For introductions to baboon social behavior, see: Strum, S., *Almost Human* (New York: Random House, 1987); Smuts, B., *Sex and Friend in Baboons* (New York: Aldine, 1985); Ransom, T., *Beach Troop of the Gombe* (Lewisburg, Pa.: Bucknell University Press, 1981).

PAGE 356 Elevated glucocorticoids and other problems in low-ranking male baboons: Sapolsky, R., "Adrenocortical function, social rank and personality among wild baboons," *Biological Psychiatry* 28 (1990): 862; Sapolsky, R., "Endocrinology alfresco: psychoendocrine studies of wild baboons," *Recent Progress in Hormone Research* 48 (1993): 437; Sapolsky, R., and Spencer, E., "Social subordinance is associated with suppression of insulin-like growth factor I in a population of wild primates," *American Journal of Physiology* 273 (1997): R1346. Similar themes with rhesus monkeys: Kaplan, J., Manuck, S., Anthony, M., and Clarkson, T., "Premenopausal social status and hormone exposure predict postmenopausal atherosclerosis in female monkeys," *Obstetrics and Gynecology* 99 (2002): 381–83.

PAGE 358 A review of rank-related differences in the stress-response of other species: Sapolsky, R., "The physiological and pathophysiological implications of social stress in mammals," in McEwen, B., ed., *Coping with the Environment.* Handbook of Physiology (Washington, D.C.: American Physiological Association Press), in press.

PAGE 358 Marmoset review: Abbott, D., Saltzman, W., Schultz-Darken, N., and Smith, T., "Specific neuroendocrine mechanisms not involving generalized stress mediate social regulation of female reproduction in cooperatively breeding marmoset monkeys," in Carter, C., Kirpatrick, B., Liederhendler, I., eds., *The Integrative Neurobiology of Affiliation* (New York: New York Academy of Sciences Press, 1997).

PAGE 358 Life for dominant wild dogs and mongooses: Creel, S., Creel, N., and Monfort, S., "Social stress and dominance," *Nature* 379 (1996): 212; Creel, S., "Social dominance and stress hormones," *Trends in Ecology and Evolution* 16 (2001): 491. The recent study with Abbott and other primatologists: Abbott, D., Keverne, E., Bercovith, F., Shively, C., Mendoza, S., Saltzman, W., Snowdon, C., Ziegler, T., Banjevic, M., Garland, T., and Sapolsky, R., "Are subordinates always stressed? A comparative analysis of rank differences in cortisol levels among primates," *Hormones and Behavior* 43 (2003): 67.

PAGE 360 For introductions to animal culture: Wrangham, R., *Chimpanzee Cultures* (Cambridge, Mass.: Harvard University Press, 1994); De Waal, F., *The Ape and the Sushi Master* (New York: Basic Books, 2001); Laland, K., and Hoppitt, W., "Do animals have culture?" *Evolutionary Anthropology* 12 (2003): 150–59.

PAGE 360 Reconciliative rhesus: Gust, D., Gordon, T., Hambright, K., and Wilson, M., "Relationship between social factors and pituitary-adrenocortical activity in female rhesus monkeys," *Hormones and Behavior* 27 (1993): 318. The benign baboon troop: Sapolsky, R., and Share, L., "A pacific culture among wild baboons, its emergence and transmission," *Public Library of Science, Biology,* (2004), in press. Baboons during a drought: Sapolsky, R., "Endocrine and behavioral correlates of drought in the wild baboon," *American Journal of Primatology* 11 (1986): 217.

PAGE 360 Social instability as a primate stressor: Sapolsky, R., "The physiology of dominance in stable versus unstable social hierarchies," in Mason, W., and

Mendoza, S., eds., *Primate Social Conflict* (New York: SUNY Press, 1993); Cohen, S., Kaplan, J., and Cunnick, J., "Chronic social stress, affiliation and cellular immune response in nonhuman primates," *Psychological Sciences* 3 (1992): 301.

PAGE 361 The immunosuppressive effects of the aggressive transfer male: Alberts, S., Altmann, J., and Sapolsky, R., "Behavioral, endocrine and immunological correlates of immigration by an aggressive male into a natural primate group," *Hormones and Behavior* 26 (1992): 167.

PAGE 362 A review of primate personality: Clarke, A., and Boinski, S., "Temperament in nonhuman primates," *American Journal of Primatology* 37 (1995): 103.

PAGE 363 Some studies of human rank: Elias, M., "Cortisol, testosterone and testosterone-binding globulin responses to competitive fighting in human males," *Aggressive Behavior* 7 (1981): 215. Meyerhoff, J., Leshansky, M., and Mougey, E., "Effects of psychological stress on pituitary hormones in man," in Chrousos, G., Loriaux, D., and Gold, P., eds., *Mechanisms of Physical and Emotional Stress* (New York: Plenum Press, 1988); Houston, B., Babyak, M., Chesney, M., Black, G., and Ragland, D., "Social dominance and 22-year all-cause mortality in men," *Psychosomatic Medicine* 59 (1997): 5; Mazur, A., and Booth, A., "Testosterone and dominance in men," *Brain and Behavioral Sciences* 21 (1997): 353–63. Hunter-gatherer history: Boehm, C., *Hierarchy in the Forest: The Evolution of Egalitarian Behavior* (Cambridge, Mass.: Harvard University Press, 1999).

PAGE 364 Endocrine consequences of winning by effort versus by luck: Mazur, A., and Lamb, T., "Testosterone, status and mood in human males," *Hormones and Behavior* 14 (1980): 236; McCaul, K., Gladue, B., and Joppa, M., "Winning, losing, mood, and testosterone," *Hormones and Behavior* 26 (1992): 486.

PAGE 364 The poor do have the most stressors: McLeod, J., and Kessler, R., "Socioeconomic status differences in vulnerability to undesirable life events," *Journal of Health, Society and Behavior* 31 (1990): 162; Cohen, S., and Wills, T., "Stress, social support and the buffering hypothesis," *Psychological Bulletin* 98 (1985): 310; Brown, G., and Harris, T., *Social Origins of Depression* (London: Tavistock, 1978).

PAGE 365 The threat of unemployment disrupts health: Beale, N., and Nethercott, S., "Job-loss and family morbidity: a study of a factory closure," *Journal of the Royal College of General Practitioners* 35 (1985): 510; Cobb, S., and Kasl, S., *Termination: The Consequences of Job Loss,* DHEW-NIOSH Publication No. 77–224 (Cincinnati, Ohio: U.S. NIOSH, 1977). The study about workers not taking their diuretics because they couldn't go to the bathroom at work: cited in Adler, N., Boyce, T., Chesney, M., Folkman, S., and Syme, S., "Socioeconomic inequalities in health: no easy solution," *Journal of the American Medical Association* 269 (1993): 3140.

PAGE 365 The poor don't cope with stressors very efficiently: Hobfoll, S., *Stress, Community and Culture* (New York: Plenum, 1998).

PAGE 366 Montreal school kids: Lupien, S., King, S., Meaney, M., and McEwen, B., "Child's stress hormone levels correlate with mother's socioeconomic status and depressive state," *Biological Psychiatry* 48 (2000): 976. Lithuanians: Kristnson et al., "Antioxidant stat and mortality from coronary heart disease in Lithuanian and Swedish men," *British Medical Journal* 314 (1997): 629. In a more recent study it was shown that the lower your SES in the British civil service (regardless of gender), the more your glucocorticoid levels rise in anticipation of work in the morning: Kunz-Ebrecht, S., Kirschbaum, C., Marmot, M., and Steptoe, A., "Differences in cortisol awakening response on work days and weekends in women and men from the Whitehall II cohort," *Psychoneuroendocrinology* 29 (2004): 516. Just to complicate things a bit, SES influences glucocorticoid levels during the workday. However, the pattern there is that, among men, the lower your SES (again, in the British civil service), the higher your glucocorticoid levels. In contrast, among women, the higher your SES, the higher your workday glucocorticoid level. See: Steptoe, A., Kunz-Ebrecht, S., Owen, N., Feldman, P., Willemsen, G., Kirschbaum, C., and Marmot, M., "Socioeconomic status and stress-related biological responses over the working day," *Psychosomatic Medicine* (2004): in press.

PAGE 366 Reviews about the SES gradient and health (these are all leaders in the field): Pincus, T., and Callahan, L., "What explains the association between socioeconomic status and health: primarily access to medical care or mind-body variables?" *Advances* 11 (1995): 4; Syme, S., and Berkman, L., "Social class, susceptibility and sickness," *American Journal of Epidemiology* 104 (1976): 1; Adler, N., Boyce, T., Chesney, M., Folkman, S., and Syme, S., "Socioeconomic inequalities in health: no easy solution," *Journal of the American Medical Association* 269 (1993): 3140; Anderson, N., and Armstead, C., "Toward understanding the association of SES and health; a new challenge for the biopsychosocial approach," *Psychosomatic Medicine* 57 (1995): 213; Evans, R., Barer, M., and Marmor, T., *Why Are Some People Healthy and Others Not? The Determinants of Health of Populations* (New York: Aldine de Gruyter, 1994); Antonovsky, A., "Social class and the major cardiovascular diseases," *Journal of Chronic Diseases* 21 (1968): 65; Marmot, M., "Stress, social and cultural variations in heart disease," *Journal of Psychosomatic Research* 27 (1983): 377; Levenstein, S., Prantera, C., Varvo, V., Arca, M., Scribano, M., Spinella, S., and Berto, E., "Long-term symptom patterns in duodenal ulcer: psychosocial factors," *Journal of Psychosomatic Research* 41 (1996): 465; Hahn, R., Eaker, E., Barker, N., Teutsch, S., Sosniak, W., and Krieger, N., "Poverty and death in the United States," *International Journal of Health Services* 26 (1996): 673. Lower birth weight: Stern, A., "Social adversity, low birth weight, and pre-term delivery," *British Medical Journal* 295 (1987): 291; Budrys, G., *Unequal Health: How Inequality Contributes to Health or Illness* (Lanham, Md.: Rowman and Littlefield, 2003).

Footnote: Diseases more prevalent among the wealthy: malignant melanoma and breast cancer: Kitagawa, E., and Hauser, P., *Differential Mortality in the United States* (Cambridge, Mass.: Harvard University Press, 1973). Multiple sclerosis: Pincus, T., and Callahan, L., "What explains the association between socioeconomic status and health: primarily access to medical care or mind-body variables?" *Advances* 11 (1995): 4. Polio: Pincus, T., in Davis, B., ed., *Microbiology, Including Immunology and Molecular Genetics*, 3d ed. (New York: Harper and Row). SES and hospitalism is reviewed in: Sapolsky, R., "How the other half heals," *Discover* (April 1998): 46.

PAGE 367 Five-to-ten-year difference in life expectancy: Wilkinson, R., *Mind the Gap: Hierarchies, Health and Human Evolution* (London: Weidenfeld and Nicolson, 2000). Decades of differences: Murray, C. J. L., Michaud, C. M., et al. *U.S. Patterns of Mortality by County and Race: 1965–1994* (Cambridge, Mass., Burden of Disease Unit, Harvard Center for Population and Development Studies, 1998).

Footnote: the *Titanic* data are discussed in Marmot, M., "Epidemiology of SES and health: are determinants within countries the same as between countries?" *Annals of the New York Academy of Sciences* 896 (1999): 16.

PAGE 367 Gradient going back centuries is discussed in: Evans, R., *Interpreting and Addressing Inequalities in Health: From Black to Acheson to Blair to . . . ?* (London: OHE Publications, 2002).

PAGE 367 SES predicts health later in life: Lynch, J., Kaplan, G., Pamuk, E., Cohen, R., Heck, K., Balfour, J., and Yen, I., "Income inequality and mortality in metropolitan areas of the United States," *American Journal of Public Health* 88 (1998): 1074. Poverty early in life: Hertzman, C., "The biological embedding of early experience and its effects on health in adulthood," *Annals of the New York Academy of Sciences* 896 (1999): 85. The nun study: Snowdon, D., Ostwald, S., and Kane, R., "Education, survival and independence in elderly Catholic sisters 1936–1988," *American Journal of Epidemiology* 120 (1989): 999; Snowdon, D., Ostwald, S., Kane, R., and Keenan, N., "Years of life with good and poor mental and physical function in the elderly," *Journal of Clinical Epidemiology* 42 (1989): 1055. Health and cumulative percentage of life spent poor: Hertzman, op. cit.

PAGE 368 SES and being resuscitated in an ambulance: Sudnow, D., *Passing On: The Social Organization of Dying* (Englewood Cliffs, N.J.: Prentice-Hall, 1967). More recently: Kapral, M., Wang, H., Mamdani, M., Tu, J., "Effect of SES on treatment and mortality after stroke," *Stroke* 33 (2002): 268; Goirnick, M., "Disparities in Medicare services: potential causes, plausible explanations, and recommendations," *Health Care Financial Review* 21 (2000): 23.

PAGE 368 A range of European countries: Cavelaars, A., "Morbidity differences by occupational class among men in seven European countries: an application of the Erikson-Goldthorpe social class scheme," *International Journal of Epidemiology* 27 (1998): 222. The SES gradient worsening in England: Susser, M., Watson, W., and Hopper, K., *Sociology in Medicine,* 3d ed. (Oxford, England: Oxford University Press, 1985).

PAGE 369 Study where poor had made more use of a prepaid health plan and still had more disease: Oakes, T., and Syme, S., "Social factors in newly discovered elevated blood pressure," *Journal of Health, Society and Behavior* 14 (1973): 198.

PAGE 369 Marmot's work: Marmot, "Epidemiology of SES and health," op. cit.

PAGE 369 Pincus's work is reviewed in Pincus, T., and Callahan, L., "What explains the association between socioeconomic status and health: primarily access to medical care or mind-body variables?" *Advances* 11 (1995): 4.

PAGE 371 People never having heard of PAP tests: Harlan, L., Bernstein, A., and Kessler, L., "Cervical cancer screening: who is not screened and why?" *American Journal of Public Health* 81 (1991): 885. Footnote: education as worsening the gradient: Asplund, K., "Down with the class society!" *Stroke* 34 (2003): 2628.

PAGE 371 Evans: Evans, "Interpreting and addressing inequalities in health," op. cit. Whitehall study: Marmot, M., and Feeney, A., "Health and socioeconomic status," in Fink, G., ed., *Encyclopedia of Stress* (San Diego: Academic Press, 2000), vol. 2, 313.

PAGE 372 International patterns of pollution: Pacala, S., Bulte, E., List, J., and

Levin, S., "False alarm over environmental false alarms," *Science* 301 (2003): 1187. No relationship between wealth and health: Marmot, "Epidemiology of SES and health," op. cit.; Kawachi, I., Kennedy, B., Lochner, K., and Prothrow-Stith, D., "Social capital, income inequality, and mortality," *American Journal of Public Health* 87 (1997): 1491. U.S. and Greek life expectancy: Bezruchka, S., "Is our society making you sick?" *Newsweek* (February 2001): 26; Wilkinson, op. cit.

Footnote: statistics on happiness: Diener, E., Oishi, S., and Lucas, R., "Personality, culture, and subjective well-being: emotional and cognitive evaluations of life," *Annual Review of Psychology* 54 (2003): 403.

PAGE 373 Adler's work: Adler, N., Epel, E., Castellazzo, G., and Ickovics, J., "Relationship of subjective and objective social status with psychological and physiological functioning: preliminary data in healthy white women," *Health Psychology* 19 (2000): 586; Adler, N., and Ostrove, J., "SES and health: what we know and what we don't," *Annals of the New York Academy of Sciences* 896 (1999): 3; Goodman, E., Adler, N., Daniels, S., Morrison, J., Slap, G., and Dolan, L., "Impact of objective and subjective social status on obesity in a biracial cohort of adolescents," *Obesity Research* 11 (2003): 1018; Singh-Manoux, A., Adler, N., Marmot, M. G., "Subjective social status: its determinants and its association with measures of ill-health in the Whitehall II study," *Social Science and Medicine* 56 (2003): 1321; Goodman, E., Adler, N. E., Kawachi, I., Frazier, A. L., Huang, B., and Colditz, G. A., "Adolescents' perceptions of social status: development and evaluation of a new indicator," *Pediatrics* 108 (2001): E31; Ostrove, J. M., Adler, N. E., Kuppermann, M., and Washington, A., "Objective and subjective assessments of socioeconomic status and their relationship to self-rated health in an ethnically diverse sample of pregnant women," *Health Psychology* 19 (2000): 613.

PAGE 374 Pictures of female models: Kenrick, D., Montello, D., Gutierres, S., and Trost, M., "Effects of physical attractiveness on affect and perceptual judgments: when social comparison overrides social reinforcement," *Perspectives in Social Psychology Bulletin* 19 (1993): 195.

PAGE 374 Building blocks of subjective SES: Singh-Manoux, op. cit.

PAGE 375 Wilkinson, op. cit. Infant mortality rates: Lynch, J., Smith, G. D., Hillemeier, M., Shaw, M., Raghunathan, T., and Kaplan, G., "Income inequality, the psychosocial environment, and health: comparisons of wealthy nations," *Lancet* 358 (2001): 194; Hales, S., "National infant mortality rates in relation to gross national product and distribution of income," *Lancet* 354 (1999): 2047; Howden-Chapman, P., and Odea, D., "Income, income inequality and health in New Zealand," in Eckersley, R., Dixon, J., and Douglas, B., eds., *The Social Origins of Health and Well-Being* (Cambridge, England: Cambridge University Press, 2001), 129. In the United States: Ross, N. A., Wolfson, M. C., Dunn, J. R., Berthelot, J. M., Kaplan, G. A., and Lynch, J. W., "Relation between income inequality and mortality in Canada and in the United States: cross sectional assessment using census data and vital statistics," *British Medical Journal* 320 (2000): 898; Lynch et al., "Income inequality and mortality," op. cit.

PAGE 376 Income inequality/health relationship not universal: Lynch et al., "Income inequality and morality," op. cit.; Osler, M., Prescott, E., Gronbaek, M., Christensen, U., Due, P., and Engholm, G., "Income inequality, individual income, and mortality in Danish adults: analysis of pooled data from two cohort studies," *British Medical Journal* 324 (2002): 13. For a very detailed review of this material, see Lynch, J., Smith, G., Harper, S., Hillemeier, M., Ross, N., Kaplan, G., and Wolfson, M., "Is income inequality a determinant of population health?: A systematic review," *The Milbank Quarterly* (2004), in press. Wealth distribution in the United States: Bezruchka, op. cit.

PAGE 377 The asymptote artifact was first pointed out in Rodgers, G. B., "Income and inequality as determinants of mortality: an international cross-section analysis," *Population Studies* 33 (1979): 343. This potential artifact contributes to the phenomenon, but doesn't explain all of it: Wolfson, M., Kaplan, G., Lynch, J., Ross, N., and Backlund, E., "Relation between income inequality and mortality: empirical demonstration," *British Medical Journal* 319 (1999): 953.

PAGE 377 Footnote: The Robin Hood index: Atkinson, A., and Micklewright, J., *Transformation in Eastern Europe and the Distribution of Income* (New York: Cambridge University Press, 1992).

PAGE 378 The concept of social capital: Coleman, J., *Foundations of Social Theory* (Cambridge, Mass.: Belknap Press of Harvard University Press, 1990). Kawachi's work: Kawachi, I., and Kennedy, B., *The Health of Nations: Why Inequality Is Harmful to Your Health* (New York: The New Press, 2002); Kawachi, I., and Berkman, L., "Social ties and mental health," *Journal of Urban Health* 78 (2001): 458. This contains the college drinking study.

PAGE 379 Being an invisible member of society: Antonovsky, A., "A sociological critique of the 'Well-Being' movement," *Advances* 10, no. 3 (1994): 6.

PAGE 379 More crime: gun ownership: Hemenway, D., Kennedy, B., Kawachi, I., and Putnam, R., "Firearm prevalence and social capital," *Annals of Epidemiology* 11 (2001): 484. Income inequality predicting crime: Kawachi, I., Kennedy, B., and Wilkinson, R., "Crime: social disorganization and relative deprivation," *Social Science and Medicine* 48 (1999): 719.

PAGE 380 Evans: Evans, "Interpreting and addressing inequalities in health," op. cit.

PAGE 381 Health in the Eastern Bloc: Evans, "Interpreting and addressing inequalities in health," op. cit. Also see Kennedy, B., Kawachi, I., and Brainerd, E., "The role of social capital in the Russian mortality crisis," *World Development* 26 (1998): 2029.

PAGE 381 And the United States: heavily armed: Hemenway et al., op. cit. Putnam's metaphor: Putnam, R., *Bowling Alone* (New York: Simon & Schuster, 2000). U.S. health worse even when matched with Canada for income inequality: Lynch, "Income inequality and mortality," op. cit. Income inequality worsening in the United States: Atkinson, A. B., Rainwater, L., and Smeeding, T. M., *Income Distribution in OECD Countries: Evidence from the Luxembourg Income Study* (Paris: OECD, 1995); Lindert, P. H., "When did inequality rise in Britain and America?" *Journal of Income Distribution* 9 (2000): 11.

PAGE 382 The conclusion by Adler and colleagues: Adler, N., Boyce, T., Chesney, M., Folkman, S., and Syme, S., "Socioeconomic inequalities in health: no easy solution," *Journal of the American Medical Association* 269 (1993): 3140.

CHAPTER 18: MANAGING STRESS

PAGE 384 Footnote: A technical description of alopecia areata can be found in Rook, A., and Dawber, R., *Diseases of the Hair and Scalp,* 2d ed. (Oxford: Blackwell Scientific Publications, 1991). In actuality, though, there is not really a change in hair color under those circumstances. Alopecia areata occurs in people who already have some degree of whitening or graying of their hair. With the onset of the trauma, hair that is not white or gray falls out, probably because the immune system attacks dark-hair bulbs. Thus, all that is left is the white or gray hair. Various experts I've consulted suggest that the phenomenon represents a bit of media hype—it is extremely rare and usually takes weeks or months, rather than occurring in a single night.

A particularly amusing account of the history of the disorder and speculations about it can be found in Jelinek, J., "Sudden whitening of the hair," *Bulletin of the New York Academy of Medicine* 48 (1972): 1003. Jelinek, a professor of dermatology, recounts many tales over the centuries of people who, condemned to be executed by their king, turn white with terror the night before the scheduled execution. The now white-haired prisoner is brought before the king and assembled court for execution the next morning. Everyone is moved with wonder and pity at the transformation, and the poor wretch is pardoned. Numerous sources claim that the hair and beard of Sir Thomas More, who had fallen out of favor with King Henry VIII and was condemned to death, turned white the day before his execution. In contrast to the general pattern of these tales, Henry, unimpressed, still had him killed and his head parboiled and displayed on London Bridge. Over the course of her imprisonment prior to her execution, Marie Antoinette's hair was also reported to have turned gray. This may not have represented a true case of alopecia areata, however. "It has cynically been conjectured that the keepers of her dungeon neglected to furnish their guest's dressing table with hair dyes. The iconoclast respects nothing, not even the grey hairs of royalty," opined the mordant Dr. Jelinek.

If you view the world in a certain myopic way, you might argue that alopecia areata plays the central role in making sense of modern life. For example, a number of media pundits commented on the noticable graying of Osama bin Laden's hair from one clandestine video to the next, taking that as a sign of the stressful toll that the (unsuccessful) U.S. hunt for him was exacting. Meanwhile, part of the documentation of mistreatment of Northern Irish political prisoners includes their hair turning white (Conroy, J., *Unspeakable Acts, Ordinary People* [New York: Knopf, 2000]). On the historical front, an injurious train wreck is credited with having turned Annie Oakley's celebrated long brown hair white within a few days (www.ormiston.com), while a recent road rage lawsuit in Palo Alto, California, involved not only charges of damage to an SUV (the rageful perpetrator dinged the car's door when he kicked it, after the woman driving the SUV nearly ran over the man and his family in a crosswalk), but additional costs for her subsequent stress-induced hair loss. Alas, for those hoping for alopecia areata to take its rightful dominant place in the American legal system, that part of the lawsuit didn't fly ("Kicking professor cops a plea," *Palo Alto Daily News* [17 December 2003]).

PAGE 384 The tendency for variability to increase in aging populations is discussed in Rowe, J., Wang, S., and Elahi, D., "Design, conduct, and analysis of human aging research," in Schneider, E., and Rowe, J., eds., *Handbook of the Biology of Aging,* 3d ed. (San Diego: Academic Press, 1990), 63.

PAGE 386 Features of Holocaust survivors are discussed in Valent, P., "Holocaust survivors, experiences of," in Fink, G., ed., *Encyclopedia of Stress* (San Diego: Academic Press, 2000), vol. 2, 396. One of the themes that comes through is encompassed in the quote by the psychotherapist and Holocaust survivor, Victor Frankl: "Everything can be taken from a man but one thing, the last of human freedoms—to choose one's attitude in any given set of circumstances," Frankl, V., *Man's Search for Meaning* (New York: Basic Books, 1985). To return to a theme emphasized at various points in the book, it is immensely impressive and moving if some people were able to withstand the hell of the Holocaust with an intact ability to choose their attitude. However, no one should ever preach to some victim about how they are expected to pull off such a miracle of coping.

PAGE 387 The encouraging topic of successful aging is reviewed in Rowe, J., and Kahn, R., "Human aging: usual and successful," *Science* 237 (1987): 143; Baltes, P., and Baltes, M., *Successful Aging* (Cambridge, England: Cambridge University Press, 1990). Also, refer back to chapter 12 for a more thorough overview of the subject.

PAGE 388 Cognitively unimpaired aged rats showed none of the usual degenerations: Issa, A., Rowe, W., Gauthier, S., and Meaney, M., "Hypothalamic-pituitary-adrenal activity in aged, cognitively impaired and cognitively unimpaired rats," *Journal of Neuroscience* 10 (1991): 3247. Neonatal handling produces similar protection in old age: Meaney, M., Aitken, D., Bhatnager, S., van Berkel, C., and Sapolsky, R., "Effect of neonatal handling on age-related impairments associated with the hippocampus," *Science* 239 (1988): 766; Meaney, M., Aitken, D., and Sapolsky, R., "Postnatal handling attenuates neuroendocrine, anatomical and cognitive dysfunctions associated with aging in female rats," *Neurobiology of Aging* 12 (1990): 31.

PAGE 388 Mother rats who lick and groom: Liu, D., Diorio, J., Tannenbaum, B., Caldji, C., Francis, D., Freedman, A., Sharma, S., Pearson, D., Plotsky, P., and Meaney, J., "Maternal care, hippocampal glucocorticoid receptors, and HPA responses to stress," *Science* 277 (1997): 1659.

PAGE 389 Vaillant, G., and Mukamal, K., "Successful aging," *American Journal of Psychiatry* 158 (2001): 839.

PAGE 390 The Oscar finding: Redelmeier, D., and Singh, S., *Annals of Internal Medicine* 134 (2001): 955. The finding is explained by the authors along the lines of its being the case that no matter how awful subsequent acting gigs might be and how utterly the movies tanked, "An Oscar is an accomplishment that no one can take away."

PAGE 390 Coping styles among parents of children with cancer: Wolff, C., Friedman, S., Hofer, M., and Mason, J., "Relationship between psychological defenses and mean urinary 17-hydroxycorticosteroid excretion rates. I. A predictive study of parents of fatally ill children," *Psychosomatic Medicine* 26 (1964): 576; Hofer, M., Wolff, E., Friedman, S., and Mason, J., "A psychoendocrine study of bereavement, parts I and II," *Psychosomatic Medicine* 34 (1972): 481.

PAGE 392 Resistance to learned helplessness is discussed in Seligman, M., *Helplessness*, 2d ed. (New York: W. H. Freeman, 1992).

PAGE 392 Sapolsky, R., "Why should an aged male baboon transfer troops?" *American Journal of Primatology* 39 (1996): 149; Sapolsky, R., "The graying of the troops," *Discover* (March 1996): 46.

PAGE 395 Change in cholesterol profiles in Type-A individuals receiving counseling: Gill, J., Price, V., and Friedman, M., "Reduction in Type A behavior in healthy middle-aged American military officers," *American Heart Journal* 110 (1985): 503. Also see Thoresen, C., and Powell, L., "Type A behavior pattern: new perspectives on theory, assessment and intervention," *Journal of Consulting and Clinical Psychology* 60 (1992): 595–604.

PAGE 395 Changing of the stress-response over time among parachuting trainees: Ursin, H., Baade, E., and Levine, S., *Psychobiology of Stress* (San Diego: Academic Press, 1978).

PAGE 396 Self-medication among acute pain patients can be conducted safely: Norman, J., White, W., and Pearce, D., "New possibilities in analgesia: the demand analgesia computer. Round table on morphinomimetics," 5th European Congress of Anaesthesiology (Paris, 1978); Jully, C., and Sibbald, A., "Control of postoperative pain by interactive demand analgesia," *British Journal of Anaesthesiology* 53 (1981): 385; Baumann, T., Bastenhorst, R., Graves, D., Foster, T., and Bennett, R., "Patient-controlled analgesia in the terminally ill cancer patient," *Drug Intelligence Clinical Pharmacology* 20 (1986): 297; Citron, M., Johnston-Early, A., Boyer, M., Krasnow, S., Hood, H., and Cohen, M., "Patient-controlled analgesia for severe cancer pain," *Archives of Internal Medicine* 146 (1986): 734. Such self-medication can be associated with an overall decrease in the amount of medication taken: Chapman, C., and Hill, H., "Prolonged morphine self-administration and addiction liability: evaluation of two theories in a bone marrow transplant unit," *Cancer* 63 (1989): 1636; Chapman, C., "Giving the patient control of opioid analgesic administration," in Hill, C., and Fields, W., eds., *Advances in Pain Research and Therapy*, vol. 11 (New York: Raven Press, 1989), 339; Chapman, C., and Hill, H., "Patient-controlled analgesia in a bone marrow transplant setting," in Foley, K., ed., *Advances in Pain Research and Therapy*, vol. 16 (New York: Raven Press, 1990), 231.

PAGE 397 Coping styles differ between young and aged humans: Folkman, S., Lazarus, R., Pimley, S., and Novacek, J., "Age differences in stress and coping processes," *Psychology and Aging* 2 (1987): 171. Manipulating psychological variables in nursing home populations: This large literature is reviewed in Rodin, J., "Aging and health: effects of the sense of control," *Science* 233 (1986): 1271; Rowe, J., and Kahn, R., "Human aging: usual and successful," *Science* 237 (1987): 143. Individual studies: Schulz, J., "Effects of control and predictability on the physical and psychological well-being of the institutionalized aged," *Journal of Personality and Social Psychology* 33 (1976): 563; Schulz, J., and Hanusa, B., "Long-term effects of control and predictability-enhancing interventions: findings and ethical issues," *Journal of Personality and Social Psychology* 36 (1978): 1194.

PAGE 400 Follow-up to cancer study: Hofer, M., Wolff, E., Friedman, S., and Mason, J., "A psychoendocrine study of bereavement, parts I and II," *Psychosomatic Medicine* 34 (1972): 481.

PAGE 400 Follow-up to nursing home study: Schulz, J., "Effects of control and predictability on the physical and psychological well-being of the institutionalized aged," op. cit.: 563.

PAGE 401 The physiological effects of exercise, and the personality profiles of exercisers: Khatri, P., and Blumenthal, J. "Exercise," in Fink, G., ed., *Encyclopedia of Stress* (San Diego: Academic Press, 2000), vol. 2, 98. The importance of exercise being voluntary: Greenwood, B., Foley, T., Day, H., Campisi, J., Hammack, S., Campeau, S., Maier, S., and Fleshner, M., "Freewheel running prevents learning helplessness/behavioral depression: role of dorsal raphe serotonergic neurons," *Journal of Neuroscience* 23 (2003): 2889.

PAGE 402 Some papers showing the salutary effects of transcendental meditation on various physiological endpoints (resting glucocorticoid levels, oxygen consumption, heart rate, and so on): Wallace, R., "Physiological effects of transcendental meditation," *Science* 167 (1970): 1751; Wallace, R., and Benson, H., "The physiology of meditation," *Scientific American* (February 1972): 84 (these two papers cover much the same material, but the latter is more accessible and gives more of an overview of the subject); Jevning, R., Wilson, A., and Davidson, J., "Adrenocortical activity during meditation," *Hormones and Behavior* 10 (1978): 54; Carlson, L. E., Speca, M., Patel, K. D., and Goodey, E., "Mindfulness-based stress reduction in relation to quality of life, mood, symptoms of stress, and immune parameters in breast and prostate cancer outpatients," *Psychosomatic Medicine* 65 (2003): 571; Newberg, A., Alavi, A., Baime, M., Pourdehnad, M., Santanna, J., d'Aquili, E., "The measurement of regional cerebral blood flow during the complex cognitive task of meditation: a preliminary SPECT study," *Psychological Research* 106 (2001): 113; Lazar, S., Bush, G., Gollub, R., Fricchione, G., Khalsa, G., and Benson, H., "Functional brain mapping of the relaxation response and meditation," *NeuroReport* 11 (2000): 1581; Carlson, L., Speca, M., Patel, K., and Goodey, E. "Mindfulness-based stress reductions in relation to quality of life, mood, symptoms of stress and levels of cortisol DNEAS and melatonin in breast and prostate cancer outpatients," *Psychoneuroendocrinology* 29 (2004): 448.

PAGE 404 John Henryism: James, S., "John Henryism and the health of African-Americans," *Culture, Medicine and Psychiatry* 18 (1994): 163. An internal locus of control in a population of Harvard grads: Peterson, C., Seligman, M., and Vaillant, G., "Pessimistic explanatory style is a risk factor for physical illness: a thirty-five-year longitudinal study," *Journal of Personality and Social Psychology* 55 (1988): 23.

PAGE 406 Immune function tends to decline in rodents socially housed: Bohus, B., and Koolhaas, J., "Psychoimmunology of social factors in rodents and other subprimate vertebrates," in Ader, R., Felten, D., and Cohen, N., eds., *Psychoneuroimmunology*, 2d ed. (San Diego: Academic Press, 1991), 807. Social housing tends to elevate glucocorticoid levels in rodents and primates: Levine, S., Wiener, S., and Coe, C., "The psychoneuroendocrinology of stress: a psychobiological perspective," in Levine, S., and Brush, F., eds., *Psychoendocrinology* (San Diego: Academic Press, 1989). This review also discusses the study showing that infant monkeys separated from their mothers are not necessarily comforted (that is, show lowered glucocorticoid secretion) merely by being put in a social group. Also see Clarke, A., Czekala, N., and Lindburg, D. "Behavioral and adrenocortical responses of male cynomolgus and lion-tailed macaques to social stimulation and group formation," *American Journal of Primatology*, submitted. Marital discord is associated with immune suppression: Kiecolt-Glaser, J., Fisher, L., Ogrocki, P., Stout, J., Speicher, C., and Glaser, R., "Marital quality, marital disruption, and immune function," *Psychosomatic Medicine* 49 (1987): 13; Kiecolt-Glaser, J., Kennedy, S., Malkoff, S., Fisher, L., Speicher, C., and Glaser, R., "Marital discord and immunity in males," *Psychosomatic Medicine* 50 (1988): 213; Kiecolt-Glaser, J., Malar, J., Chee, M., Newton, T., Cacioppo, J., Mao, H., and Glaser, R., "Negative behavior during martial conflict is associated with immunological down-regulation," *Psychosomatic Medicine* 55 (1993): 395; The health dangers of a bad marriage: Robles, T., and Kiecolt-Glaser, J., "The physiology of marriage: pathways to health," *Physiology and Behavior* 79 (2003): 409.

PAGE 407 Religion and health. Religiosity versus spirituality: Hill, P., and Pargament, K., "Advances in the conceptualization and measurement of religion and spirituality," *American Psychologist* 58 (2003): 64. Thoresen's work can be found in: Thoresen, C., "Spirituality and health: is there a relationship?" *Journal of Health Psychology* 4 (1999): 291; McCullough, M., Hoyt, W., Larson, D., Koenig, H., and Thoressen, C., "Religious involvement and mortality: a meta-analytic review," *Health Psychology* 19 (2000): 211; Miller, W., and Thoresen, C., "Spirituality, religion, and health," *American Psychologist* 58 (2003): 24; Powell, L., Shahabi, L., and Thoresen, C., "Religion and spirituality: linkages to physical health," *American Psychologist* 58 (2003): 36. I found the final one to be particularly useful. Sloan's work: Sloan, R., and Bagiella, E., "Claims about religious involvement and health outcomes," *Annals of Behavioral Medicine* 24 (2002): 14–21. Galton's observation is noted in Brown, A., *The Darwin Wars* (New York: Simon and Schuster, 1999). Decreased risk of depression and cardiovascular disease: Luskin, F., "Review of the effect of spiritual and religious factors on mortality and morbidity with a focus on cardiovascular and pulmonary disease," *Journal of Cardiopulmonary Rehabilitation* 20 (2000): 8; Koenig, H., McCullough, M., and Larson, D., *Handbook of Religion and Health* (New York: Oxford University Press, 2001); Larson, D., Swyers, J., and McCullough, M., *Scientific Research on Spirituality and Health: A Consensus Report* (Rockville, Md.: National Institutes of Health, 1998).

PAGE 410 Responses to Sloan's critique: McCullough, M., Hoyt, W., Larson, D., "Small, robust, and important: reply to Sloan and Gabiella 2001," *Health Psychology* 20 (2001): 228.

PAGE 410 Some extraordinary examples of such sources of comfort can be found in: Van Biema, D., *Time* (16 July 2001): 62.

PAGE 411 Packer, S., "Religion and stress," in Fink, G., ed., *Encyclopedia of Stress* (San Diego: Academic Press, 2000), vol. 3, 348.

PAGE 411 Footnote; Tannen's book: Tannen, D., *You Just Don't Understand* (New York: Morrow, 1990). The notion of the right coping style for the right stressor dominated the work of the late Richard Lazarus of the University of California, Berkeley. A good summary can be found in: Lazarus, R., "Toward better research on stress and coping," *American Psychologist* 55 (2000): 665; Lazarus, R., "Coping theory and research: past, present, and future," *Psychosomatic Medicine* 55 (1993): 234. The differences among coping strategies is discussed in Rahe, R., "Coping, stress and," in Fink, G., ed., *Encyclopedia of Stress* (San Diego: Academic Press, 2000), vol. 1, 541.

PAGE 412 Seligman, M., *Learned Optimism* (New York: Knopf, 1991).

PAGE 412 Antonovsky's work is summarized in: Antonovsky, A., "A sociological critique of the 'Well-Being' movement," *Advances* 10, no. 3 (1994): 6.

PAGE 415 Some caveats embedded in the final section: Warning against over-loading aged individuals with too much control and responsibility: Rodin, J., "Aging and health: effects of the sense of control," *Science* 233 (1986): 1271; Langer, E., *The Psychology of Control* (Beverly Hills, Calif.: Sage, 1983); Langer, E., *Mindfulness* (Reading, Mass.: Addison Wesley, 1989).

The dangers of unrealistic anger: Williams, R., *The Trusting Heart: Great News about Type A Behavior* (New York: Random House, 1989). Also Williams, R., and Williams, V., *Anger Kills: Seventeen Strategies for Controlling the Hostility That Can Harm Your Health* (New York: Times/Random House, 1993).

The advantages of denial: Lazarus, R., "The costs and benefits of denial," in Breznitz, S., ed., *The Denial of Stress* (New York: International Universities Press, 1983), 1.

THE FAR SIDE   By GARY LARSON

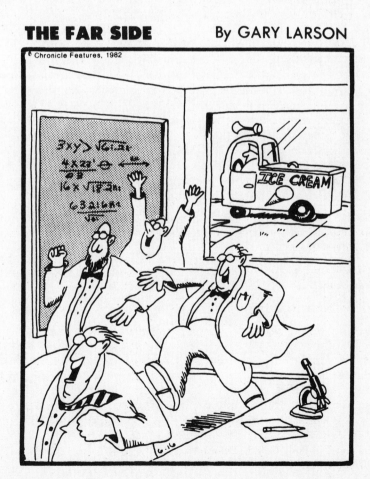

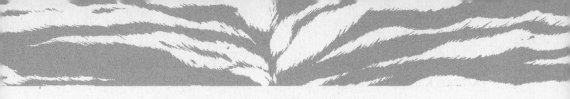

ILLUSTRATION CREDITS

PAGE 128 Courtesy of Laurance Frank, University of California, Berkeley.

PAGE 133 Konner/Anthro-Photo.

PAGE 151 Courtesy of Gilla Kaplan, The Rockefeller University.

PAGE 188 Philadelphia Museum of Art, SmithKline Beckman Corporation Fund.

PAGE 199 Courtesy of Vic Boff.

PAGE 204 Alfred Eisenstaedt, *Life* magazine.

PAGE 212 *The Far Side* © 1984 Farworks, Inc., used by permission of Universal Press Syndicate. All Rights Reserved.

PAGE 214 By permission of Jerry Van Amerongen and Creators Syndicate.

PAGE 216 Courtesy of Dr. Ana María Magariños and Dr. Bruce S. McEwen, Rockefeller University, New York.

PAGE 228 © Bryan & Cherry Alexander Photography. Reprinted by permission.

PAGE 230 Courtesy of Mary-Anne Martin/Fine Art, New York; © 1999 Alfredo Castañeda.

PAGE 237 Courtesy of the artist; © 1994 Jeff Wall.

PAGE 240 Courtesy of Morris Zlapo.

PAGE 241 DeVore/Anthro-Photo.

PAGE 242 Anthony Taber © 1983 from *The New Yorker* Collection. All Rights Reserved.

PAGE 246 Rick Backlaws/Image West Photography.

PAGE 250 Courtesy of Sidney Janis Gallery, New York; © 1993 George Segal/VAGA, New York.

PAGE 257 Private collection; courtesy of George Tooker and Chameleon Books, Inc.

PAGE 265 Drawing by Roz Chast.

PAGE 273 New Britain Museum of American Art, Gift of Olga H. Knoepke; courtesy of George Tooker and Chameleon Books, Inc.

PAGE 311 Robert Sapolsky, Stanford University.

PAGE 321 Mick Stevens © 1982 from *The New Yorker* Collection. All Rights Reserved.

PAGE 326 Courtesy of Gerald W. Friedland, Stanford University Department of Radiology.

PAGE 330 Dr. Meyer Friedman, Meyer Friedman Institute.

PAGE 332 Clifford Goodenough, Davidson Galleries, Seattle.

PAGE 338 © 1970 Philip Guston.

PAGE 344 Courtesy of Mary Boone Gallery, New York; © 2003 Toland Grinnell.

PAGE 351 Courtesy of Leslie Muth Gallery; © 1994 Leroy Almon.

PAGE 357 Robert Sapolsky, Stanford University.

PAGE 359 Robert Sapolsky, Stanford University.

PAGE 385 Hermitage Museum, St. Petersburg, Russia; Scala Art Resource, New York; © 1998 Succession H. Matisse/Artists Rights Society (ARS), New York.

INDEX

ABOUT THE AUTHOR

ROBERT M. SAPOLSKY is a professor of biology and neurology at Stanford University and a research associate with the Institute of Primate Research, National Museum of Kenya. He is the author of *A Primate's Memoir* and *The Trouble with Testosterone*, which was a *Los Angeles Times* Book Award finalist. A regular contributor to *Discover* and *The Sciences*, and a recipient of a MacArthur Foundation "genius" grant, he lives in San Francisco.